术后疼痛管理
——循证实践指导——

Postoperative Pain Management: an evidence-based guide to practice

注 意

医学领域的知识和最佳临床实践在不断发展。由于新的研究与临床经验不断扩展着我们的知识,在治疗和用药方面做出某些改变也许是必需的或适宜的。建议读者核对所处方每种药品其生产厂家所提供的最新产品信息,以确定药物的推荐剂量、服用方法、持续时间及相关禁忌证。根据自己的经验和患者的病情,决定每一位病人的服药剂量和最佳治疗方法,是经治医师的责任。不论是出版商还是著者,对于由于本出版物引起的任何个人或财产的损伤或损失,均不承担任何责任。

出版者

术后疼痛管理
——循证实践指导——

Postoperative Pain Management: an evidence-based guide to practice

主　编　George Shorten
　　　　Daniel B. Carr
　　　　Dominic Harmon
　　　　Margarita M. Puig
　　　　John Browne

主　译　邓小明　熊源长
副主译　许　华　朱科明

北京大学医学出版社
Peking University Medical Press

图书在版编目（CIP）数据

术后疼痛管理：循证实践指导/（美）肖特（Shorten, G.）等著；邓小明等译. —北京：北京大学医学出版社，2008

书名原文：Postoperative Pain Management：An Evidence-based Guide to Practice

ISBN 978-7-81116-604-0

Ⅰ. 术… Ⅱ. ①肖…②邓… Ⅲ. 外科手术—疼痛—治疗 Ⅳ. R619

中国版本图书馆 CIP 数据核字（2008）第 102575 号

北京市版权局著作权合同登记号：图字：1-2007-3924

Postoperative Pain Management：an evidence-based guide to practice
George Shorten et al.
ISBN-13：978-1-4160-2454-5
ISBN-10：1-4160-2454-9
Copyright © 2006 by Saunders, an imprint of Elsevier Inc.

Authorized Simplified Chinese translation from English language edition published by the Proprietor.
978-981-272-045-0
981-272-045-6

Elsevier (Singapore) Pte Ltd.
3 Killiney Road, #08-01 Winsland House I, Singapore 239519
Tel：(65) 6349-0200, Fax：(65) 6733-1817
First Published 2008
2009 年初版

Simplified Chinese translation Copyright © 2009 by Elsevier (Singapore) Pte Ltd and Peking University Medical Press. All rights reserved.

Published in China by Peking University Medical Press under special agreement with Elsevier (Singapore) Pte Ltd. This edition is authorized for sale in China only, excluding Hong Kong SAR and Taiwan. Unauthorized export of this edition is a violation of the Copyright Act. Violation of this Law is subject to Civil and Criminal Penalties.

本书简体中文版由北京大学医学出版社与 Elsevier (Singapore) Pte Ltd. 在中国境内（不包括香港特别行政区及台湾）协议出版。本版仅限在中国境内（不包括香港特别行政区及台湾）出版及标价销售。未经许可之出口，是为违反著作权法，将受法律之制裁。

术后疼痛管理：循证实践指导

主　　译：	邓小明　熊源长
出版发行：	北京大学医学出版社（电话：010-82802230）
地　　址：	(100191) 北京市海淀区学院路 38 号 北京大学医学部院内
网　　址：	http://www.pumpress.com.cn
E - mail：	booksale@bjmu.edu.cn
印　　刷：	北京佳信达欣艺术印刷有限公司
经　　销：	新华书店
责任编辑：	李海燕　　责任校对：杜悦　　责任印制：郭桂兰
开　　本：	889mm×1194mm　1/16　　印张：18.5　　字数：581 千字
版　　次：	2009 年 7 月第 1 版　2009 年 7 月第 1 次印刷
书　　号：	ISBN 978-7-81116-604-0
定　　价：	86.00 元

版权所有，违者必究
（凡属质量问题请与本社发行部联系退换）

译校人员名单

主　译　邓小明　熊源长

副主译　许　华　朱科明

审校者（按姓氏拼音字母为序）

卞金俊	包　睿	陈　辉	杜健儿
范晓华	侯　炯	李金宝	李文献
刘　毅	马　宇	孟　岩	倪　文
汤　媛	万小健	王天舒	王晓琳
许　华	许　涛	严晓晴	杨　涛
朱科明	朱文忠	翟　蓉	张伟时
邹毅清			

译　者（按姓氏拼音字母为序）

陈　芳	晨　光	陈界石	程　琛
傅　冬	葛建云	韩　烨	李斌本
李　杰	李双双	李卫星	刘　佳
毛燕飞	倪丽亚	圣　奎	盛　颖
水恒兵	吴　倩	汪鼎鼎	王　薇
王玮玮	项明琼	许小平	杨宇光
余喜亚	张　杰	张　瑛	张庆兵
赵晓虹	周　懿	周英杰	

著者名单

Salahadin Abdi, MD, PhD
Associate Professor of Anesthesiology
Harvard Medical School
Director, Massachusetts General Hospital Pain Center
Boston, Massachusetts
The Principles of Evidence-Based Practice

Donal Buggy, MD, MSc, DME, FRCPI, FFARCSI, FRCA
Senior Lecturer in Anaesthesia and Intensive Care Medicine
University College Dublin
Consultant in Anaesthesia and Intensive Care Medicine
Mater Misericordiae University Hospital
Dublin, Ireland
Nonconventional and Adjunctive Analgesia

Daniel B. Carr, MD, FABPM, FFPMANZCA(Hon)
Professor of Anesthesiology and Medicine (Adjunct)
Tufts University School of Medicine
Saltonstall Professor of Pain Research
Tufts New England Medical Center
Boston, Massachusetts
Chief Executive Officer and Chief Medical Officer
Javelin Pharmaceuticals, Inc.
Cambridge, Massachusetts
Accessing and Assessing Medical Evidence

Jeremy N. Cashman, BSc, MB,BS, MD, FRCA
Honorary Senior Lecturer
St. George's Hospital Medical School
Consultant Anaesthetist
St. George's Hospital
Department of Anaesthetics
London, England
Patient-Controlled Analgesia

Rachel A. Farragher, MB, FCARCSI
Lecturer in Anaesthesia
University College Hospital Galway
Galway, Ireland
Postoperative Pain Management after Cesarean Section

Kate Fitzgerald, MSc, FCARCSI, SpR in Anaesthesia
Specialist Registrar in Anaesthesia
University College Dublin
Mater Misericordiae University Hospital
Dublin, Ireland
Nonconventional and Adjunctive Analgesia

Henry Frizelle, MD, FFARCSI
Consultant Anaesthetist
Mater Misericordiae University Hospital
Dublin, Ireland
Mechanisms of Postoperative Pain-Nociceptive

Dominic Harmon, MD, FRCA, FFARCSI
Consultant Anaesthesia/Pain Medicine
Mid-Western Regional Hospital
Dooradoyle
Limerick, Ireland
Regional and Peripheral Techniques; Postoperative Pain Management in the Elderly; Postoperative Pain Management in the Ambulatory Setting

James Helstrom, MD
Instructor
Harvard Medical School
Assistant in Anesthesia
Massachusetts General Hospital
Boston, Massachusetts
Nonsteroidal Anti-inflammatory Drugs in Postoperative Pain

Robert W. Hurley, MD, PhD
Fellow in Pain Medicine
Johns Hopkins Medical Institutions
Baltimore, Maryland
Postoperative Pain Management and Patient Outcome

Gabriella Iohom, MD, PhD
Senior Lecturer
National University of Ireland
University College Cork
Consultant Anaesthetist
Cork University Hospital
Cork, Ireland
Clinical Assessment of Postoperative Pain

Shyamala Karuvannur, MD
Assistant Professor
State University of New York at Stony Brook
Stony Brook School of Medicine
Stony Brook, New York
Medical Director of Women's Health
Department of Veterans Affairs
Northport, New York
Postoperative Pain Management in the Ambulatory Setting

Joel Katz, PhD
Professor and Canada Research Chair in Health Psychology
Department of Psychology
York University
Director, Acute Pain Research Unit
Department of Anesthesia and Pain Management
Toronto General Hospital and Mount Sinai Hospital
Toronto, Ontario
Canada
Prediction and Prevention of Acute Postoperative Pain: Moving Beyond Preemptive Analgesia

Brian Kinirons, MB, FFARCSI
Consultant Anaesthetist
Department of Anaesthesia and Intensive Care
University College Hospital Galway
Consultant Anaesthesiologist
Galway Regional Hospitals
Galway, Ireland
Regional and Peripheral Techniques

John G. Laffey, MD, MA, BSc, FFARCSI
Clinical Lecturer
Department of Anaesthesia
National University of Ireland
Consultant Anaesthetist
University College Hospital Galway
Galway, Ireland
Postoperative Pain Management after Cesarean Section

Yuan-Chi Lin, MD, MPH
Associate Professor of Anaesthesia and Pediatrics
Harvard Medical School
Senior Associate in Anesthesia and Pain Medicine
Department of Anesthesiology, Perioperative and Pain Medicine
Children's Hospital Boston
Boston, Massachusetts
Postoperative Pain Management in Infants and Children

William A. Macrae, MB,ChB, FRCA
Honorary Senior Lecturer
University of Dundee
University of St. Andrews
Consultant Anesthetist and Pain Specialist
Ninewells Hospital
Dundee, Scotland
Can We Prevent Chronic Pain after Surgery?

Laxmaiah Manchikanti, MD
Department of Anesthesiology
University of Louisville School of Medicine
Louisville, Kentucky
Medical Director, Pain Management Center of Paducah
Paducah, Kentucky
The Principles of Evidence-Based Practice

Colin J. L. McCartney, MB,ChB, FCARCSI, FRCA, FRCPC
Assistant Professor of Anesthesia
University of Toronto Faculty of Medicine
Staff Anesthesiologist
Toronto Western Hospital
Toronto, Ontario
Canada
Use of Opioid Analgesics in the Perioperative Period

Diarmuid McCoy, FFARCSI, FFPMANZCA, DPM (CARCSI)
Consultant in Anaesthesia and Pain Medicine
Department of Anaesthesia, Perioperative Care and Pain Medicine
The Geelong Hospital
Barworth Health
Geelong, Victoria
Australia
Postoperative Pain Management in the Elderly

Connail R. McCrory, LRCP&SI, FFARCSI, FIPP, MD
Clinical Lecturer
Department of Surgery
Trinity College
Consultant Anaesthetist and Pain Specialist
Lead Clinician Pain Medicine
Department of Anaesthesia, Intensive Care and Pain Medicine
St. James's Hospital
Dublin, Ireland
Mechanisms of Postoperative Pain-Neuropathic

Peter G. Moore, MD, PhD
Professor and Chair
Department of Anesthesiology and Pain Medicine
University of California, Davis, School of Medicine
Sacramento, California
Defining Pain Management Objectives

Marcus M llner, MD, MSc (Epidemiol)
Associate Professor
Department of Emergency Medicine
Medizinuniversit t Wien/Allgemeines Krankenhaus Wien
Vienna, Austria
Accessing and Assessing Medical Evidence

Damian Murphy, FFARCSI, MD
Consultant Anaesthetist
Department of Anaesthesia, Intensive Care, and Pain Relief Service
Cork University Hospital
Wilton, Cork
Ireland
Applied Clinical Pharmacology of Opioids

Srdjan S. Nedeljković, MD
Assistant Professor of Anaesthesia
Harvard Medical School
Director, Fellowship Education
Pan Management Center
Department of Anesthesiology
Perioperative and Pain Medicine
Brigham and Women's Hospital
Boston, Massachusetts
Postoperative Pain Management for Patients with Drug Dependence

Ahtsham Niazi, FCARCSI
Consultant Anaesthetist
Our Lady's Hospital
Navan, County Meath
Ireland
Use of Opioid Analgesics in the Perioperative Period

Joseph Pergolizzi, MD
Adjunct Assistant Professor
Department of Medicine
Johns Hopkins University School of Medicine
Baltimore, Maryland
Board of Directors, Coalition for Pain Education
New York, New York
Senior Partner, Naples Anesthesia and Pain Associates
Naples, Florida
Multimodal Analgesic Therapy

Narinder Rawal, MD, PhD
Professor of Anesthesiology and Intensive Care
University Hospital
rebro, Sweden
Acute Pain Services

H. Paul Redmond, BSc, MCh, FRCSI
Professor and Head, Department of Surgery
National University of Ireland (Cork)
Professor of Surgery
Cork University Hospital
Wilton, Cork
Ireland
The Neurohumoral, Inflammatory, and Coagulation Responses to Surgery

Carl E. Rosow, MD, PhD
Professor of Anaesthesia
Harvard Medical School
Anesthetist
Department of Anesthesia and Critical Care
Massachusetts General Hospital
Boston, Massachusetts
Nonsteroidal Anti-inflammatory Drugs in Postoperative Pain

Navparkash Sandhu, MS (Surg), MD
Assistant Professor of Anesthesiology
New York University School of Medicine
Associate Attending
Bellevue Hospital Center
Assistant Attending
New York University Medical Center
New York, New York
Postoperative Pain Management in the Ambulatory Setting

Conor J. Shields, MD, AFRCSI
Senior Specialist Registrar in Surgery
Cork University Hospital and National University of Ireland (Cork)
Wilton, Cork
Ireland
The Neurohumoral, Inflammatory, and Coagulation Responses to Surgery

Ulrike M. Stamer, MD
Associate Professor of Anesthesiology and Pain Medicine
Department of Anesthesiology and Intensive Care Medicine
University of Bonn
University Hospital Bonn
Bonn, Germany
Postoperative Pain-Genetics and Genomics

Frank Stüber, MD
Professor of Anesthesiology and Intensive Care Medicine
Department of Anesthesiology and Intensive Care Medicine
University of Bonn
Bonn, Germany
Postoperative Pain-Genetics and Genomics

Richard M. Talbot, FCARCSI
Clinical Research Fellow
School of Biomolecular and Biomedical Science
The Conway Institute of Biomolecular and Biomedical Research
University College Dublin
Specialist Registrar
Department of Anaesthesia, Intensive Care and Pain Medicine
St. James's Hospital
Dublin, Ireland
Mechanisms of Postoperative Pain-Neuropathic

Jeffrey Uppington, MB, BS, FRCA
Professor of Anesthesiology and Pain Medicine
University of California, Davis, School of Medicine
Vice Chairman, Department of Anesthesiology and Pain Medicine
University of California, Davis, Medical Center
Sacramento, California
Guidelines, Recommendations, Protocols, and Practice

Ajay D. Wasan, MD, MSc
Instructor, Departments of Anesthesiology and Psychiatry
Harvard Medical School
Instructor, Department of Psychiatry
Brigham and Women's Hospital
Boston, Massachusetts
Postoperative Pain Management for Patients with Drug Dependence

Oliver H. G. Wilder-Smith, MD, PhD
Associate Professor for Nociception and Pain
Radboud University
Consultant in Anesthesiology and Pain Medicine
Nijmegen Medical Centre
Nijmegen, The Netherlands
Opioids: Excitatory Effects-Hyperalgesia, Tolerance, and the Postoperative Period

Leonard M. Wills, BSc
Remedica Medical Education and Publishing
London, England
Multimodal Analgesic Therapy

Christopher L. Wu, MD
Associate Professor of Anesthesiology and Critical Care Medicine
Johns Hopkins University School of Medicine
Baltimore, Maryland
Postoperative Pain Management and Patient Outcome

译者前言

良好的术后镇痛可以影响外科手术患者的围手术期转归，对降低患者手术后慢性疼痛的发生率及远期死亡率也有一定的作用。10余年前，国内引入了患者自控镇痛（patient-controlled analgesia, PCA）的概念和技术，使我国术后镇痛的理念和技术前进了一大步。患者用上一个"镇痛泵"即能免除手术后剧烈疼痛，这无疑是一大幸事，还大大降低了患者对手术治疗的恐惧，增加了其配合治疗、战胜疾病的勇气和信心。但由于对术后疼痛的发生机制、镇痛药物的合理使用、镇痛技术的优化选择以及患者个体化差异等方面认识的不足，尽管引进了PCA技术，却仍远远没有达到患者所期望的"一痛就按，一按就不痛"的理想境界。时常出现患者术后镇痛不足或过度，或因为镇痛方法或镇痛药物选择不当，患者难以耐受其副作用，甚或出现危及生命的并发症等，引起患者和相关医护人员的猜疑或不满。所以，对术后疼痛及其治疗进行更广泛、深入的研究和提高术后镇痛质量是迫在眉睫的任务。

由于术后疼痛是患者的"第五大生命体征"，对患者影响重大，又涉及患者住院日及ICU滞留时间等社会经济问题，所以术后疼痛及其治疗的研究已成为国际上疼痛研究最热门的专题之一。随着国人生活水平的提高、人口的老龄化和手术指征的扩大，患者及其家属对术后镇痛的要求越来越高，而降低患者住院日和控制医疗费用已成为医院和科室质量考评的重要指标。国内各级相关医疗机构和科研机构也进一步认识到术后镇痛的重要性，这对术后疼痛管理的研究及临床应用带来了新的机遇和挑战。

目前国内关于术后疼痛管理的专著很少，尚没有结合国际最新进展对术后疼痛及治疗进行全方位深入探讨的专著。对麻醉与镇痛专业队伍建设和人员培训而言，更缺少一本理论探讨深入浅出、实践操作切实可行的参考书。

为此，我们集全科之力，在繁忙的临床工作之余，将Postoperation Pain Management一书翻译成中文，并在相关各方面支持下得以出版。

本书论述了手术创伤对机体的影响，并从遗传学及基因组学等多层面阐述了术后疼痛发生的机制及对机体的影响。根据循证医学的原则，客观评价和讨论了目前临床常用镇痛药物及方法的应用原则、治疗效果和优缺点。对疼痛评估、超前镇痛及预防镇痛、多模式镇痛也进行了深入论述，同时兼顾了小儿患者、老年患者、药物滥用者、剖宫产产妇、门诊手术患者等特殊患者或情况下的术后镇痛。全书内容翔实而全面，相信一定会使读者获益匪浅。

本书以从事麻醉镇痛专业、疼痛研究的专业人员及对疼痛治疗感兴趣的医师为主要阅读对象，并兼顾了基层医院的医师和相关专业的实习医师、研究生等。

鉴于译者水平有限，加之翻译时间较短，译文中难免有诸多不足乃至错误之处，敬请同行不吝指正。

邓小明
2008年4月16日

序

本书主题即急性疼痛的管理发展到今天已日趋成熟。早在1971年,我发表了第一篇关于急性疼痛有效管理对预后相关客观指标影响的文章[1]。但是,当时人们几乎根本不去关心如何改善急性疼痛管理,也谈不上运用精确的方法去评估治疗的有效性、副作用及预后。因此,1984年受命组织编写危重病医学中有关急性疼痛管理的专著时,我发现急性疼痛的管理进步甚微[2]。令人惊奇的是,尽管目前关于术后疼痛的管理已经取得到了长足的进步,但是直至今日,危重医学中的疼痛管理方面仍缺乏高质量的研究工作。

负责疼痛领域研究的主要国际组织——国际疼痛研究协会(International Association for the Study of Pain,IASP)成立于1974年,该学会一直以来主要致力于慢性非癌性疼痛的治疗工作。1987年,我开始担任IASP主席一职,我将急性疼痛管理列为IASP未来发展的一项新的重要工作,并制定了一项重要的IASP原则性文件,即建立改善急性疼痛管理的临床组织[3]。然而,这个文件并没有对迅速积累起来的急性疼痛管理研究文献进行严格的分析。1992年,本书的编者之一,IASP主席Dan Carr教授[4]第一次提出了有关急性疼痛管理的循证医学临床实践指南,这是急性疼痛管理的一个里程碑。美国卫生保健政策与研究署(Agency for Health Care Policy and Research,AHCPR)公报是第一个大范围制定临床医疗指南的项目,因此将急性疼痛选入该项目显得极为重要。

1995年,我负责主持澳大利亚国家健康与医疗研究委员会(National Health and Medical Research Council,NHMRC)工作组;1998年,NHMRC制定了一个极为广泛的临床实践指南,该指南涵盖了内科和外科急性疼痛管理的所有方面[5]。该NHMRC文件在2005年中期由澳大利亚-新西兰麻醉医师学院修订出版[6]。目前这个时代的一个重要变化是有较高质量的研究,且可获得医学证据并对其进行严格评估,为急性疼痛治疗的改善提供基础。同时,编者呼吁转变对急性疼痛的处理态度和临床实践方式,并提出急性疼痛管理是一项基本人权[7,8]。

正是在这个背景下,出版了《术后疼痛管理:循证实践指导》一书。编者George Shorten、Daniel Carr、Dominic Harmon、Margarita Puig和John Browne对改善术后疼痛管理作出了巨大贡献,并不断超越自我。此书涵盖了急性疼痛循证管理的所有重要方面,并将急性疼痛循证管理纳入循证医学的大范畴之中。

为了便于读者更好解读,正文的编排更像是一本教科书,而不像以前发表的那些实践指南。为临床医师衔接当代知识与临床实践也是此书重点内容之一。前3章介绍了循证实践的概念、怎样获得和评估医学证据以及指南(guideline)、标准(standard)、协议(protocol)与政策(policy)之间的区别。第1章重点区分了术语"循证医学"与"循证实践"的不同之处,后者针对个体化患者所有最佳有效证据决定的最佳治疗方案。二者的不同也突出了本书重点面向临床医师的特点。因此,本书重点阐述了如何获取和评估医学证据,并如何将其整合到指南、建议、协议和实践中去。

所有医务工作者将会从本书第2部分受益,此部分全面地描述了目前术后疼痛与镇痛的科学基础。尽管其他地方也有这方面的论述,但是该部分特别清晰地阐述了外科手术的损伤反应以及术后伤害性与神经病理性疼痛的机制。有关遗传学和基因组学的章节从当前最为前沿的角度解释了目前遗传学可能如何影响术后疼痛管理,以及将来可能影响更大。这当然是一个令人激动的展望。本书另外一个重要议题是有效的术后疼痛管理对于患者结局的影响。

第3部分非常全面地介绍了术后疼痛管理的各种方法,并恰当地引出了临床实践指南和其他方法的应用。表示不同治疗方法的证据强度方面,一些章节(如第16章,患者自控镇痛)采用"证据等级"方式,但其他章节更多地采用描述性方式。不管何种方式,读者对所有治疗方法均能得出一个清晰的证据强度。

还有重要的一章讨论了急性术后疼痛"预测和预防"(prediction and prevention)的现代新概念,而不是以前"超前镇痛"(preemptive analgesia)的概念。同样,多模式镇痛一章非常明确地论述了多模式镇痛已经成为改善术后疼痛管理的一种重要的新方法。正如新近临床实践指南所关注的，本书也适当关注了一些特殊情形的术后临床疼痛管理，如小儿与老年人、药物依赖患者、剖宫产患者以及门诊手术患者。最后讨论了慢性疼痛的主要人道主义和经济问题。本书所描述的新的疼痛机制和改进的管理方式给人们带来了新的曙光，预防手术后持续性疼痛的目标或许能够成为现实。越来越多的证据显示，手术后持续性疼痛的发生率远比我们以前预想的要高得多，因此，本书以相当篇幅讨论了持续性或慢性疼痛的主要问题。

我认为，本书对急性疼痛领域作出了重要贡献，在此，谨对编委和作者表示衷心的祝贺。

Michael J. Cousins AM, MD
Professor and Director
Pain Management Research Institute
University of Sydney at Royal North Shore Hospital
St. Leonards, New South Wales
Australia

（毛燕飞译　邓小明校）

参考文献

1. Cousins MJ, Wright CJ: Graft, muscle and skin blood flow changes after epidural block in vascular surgery. Surg Obstet Gynecol 1971;133:59–65.
2. Cousins MJ, Phillips GD: Acute Pain Management. Clinics in Critical Care Medicine. London, Churchill Livingstone, 1986.
3. Ready LB, Edwards WT: Management of Acute Pain: A Practical Guide. Seattle, Wash, IASP Publications, 1992.
4. Carr DB, Jacox AK, Chapman CR, et al: Acute Pain Management: Operative or Medical Procedures and Trauma. Clinical Practice Guideline No.1; AHCPR Publication No. 92-0032. Rockville, Md, AHCPR, 1992.
5. Acute Pain Management: Scientific Evidence (1st ed). Canberra, Australia, NHMRC, 1998, http://www.nhmrc.gov.au/publications/synopses/cp104syn.htm.
6. Acute Pain Management: Scientific Evidence (2nd ed). Melbourne, Australia, ANZCA, 2005, http://www.nhmrc.gov.au/publications/synopses/cp104syn.htm..
7. Cousins MJ: Relief of acute pain: A basic human right? Med J Aust 2000;172:3–4.
8. Cousins MJ, Brennan F, Carr DB: Pain relief: A universal human right. Pain 2004;112:1–4.

著者前言

1906年，George Bernard Shaw 在《医师的困境》（The Doctor's Dilemma）一书中写道："当医师面对公众著书立说或谈论手术时，他们暗示氯仿已经使外科手术变得无痛。经历了手术的患者体会更深。"令人惊奇的是，在随后的一个世纪里，术后疼痛的控制却几无进展，这种状态一直持续到人们因诸多因素集中关注到术后疼痛控制差的时候。首先，人们对疼痛神经生物学的了解以及对疼痛控制差与术后并发症如呼吸功能不全和心肌梗死风险之间的关系有了新的认识。其次，人们越来越认识到疼痛控制应作为一项人权和医疗保健标准，体现消费者权益的提高。第三，世界范围内医疗卫生系统经济压力不断增加，由此倡导术后尽早出院。疼痛控制不充分可导致病人延迟出院或增加再次入院的可能性，因此，这就增强了择期手术期间有效控制疼痛的动机。

对急性疼痛控制关注的增加促进了麻醉科急性疼痛服务的发展，并吸引学者将兴趣转移到原本忽略的术后疼痛控制方面。成百上千的各种技术不断涌现，临床医师发现自身受到这些新信息数量庞大和质量不一的挑战。20世纪90年代早期就出现了有关急性疼痛控制的循证指南，从此后，专业组织和政府组织已经开始准备各种实践指南，并对证据进行综述，以不断提高到更高标准。然而，目前的质量评估指出，按最佳实践进行临床实践所达到的预期效果与实际效果之间一直存在着差距。

尽管术后疼痛管理方面的科学技术研究在近十年来取得了重大进步，但是其对临床实践的影响一直受一些因素所限：①新信息的增长速度飞快（信息膨胀）；②对新技术或新药品方面的培训与教育不充分或不可持续；③临床医师不确定何种改进适于临床实践（即被可靠的证据所支持）；④实践或后勤方面，如价格、局部因素（可用的设备或技术）、患者期望值以及医务人员不足等。

本书具有如下特色：

- 提出了一种构架，在这个构架内读者能够根据当前所得到的最好证据来判定实践是否可行。
- 以所有参与术后疼痛管理的医护人员都能接受的方式提供这些信息。这些医护人员包括麻醉医师、麻醉护士、外科医师、临床护理专家、恢复室（PACU）护士以及外科病房工作人员。
- 适于期望采用当前最佳实践的受训者和执业者。

自从1992年Guyatt及其同事首次使用"循证医学"这一术语，并在同年该术语被纳入有关急性术后疼痛管理的第一个官方临床实践指南中以来，"循证医学"的观点得到世界理论界同行的广泛认可（但在实践中较缓慢）。作为临床医师，本书的主编们结合自己的经验处理过成千上万的术后疼痛患者。我们强烈支持以循证的方式来预防和治疗术后疼痛，而不建议也不介绍那些不切实际的不可行方法。我们相信"知识到实践"之间的距离会越来越小，从而不会错过任何一例患者。术后疼痛不允许延迟治疗或治疗不充分。我们有效介入的时间窗较短；如果我们没有进行及时有效的处理，结果可影响患者终生。

目前提供给我们的证据基础还不完善，但是其数量和质量正在提高。缺乏可信度的调查研究仍占有很大的比例。通过"处方"处理术后疼痛的方法仍到处可见。另外，许多重要的临床问题直到被发现后才会引起关注。

将最佳证据与个体患者的偏爱、环境及所遭受的痛苦整合起来，这在疼痛管理中比其他几乎所有的临床问题都显得更为重要，也更为困难。这些困难包括术前患者对阿片类药物耐受或依赖、患者使用抗凝剂后禁忌某些区域麻醉技术、患者失眠或手术结果不佳导致的悲伤和焦虑情绪等。遗憾的是，一些人认为，相对他（她）的主要"职责"来讲，术后疼痛是偶然的、不重要的或事不关己的事情，因此不负责任地将术后疼痛管理搁置。在其他病例中，疼痛处理不充分可能并不是由于缺乏疼痛处理的意识，而是由于缺乏专业技术（如周围神经阻滞）或由于经济或管理因素（如无力承担急性疼痛管理团队的费用）。

本书的主编和作者坚信循证实践的原则能应用于"真实世界"中的术后疼痛管理。这个观点能够得到其他学者的认可是本书编者们的殷切期望；实际上，它已得到全世界疼痛组织领导们的支持。我们希望您，亲爱的读者，将会发现花点时间阅读本书能够使您获益匪浅。

George Shorten
Daniel B. Carr
Dominic Harmon
Margarita M. Puig
John Browne

(毛燕飞　刘双庆译　邓小明校)

致谢

Shorten 医师衷心感谢 Bronagh、Geraldine 和 Jack 三位不辞辛苦的帮助,还要感谢帮助解决问题的专家 Renee Mooney 女士。

Carr 医师诚挚感谢 Tufts 新英格兰医学中心 Evelyn Hall 在行政管理上的支持;感谢 Tufts 新英格兰医学中心疼痛研究 Saltonstall 基金会目前进行的学术活动的支持;衷心感谢其家人和 Javelin 制药有限公司的同事对其完成本书所给予的鼓励和理解。

Shorten 和 Carr 还衷心感谢 Richard J. Kitz 医师对他们早期学术研究的支持和鼓励。

(毛燕飞译 邓小明校)

目录

第1部分 循证实践

1 循证医学实施原则 ············· 1
2 医学证据的获取与评估 ············ 5
3 指南、建议、草案和实践 ············ 12

第2部分 术后疼痛与镇痛的科学基础

4 手术对神经内分泌反应、炎症反应和凝血反应的影响 ············ 29
5 术后伤害性疼痛的机制 ············ 36
6 术后神经性疼痛的机制 ············ 42
7 术后疼痛：遗传学和基因组学 ············ 65
8 术后疼痛处理与患者结局 ············ 73
9 阿片类药物的异化效应（痛觉过敏和耐受）及其对术后镇痛的影响 ············ 86

第3部分 术后疼痛管理

10 疼痛管理目标的制定 ············ 97
11 术后疼痛的临床评估 ············ 104
12 术后急性疼痛的预测和预防：超前镇痛新进展 ············ 111
13 急性疼痛服务 ············ 120
14 阿片类药物的应用临床药理学 ············ 129
15 阿片类镇痛药在围手术期的应用 ············ 139
16 患者自控镇痛 ············ 150
17 区域麻醉和外周神经阻滞技术 ············ 157
18 非甾体类抗炎药在术后镇痛中的应用 ············ 165
19 多模式镇痛疗法 ············ 188
20 非常规及辅助镇痛 ············ 204

第4部分 临床特殊人群的术后疼痛管理

21 婴儿与儿童术后疼痛管理 ············ 219
22 老年患者术后疼痛管理 ············ 227
23 剖宫产术后疼痛的处理 ············ 233
24 药物依赖性患者的术后疼痛管理 ············ 247
25 门诊手术的术后疼痛管理 ············ 258
26 术后慢性疼痛的预防 ············ 268

# 第1部分 循证实践

1 循证医学实施原则

SALAHADIN ABDI · LAXMAIAH MANCHIKANTI

循证医学（evidence-based medicine）是指对个体患者所作出的最为明智、确定和最负责任的治疗决定[1]。近10年来最引人注目的事件是对循证医学所产生的空前兴趣以及所出现的各种能够为医疗保健及临床实践所提供的真实可靠的信息资源，其中包括各种临床指南。因此，临床决策越来越倾向于依据基于研究的证据，而非单纯依据专家意见或临床经验。

20世纪后期，对临床实践的科学评估日益成为关注的焦点。医疗保险和医疗辅助服务中心及卫生保健研究和质量评估机构的Tunis等[2]描述，临床实践中普遍而持续存在却又未能解释的差异以及不恰当的治疗措施[3]，加上不断增加的医疗开支[4]，使人们越来越渴望得到关于临床治疗有效性的确实证据。有理由相信，高质量证据的缺乏是产生地区差异、不当医疗及错误诊断的部分原因[5,6]。某一结果借助于网络传播可以使得生物医学信息的获取和检索越来越便捷，这使得指南制定者、临床医师以及患者和家属对于在日常医疗卫生服务的选择中更加重视获取有效而可靠的信息。

循证医学的实施要求将患者个体的临床成功实践与系统研究所能获得的最好证据加以整合，使得所做出的治疗决策充分考虑所有能够获取到的相关有效信息，这包括随机对照试验得到的有效临床证据以及其他各种类型的证据、患者信息和资源。所有这些意味着：一项有效的研究必须建立在所有相关和有效的信息之上，而针对某一问题的结论必须考虑所有信息的准确度和证据的适用性。另一方面，循证的实施使得那些无偏倚的证据相对于有偏倚者更受重视。

以下4个基本要素可以对循证实践加以定义[7]：

1. 认识患者的疾病并形成一个临床问题的架构；
2. 具备有效调查医学文献和检索最佳可用证据的能力，以对临床问题作出回答；
3. 严肃评价所获得的证据；
4. 将所得证据与个体患者的各个因素进行比较，得到针对该个体的最佳临床治疗决策。

因此，循证医学实际上是一个松散的概念，其在不同时期的应用不仅体现了某些特殊观点，而且还展现了个人的观念、喜好和猜想。这些动机和方法的偏差也引出了关于循证医学是否能真正基于证据的疑问。

寻找证据

为了完成疼痛治疗方面的循证医学研究及找到所有相关证据，研究者必须阅读所有各类证据的文献，后者不仅包括系统综述和随机临床研究，还包括所有已发表的观察性研究和诊断性试验报告。文献检索的策略应该包括所有能够获取的文献资料。另一方面，因为已发表的许多有关疼痛治疗的文献在重要性和连贯性上存在差异，所以许多专家提倡用独立的标准来衡量各个证据的重要性和相关性。例如，通过两个较弱权重、低质量的随机对照试验所得出的相反结论，总体上就不如一项大样本并且严谨的观察性试验所得出的结论更具说服力。

由于地区和特殊问题的差异，如果仅仅运用MEDLINE搜索文献，大概仅能搜索到半数已发表的随机对照试验研究[1]。关于止痛试验的系统回顾和其他研究已经显示，在 MEDLINE 的检索结果低估了非英语文献资源并且仅仅包含已发表的文章[1]，因此存在研究发表的偏倚性和发表语言的偏倚性。另外，从文献发表的国家来看，还存在地理上的差异。例如，关于针灸治疗有效性的研究，来自中国的结果明显高于其他国家。

另一个问题是，如果仅仅利用数据库查找文献，即使像 MEDLINE 这样包含很多文献的数据库，也很难鉴别所有的结果都是相关研究。这种粗略的检索可能在于：①检索范围狭窄；②MEDLINE 索引不合适；③最初的报告本身比较模糊。同样，对于 EMBASE 也是如此。一般而言，MEDLINE 包含大多数英文杂志，而 EMBASE 则可提高对于欧洲各种语言杂志的覆盖范围。虽然 MEDLINE 和 EMBASE 的检索结果有 34% 左右的重叠率，但针对某一特殊问题则可能有 10%～75% 的差异。因此，如果想要广泛了解某一内容的文献，绝不能仅仅依靠某一种数据库，否则就可能会丢失那些没有被索引的杂志、科学会议记录和科学通讯上的同行评审的文章。通过数据库查询参考文献的清单可更进一步地确认相关研究。事实上，Cochrane 协作组（www.cochrane.org）建议评审者查看通过数据库搜索获得的所有相关文章的参考文献，对于可能相关的文献均应考虑和评估其是否应包含在综述中。当利用此种搜索方法时，必须谨记其潜在有参考偏倚和仅代表个人观点的可能性，这一缺陷有可能通过大量搜索策略加以避免。

评价初始报告

最佳临床研究是随机、双盲、对照试验。20 世纪 40 年代，在对于链霉素治疗结核病的疗效评估中，随机对照试验被引入临床医学[8]。随后，随机对照试验在评估治疗因素疗效方面成为金标准[9-11]。1982 年，Sacks 等[12]比较了已发表的随机对照研究与过去的观察性研究之间的区别。这项里程碑式的评估指出，利用历史对照的观察性研究中，有 44 项认为有效（79%），而 50 项随机对照研究中仅 10 项有效，占 20%。因此，研究人员指出，病例选择的偏倚对于观察性研究所得出的支持新疗法的结果可能发挥了至关重要的作用。

然而，2002 年 Kjaergard 和 Als-Nielsen[13]在《英国医学杂志》发表的一项关于商业利益和作者结论之间关系的研究显示，研究者对于随机临床试验结果的解释倾向于支持具有商业利益（即当试验资金由营利性机构提供时）的研究目标。该结论是基于对 12 个医学专业共 159 项研究结果所做的分析，但这些研究的作者均申明其他商业因素（个人、机构或党派等）与作者的结论间并无显著相关性。Djulbegovic 等[14]考察关于多发性骨髓瘤的研究报告得出了相似结论，认为在与传统疗法的比较中，那些由医药公司赞助的研究相对于由非营利组织赞助者更易得出支持研究目标的结果。

随机分配研究对象无论对于对照组或试验组在科学性上均被认为无可挑剔，但随机分配并不能绝对避免偏倚的发生，而只是减少发生偏倚的概率。由于实施随机对照试验的困难和复杂性，通常只能在十分同质的患者中实施。通常，研究者并不积极关注研究对象的来源，而只是关注如何能够将差异均衡地分配在两组中。其结果是，随机化通常是用其内部的一致性（试验组和对照组相似的人口学资料和可比性）换取外部的可靠性（普遍化）[15]。因此，随机化并不能带来一些人认为的保护性屏障。此外，许多患者拒绝参加此种分配过程，因为他们认为随机化有可能将其分配在对照组。因此，对于所有或者大多数将医疗方法与结果相关联的经验性临床治疗数据，单单依靠随机对照试验似乎并不可行[16]。

在这种情况下，特别在无随机对照试验时，就必须依赖结局研究。通常，导致治疗组与对照组结果不同的原因可能来源于偶然因素、混杂因素或组间差异所致的偏倚和两组处理上的差别，当然也可能是两组间干预措施的真实效应。混杂和偏倚可以通过随机取样、单盲法或双盲法加以避免。因此，随机化被认为是避免偏倚和维持试验组与对照组相似性的基石。类似于投掷硬币（或任何其他相当方法）的随机化处理可以保证医师们不会有意无意地将特殊患者分到某一组中。而若不进行随机化，诸如外科与内科治疗的对比就易出现选择性偏倚。假设低危者更可能被分到外科组，只留下高危患者进入内科治疗组。同样，如果将志愿者分配到治疗组，而非志愿者进入对照组，也可能导致偏倚性，因为志愿者与非志愿者本身就可能具有许多方面的差异[17]。根据隔日、隔号或应用其他"预先确定的"分配方法来分配患者至治疗组或对照组，人们也一直持批评态度。即使认为随机化能够保证两组之间只有偶然因素才会带来差异，但其结果仍不能确保适用于临床实践。

目前认为，通过系统回顾和荟萃分析来解答关于临床诊断和治疗的问题是严谨的科学方法。这两种分析方法中，方法学标准和对照是最为关键的部分。除两者之外，共识同样也被认为是证据之一。然而，单独发表的研究并不能提供有关临床实践所必需而完整的相关内容，这使得有必要寻找其他相关的信息和证据来源以及有关共识。共识通常从专家委员会获得，也可以来自于其他擅长于此领域的专家或者从公开讨论会上获取。与荟萃分析或系统回顾相似，卫生技术评定（health technology assessment，HTA）是另一种较常见的证据评价方法。HTA通过系统分析得出相关治疗建议，来帮助医师和患者在卫生保健方面做出决策。通常根据保健的需要或条件限制而被接受、调整或完全拒绝这些建议。

大量证据的强度分级

用于大量证据强度分级的系统有多种，相比较而言，它们在一致性和连贯性上不如用于评定研究质量等级的系统[18]。在质量等级评定系统中，选择何种证据分级系统取决于所测定证据强度的理由、所综述的研究类型以及综述小组的架构。用于大量证据强度评定的总体项目列于表1-1。国家卫生与医学研究委员会（National Health and Medical Research Council，NHMRC）[19]描述的有关证据等级的5个要点列于表1-2中。有些系统需要大量资源，使用起来十分麻烦，

表1-1　评定大量证据的普遍标准

标准	定义
质量	对一既定课题所有相关研究的质量，这里的"质量"是指此研究的设计、实施和分析已将选择性偏倚、测量偏倚及混杂偏倚的程度降到最低
数量	疗效的大小 评估该课题的相关研究的数目 适用于所有相关研究的总体样本量
一致性	对于任何给定课题，用相似或不同研究设计所得到的结果相似

Adapted from West S, King V, Carey TS, et al: Systems to Rate the Strength of Scientific Evidence. Evidence Report/Technology Assessment No. 47; AHRQ Publication No. 02-E016. Rockville, Md, University of North Carolina and Agency for Healthcare Research and Quality, 2002.

表1-2　证据等级评定中的关键要点

- 研究同一等级证据内或不同等级证据间有关某一治疗效应的结论，分析其差别
- 在证据汇总的编辑中，分析偏差尤其重要
- 在某些资料由于认为其存在对于做出某项结论有不合理偏倚而被拒绝时，应该应用包括生物统计学和流行病学的方法来寻找造成这种不合理偏倚的可能原因
- 需承认并非所有的情况都适合应用随机对照试验这一事实。有最佳证据的情况下，应该应用指南
- 认识这样的事实，即可能需要利用来自不同科研设计的证据来认识不同治疗效应的各个方面

Adapted from How to Use the Evidence: Assessment and Application of Scientific Evidence. Canberra, Commonwealth of Australia, National Health and Medical Research Council, 2000, pp 1-84.

表1-3　证据分级

I级	明确的：来自多个相关和高质量科学研究或对荟萃分析进行的一致性综述的证据
II级	有力的：研究证据至少来自一项设计合理的随机对照试验；或来自多个设计合理的小样本研究或多个低质量研究
III级	中度的：（a）证据来自精心设计的不严格的随机对照试验（轮流分配或其他方法分配）；（b）证据来自同期对照和非随机法分配的比较性试验（群组研究、病例对照研究或有对照组的间断时间序列研究）；（c）证据来自与历史对照的比较性研究、两个或多个单臂研究，或无平行对照组的间断时间序列研究
IV级	限制的：证据来自多个中心或研究小组精心设计的非试验性研究；或者在不同试验中产生矛盾结果的证据
V级	不确定的：受尊敬的权威意见、基于临床证据、描述性研究或专家委员会的报告

Adapted and modified from Australian and New Zealand College of Anaesthetists and Faculty of Pain Medicine: Acute Pain Management: Scientific Evidence, 2nd ed. Canberra, Australia, National Health and Medical Research Council, 2005, pp v-vii.

而另外一些则不够完善或缺乏包容性。表 1.3 显示证据设计水平为Ⅰ～Ⅴ级的标准[20,21]。关于个别报道或大量证据的价值将在第 2 章中充分讨论。

结论

循证医学的实施是通过对最佳证据的评估和综合处理来完成的。在此之后，通过对无偏倚文献的综合评估，操作指南、参数以及临床处理路线得以形成，以此来帮助医患双方作出有关医疗保健的最终决策。推荐的操作方法可能根据具体的临床需要或条件限制而被采纳、调整或被拒绝。显然，循证医学提供了超越个体局限的可能性，如临床经验的不足、某种干预措施由于出现某种反应而被错误记忆夸大以及那些需要通过大量临床观察才能得出的一系列具有临床信号标志的特征。第一份建立于循证医学基础上关于术后急性疼痛临床实践指南的发表成为该领域应用循证医学技术的标志性事件[22]。正如法庭虽然会辩论某项证据是否应被采纳以及怎样衡量其优劣，但却绝不会在缺乏证据的情况下作出判决，临床医师已经认识到在日常工作中采用无偏倚临床证据的重要性。改善因特网上证据库访问的途径将会加速这种业已强大的发展趋势。

（李斌本译　李文献　邓小明校）

参考文献

1. McQuay H, Moore A (eds): An Evidence Based Resource for Pain Relief. New York, Oxford University Press, 1998.
2. Tunis SR, Stryer DB, Clancy CM: Practical clinical trials: Increasing the value of clinical research for decision making in clinical and health policy. JAMA 2003;290:1624–1632.
3. Wennberg J, Gittelsohn A: Small area variation in health care delivery. Sci Am 1973;182:1102–1108.
4. Schuster MA, McGlynn EA, Brook RH: How good is the quality of health care in the United States? Milbank Q 1998;76:517–563.
5. Eddy DM, Billings J: The quality of medical evidence: Implications for quality of care. Health Aff (Milwood) 1988;7:19–32.
6. McNeil BJ. Shattuck lecture—Hidden barriers to improvement in the quality of care. N Engl J Med 2001;345:1612–1620.
7. Hatala R, Guyatt G: Evaluating the teaching of evidence-based medicine. JAMA 2002;288:1110–1112.
8. Medical Research Council: Streptomycin treatment of pulmonary tuberculosis. BMJ 1948;2:769–782.
9. Byar DP, Simon RM, Friedewald WT, et al: Randomized clinical trials: Perspectives on some recent ideas. N Engl J Med 1976;295:74–80.
10. Feinstein AR: Current problems and future challenges in randomized clinical trials. Circulation 1984;70:767–774.
11. Abel U, Koch A: The role of randomization in clinical studies: Myths and beliefs. J Clin Epidemiol 1999;52:487–497.
12. Sacks H, Chalmers TC, Smith H Jr: Randomized versus historical controls for clinical trials. Am J Med 1982;72:233–240.
13. Kjaergard LK, Als-Nielsen B: Association between competing interests and authors' conclusions: Epidemiological study of randomized clinical trials published in the BMJ. BMJ 2002;325:1–4.
14. Djulbegovic B, Lacevic M, Cantor A, et al: The uncertainty principle and industry sponsored research. Lancet 2000; 356:635–638.
15. Kane RL: Approaching the outcome question. In Kane RL (ed): Understanding Health Care Outcomes Research. Gaithersburg, Md, Aspen Publishers, 1997, pp 1–15.
16. Concato J, Shah N, Horwitz RI: Randomized, controlled trials, observational studies, and the hierarchy of research designs [see comment]. N Engl J Med 2000;342:1887–1892.
17. Daly LE, Bourke GJ: Epidemiological and clinical research methods. In Daly LE, Bourke GJ (eds): Interpretation and Uses of Medical Statistics. Oxford, Blackwell Science, 2000, pp 143–201.
18. West S, King V, Carey TS, et al: Systems to Rate the Strength of Scientific Evidence. Evidence Report/Technology Assessment No. 47; AHRQ Publication No. 02-E016. Rockville, Md, University of North Carolina and Agency for Healthcare Research and Quality, 2002.
19. How to Use the Evidence: Assessment and Application of Scientific Evidence. Canberra, Australia, National Health and Medical Research Council, 2000, pp 1–84.
20. Australian and New Zealand College of Anaesthetists and Faculty of Pain Medicine: Acute Pain Management: Scientific Evidence, 2nd ed. Canberra, Australia, National Health and Medical Research Council, 2005, pp v–vii.
21. Manchikanti L, Heavner JE, Racz GB, et al; Methods for evidence synthesis in interventional pain management. Pain Physician 2003;6: 89–111.
22. Carr DB, Jacox AK, Chapman CR, et al: Acute Pain Management: Operative or Medical Procedures and Trauma. Clinical Practice Guidline No. 1; AHCPR Publication No. 92-0023. Rockville, Md, AHCPR, 1992.

2 医学证据的获取与评估

MARCUS MüLLNER · DANIEL B. CARR

我们每天在处理病人的时候，都需要作出无数个决定：是否需要使用这项诊断程序？如何解释这些结果？对这一特定患者的最佳治疗方法是什么？床旁决策过程主要聚焦于对特殊状况和个体患者的特定认知。这一以日常工作为基础、用于个体患者的工作经验，它的产生常常结合了来自大量人群或至少是一个或多个临床试验中多组患者的普遍性结论[1]。因此在实践中，定性知识在与定量知识的整合过程中常会受到临床医师偏倚的影响[2]。本章将集中讨论愈来愈能指导临床决策的定量认知。在当前这个倡导循证医学的年代，与临床相关的诸多方面，例如说服保险公司为我们所提供的治疗买单、使陪审团认定我们所采取的措施适当，如此种种，我们均希望能定量测定我们所作出的决定。为了作出针对特定患者的个性化决定，我们首先需要了解一些普遍的影响因素。一些典型的例子包括：对某一特殊治疗，我们所能期望达到的平均治疗效果是什么？特殊治疗有何风险？能用这一诊断程序检测病情状况吗？阴性测试结果是否真的意味着患者不存在该病情？

本章阐述如何获取和评估科学文献，尤其是与急性疼痛有关的文献。为了简洁起见，我们仅重点讨论干预治疗。诸如那些与预后、诊断性检查的价值和经济学分析有关的其他问题，在牛津的循证医学国家健康服务中心网站上有详细讨论[1]。这里我们所采用的是最广泛意义上的"干预治疗"概念，范围包括从药物治疗到手术治疗再到行为干预，其实是指能对病程产生有益影响的任何干预措施。

在讨论如何获取文献之前，我们首先来描述一下如何评估文献，因为某些类型的研究不适用于循证医学实践，故不必为繁忙的临床医师所掌握。

我们从科研中能学到多少知识？

在研究具体方法前，首先，我们必须提出一个哲学观点。本文作者之一（MM）曾在维也纳学习医学，那里的学生在医学院学习期间没有接触科学哲学这一学科；也许世界上的医学院校大都如此，但这一事实的确令人遗憾，因为这一学科会使我们理解我们实际上知道并理解的东西是多么的少，而我们所谓的"知识"周围又包绕着多少的不确定性[2]。事实上，我们必须意识到临床真相的全部细节将永远是不可知的。真相涉及太多方面，以致于没人能了解它，即使是最著名的专家仅在其专业内也做不到。以双氯芬酸（和其他非类固醇类镇痛药）为例，必须承认，我们永远也不会知道它是否能真正缓解关节炎患者的疼痛。但现有的证据是如此具有说服力，以致于我们乃至整个社会都毫不怀疑它的镇痛效果。但当我们提出"双氯芬酸在骨关节炎患者中的平均效果有多大"这一问题时，就引发了另外一个疑问："为减轻关节炎疼痛而连续服用双氯芬酸数月至数年的患者会产生什么副作用？"。再完美的研究也无法精确地回答这些问题，但我们如果有足够（以质量和数量方式表示）的证据，就可以得出结论，认为我们的结果是十分合理并且接近自然真相的临床事实。

遗憾的是，许多医学研究的质量较差或者漏洞百出[3]。质量差的研究不仅浪费资源，而且使我们远离真相。更多的是，有缺陷的试验夸大了干预治疗的有效性[4]，有时可能掩盖这些治疗的有害作用[5-7]。但这一令人失望的状况在疼痛治疗领域尤其明显，尽管在这个广泛的领域中，关于急性疼痛治疗的文献比癌性疼痛或慢性非癌性疼痛治疗包含更多高质量的临床证据[9]。

考虑到"认识"的微妙及其难以捉摸的特性，任何所获得的文献都有存在缺陷的可能。读者在利用这些文献影响临床决策前，必须对这一研究进行全面而严格的评估。

评估医学文献

证据分层

在详细论述之前，我们先介绍一下著名的证据水平分层系统。这一体系有不同的表达形式，有些只是用不同的简单数字表示分层。关于这些不同水平的分层系统，复杂程度不一[1]，图 2-1 列出的一个简明提纲更有帮助。

若想知道某项干预是否有效，最低层次的依据就是专家意见。建立在某一观点和个体经验之上的认知常常存在缺陷。大部分新的治疗方法所带来的好处太过于细微，单靠个人或一组人（如一个科室）的经验很难感受得到它。例如，若要了解急性心肌梗死溶栓疗法的生存效果，专家意见都来自于个案报道或病例总结，常存在患者选择的偏倚，因而可能不具有代表性；此外，这类报道常常都没有设立对照组。没有对照组的观察性研究，例如病例对照研究和群组研究，显然比个人观点或病例报道要好，但仍属于低层次证据。此类研究设计可能存在各种问题，但最主要的问题是，常因为某种原因（往往是不明显的原因），一个患者适合接受某种治疗，而另一个患者则不适合。治疗组和非治疗组间的比较只有在对每个患者进行随机分组的条件下才是合理的。单纯随机分组就能排除一些隐蔽因素对治疗结果判定的影响。事实上，非随机化研究常常会过分夸大干预效果[10]。所以，随机对照试验（randomized controlled trial，RCT）在这一体系中处于较高层次。但我们也要意识到，单个试验仅能反应全局中的一点。谁能只根据一张瑞士保险总部大楼的图片而描绘出整个伦敦城的面貌呢（图 2-2）？

若某人看了朋友近期访问伦敦时拍摄的一系列照片，他是否能更好地了解伦敦呢？想象一下这些照片所展示的内容。其中大部分肯定是他朋友认为有吸引力的、值得纪念的地方。这些照片会使他相信伦敦是个有魅力的城市，但显然他无法看到能代表整个伦敦的照片。这就需要一个更客观、更系统的途径——一张全市街道地图，还要附上有关该市居民如何生活、如何与人相处、如何形成多元化社会的经济和社会学数据。这一方法带领我们达到了证据体系的最高层次：RCT 的系统综述。若干个总体近似的试验结果用数学方法整合起来，这一过程即是荟萃分析。我们通过非正式途径收集的证据就像在旅途中所拍摄的照片。我

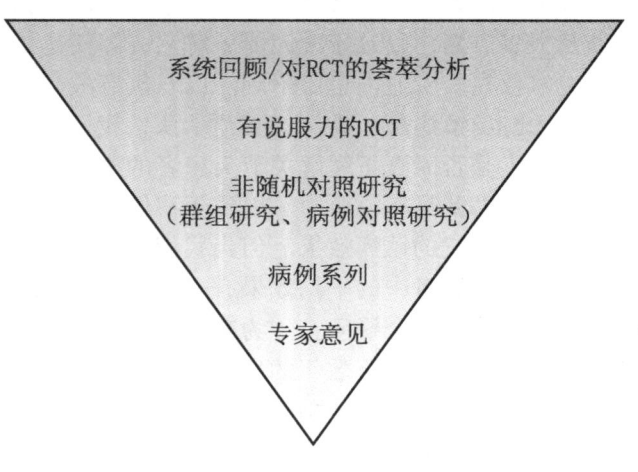

图 2-1　证据分层（RCT，随机对照试验）。

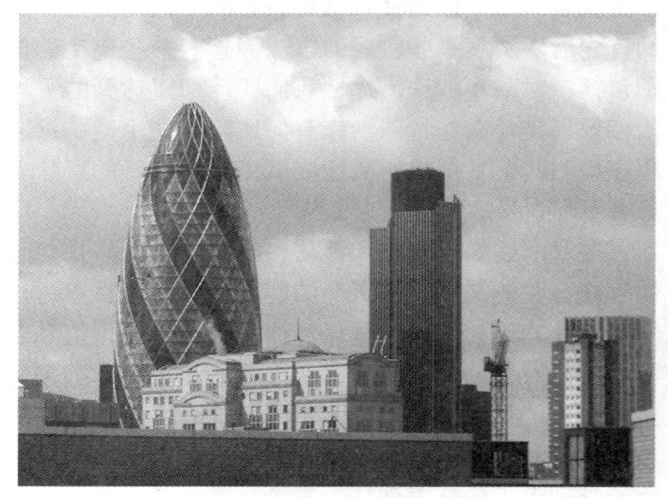

图 2-2　伦敦瑞士保险总部大楼。

们只收集最符合自己需要的证据，一方面是因为它们容易获得；另一方面它也符合我们的喜好（通常我们都有所偏爱，尤其是见到这些证据已得到证实时）。

对随机对照试验严格评估

为了证实某一干预是否有效，相关研究必须符合下面两项标准：①要设立试验组和对照组，②对患者随机分组。如果你有丰富经验和思辨能力且时间充裕，也可以评估一些非随机对照试验，以作为补充证据。令人遗憾的是，临床医师都很忙，他们的专业知识都是建立在临床实践之上，没有详细的方法学知识。如果没有足够的时间，那你就直接忽略掉所有的非随机化研究。

随机分组尽管很重要，但它也只是一个必要条件，其他一些质量标准也会影响试验结果的评估。接下来讨论在评估有关治疗效果的随机对照试验时，读者应考虑的一系列问题。

此项干预与我感兴趣的措施是否类似？

这一问题看似简单，但许多情况下我们自认为所评估的某项干预措施与自己所关心的干预措施很相似，而实际上还是有所区别的。在某项特殊干预缺乏证据时，这一现象更为常见。例如，对已行胸部或上腹部手术的患者，外科医师必然决定是否需要硬膜外注入氢吗啡酮和布比卡因的混合液以改善其呼吸功能[11]。也许他准备在手术示教室和术后病房实施这一技术。他最初找到的文献都是运用布比卡因混合其他阿片类（例如吗啡）的随机对照试验[12,13]，通过这些研究似乎可以得出推论：运用实质上相同的硬膜外药物可以产生相似的效果。

是否设有对照组？

如前所述。

治疗是否为随机分配？

如前所述。

随机化分组是否不可预见？

这就是所谓的"分配隐藏"问题。这是一个棘手的概念。就如同上文所说，人们总有偏好。按隔日分组、按生日的奇偶数分组或按贴出来的随机化表分组等，这些方法都能事先知道分组。这样也会得到一个类似随机化的分配顺序。问题是参加试验的医师可能会选择性地引导患者进入这一组或另一组。有足够的证据表明，不隐蔽分组就会夸大对疗效的评价[14]。我们永远无法知道某一特定试验是否夸大了疗效以及究竟夸大了多少，但平均来说会夸大疗效30%～40%[14]。遗憾的是，许多研究都没有交待其试验分组是否隐藏。若缺少这一信息，那么除非能得到证实，否则读者就应假定其分配方案没有被隐藏。这种悲观的态度也适用于本文讨论的其他观点。

评估者是否将每例患者盲选进入试验组或对照组？

这一点与其前后的问题都紧密相关。假设要求患者在视觉模拟评分标度尺上记录疼痛的程度，而此项研究没有设空白对照组。显然，效果评估者（患者）就会知道干预措施。这就会影响治疗效果，通常是使其增强。盲法是个难题。理想的是，每个涉及试验者（患者、治疗医师、结果评估者和统计者）都应不知道分组。若一项研究自称是双盲，但没有解释如何实施盲法，那么读者就可以猜猜谁知道分组而谁不知道。Schultz和Grimes对此有更深入的讨论[15]。

试验是"软终点"还是"硬终点"？

在疼痛治疗的研究领域，大部分试验终点都是主观的，即所谓的"软终点"。对于盲法研究，采用"软终点"是可以接受的，但如果是非盲法研究，这就会有大问题了。例如，在欧洲或美国医药公司为取得某一药物的销售权而进行非盲法研究通常是不允许的。

"硬终点"就是即使不是盲法也不会导致对结果的误判。最客观的硬终点就是死亡率。许多专业测量结果，例如实验室指标虽然也是客观的，但所有主观终点都是软终点。由患者口头或在一个100 mm的刻度尺上做出标记，对疼痛程度按0～100分级，都是很慎重、很有效的方法，至少对于其他精神方面正常的成人是这样的[16]。患者对院内疼痛治疗的满意度除了取决于疼痛治疗的效果外，还受多种个体差异因素影响，且患者对并不理想的急性疼痛治疗普遍都抱有宽容的态度[17]。

怎样设置对照组？

理想情况下，对照组接受的是安慰剂——没有药效的替代药。这样的安慰剂在外观、质地和味道上都要与试验药相似，以保证患者或结果评估者的主观看法不会影响到结果。某些疼痛研究可能会选用所谓的"标准治疗药"作为安慰剂，这些无镇痛作用的药物可产生预知的副作用如口干或嗜睡，而这些副作用正是试验药物预计应该出现的。运用了安慰剂的疼痛研究都说明了安慰效应在疼痛试验中极其重要。某些疼痛干预措施是无法设安慰剂对照的，例如研究其他一些围手术期用药时PCA泵中加入的吗啡，常是作为一种"急救性"用药来准备的。即使使用安慰针灸[18]或伪手术[19]等方法，这类研究仍要是开放性的（即不设安慰剂对照）。例如，若在前期的盲法研究中，患者对试验药物呈阳性反应，那他就可以进入持续性研究，这类研究以开放性方式继续给予药物，以获取有关持续使用同一种药所产生的不良反应的数据。

研究人群是否与我的患者足够相似？

很明显，这也是个要点。但要对研究人群和自己的患者进行比较，有时也很棘手。年龄、性别、种族、病种和其他重要的基本特征都要匹配。这个概念也被称为外部条件的有效性。若某项研究是在大学的附属医院进行的，而临床医师在没有教学和科研条件的医院工作，那么他就要意识到文献中的患者和他自己的患者有很大区别。众所周知，教学医院进行临床试验所选择的患者都比较年轻，很少有并发症，也更能坚持治疗。高血压治疗在教学医院中就比在基层医院更有效。在疼痛治疗领域，临床试验通常会排除掉一些患者，包括患有重大伴发疾病、高龄、可能在接受多种药物治疗等。但是，此类患者在医院和家庭诊室接受急性术后疼痛治疗中所占的比例正越来越高。

患者的最终分析是否随机化？

这是"意向性治疗"原则。意向性治疗分析是个难懂的概念。它是指患者无论在研究中实际接受了何种处理，均按其最初分组情况进行结果分析。

为了说明这个问题，我们还是以上述硬膜外给予阿片类药物改善术后呼吸功能为例[20,21]。通常在硬膜外给予阿片类药物产生良好术后镇痛的同时，患者也会出现不良反应，若不良反应太严重患者就会要求进行干预（例如注射小剂量纳洛酮以拮抗通气不足或治疗顽固性瘙痒，留置导尿管以处理尿潴留）。此类干预会使这些患者被排除在进一步的试验之外。对于退出试验的患者或因其他种种原因而未能记录下数值的患者，通常记录其前一次评分值作为疼痛强度评分。理论上，患者的疼痛被很好地控制了，但对副作用很不满意，此时继续观察则可能曲解措施所带来的益处，而忽视其潜在风险。把这些患者留在术后镇痛试验中，若他们要求使用纳洛酮治疗不良反应，就会增加对疼痛治疗的总体评分；若不得已进行其他干预措施，如留置导尿管，则会降低患者的满意度。这种方法可能会降低干预的镇痛效果，但现实中却能做出效果评估。在日常临床实践中，所使用的装置（此处是硬膜外导管）常常会失效，如果某个装置理论上是有效的，但实际中因为常常失效而变得无效，那么只能不再使用。若只分析来自按原方案完成试验的患者数据，即按方案分析，则会夸大效果。按方案分析反映的是生物学效应，意向性治疗分析则反映的是临床效应。

对研究的评估

一名有经验的评估者用1个小时就能评估出一份研究报告的所有信息。读者可能认为自己由于缺少时间和经验，而无法运用这些标准。值得庆幸的是，我们可以走些捷径。RCT的质量主要取决于三大因素：①分配隐藏；②意向性治疗分析；③盲法评估结果。若时间紧张，我们只需思考这3个问题。

对系统回顾的严格评估

要写出好的系统综述，作者需要为读者做好上述所有的质量评估，并由读者判断。这就意味着对系统综述的评估更为困难，且仅集中讨论关键问题。读者需要分辨出一个系统综述是否有用。在评估一份系统综述和荟萃分析时要考虑以下问题：

回顾性研究是否有明确的假设或目标？

这是区分一般综述和系统综述的关键点。

回顾性研究是否包含非随机试验？

有关医学干预有效性的系统综述理论上应只能包括RCT。若涉及了非随机试验，则要单独列出分析，这些试验只能作为佐证。尽管一份评价有时运用所谓的近似随机试验（例如按隔日分组）是有意义的，但只要它涉及了非随机化试验，我还是建议临床医师在只能做出快速判断时不要把它列为系统综述。

是否明确描述了干预措施？

这一问题的用意很明显。

是否明确描述了试验终点？

这一问题的用意很明显。

是否明确定义了目标人群？

这一问题的用意也很明显。

是否明确描述了检索策略？

通过细节描述，理论上任何人都能重复此项研究并得出相同结果。就是说他们使用的搜索词和数据库都应该详细加以说明。

怎样采集数据？

我我们所有的行为都会出错（质量上和数量上都会有），可以预见有5%的数据是错误的。如果在数据采集中加入了一些判断，则出错的风险更大[2]。在进行系统综述时，需要进行大量判断，尤其决定试验质量时（见下一个问题）。所以，要由两个人分别采集数据并进行比较。通过讨论或由经验丰富的方法学家来解决分歧。

研究者是否了解试验质量？

如上所述，系统综述至少要有3个决定试验质量的要点：分配方案隐藏、意向性治疗分析和盲法评估结果。系统综述的领导者在处理试验质量时可以使用多种方法，统称为"灵敏度分析"。通常的做法是，把低质量的试验去除后重新分析。理论上，结果应保持不变，就是说其对质量偏倚的影响是稳定的。可惜的是，现在大部分有效试验都缺少一个或多个要点，一旦它们都被排除，就没有多少可供评价的试验了。

评估

评估系统综述和荟萃分析会涉及更多方面，但进行快速评估时掌握以上所述方法就足够了。而且其他方面需要更多的方法学细节，这也超出了本综述的范围。实际上，评估系统综述质量的方法有很多[22]。

若读者有兴趣了解更多，我们推荐Cochrane协作网的自学材料[23]。要知道，并非每个RCT都是高质量的，做临床决定时，RCT并非就比非随机试验有价值[24]。例如，一个RCT的两组中各有12名患者，仅使用单次剂量的治疗药物（而临床上这一药物可能要持续使用数周或数月）来判断对患者疼痛治疗的效果及对生活质量和生理功能的影响，它所能提供的信息可能就不如一项经严格控制的病例对照研究（每组包含数千例患者，且用药时间持续3个月）多。遗憾的是，对于急性疼痛、癌性疼痛或慢性疼痛的临床试验，前者都是不标准的。此外，有关某一临床问题的证据，我们除了要记住证据的类型，还要记住其强度和连贯性[25]。

一名经验丰富的评估者用半小时就能从一份研究报告中得到其他方面的信息。读者可能认为由于缺少时间和缺乏经验，自己无法运用这些标准分析RCT，所以最好由他人做出评估，而读者只需使用这些资源，这就是下一课题。

获取医学证据

理论上，除非临床医师要做一次彻底的系统综述，否则就不需要进行文献检索。任何人要为系统综述做文献检索都需要具有更多的背景知识，只看本章内容是不够的。许多情况下，对于一名医师来说，寻找临床问题的相关试验只是浪费资源，而且更糟糕的是会错误地把某项并不适合的试验运用到临床中。重要的是使用那些他人已经严格评估过的资源。证据资源数量巨大，且不断增加，已经根据预定质控程序进行了严格判读。表2-1列出了一些常见的资源，在各自的网站上都提供了详尽的信息。

以下是一位急诊医师搜集依据的情景：

一名年轻人因自行车事故来到急诊室，其肘部骨折已得到控制，但疼痛由轻微变成剧烈。在进行骨折

表2-1　循证医学的常见资源

数据库	网址
Cochrane 图书馆	http://www.cochrane.org
ACP 杂志俱乐部	http://www.acpjc.org
循证医学	http://ebm.bmjjournals.com
护理循证医学	http://ebn.bmjjournals.com
临床证据	http://www.clinicalevidence.com
Trip 数据库	http://www.tripdatabase.com
医疗保健机构质控与研究（前称医疗保健质量机构与研究）	http://www.ahrq.gov

闭合复位过程中，患者注射了短效静脉麻醉剂（丙泊酚），但随后不久其"因为疼痛"而出现呕吐。他声称既往在拔牙后口服阿片类药也曾呕吐过。

那么医师现在应如何处理？①口服非甾体类抗炎药（nonsteroidal anti-inflammatory drug，NSAID），②口服阿片类镇痛药，③注射非甾体类抗炎药，④注射阿片类镇痛药，⑤镇吐，或者⑥包括物理方法在内的非药物治疗(如冰敷)，应该选择哪种治疗方案呢？除非患者至少能够喝下清水，否则按其目前的呕吐情况是无法口服用药的，并且他有使用阿片类镇痛药后出现恶心反应的病史，所以医师只能使用非甾体类抗炎药镇痛。由于医师希望该患者在离开急诊室时疼痛能得到有效控制，因此他决定检索一下已发表的证据是否支持他在急诊室内给患者胃肠外使用非甾体类抗炎药，或者能否在使用了止吐剂后给患者口服给药。

通过 google 学术搜索引擎[26]，医师能够找到一份关于这个问题的系统综述。在搜索空格中键入单词"NSAID"、"efficacy" 和 "route"，医师在 Oxford Bandolier 网站[27]找到 1 篇系统综述。这份评价显示，除了肾绞痛外，还缺乏证据能证明注射非甾体类抗炎药优于口服用药[5]。另一方面，作者们也提醒，缺乏证据并不等于证据无效，也即他们并没有断言对于包括肾绞痛在内的情况下，各种给药途径间不存在效果差异。

医师认为，当时患者有过恶心呕吐，最好还是采取注射非甾体类抗炎药。于是，医师就想知道哪种非甾体类抗炎药更为有效。他再次访问 Oxford Bandolier 网站[27]，并且点击了"急性疼痛"链接图标后，找到一张关于 NSAID 用于急性疼痛的镇痛效果评价表，此表根据功效列出了各种非选择性 NSAID 以及环氧合酶-2（cyclooxygenase-2，Cox-2）抑制剂。此表表明，在单剂量药物研究中，40mg 伐地考昔（环氧合酶-2 抑制剂）是治疗术后急性疼痛最有效的注射制剂(包括与注射用阿片类药比较)。其中一位同事表示质疑，考虑到严重心脏意外、手术部位出血和其他副作用，以及他最近听说的骨骼愈合欠佳，那么使用昔布类药是否安全。因此，这位医师查询了 Oxford Bandolier 网站，结果发现，没有证据表明短时期使用 NSAID 和环氧合酶抑制剂会使骨骼愈合不良。同时，此评价提到了吸烟无疑是骨骼愈合不良的危险因素；医师发现该患者正是一个吸烟者。回想起最近关于昔布类药安全性的争论以及顾问团为美国食品与药品监督管理局（Food and Drug Administration，FDA）所做的一次听证会（其目的在于衡量使用昔布类药安全性的正反两方面证据），医师去查询了 PubMed 医学生物文献数据库[28]，输入关键词"昔布类药心血管安全性（coxib cardiovascular safety）"。第 2 次查询找到了 2005 年 FDA 所做的相关听证会。现在，医师已经在互联网上浏览 5 分钟。医师点击了那个标题，却发现由于他不是该文章所发表杂志的订阅者，无法看到摘要，只能看到文章开头的 100 个字。这些文字表明，环氧合酶抑制剂可增加心血管相关并发症的危险性，但是并没有说何时或者何种特定情况下，这种危险性更明显。然后，医师转向 google 学术搜索引擎，输入关键词"NSAID 安全性 手术（NSAID safety surgery）"，所找到的第 1 条是一个关于环氧合酶抑制剂安全性的文献综合数据库，后者是 2005 年由一家大型整形外科中心的医师们所创办的[29]。他惊奇地发现，虽然研究非常有限，但无论临床试验还是动物试验都表明：NSAID 和环氧合酶抑制剂都可能延缓骨折的愈合。

医师把冰袋放置在骨折部位，观察到患者的疼痛得到缓解的同时，其恶心也有显著减轻。患者喝清水时也不再恶心了。医师又来到 google 学术搜索引擎上，输入关键词"疼痛导致恶心（pain cause nausea）"。找到的前两条结果都支持这种联系，这两条结果都来自牛津的 McQuay 所著的文章[30]。医师建议这位患者继续使用冰袋，并开了曲马多（一种非阿片类镇痛药）处方，48 小时的用量。搜索这一信息断断续续用了 15 分钟。

结论

医学证据的获取与评估不是一项简单的技能。理论上，只应查阅那些所有文章都已经过严格判读的资源。1906 年，萧伯纳写了戏剧《医师的窘境》(The Doctor's Dilemma)，他在戏中预言，需要分配稀缺而又有效的医疗资源时就会产生伦理问题。萧伯纳是胫骨骨髓炎患者，经历了无数次手术。他写到，尽管全麻能使手术无痛，但"患者为麻醉付出的代价是数小时可怜的呕吐；而此后就是手术伤口的疼痛，这些伤口最终也会像其他伤口一样愈合"。他更发现"因为没有接受过相关方面的训练，医师不会使用医学证据，没有生物统计学知识，不了解人文倾向和经济压力。

基本上，医师们必须想患者所想，这就是所谓的旁观者清"。

2000年以前，圣经旧约丹尼尔卷中记载了人类最早的有记录的临床试验。(圣经中的试验为不设安慰剂组的非随机化平行队列试验。结果发现，简单的素食饮食要优于偏食一种营养食品。)今天，临床实践和社会大众都普遍认同，临床试验是非常有效的工具。尽管循证医学中有关特定问题的争论仍将继续，可立法者、政策制定者、保险公司以及患者现在都能够迅速而广泛地搜集医学证据，这一事实已彻底地改变了临床实践。在21世纪，为满足患者及其家属的期望而需要实施高质量的疼痛治疗，每位医学工作者必须在日常工作中学会获取和评估医学证据。

(盛　颖译　朱文忠　李文献校)

参考文献

1. National Health Service (NHS) Center for Evidence-Based Medicine. Available at www.cebm.net/
2. Carr DB: On the silent "l" in "qualntitative." In Carr DB, Loeser J, Morris D (eds). Narrative, Pain and Suffering. Seattle, IASP Press, 2005, pp 325–354.
3. Altman DG: The scandal of poor medical research. BMJ 1994;308:283–284.
4. Kjaergard LL, Villumsen J, Gluud CL: Reported methodologic quality and discrepancies between large and small randomized trials in meta-analyses. Ann Intern Med 2001;135:982–989.
5. Tramer MR, Moore RA, Reynolds DJM, McQuay HJ: Quantitative estimation of rare adverse events which follow a biological progression: A new model applied to chronic NSAID use. Pain 2000;85:169–182.
6. Koreny M, Riedmuller E, Nikfardjam M, et al: Arterial puncture closing devices compared with standard manual compression after cardiac catheterization: Systematic review and meta-analysis. JAMA 2004;291:350–357.
7. Edwards JE, McQuay HJ, Moore RA, Collins SL: Reporting of adverse effects in clinical trials should be improved: Lessons from acute postoperative pain. J Pain Symptom Manage 1999;18:427–437.
8. Haynes B: Bridging the Gaps between The Cochrane Collaboration and Clinical Practice. Plenary session presentation at Cochrane Colloquium, Oct. 2–6, 2004, Ottawa, Canada. Available at www.cochrane.mcmaster.ca/Colloquium/PPTs/Oct3/Plenary1_CCConHallABEF_1100_Haynes.ppt#1 (accessed November 22, 2004).
9. Carr DB, Goudas LC, Balk EM, et al: Evidence report on the treatment of pain in cancer patients. J Natl Cancer Inst Monogr 2004;32:23–31.
10. Ioannidis JP, Haidich AB, Pappa M, et al: Comparison of evidence of treatment effects in randomized and nonrandomized studies. JAMA 2001;286:821–830.
11. Ballantyne JC, Carr DB, deFerranti S, et al: The comparative effects of postoperative analgesic therapies on pulmonary outcome: Cumulative meta-analyses of randomized, controlled trials. Anesth Analg 1998;86:598–612.
12. Block BM, Liu SS, Rowlingson AJ, et al: Efficacy of postoperative epidural analgesia: A meta-analysis. JAMA 2004;291:1197–1198.
13. Choi PT, Bhandari M, Scott J, Douketis J: Epidural analgesia for pain relief following hip or knee replacement (Cochrane Review). In The Cochrane Library, issue 2. Chichester, UK, John Wiley & Sons, 2005.
14. Schulz KF, Chalmers I, Hayes RJ, Altman DG: Empirical evidence of bias: Dimensions of methodological quality associated with estimates of treatment effects in controlled trials. JAMA 1995;273:408–412.
15. Schulz KF, Grimes DA: Blinding in randomised trials: Hiding who got what. Lancet 2002;359:696–700.
16. Carr DB, Goudas LC, Lawrence D, et al: Management of Cancer Symptoms: Pain, Depression, and Fatigue. Evidence Report/Technology Assessment No. 61. AHRQ Publication No. 02-E032. Rockville, Md, Agency for Healthcare Research and Quality, 2002.
17. Miaskowski, C, Nichols R, Brody R, Synold T: Assessment of patient satisfaction utilizing the American Pain Society's Quality Assurance Standard on acute and cancer-related pain. J Pain Symptom Manage 1994;9:5–11.
18. Streitberger K, Kleinhenz J: Introducing a placebo needle into acupuncture research. Lancet 1998;352:364–365.
19. Moseley JB, O'Malley K, Petersen NJ, et al: A controlled trial of arthroscopic surgery for osteoarthritis of the knee. N Engl J Med 2002;347:81–88.
20. Dolin, SJ, Cashman JN, Bland JM: Effectiveness of acute postoperative pain management: I. Evidence from published data. Br J Anaesth 2002;89:409–423.
21. Viscusi ER, Gavia M, Hartrick CT, et al: Forty-eight hours of postoperative pain relief after total hip arthroplasty with a novel, extended-release epidural morphine formulation. Anesthesiology 2005;102:1014–1022.
22. West S, King V, Carey TS, et al: Systems to date the strength of scientific evidence. Evidence Report/Technology Assessment No. 47. AHRQ Publication No. 02-E016. Rockville, Md, Agency for Healthcare Research and Quality, 2002.
23. Cochrane Collaboration Open Learning Material. Available at www.cochranenet.org/openlearning/HTML/mod0.htm/
24. Jadad AR, Cepeda MS: Clinical trials in pain relief: 10 challenges. Pain Clinical Updates 1999;7:1–4.
25. Jacox AK, Carr DB, Payne R, et al: Management of Cancer Pain. Clinical Practice Guideline No. 9; AHCPR Pub. No. 94-0592. Rockville, Md, Agency for Health Care Policy and Research, 1994.
26. Google Scholar Search. Available at http://scholar.google.com/
27. Oxford Pain Internet Site. Available at http://www.jr2.ox.ac.uk/bandolier/booth/painpag/
28. PubMed. Available at http://www.ncbi.nlm.nih.gov/entrez/query.fcgi?CMD=Limits&DB=pubmed/
29. Urban MK, Markenson JA, Lane JM: HSS physicians review literature on the safety of COX-2 inhibitors. Available at http://www.hss.edu/Professionals/Conditions/Arthritis/Safety-of-Cox-2-Inhibitors/
30. McQuay H: Opioids in pain management. Lancet 1999;353:2229–2232.

3 指南、建议、草案和实践

JEFFREY UPPINGTON

许多术语被纳入指南的一般词汇表。除了建议和草案，还有政策、标准、参数、建议、警告、流程、选择和公告等。这些定义和用法相互重叠，很多术语可以互换使用。

Eddy[1]在实践策略这一项下，基于各种实践策略的严格程度，定义了3类最基本的策略（旁注3-1）。美国麻醉医师学会（American Society of Anesthesiologist，ASA）对实践参考策略陈述中所用的一些术语进行了定义（旁注3-2）[2]。遵循实践标准的规定或要求是一种潜在的义务。医学会将指南定义为"一种为协助从业者和患者对特定临床情况给予合适医疗保健决策的系统性成熟陈述"[3]，而且这一定义被许多权威专家所认可和使用[4-6]。因为这一定义所指的指南是"协助"决策，而非做出决策，所以指南并没有强制执行标准或草案的性质。本章主要讨论由 Eddy[1]和医学会[3]定义的草案（标准）和指南。一般认为，其他术语可与这些术语互换使用。

指南发展和使用的历史

对指南发展历程的简单回顾可以帮助我们理解当前实践指南的地位。公元前4世纪，Plato讨论了医师根据实践经验从业和根据严格规定[7]来从业的不同之处。Plato 的观点是，具有专门经验的重要标志包括反应能力和即刻处理能力，使用指南会减弱后一种实践能力[7]。尽管 Plato 准备退一步承认指南的作用，但他认为实践中指南的使用仍是有争议的，因为指南并没有考虑到特定的个体，而是根据患者的平均情况制订的[8]。对指南的这种批评一直延续至今。现代，有很多国家军队已经使用了临床应急预案，在转运到更完备的医院之前，指南帮助指导前方随军医务人员对受伤的士兵进行诊断和处理[9]。后来指南为训练中的医师以及内科医师提供参考意见[10]。

然而，在20世纪80年代的美国，以下的三大主要因素在重大改变中起决定作用[11]：

(1) 提高医疗保健经费，包括医师的工资[12-14]。

(2) 实践的差异。很多实例有力地证实了临床实践中的差异[15-20]。尽管它不是很明确，但其中一些差异可以由患者人群、当地资源、患者的偏爱[21-23]等来解释，但仍持续存在实践差异的问题[24-26]，直到今天[27]。它仍然处于医疗保险经费努力缩减的最前列[28,29]。

(3) 关于不必要的治疗和医疗操作的报告。最常被引用的是 RAND 社团的研究[30]，但是推断需要一个非常大的涉及面[31,32]。

美国健康与人类服务部（Department of Health and Human Service，DHHS）带头采取了有效行动[33]，其他联邦卫生部门也成立了鉴定组，他们和院校研究人员研

旁注3-1　实践策略

标准：严格使用，在所有实际情况中必须遵守
指南：较弹性，在大多数情况下遵守
选择：就推荐而言是中性，只表示可应用的不同选择

Adapted from Eddy DM: Designing a practice policy: Standards, guidelines and options. JAMA 1990;263:3077-3084.

旁注 3-2	关于实践参考的政策陈述 *
实践参考	就特定问题发展的提供诊断和治疗的指导和方向，可能包括标准、指南或警告
实践标准	临床实践的规则或最低要求，对健全的患者治疗方案而言代表可普遍接受的原则。可以包括实践方针的陈述、草案、患者治疗的特殊推荐
实践指南	关于患者诊疗的系统发展的推荐，为一种基本诊疗对策或者基本诊疗对策范围
实践忠告	系统发展的报告，旨在对科学依据不充分的患者保健领域协助决策
实践警告	旨在协助患者进行保健领域决策的报告，帮助对特殊问题警觉
陈述、状况、记录	代表政府在很多主题上的观点，并不从属于同样水平的科学综述，例如标准、指南、忠告、警报等

*Approved by House of Delegates October 13, 1993, and last amended October 27, 2004.

Adapted from American Society of Anesthesiologists: Policy Statement on? Practice Parameters. Available at http://www.asahq.org/publicationsAndServices/sgstoc.htm (accessed March 2, 2005).

旁注 3-3	专业团体建立实践指南示例
美国变态反应与免疫学学会	
美国儿童和青少年精神病学学会	
美国眼科学学会	
美国矫形外科学会	
耳鼻喉头颈外科学会	
美国儿科学会	
美国肌电描记术和电诊断法协会	
美国心脏病学会	
美国急救医师学会	
美国妇产科医师学会	
美国职业医学学院	
美国内科医师学会	
美国预防医学会	
美国放射学会	
美国风湿病学会	
美国外科医师学会	
美国老年医学会	
美国医学会	
美国精神病学协会	
美国胃肠内镜检查学会	
美国麻醉医师学会	
美国泌尿外科学会	
美国病理学家学会	

Adapted from the Office of Quality Assurance, American Medical Association: Listings of Practice Parameters, Guidelines, and Technology Assessments. Chicago, American Medical Association, 1989; and Woolf SH: Practice guidelines: A new reality in medicine. 1: Recent developments. Arch Intern Med 1990;150:1811-1818.

究具有显著差异的操作的适用性和有效性[11]。到1988年，为了减少实践的差异，明确建议使用实践指南。

因为政府并没有推出一个统一的版本[37-38]，许多公共卫生服务机构开始推出各自的指南[34-36]。医师有偿回顾报告经常把操作指南作为其实现报告内容的主线[39]。同时，医师组织继续从事指南的发展[40]。许多专业团体提供实践指南（见旁注3-3）[11,41]。卫生保健组织[43]、各州和地方政府也发布各种指南[42]。

国际指南

指南及其发展受到国际上的普遍关注（旁注3-4）[44]。在英国，对使用证据评估的指南的发展越来越关注[45]，包括护理实践[46]。苏格兰大学指南合作网络使用系统多学科路径来制定和传播循证指南[47]。他们网页的主机站点包含了指向其他国际互联网址的链接。澳大利亚知名网站IMPACT（Interdisciplinary Maternal Perinatal Australasian Clinical Trials）有许多指南发展成果的资源[48]。全世界的杂志现在专门热衷于医疗保健的循证研究[49-51]。

指南的益处

使用指南的主要益处在于使患者的治疗质量更好。然而，在后来的讨论中，不同团体（医师、支付者和管理者）规定的质量标准也不一样[44]。但是在这些支持者中至少有一个共识，指南拥有几个潜在的益处。

对患者的益处

已证实指南在实践中拥有以下潜在的鼓舞人心的效果，即减少发病率和病死率，在某些条件下改善生活质量[44]。它们具有减少医疗差异的潜在优势。如果Archie Cochrane关于"如果实践与指南有很大程度偏离的话，你将不可能都正确"[52]的观察报告是正确的，指南将是有益的。没有更好的试验证据表明不同变化

旁注 3-4	国际上关于指南的一般看法
欧洲	英国——在国家健康服务机构、专业组织、研究者的促进下,指南已经存在数十年,正引起许多人的兴趣。 荷兰——Dutch 大学普通行医者从 1987 年起每 8~10 年就对指南提出一些更新。指南主要由 Dutch 大学健康中心完成。 芬兰和瑞典——芬兰自从 1989 年已经产生了 700 余部指南,已经进入循证医学时代。在瑞典,瑞典科学技术委员会和其他政府团体已经提出瑞典实践指南。 法国——国家健康机构通过沿袭或修改其他国家的指南而出版了 100 部以上的实践指南,这些指南被普通行医者通过网络传播同时接受大众的评价。 德国、意大利和西班牙——指南在这些国家正在引起重视。在西班牙,健康技术委员会正筹备指南并教授指南发展方法。
北美	美国——在美国的医院及健康计划中"指南、方案和保健通道"一般用于提高质量和降低费用。尽管循证医学已经引起重视,但很多健康保健组织制定实践指南主要是为了缩短住院日和其他费用。 加拿大——加拿大健康保健大多由各州提供资金,但采用指南的机构的比例同美国相似。
澳大利亚和新西兰	澳大利亚——指南源于 20 世纪 70 年代晚期,当时州健康部门开始认可指南的小册子,强调了对循证指南的需求。 新西兰——指南直接源于政府健康政策。新西兰政府通过指南选择性地限制健康服务的政策引起了国际上的注意。新西兰心脏基金会的一项高血压指南和随后的胆固醇控制指南采用了新的方法学而有所突破,是将建议与患者绝对风险概率相关联,而非与一般治疗标准相关联。

Adapted from Woolf SH, Grol R, Hutchinson A, et al: Potential benefits, limitations, and harms of clinical guidelines. BMJ 1999;318:527-530.

的医疗方式能够改变和促进医护质量,所以许多人和政府机构的假设是:这个观察报告是正确的。操作指南也具有改善预后的潜在可能[53-56]。他们通过传单、录音磁带或其他教育性资料帮助患者,尤其是那些评估不同结局概率的资料[57]。这些项目帮助医师和患者了解合理的医疗保健选择。当指南通过唤起人们注意未被承认的或资金不足的健康问题而影响国家政策方针时,患者也能在这方面受益。

对医疗保健提供者的益处

好的操作指南可以提高临床治疗的质量。当尚无恰当的治疗方式时,指南是有益的,它有助于推翻过时的习惯,提供令人放心的恰当的临床行为,并改善治疗的连贯性[44]。如果有循证医学的实践支持,操作指南可以提醒临床医师进行由良好科学证据支持的治疗。指南可显示出医学文献间的差距,可帮助医学研究者改进文献质量。临床医师和付款者均可为他们各自的利益而使用指南,比如法医学上的保护、赔付比例等[44]。当然,以上这些益处也存在一些不尽如人意的方面。

对医疗保健体系的益处

通过标准化治疗,临床操作指南在提高金钱的有效性和价值方面是有效的[44,58,59]。指南在危急情况处理方面发挥了主要作用,包括患者的目标以及达到目标的必要步骤和时间[60]。指南还被用作另一种工具来提高工作效率和改善工作质量[61]。指南和紧急处理步骤可以降低成本,并具有额外益处,即通过发送治疗质量并承诺优良效果的信息提高采用指南的人员的公众形象[44]。

指南的不足

关于指南的使用已经出现许多批评。指南存在以下几个方面的缺点:那些被推荐的操作指南缺乏科学证据、存在误导或可能被误解[44];指南制定者的观点影响指南的推荐,而这些观点可能基于错误的认识;患者可能并不是指南惟一的优先考虑的对象[62];推荐的操作指南可能集中注意在控制费用或者保护特殊群体(比如医师、公司经理、政治人物等)利益上,而危害患者的需求[44]。

有缺陷的指南存在的潜在危害将在下面部分进行讨论。

对患者的危害

有缺陷的指南其最大风险是对患者的危害。它存在这样的风险：忽略患者优先和特殊情况，而减少患者的个体化治疗[63]。对多种病情的患者采用特定疾病的指南是靠不住的，因为适用的指南不止一个[64]。还有的风险是指南可能是无效的[65-67]。指南能够改变实践的证据已有报道[68-69]，但其影响很小且很短暂[70]。

对医疗保健提供者的危害

有缺陷的指南能够降低医方提供的医护质量。临床指南质量的发展并不像它应有的那样严格[71,72]，从而要求其改善[73]。指南之间可能会有冲突[74,75]，这种情况可能会导致混乱和妨碍合适的医疗行为。指南过剩的情况造成信息传播困难和目的不清[76,77]。临床医师可能因为职业因素反而会受累。被视为"食谱医学"实践[78]并不吸引人，但指南不是食谱医学[5]。许多医师不信任指南，认为它们会增加成本，可用于医师的训练，但在医疗行为中产生的满意度有限[79]。

对医疗保健系统的危害

如果指南导致成本增加，疗效减少，或者有限资源的浪费，这样就会产生危害[44]。

指南的法律因素

医疗疏忽的定义包含许多基本要素（旁注 3-5）[80]，而临床指南能够影响医护标准的定义。临床医师担心指南过细会增加他们在法医学上的不利[81]。然而，至少在 1995 年的美国，指南只在很少的医疗事故行为中起到主导作用[82]。虽然如此，这个局面并非如此简单。

旁注 3-5　医疗疏忽

医疗疏忽是复合的法律裁决，包括三个重要组成部分。提出诉讼者，即原告，必须提供：
1. 被告的医师对原告存在失职。
2. 该医师没有提供标准的医疗监护，没能履行医疗的职责。
3. 其失职导致原告的伤害，而该伤害是可预见和可避免的。

循证指南能影响法庭对第二条进行裁决的方式。

Adapted from Hurwitz B: How does evidence-based guidance influence determinations of medical negligence? BMJ 2004;328:1024-1028.

法国在 1993 年的法令中制定了许多强制性实践指南。一旦发布出来，指南就成为医师和国家社会保健机构之间的强制性协定[83,84]。正式控告，即指控参与者实施了与指南不相适应的行为，曾被送往法国欺诈行为调查委员会[83]。

英国的法定监护标准根据 Bolam 学说定义为：这是一个能实施并声称具有某项特殊技能的一般熟练人员的标准[85]。美国的标准也相似，它包含"合理与审慎"的概念[86]。虽然指南被专家引入法庭当作"可接受和典型的监护标准"证据，但它们仍不能替代专家意见[79]。没达到质量标准[87]的指南不应成为法定标准，但由于法庭一般不请专家评价指南的可靠性，这种可能最终会变成现实[88]。

目前在美国，指南在法庭纠纷上并未发挥主要作用。一个在美国广为报道的例子，某医师尽管依据国家临床指南未给患者开具选择性前列腺抗原（PSA）检查，其门诊部依然被认为负有责任，且该医师被认为不负责任[89]。这一裁决引发医师们的进一步议论[90,91]，但遵循指南并不总是能保证良好的医疗，而偏离指南的行为也并不视为一定引起较差的医疗效果，这才是合理的态度[92]。Hurwitz[80]概括了指南的法律立场："指南并非医疗工作的法定标准，但它确实给法庭提供了判决临床行为的标尺[80]"。

循证医学（evidence-based medicine, EBM）

EBM 的定义在第 2 章讨论过，但一个关于它的简要综述与指南有关。EBM 是指"在给每个不同患者作出医护决定时，尽责、清楚和明智的使用当前最佳证据"[93]。该词最初在 20 世纪 90 年代早期的文献中出现过[94,95]，起初也只被设计用于住院医师的教学[96]。Archie Cochrane、Alvan Feinstein 和 David Sackett[97]这些权威人士奠定了 EBM 的基础，但 David Eddy 在 10 年前已经在论述类似问题。对于 EBM，有许多支持者[97-100]，也有许多反对者[101-103]和怀疑者[104]。一些作者在讽刺和幽默中表达了他们的反对[105,106]，其他一些人则提供了诙谐的选择[107]。还有人则对将 EBM 应用于健康政策[108]以及怎样应用于医院管理和作出伦理上的决定持谨慎态度[109]。EBM 可用于患者个体[110]，而指南发展中 EBM 的应用则与本章有关[111]。尽管有人支持将 EBM 用于麻醉[111]，但其他人则强调将其用于麻醉实践的困难[112-114]。疼痛治疗中正在逐步应用EBM[115-117]，但并不常用。Merrill[118]已经尝试评估疼痛介入治疗方面的文献，作为慢性非癌性疼痛治疗循证指南的资源。

指南的发展

循证指南是循证医学的自然进程，因为它们都致力于将经验教训推广实施。尽管如此，指南发表一般要早于循证医学，而且现在公布的许多指南都是旧指南再加上新的进展。Eddy[119]已阐明了传统和新近政策的实施方式，并就他所强调的指南应涵盖的特殊任务方面做了比较（旁注3-6）。这包括了很多关键部分，比如在旁注3-7中所建议的一个问题，它建议指南应该包括一个特殊的权衡表格，即利害关系的比较[120]。这样临床医师可以据此权衡每位患者的损失和受益情况[121]。Woolf[122]也提出了一些类似于Eddy的指南类型（旁注3-8）。医疗工作者在阅读指南时应该了解指南是如何形成的，这样才能更有效地接受并正确使用指南[123]。因此，指南或政策应该容纳这些内容，最好能包括旁注3-9所列出的内容。

旁注3-10总结了有关指南发展的一种方法[122]。其他方法在本质上与其类似[45,124]并包含相同的步骤[125-129]。尽管有些差异，但也仅限于如何评估指南所基于的证据，以及如何对基于这些证据的建议按照其有效性和合法性分类。美国卫生保健质量与研究中心（Agency for Healthcare Research and Quality，AHRQ）已经推出了一个被广泛接受的研究类型（见旁注3-11）[130]。加拿大预防保健办公室也推出了一套被广大权威人士所认可的有关提议和研究的分类设计[131]（表3-1）。这些方法已经被其他一些专业人士采用并进一步修改，具体列于表3-2至表3-4[45,129,132]。

众多有关各种证据、循证医学、回顾性研究、荟萃分析及指南的信息均可以在互联网上获取[99,127,133]。

旁注3-6	指南任务和方法
指南的任务	明确重要的健康结局 行为效果的证据分析 评估这些结果的重要性（受益和伤害） 比较受益和伤害，评估成本 比较健康结局和成本；比较可选的实践行为，决定优先采取哪种
传统方法	明确医疗行为是标准化和可接受的 该实践在通常应用中是必需的 政策没有制定，仅仅来源于教科书、讲话、信件、主席或会谈 任务非明确提出，而是隐晦地出现 无正式的结局分析
新方法	
总体主观性判断	决策者试图考虑所有（整体）因素（主观的）形成意见（判断） 不做任何指南性任务 接近传统方法 最简单、最快速、最便宜 被美国医学会诊断和治疗技术评价计划所采用
基于证据	描述可用的证据 将政策关联于证据 不明确评估数量和范围 被蓝十字蓝盾协会和美国预防服务部的技术覆盖计划所采用
基于结果	政策有证据可依 明确评估可选程序的结果 强调对有效性证据存在与否进行量化 被技术评估国会部的有些政策所采用
基于优先	明确实施所有任务 包括患者优先顺序评估

Adapted from Eddy DM: Practice policies: Where do they come from? JAMA 1990;263:1265, 1269, 1272, 1275.

旁注 3-7　有用的临床指南的关键组成

关键决定及其结果的鉴定

作出诊断
估计预后
评估相关结果
- 受益
- 成本
- 治疗选择的风险

在每个关键决定点作出明确决定时所必需的有关有效证据的回顾分析

证据跟患者个体相关
指南制定者应尽可能依据绝对风险和收益作指导
每年计算 100 位治疗（或未治疗）患者的事件
如能得到数据，结算成本效益率
根据患者的偏好和可用资源权衡明确的陈述

介绍：证据和建议以简洁可行的方式进行表达

形式灵活，适用于特定的患者或情况
信息必须可被检索到，能被迅速吸收

Adapted from Jackson R, Feder G: Guidelines for clinical guidelines. BMJ 1998;317:427-428.

旁注 3-8　建立实践指南的方法

形成非正式的一致意见

同总体主观性发展一样（参见表 3-6）

形成正式的一致意见

形成于数天的专家组正式会议。被国家健康发展工程研究院采纳，被 RAND 公司采纳

循证指南之形成

同基于证据的方式一样（见表 3-6）

明确的指南形成

确定伤害和收益
介入成本估计
明确估计结局发生的可能性
评估出自专家意见，但评估的来源记录于文档
所有假定制成表格
作出判断，包括患者选择——同基优先原则的指南（见表 3-6）

Adapted from Woolf SH: Practice guidelines, a new reality in medicine. II: Methods of developing guidelines. Arch Intern Med 1992;152:946-952.

旁注 3-9　政策陈述：以明确的方式

1. 政策概要	陈述短小简明，充分准确，各自可被理解
2. 背景	理解政策所需的任何信息 回答"为何颁布政策"
3. 健康问题	定义被关注的临床问题和健康隐患 作为政策目的的干预和其他用于比较的备选干预 对执业者（如训练）或设置或运用（如设备）的形式的任何限制
4. 健康和经济上的结果	列出健康结果 列出考虑的经济成本
5. 证据	描述政策依据的证据 它是如何解释的 采用何种主观判断
6. 对健康和经济结果的影响	健康和经济结果的量化评估 如可应用，其不确定的范围
7. 获得结果评估的方法	上述评估是如何作出的 如可应用，包括统计学方法和模型
8. 优先的判断	关于结果期望的判断 比较收益和伤害 描述意见一致的程度 描述优先判断的来源（如患者调查）
9. 修正指南——灵活政策的说明	描述使用指南时的考虑因素 用于不同患者和情况的说明
10. 与其他政策的冲突	解释与解决与其他政策在同样健康问题方面的冲突
11. 同其他干预的比较	与其他干预结合制定的政策
12. 警戒	政策没有最终版；描述可能改变之的人们期望的发展；建议进行回顾或更新的日期
13. 政策的制订者	人名和任何利益冲突

Adapted from Eddy DM: Guidelines for policy statement: The explicit approach. JAMA 1990;263:2239-2240, 2243.

旁注 3-10	指南发展的方法的问题
1. 初步决策	主题的选择： • 可以是患者情况、患者主诉（如疼痛）或操作（如硬膜外） • 优先推荐正规的操作方法[124] 专家小组成员的选择： • 不同专科的医师 • 其他人员，包括方法论学者、健康经济学家、患者和消费者代表 目的说明： • 主题的详细说明、设置和供者类型
2. 临床适用性的评估	临床利害评估 临床证据评估： • 从文献、书籍[125,126]或电子文献[126]中重新获取证据 • 个体研究的评估 • 证据的综合
3. 专家意见的评估	非正式的方法、讨论和投票 正式的方法，比如名义群体技术（NGT 法）和 Delphi 法[127] 利害概要[21] 适当的决策；许多政策可灵活应用
4. 公共政策的评估	资源有限性 可行性问题
5. 指南文件的发展和评估	同行评审和试行性研究 对指南公布、评估和更新的建议 对研究的建议

Adapted from Woolf SH: Practice guidelines, a new reality in medicine. II: Methods of developing guidelines. Arch Intern Med 1992;152:946-952.

指南相关性证据被列于表 3-5，循证医学的部分则列于表 3-6。

对任何资源来源及其产生的数据都需要彻底地批判审查。区分系统性回顾研究十分重要，它利用统计学方法对类似设计的众多研究结果进行汇总及荟萃分析[134-136]，是对直观、可重复进行的初级研究中最佳证据的简要概括[137]。每一项随机对照试验的结果都必须经过严格而精确的检验。同样，每个荟萃分析的结果也必须经过彻底检验，这是因为存在偏倚[139]等很多已报道[138]的问题。另一个普遍存在的问题是对同一研究的双荟萃或多荟萃分析常常可以得出不同的结论[140-143]。Lelorier[144]等研究也发现，大型随机对照研究的结局有 35%经荟萃分析未得到准确预测。

旁注 3-11	研究类型的划分
	1. 系统性回顾和随机对照试验 2. 随机对照试验 3. 非随机干预试验 4. 观察性研究 5. 非试验性研究 6. 专家意见

Adapted from Carr DB, Jacox AK, Chapman CR, et al: Acute Pain Management: Operative or Medical Procedures and Trauma. (Clinical Practice Guideline No 1; AHCPR Publication No 92-0023.) Rockville, MD, Agency for Health Care Policy Research, 1993, p 107.

指南的评估

对指南评估而言，严格评估是非常重要的。对指南所依据证据的一些评估方法也同样适用于指南本身[132,145,146]。而与新指南的评估相比，对已制定的旧指南则可以略微降低要求[147,148]，因为它们已经过其他作者的讨论[149]。

表 3-1	加拿大预防保健办公室关于建议和研究设计的分类
分类	描述
建议	
A	有有效证据支持的在定期健康检查中被特别考虑的建议
B	有合理证据支持的在定期健康检查中被特别考虑的建议
C	虽然在定期健康检查中缺乏支持提议的证据，但提议可能在其他背景下产生
D	有合理证据支持的在定期健康检查中被剔除的提议
E	有有效证据支持的在定期健康检查中不予考虑的建议
研究设计	
I	证据来源于至少 1 项设计合理的随机对照研究
II-1	证据来源于设计良好的非随机对照研究
II-2	证据来源于设计良好的队列研究或病例对照分析研究，尤其是来源于多中心或研究组织者更佳
II-3	证据来源于有或无干预的不同时间或地点间的比较；非对照试验中出人意料的结果
III	基于临床经验、描述性研究或专家委员会报告的权威专家意见

Adapted from The periodic health examination. Canadian Task Force on the Periodic Health Examination. Can Med Assoc J 1979;121:1193-1254; and Woolf SH: Practice guidelines, a new reality in medicine. II: Methods of developing guidelines. Arch Intern Med 1992;152:946-952.

表 3-2	分类图解
证据的分类	
Ia	证据来源于随机对照研究的荟萃分析
Ib	证据来源于至少一项随机对照研究
IIa	证据来源于至少一项非随机对照研究
IIb	证据来源于一项其他类型的预试验研究
III	证据来源于非实验性描述性研究，如比较性研究、相关性研究和病例对照研究
IV	证据来源于专家委员会的意见或报告、权威专家的临床经验
提议的强度	
A	直接基于 I 类证据的提议
B	直接基于 II 类证据或由 I 类证据推导而来的提议
C	直接基于 III 类证据或由 I、II 类证据推导而来的提议
D	直接基于 IV 类证据或由 I、II、III 类证据推导而来的提议

Adapted from Shekelle PG, Woolf SH, Eccles M, Grimshaw J: Clinical guidelines: Developing guidelines. BMJ 1999;318:593-596.

表 3-3	其他有关提议和证据的分类设计
证据的分类	
I	基于设计良好的随机对照研究、荟萃分析或系统回顾
II	基于设计良好的队列研究或病例对照研究
III	基于非对照研究或共识
提议的强度	
A	直接基于 I 类证据的提议
B	直接基于 II 类证据或由 I 类证据推导而来的提议
C	直接基于 III 类证据或由 I、II 类证据推导而来的提议

Adapted from Eccles M, Clapp Z, Grimshaw J, et al: North of England evidence based guidelines development project: Methods of guideline development. BMJ 1996;312:760-762.

表 3-4	循证指南中提议分级校正*
证据水平	
1++	高质量随机对照试验（RCT）的荟萃分析、系统回顾或低偏倚风险的随机对照试验
1+	控制得当 RCT 的荟萃分析、系统回顾或低偏倚风险的随机对照试验
1-	RCT 荟萃分析、系统回顾或高偏倚风险的随机对照试验
2++	高质量病例对照研究或队列研究的系统回顾 或者低混杂偏倚或概率风险的高质量病例对照研究或队列研究，且呈高度因果相关
2+	低混杂偏倚或概率风险且控制得当的病例对照研究或队列研究，且结果呈中度因果相关
2-	高混杂偏倚或概率风险的病例对照研究或队列研究，且有无因果关系的显著风险
3	非分析性研究，如单个或系列病例研究
4	专家意见
提议的等级	
A	至少 1 项荟萃分析、系统回顾或随机对照试验归为 1++，可直接应用于目标人群；或 RCT 系统回顾或主要包含 1+ 级研究的大量证据，可直接应用于目标人群且所有试验结果一致
B	主要包含 2++ 级研究的大量证据，可直接应用于目标人群且已证实结果的总体一致性或由 1++ 或 1+ 证据推导而来的证据
C	主要包含 2+ 级研究的大量证据，可直接应用于目标人群且已证实结果的整体一致或由 2++ 证据推导而来的证据
D	3 或 4 级证据或由 2+ 研究推导而来的证据

*Revised from Agency for Health Care Policy and Research System.
Adapted from Harbour R, Miller J: A new system for grading recommendations in evidence based guidelines. BMJ 2001;323:334□336.

指南的执行

一部指南投入使用需要两个步骤，即公布和执行[46]。公布的方法包括专业渠道传播、会议、报告和咨询等示教性传播，以及散发到个人等，这些方法可以同时在地区和国家进行。公开出版发行和直接邮件投递等公布方法虽然不太成功[150-152]，但对于明确指导教育更加有益[153]。

患者预后的明确反馈可以帮助提高指南的依从性[154]。指南是在医院内执行的，因此坚强的管理支持、强而有力的管理阶层、共同改进的奋斗目标和可靠的反馈信息都可以帮助提高指南的依从性[155]。在医院，护士资源也有促进作用[156]。

新指南的遵守和实践上的改变还存在一些障碍[151,157]，譬如对指南通晓或熟悉的程度不够、对指南指导作用的认同不够、缺乏自身说服力和前指南的惯性使用，以及来自患者和医疗环境等各种外部的阻碍因素[158]。患者选择可能不太符合严格的指南说明，这同样可以降低指南的依从性[159]。在普通操作或初级护理方面，决定何种操作都是按照"共识-内在认知-默认"这条思路进行的[160]，而这种思维方式是很难改变的。

指南的执行策略必须将以上因素考虑在内，开发利用[160,161]、聚焦障碍、制度纳入、集中推广[155]等都不失为好的方法[151]。一个执行计划必须涵盖以下几方面，即提出变化的具体方面，分析障碍的背景和组织，将需求与干预相关联，并利用推动者去实施该项计划并监控进程[162]。

对某些指南来说，强制执行也是一种实施的方法。比如，某些州立法机构规定必须遵守麻醉管理条例[163,164]。而一些不负责任的保险公司也被要求必须遵从指南的规定[165]。指南的执行度已经被提出作为医院质量的指标[166,167]，美国医疗保险和公共医疗补助制度（Centers for Medicare and Medicaid Services, CMS）和其他的一些医疗支付机构已经制定了针对医院和临床医师的不同的支付金额的程序，其中部分取决于他

表 3-5	循证指南的数据来源：指南数据库
数据库	网址
欧洲指南评估研究 AGREE（Appraisal of Guidelines, Research and Evaluation for Europe）	http://www.agreecollaboration.org
美国临床内分泌学家协会 American Association of Clinical Endocrinologists	http://www.aace.com/clin/
美国胸科医师学会 American College of Chest Physicians	http://www.chestnet.org
美国医师学会 American College of Physicians	http://www.acponline.org
澳大利亚国家健康与医学研究委员会 Australian National Health and Medical Research Council（NHMRC）	http://www.health.gov.au/nhmrc/publications
健康服务研究中心 Center for Health Services Research（CHSR）	http://www.ncl.ac.uk.pahs/research/services
临床效果评估计划 Clinical Efficacy Assessment Project（CEAP）	http://www.acponline.org/sci-policy/guidelines/ceap.htm
CDC 社区预防服务组织 CDC Task Force on Community Preventative Services	thecommunityguide.org
临床实践指南 Clinical Practice Guidelines	http://www.kurucz.ca/sue/clinicalpracticeguidelines.com
临床实践指南 Clinical Practice Guidelines	http://www.cam.ca/cpgs
欧洲心脏学会 European Society of Cardiology	http://www.escardio.org
Finnish 指南（英文版） Finnish Guidelines（in English）	http://www.ebm-guidelines.com
德国医疗质量机构 German Agency for Quality in Medicine	www.aezq.de
指南信息服务 Guideline Information Service	www.leitlinien.de
国际指南网络 Guidelines-International-Network	http://www.g-i-n.net
健康服务技术评估 Health Services Technology Assessment	http://hstat.nlm.nih.gov/hq/Hquest
健康技术评估数据库 Health Technology Assessment databases	http://www.hta.nhsweb.nhs/htapubs.htm http://www.inahta.org http://www.shef.ac.uk/~scharr/ir/htaorg.html
新西兰指南小组 New Zealand Guidelines Group	http://www.nzgg.org.nz
英国临床卓越学会 NHS National Institute for Clinical Excellence	http://www.nice.org.uk
SCHARR 数据库 SCHARR database □	http://www.shef.ac.uk/~scharr/ir/guidelin/html
苏格兰学院指南网络 Scottish Intercollegiate Guidelines Network（SIGN）	http://www.sign.ac.uk
美国卫生保健质量与研究机构 U.S. Agency for Healthcare Research and Quality	http://www.ahrq.com
美国国家清算所 U.S. National Guideline Clearing House	http://www.guideline.gov
美国预防服务组织 U.S. Preventative Services Task Force	http://www.ahspr.gov/clinic/cps3dix.htm#Background

Adapted from Oosterhuis WP, Bruns DE, Watine J, et al: Evidence-based guidelines in laboratory medicines: Principles and methods. Clin Chem 2004;50: 806-818; and Hunt DL, Jaeschke R, McKibbon KA: User's guides to the medical literature. XXI: Using electronic health information resources in evidence-based practice. Evidence-Based Medicine Group. JAMA 2000;283:1875-1879.

表 3-6　循证指南的数据来源：系统回顾和循证资源

数据库	网址
ACP 杂志俱乐部　ACP Journal Club	http://www.hiru.mcmaster.ca/acpjc/default.htm
澳大利亚 Cochrane 中心　Australasian Cochrane's Center	http://som.Flinders.edu.au/FUSA/COCHRANE
循证卫生保健　Bandolier: Evidence-Based Healthcare	http://www.ebandolier.com
最佳证据　Best Evidence	http://www.acponline.org/catalog/electronic/best_evidence.htm
临床证据　Clinical Evidence	http://www.evidence.org/index-welcome.htm
Cochrane 图书馆　Cochrane Library	http://www.cochrane.org
系统筛选和诊断实验 Cochrane 方法研究小组　Cochrane Methods Working Group on Systematic Review of Screening and Diagnostic Tests	http://www.cochrane.org/cochrane/sadtdoc1.htm
有效回顾摘要数据库　Database of Abstracts of Reviews of Effectiveness（DARE）	http://www.agatha.york.ac.uk
循证医学回顾　EBMR Reviews（OVID）	http://www.ovid.com/products/cip/ebmr.cfm
EMedicine	http://www.emedicine.com
循证医学　Evidence-Based Medicine	http://www.bmjpg.com/template.cfm?name=specjou_be
哈里斯热线：最佳证据　Harrison's Online: Best Evidence	http://www.harrisonsonline.com
IFCC 委员会循证医学试验室数据库　IFCC Committee on Evidence-Based Laboratory Medicine（C-EBLM） database	http://www.ckchlmb.nl/ifcc
感恩医疗互联网　Internet Grateful Med	http://www.igm.nlm.nih.gov
医学博士参考　MD Consult	http://www.mdconsult.com
医疗矩阵　Medical Matrix	http://www.medmatrix.org/info/medlinetable.asp
医学世界探秘　Medical World Search	http://www.mwsearch.com
MEDION 数据库　MEDION database	http://www.mediondatabase.nl
英国国民健康保险制度循证医学中心　National Health Service (NHS) Center for Evidence-Based Medicine	http://www.cebm.net
证据等级及提议评分　Levels of evidence and grades of recommendations	http://www.cebm.net/levels_of_evidence.asp
国家健康图书馆　National Library for Health	http://www.nelh.nhs.uk/guidelinesdb/html/glframes.htm
美国国位医学图书馆　National Library of Medicine	http://text.nlm.nih.gov
NHS 回顾与公布中心　NHS Center for Reviews and Dissemination	http://www.york.ac.uk/inst/crd
NHS 循证医学研究和发展中心　NHS Research and Development Center for Evidence-Based Medicine	http://www.cebm.jr2.ox.ac.uk
公共医学　PubMed	http://www.ncbi.nlm.nih.gov/PubMed
SCHARR 数据库　SCHARR database	http://www.shef.ac.uk/~scharr/ir/netting
Alberta 循证医学大学　University of Alberta EBM Toolkit	http://www.med.ualberta.ca/ebm
最新进展　UpToDate	http://www.uptodate.com

Adapted from Oosterhuis WP, Bruns DE, Watine J, et al: Evidence-based guidelines in laboratory medicines: Principles and methods. Clin Chem 2004;50: 806-818; Hunt DL, Jaeschke R, McKibbon KA: User's guides to the medical literature. XXI: Using electronic health information resources in evidence-based practice. Evidence-Based Medicine Group. JAMA 2000;283:1875-1879; and McQueen MJ: Overview of evidence-based medicine: Challenge for evidence-based laboratory medicine. Clin Chem 2001;47:1536-1546.

们对临床指南的依从性[168]。

指南的维护

前面已经很详细地介绍了指南的发展程序，而对于应该何时回顾更新指南、采取何种程序来完善指南，在任务中却表述得不太清楚。表 3-12 列出了可能需要更新指南的一些情况[169]。在 2001 年的一次报告中 Shekelle 等[170]用聚焦文献综述的方式回顾了 AHRQ 所制定的 17 项指南，发现其中 7 部指南需要较大的改动，6 部需要小范围的更新，只有 3 部仍旧有效，而最后 1 部的有效性不能完全肯定。借此他们建议指南需要每 3 年更新 1 次。另有一些人也提出指南应采用更为实用的方法，并应根据更有说服力的（Ⅰ级）证据做出相应的更新[171]。

Gartlehner 等[172]则对指南的回顾方法方面做了比较。传统的回顾方法是由 RTI 国际-北卡罗莱纳州立大学循证实践中心制定的，检索可解答关键问题、符合入选标准且方法学合理的研究[172]。研究人员对这种传统方法和前述改进的回顾方法做了对比研究[170]，结果显示改进的方法能够提供更好的时效性，详见旁注 3-13。

旁注 3-12	可能需要更新临床指南的情况
干预手段中已存在的利害证据改变	众多利害关系的新信息 新的利害关系信息
既往重要结论改变	新证据证实既往被低估或未预料到的结局 关于患者偏好的新证据（如临终关怀）
有效干预改变	新的预防、诊断或治疗措施
当前最佳操作证据改变	发展指南是用来帮助减少理想操作与当前实际实践之间的差距，这种差距会不断减小，直至指南不再被需要
结局价值改变	经济学利益可能改变 伦理学问题可能被重新定义
可利用卫生保健资源改变	可利用资源可能增加 可利用资源同样可能减少

Adapted from Shekelle P, Eccles MP, Grimshaw JM, Woolf SH: When should clinical guidelines be updated? BMJ 2001;323:155-157.

旁注 3-13	指南更新的精确性回顾方法

1. 文献查询
   - 在 medline 上查找医师简要索引（AIM）
   - 限定于综述类文章、社论、指南和评论
   - 在 Premedline、美国卫生服务技术评估网站（HSTAT）、Cochrane 图书馆和 NIH 上查找
2. 创建所有可找到引用文献的数据库
3. 一号评估者阅读所有摘要，并接收相关部分的资料
4. 二号评估者阅读被一号所否定的所有摘要
5. 如果两人同时否决，则在数据库中标记被否决的摘要
6. 接收余下其他所有摘要
7. 一号评估者快速浏览所有全文，并确认相关文章
8. 二号评估者阅读被一号评估者否定的所有全文，并确认相关文章
9. 被两者同时否决的文章也同样在数据库中标为否决
10. 接收余下所有文章
11. 按参考书目汇编被接收的全文文章和研究
12. 一号评估者阅读并接受符合入选标准的相关研究
13. 二号评估者阅读并接受符合入选标准的相关研究
14. 汇总评估者意见，接收两者均认可的研究
15. 利用已认可研究精炼指南

Adapted from Gartlehner G, West SL, Lohr KN, et al: Assessing the need to update prevention guidelines: A comparison of two methods. Int J Qual Health Care 2004;16:399-406.

临床指南的评估

指南有效与否取决于判断成功的那个人以及他是如何定义其有效性的[173]。指南对临床医师、患者、医疗支付者、决策者、管理者以及律师提供了不同的收益。表 3-7 从知识、态度、行为和结果四种相关类别列出了指南的潜在利益。

部分调查显示，大多数临床医师都知道全国性指南[174,175]，但另有部分调查显示，仅少数人能讲出所推荐操作的任一具体名称[176]。没有证据显示仅仅公开发行指南就可以改变临床医师对待指南的态度[151,175]，而在指南的执行部分也已经讨论过临床医师无法依从指南的原因。尽管对于指南能否改善临床患者的预后一直都存在着疑问[177]，但一些研究的结果却提示了确实存在改善[178-180]。总而言之，指南将仍有希望改善临床结局[181]。

表 3-7	操作指南的潜在利益
种类	利益
知识	提升医学教育（医学院校、住院培训、继续医学教育）；解释如何评估证据；阐明未来有效研究的调查日程
态度	护理新标准的接受；技术水平、专业水准和健康状况的强力可信度*
行为	对所推荐操作的依从性提高；降低操作变异性*
结果	改善临床结局（如死亡率、发病率等）；降低成本*，增强卫生保健的价值；增加医疗赔偿服务*；减少法医学责任*

*利益寻求者主要是一些特殊群体，如临床医师（增加医疗赔付、减少法医学责任）、社会学专家（提高医疗行业可信度）、医疗支付者（降低消费）和决策者（降低操作变异）。

Adapted from Woolf SH: Practice guidelines: A new reality in medicine. III: Impact on patient care. Arch Intern Med 1993;153:2646-2655.

急性痛的操作指南

AHCPR（目前为 AHRQ）早期曾制定过一个有关急性疼痛处理的指南[130]。它的目的在于改进术后急性痛的处理和药物使用方法，减少治疗中的变异性。该机构采用现有的知识基础、评估报告及来自各个不同领域的专家小组成员们的意见，有时甚至是一些并未获得一致通过的意见。这个指南就是上文所提到的由 Shekelle 等在 2001 年所发现的需要更新的指南之一[170]。尽管如此，直到 2005 年它才不再被视作医学实践的指南[182]。该指南以及其他全球性疼痛处理指南的制定原则已在其他部分做了总结[183]。

美国麻醉医师学会（American Society of Anesthesiologists，ASA）已制定了一套围手术期急性痛处理的操作指南[184]，它在 1995 年首次出版发行并在 2003 年修订。专家小组由麻醉学家、疼痛治疗专家组成，而信息则来源于 ASA 的成员们。证据经过评估区分为支持性证据、建议性证据、可疑性证据和沉默证据。这部指南公布在 ASA 的官方网站上[184]。

随着急性痛回顾性研究的数据日益增多，澳大利亚国家健康与医学研究委员会所制定的一套内容全面，综合性高的指南脱颖而出。这套指南在 1998 年初次制定并在 2005 年再次更新[185]，也发布在委员会的官方网站上。

小结

尽管存在争论，但循证指南就此确立并将越来越多。对临床工作者和疼痛治疗师而言，了解指南的来源、知道如何去评价并完善指南以及如何运用并执行指南，无疑是非常重要的。这就是本章的目的所在。

（许小平 李卫星译 严晓晴 熊源长校）

参考文献

1. Eddy DM: Designing a practice policy: Standards, guidelines and options. JAMA 1990;263:3077–3084.
2. Policy Statement on Practice Parameters. Available at www.asahq.org/publicationsAndServices/sgstoc.htm (accessed March 2, 2005).
3. Field MJ, Lohr KN (eds): Guidelines for Clinical Practice: From Development to Use. Washington, DC, National Academy Press, 1992.
4. Woolf SH, Grol R, Hutchinson A, et al: Potential benefits, limitations, and harms of clinical guidelines. BMJ 1999;318:527–530.
5. Heffner JE: The overarching challenge. Chest 2000;118:1S–3S.
6. Cluzeau FA, Littlejohns P: Appraising clinical practice guidelines in England and Wales: The development of a methodologic framework and its application to policy. Jt Comm J Qual Improv 1999;25:514–521.
7. Annas J, Waterfield R (eds): Plato: Statesman. Cambridge, Cambridge University Press, 1995.
8. Hurwitz B: Legal and political considerations of clinical practice guidelines. BMJ 1999;318:661–664.
9. Bargar RJ: Introduction. In Casanova JE (ed): Tools for the Task: The Role of Clinical Guidelines. Tampa, Fla, American College of Physician Executives, 1997, pp 1–2.
10. Farmer A: Medical practice guidelines: Lessons from the United States. BMJ 1993;307:313–317.
11. Woolf SH: Practice guidelines: A new reality in medicine. 1: Recent developments. Arch Intern Med 1990;150:1811–1818.
12. Vicenzio JV: Trends in medical care costs: A look at the 1990s. Stat Bull Metrop Insur Co. 1990;January–March:28–35.
13. Iglehart JK: Payment of physicians under Medicare. N Engl J Med. 1988;318:863–868.
14. Iglehart JK: The recommendation of the Physician Payment Review Commission. N Engl J Med 1989;320:1156–1160.
15. Wennberg JE, Gittelsohn A: Small-area variation in health care delivery. Science 1973;182:1102–1108.
16. Wennberg JE, Freeman JL, Culp WJ: Are hospital services rationed in New Haven or over-utilized in Boston? Lancet 1987;1(8543):1185–1189.
17. Perrin JM, Homer CJ, Berwick DM, et al: Variation in rates of hospitalization of children in three urban communities. N Engl J Med 1989;320:1183–1187.
18. Lewis CE: Variations in the incidence of surgery. N Engl J Med 1969;281:880–885.
19. Chassin M, Brook R, Park R, et al: Variations in the use of medical and surgical services by the Medicare population. N Engl J Med 1968;314:285–290.
20. McLaughlin LF, Wolfe RA, Tedeschi PJ: Variation in hospital admissions among small area: A comparison of Maine and Michigan. Med Care 1989;27:623–631.
21. Eddy DM: The challenge. JAMA 1990;263:287–290.
22. Smits HL: Medical practice variations revisited. Health Aff (Millwood) 1986;5:91–96.
23. Leape LL, Park RE, Solomon DH, et al: Does inappropriate use explain small-area variations in the use of health care services? JAMA 1990;263:669–672.
24. Blumenthal D: The variation phenomenon in 1994. N Engl J Med 1994;331:1017–1018.

25. Fisher ES, Wennberg JE, Stukel TA, Sharp SM: Hospital readmission rates for cohorts of Medicare beneficiaries in Boston and New Haven. N Engl J Med 1994;331:989–995.
26. Chassin MR: Explaining geographic variations: The enthusiasm hypothesis. Med Care 1993;31(Suppl 5):YS37–YS44.
27. Wennberg DE, Wennberg JE: Addressing variations: Is there hope for the future? Health Aff (Millwood) 2003;Jul–Dec;Suppl Web Exclusives:W3–614–7.December 10, 2003.
28. Berenson RA: Getting serious about excessive Medicare spending: A purchasing model. Health Aff (Millwood). 2003 Jul–Dec;Suppl Web Exclusives:W3–586–602. December 10, 2003.
29. Lieberman SM, Lee J, Anderson T, Crippen DL: Reducing the growth of Medicare spending: Geographic versus patient-based strategies. Health Aff (Millwood). 2003;Jul–Dec;Suppl Web Exclusives:W3-603-613. December 10, 2003.
30. Chassin MR, Kosecoff J, Park RE, et al: Does inappropriate use explain geographic variations in the use of health care services? A study of three procedures JAMA 1987;258:2533–2537.
31. Holoweiko M: What cookbook medicine will mean for you. Med Econ 1989;66:118–133.
32. National Center for Health Services Research and Health Care Technology Assessment. Research Activities: DHHS Secretary Sullivan Announces NCHRS Grants Totaling $4 Million for Patient Outcomes Research Assessment Teams. Special Release. Publication 241–274–00054. Rockville, Md, National Center for Health Services Research and Health Care Technology Assessment, September 11, 1989.
33. Roper WL, Winkenwerder W, Hackbarth GM, Krakauer H: Effectiveness in health care: An initiative to evaluate and improve medical practice. N Engl J Med 1988;319:1197–1202.
34. Report of the National Cholesterol Education Program Expert Panel on Detection, Evaluation and Treatment of High Blood Cholesterol in Adults. Arch Intern Med 1988;148:36–39.
35. Immunization Practices Advisory Committee: General recommendations on immunization. MMWR Morbid Mortal Wkly Rep 1989;38:205–214, 219–227.
36. Jacoby I: The consensus development program of the National Institutes of Health: Current practices and historical perspectives. Int J Technol Assess Health Care 1985;1:420–432.
37. US Preventive Services Task Force: Guide to Clinical Preventive Services: An Assessment of the Effectiveness of 169 Interventions. Baltimore, Md, Williams & Wilkins, 1989.
38. Woolf SH, Battista RN, Anderson GM, et al: Assessing the clinical effectiveness of preventive maneuvers: Analytic principles and systematic methods in reviewing evidence and developing clinical practice recommendations. A report by the Canadian Task Force on the Periodic Health Examination. J Clin Epidemiol 1990;43:891–905.
39. Physician Payment Review Commission: Annual Report to Congress. Washington, DC, Physician Payment Review Commission, 1990.
40. Kelly JT, Swartwout JE: Development of practice parameters by physician organizations. QRB Qual Rev Bull 1990;February:54–57.
41. Office of Quality Assurance, American Medical Association: Listings of Practice Parameters: Guidelines, and Technology Assessments. Chicago, American Medical Association, 1989.
42. Pierce EC Jr: The development of anesthesia guidelines and standards. QRB Qual Rev Bull 1990;February:61–64.
43. Schoenbaum SC, Gottlieb LK: Algorithm based improvement of clinical quality. BMJ 1990;301:1374–1376.
44. Woolf SH, Grol R, Hutchinson A, et al: Potential benefits, limitations, and harms of clinical guidelines. BMJ 1999;318:527–530.
45. Eccles M, Clapp Z, Grimshaw J, et al: North of England evidence based guideline development project: Methods of guideline development. BMJ 1996;312:760–762.
46. Thomas L: Clinical practice guidelines. Evidence Based Nursing 1999;2:38–39.
47. Scottish Intercollegiate Guideline Network. Available at www.sign.ac.uk/index.html (accessed March 4, 2005).
48. Bandolier. Available at www.jr2.ox.ac.uk/bandolier/index.html (accessed March 4, 2005).
49. Interdisciplinary Maternal Perinatal Australasian Clinical trials. Available at http://128.250.188.72/psanz/IMPACT/impact_links.htm (accessed March 7, 2005).
50. ACP Journal Club. Available at www.acpjc.org/ (accessed March 4, 2005).
51. EBM on Line. Available at http://ebm.bmjjournals.com/ (accessed March 4, 2005).
52. Cochrane AL: quoted in West RR: Evidence based medicine overviews, bulletins, guidelines and the new consensus. Postgrad Med J 2000; 76:383–389.
53. Grimshaw JM, Russel IT: Effect of clinical guidelines on medical practice: Systematic review of rigorous evaluations. Lancet 1993;342:1317–1322.
54. Grimshaw JM, Russel IT: Achieving health care gains through clinical guidelines. I: Developing scientifically valid guidelines. Qual Health Care 1993;2:243–248.
55. Grimshaw JM, Russell IT: Achieving health care gains through clinical guidelines. II: Ensuring guidelines change medical practice. Qual Health Care 1994;3:45–52.
56. Effective health care. In Implementing Clinical Guidelines. Bulletin No 8. Leeds, UK, University of Leeds, 1994.
57. Entwistle VA, Watt IS, Davis H, et al: Developing information materials to present the findings of technology assessments to consumers: The experience of the NHS Center for Reviews and Dissemination. Int J Tech Assess Health Care 1998;14:47–70.
58. Shapiro DW, Lasker RD, Bindman AB, Lee PR: Containing costs while improving the quality of care: The role of profiling and practice guidelines. Annu Rev Public Health 1993;14:219–241.
59. Eisenberg JM, Williams SV: Cost containment and changing physicians' practice behavior: Can the fox learn to guard the chicken coop? JAMA 1981;246:2195–2201.
60. Pearson SD, Goulart-Fisher D, Lee TH: Critical pathways as a strategy for improving health care: Problems and potential. Ann Intern Med 1995;123:941–948.
61. Nathan RE, Hochman J, Becker R, et al: Critical pathways: A review. Circulation 2000;101:461–467.
62. Kane RL: Creating practice guidelines: The dangers of over-reliance on expert judgment. J Law Med Ethics 1995;23:62–64.
63. Woolf SH: Shared decision-making: The case for letting patients decide which choice is best. J Fam Pract 1997;45:205–208.
64. Tinetti ME, Bogardus ST, Agostini JV: Potential pitfalls of disease specific guidelines for patients with multiple conditions. N Engl J Med 2004;351:2870–2874.
65. Lomas J, Anderson GM, Domnick-Pierre K, et al: Do practice guidelines guide practice? The effect of a consensus statement on the practice of physicians. N Engl J Med 1989;321:1306–1311.
66. Kosecoff J, Kanouse DE, Rogers WH, et al: Effects of the National Institutes of Health Consensus Development Program on physician practice. JAMA 1987;258:2708–2713.
67. Hirani NA, Macfarlance JT: Impact of management guidelines on the outcome of severe community acquired pneumonia. Thorax 1997;52:17–21.
68. Sarasin FP, Maschiangelo M-L, Schaller M-D, et al: Successful implementation of guidelines for encouraging the use of beta blockers in patients after acute myocardial infarction. Am J Med 1999;106:499–505.
69. Weingarten S, Riedinger MAS, Sandhu M, et al: Can practice guidelines safely reduce hospital length of stay? Results from a multicenter interventional study. Am J Med 1998;105:33–40.
70. Grimshaw JM, Russell IT: Effect of clinical guidelines on medical practice: A systematic review of rigorous evaluations. Lancet 1993;342:1317–1322.
71. Graham ID, Beardall S, Carter AO, et al: What is the quality of drug therapy clinical practice guidelines in Canada? CMAJ 2001;165:157–163.
72. Shaneyfelt TM, Mayo-Smith MF, Rothwangl J: Are guidelines following guidelines? The methodological quality of clinical practice guidelines in the peer reviewed medical literature. JAMA 1999;281:1900–1905.
73. Lewis SJ: Further disquiet on the guidelines front. CMAJ 2001;165:180–181.
74. Feder G: Management of mild hypertension: Which guideline to follow? BMJ 1994;308:470–471.
75. Robinson L: Guidelines for the treatment of hypertension: A critical review. Cardiovasc Drugs Ther 1994;8:665–672.
76. Hibble A, Kanka D, Pencheon D, Pooles F: Guidelines in general practice: The new tower of Babel? BMJ 1998;317:862–863.
77. Gray JAM: Data, data, data: Give me peace and knowledge. BMJ 1998;317:832–834.
78. Ellwood PM: Outcomes management, a technology of patient experience. N Engl J Med 1988;318:1549–1556.

79. Tunis SR, Hayward RSA, Wilson MC, et al: Internist's attitudes about clinical practice guidelines. Ann Intern Med 1994;120:956–963.
80. Hurwitz B: How does evidence based guidance influence determinations of medical negligence? BMJ 2004;328:1024–1028.
81. Newton J, Knight D, Woolhead G: General practitioners and clinical guidelines: A survey of knowledge, use and beliefs. Br J Gen Pract 1996;46:513–517.
82. Hyams AL, Brandenberg JA, Lipsitz SR, et al: Practice guidelines and malpractice litigation: A two way street. Ann Intern Med 1995;122:450–455.
83. Maisonneuve H, Codier H, Durocher A, Matillon Y: The French clinical guideline and medical references program: Development of 48 guidelines for private practice over a period of 18 months. J Eval Clin Pract 1997;3:3–13.
84. Durand-Zaleski I, Colin C, Blum-Boisgard C: An attempt to save money using mandatory practice guidelines in France. BMJ 1997;315:943–946.
85. Bolam v Friern Hospital Management Committee. 2 All ER 118–28 (1957).
86. Posner KL, Cheney FW, Kroll DA: Professional Liability, Risk Management, and Quality Improvement. In Barash PG, Cullen BF, Stoelting RK (eds): Clinical Anesthesia, 3rd ed. Philadelphia, Lippincott-Raven, 1997, p 93.
87. Grilli R, Magrini N, Penna A, et al: Practice guidelines developed by specialist societies: The need for critical appraisal. Lancet 2000;355:103–106.
88. McDonagh RJ, Hurwitz B: Lying in the bed we've made: Reflections on some unintended consequences of clinical practice guidelines in the courts. J Obstet Gynaecol Can 2003;25:139–143.
89. Merenstein D: Winners and losers. JAMA 2004;291:15–16.
90. Hall MA, Green MD, Hartz A: Evidence-based medicine on trial. Letter. JAMA 2004;291:1697.
91. Fleming M: Evidence-based medicine on trial. Letter. JAMA 2004;291:1697–1698.
92. Mulrow CD, Lohr K: Proof and policy from medical research evidence. J Health Polit Policy Law 2001;26:249–266.
93. Sackett DL, Rosenberg WMC, Muir Gray JA, et al: Evidence based medicine: What it is and what it isn't. BMJ 1996;312:71–72.
94. Guyatt GH: Evidence based medicine. ACP J Club 1991;114:A-16.
95. Evidence-Based Medicine Working Group: Evidence-based medicine: A new approach to teaching the practice of medicine. JAMA 1992;268;2420–2425.
96. Druss B: Evidence based medicine: Does it make a difference? BMJ 2005;330:92.
97. Guyatt G, Cook D, Haynes B: Evidence based medicine has come a long way. BMJ 2004;329:990–991.
98. Straus SE, Jones G: What has evidence based medicine done for us? BMJ 2004;329:987–988.
99. McQueen MJ: Overview of evidence-based medicine: Challenge for evidence-based laboratory medicine. Clin Chem 2001;47:1536–1546.
100. Sackett DL, Haynes RB: Evidence base of clinical diagnosis: The architecture of diagnostic research. BMJ 2002;324:539–541.
101. Saani SI, Gylling HA: Evidence based medicine guidelines: A solution to rationing or politics disguised as science? J Med Ethics 2004;30:171–175.
102. Feinstein AR, Horwitz RI: Problems in the "evidence" of "evidence-based medicine. Am J Med 1997;103:529–535.
103. Grahame-Smith D: Evidence based medicine: Socratic dissent. BMJ 1995;310:1126–1127.
104. Adams CE, Gilbody S: "Nobody ever expects the Spanish Inquisition." Psych Bull 2001;25:291–292.
105. Molesworth N: Down with EBM! BMJ 1998;317:1720–1721.
106. Clinicians for the Restoration of Autonomous Practice (CRAP) Writing Group: EMB: Unmasking the ugly truth. BMJ 2002;325:1496–1498.
107. Isaacs D, Fitzgerald D: Seven alternatives to evidence based medicine. BMJ 1999;319:1618.
108. Black N: Evidence based policy: Proceed with care. BMJ 2001;323:275–279.
109. Biller-Andorno N, Lenk C, Leititis J: Ethics, EBM, and hospital management. J Med Ethics 2004;30:136–140.
110. Pronovost PJ, Berenholtz SM, Dorman T, et al: Evidence-based medicine in anesthesiology. Anesth Analg 2001;92:787–794.
111. Steinberg EP, Luce BR: Evidence based? Caveat emptor! Health Aff 2005;24:80–92.
112. Horan BF: Evidence-based medicine and anaesthesia: Uneasy bedfellows? Anaesth Intensive Care 1997;25:679–685.
113. Goodman NW: Anesthesia and evidence-based medicine. Anaesthesia 1998;53:353–368.
114. Goodman NW: Evidence-based medicine needs proper critical review. Anesth Analg 2002;95:1817–1818.
115. Rathmell JP, Carr DB: The scientific method, evidence-based medicine, and the rational use of interventional pain treatments. Reg Anesth Pain Med 2003;28:498–501.
116. McQuay HJ, Moore A: An Evidence-Based Resource for Pain Relief. Oxford, Oxford University Press, 2002.
117. Tramer MR (ed): Evidence Based Resource in Anaesthesia and Analgesia. London, BMJ Books, 2000.
118. Merrill DG: Hoffman's glasses: Evidence-based medicine and the search for quality in the literature of interventional pain medicine. Reg Anesth Pain Med 2003;28:547–560.
119. Eddy DM: Practice policies: Where do they come from? JAMA 1990;263:1265, 1269, 1272, 1275.
120. Jackson R, Feder G: Guidelines for clinical guidelines. BMJ 1998;317:427–428.
121. Eddy DM: Comparing benefits and harms: The balance sheet. JAMA 1990;263:2493, 2498, 2501, 2505.
122. Woolf SH: Practice guidelines, a new reality in medicine. II: Methods of developing guidelines. Arch Intern Med 1992;152:946–952.
123. Eddy DM: Guidelines for policy statement: The explicit approach. JAMA 1990;263:2239–2240, 2243.
124. Shekelle PG, Woolf SH, Eccles M, Grimshaw J: Clinical guidelines: Developing guidelines. BMJ 1999;318:593–596.
125. Institute of Medicine, Committee on Health and Technology, Priority-Setting Group: National Priorities for the Assessment of Clinical Conditions and Medical Technologies: Report of a Pilot Study. Washington, DC, National Academy Press, 1990.
126. Jaeschke R, Sackett DL: Research methods for obtaining primary evidence. Int J Technol Assess Health Care 1989;5:503–519.
127. Chalmers TC, Hewett P, Reitman D, Sacks HS: Selection and evaluation of empirical research in technology assessment. Int J Technol Assess Health Care 1989;5:521–536.
128. Hunt DL, Jaeschke R, McKibbon KA: Users' guides to the medical literature. XXI: Using electronic health information resources in evidence-based practice. Evidence-Based Medicine Group. JAMA 2000;283:1875–1879.
129. Fink A, Kosecoff J, Chassin M, Brook RH: Consensus methods: Characteristics and guidelines for use. Am J Public Health I 1984;74:979–983.
130. Carr DB, Jacox AK, Chapman CR, et al: Acute pain management: Operative or medical procedures and trauma. Clinical practice guideline No 1; AHCPR Publication No 92-0023. Rockville, Md, AHCPR, 1993, p 107.
131. The periodic health examination. Canadian Task Force on the Periodic Health Examination. Can Med Assoc J 1979;121:1193–1254.
132. Harbour R, Miller J: A new system for grading recommendations in evidence based guidelines. BMJ 2001;323:334–336.
133. Oosterhuis WP, Bruns DE, Watine J, et al: Evidence-based guidelines in laboratory medicines: Principles and methods. Clin Chem 2004;50:806–818.
134. Chambers I, Altman DG (eds): Systematic Reviews. London, BMJ, 1995.
135. Cook DJ, Mulrow CD, Haynes RB: Systematic reviews: Synthesis of best evidence for clinical decisions. Ann Intern Med 1997;126:376–380.
136. Grennhalgh T: How to read a paper: Papers that summarize other papers (systematic reviews and meta-analysis). BMJ 1997;315:672–675.
137. Glass G: Primary, secondary and meta-analysis of research. Educ Res 1976;5:3–8.
138. Bailar JC III: The practice of meta-analysis. J Clin Epidemiol 1995;48:149–157.
139. Bailar JC III: The promise and problems of meta-analysis. N Engl J Med 1997;337:559–561.
140. Kerikowske K, Grady D, Rubin SM, et al: Efficacy of screening mammography: A meta-analysis. JAMA 1995;273:149–154.

141. Smart CR, Hendrick RE, Rutledge JH III, Smith RA: Benefit of mammography screening in women ages 40 to 49 years: Current evidence from randomized controlled trials. Cancer 1995;75:1619–1626.
142. Rosenfeld RM, Post JC: Meta-analysis of antibiotics for the treatment of otitis media with effusion. Otolaryngol Head Neck Surg 1992;106:378–386.
143. Williams RL, Chalmers TC, Strange KC, et al: Use of antibiotics in preventing recurrent acute otitis media and treating otitis media with effusion: A meta-analytic attempt to resolve the brouhaha [erratum in JAMA 1994;271:430]. JAMA 1993;270:1344–1351.
144. Lelorier J, Grégoire G, Benhaddad A, et al: Discrepancies between meta-analysis and subsequent large, randomized, controlled trials. N Engl J Med 1997;337:536–542.
145. Hayward RSA, Wilson MC, Tunis SR, et al: Users' guides to the medical literature. VIII. How to use clinical practice guidelines. A: Are the recommendations valid? The Evidence-Based Medicine Working Group. JAMA 1995;274:570–574.
146. Hayward RSA, Wilson MC, Tunis SR, et al: Users' guides to the medical literature. VIII. How to use clinical practice guidelines. B: What are the recommendations and will they help you in caring for your patients? The Evidence-Based Medicine Working Group. JAMA 1995;274:1630–1632.
147. Graham ID, Beardall S, Carter AO, et al: What is the quality of drug therapy clinical practice guidelines in Canada? CMAJ 2001;165:157–163.
148. Grilli R, Magrini N, Penna A, et al: Practice guidelines developed by specialist societies: The need for a critical appraisal. Lancet 2000;355:103–106.
149. Lewis SJ: Further disquiet on the guideline front. CMAJ 2001;165:180–181.
150. Grol R: Implementing guidelines in general practice care. Quality in Health Care 1992;1:184–191.
151. Lomas J, Anderson GM, Domnick-Pierre K, et al: Do practice guidelines guide practice? The effect of a consensus statement on the practice of physicians. N Engl J Med 1989;321:1306–1311.
152. Freemantle N, Harvey EL, Wolf F, et al: Printed educational materials: Effects on professional practice and health care outcomes (Cochrane Review 2000). In The Cochrane Library, issue 3. Chichester, UK: John Wiley & Sons, 2003.
153. Lomas J, Enkin M, Anderson GM, et al: Opinion leaders vs audit and feedback to implement practice guidelines: Delivery after previous Cesarean section. JAMA 1991;265:2202–2207.
154. Martens WC, Higby DJ, Brown D, et al: Improving the care of patients with regard to chemotherapy-induced nausea and emesis: The effect of feedback to clinicians on adherence to antiemetic prescription guidelines. J Clin Oncol 2003;21:1373–1378.
155. Bradley EH, Holmboe ES, Mattera JA, et al: A qualitative study on increasing β-blocker use after myocardial infarction: Why do some hospitals succeed? JAMA 2001;285:2604–2611.
156. Ansari M, Shlipak MG, Heidenreich PA, et al: Improving guideline adherence: A randomizes trial evaluating strategies to increase β-blocker use in heart failure. Circulation 2003;107:2799–2807.
157. Phillips LS, Branch WT Jr, Cook CB, et al: Clinical inertia. Ann Intern Med 2001;135:825–834.
158. Cabana MD, Rand CS, Powe NR, et al: Why don't physicians follow clinical practice guidelines? A framework for improvement. JAMA 1999;282:1458–1465.
159. Haynes RB, Devereaux PJ, Guyatt GH: Physicians' and patients' choices in evidence based practice: Evidence does not make decisions, people do. BMJ 2002;324:1350.
160. Gabbay J, le May A: Evidence based guidelines or collectively constructed "mindlines"? Ethnographic study of knowledge management in primary care. BMJ 2004;329:1013–1018.
161. Grol R, Dalhuijsen J, Thomas S, et al: Attributes of clinical guidelines that influence use of guidelines on general practice: Observational study. BMJ 1998;317:858–861.
162. Grol R, Grimshaw J: Evidence-based implementation of evidence-based medicine. Jt Comm J Qual Improv 1999;25:503–513.
163. Pierce EC Jr: The development of anesthesia guidelines and standards. QRB Qual Rev Bull 1990;16:61–64.
164. Pomeranz D: Practice parameters: Massachusetts Medical Society studies potential. Penn Med 1991;94:16,18.
165. Holzer JF: The advent of clinical standards for professional liability. QRB Qual Rev Bull 1990;16:71–79.
166. Kelly JT, Kellie SE: Medicare peer review organization preprocedure review criteria. JAMA 1991;265:1265–1270.
167. Larson EB: Evidence-based medicine: Is translating evidence into practice a solution to the cost-quality challenges facing medicine? Jt Comm J Qual Improv 1999;25:480–485.
168. Strunk BC, Hurley RE: Paying for quality: Health plans try carrots instead of sticks. Issue Brief Cent Stud Health Syst Change 2004 May;(82):1–4.
169. Shekelle P, Eccles MP, Grimshaw JM, Woolf SH: When should clinical guidelines be updated? BMJ 2001;323:155–157.
170. Shekelle PG, Ortiz E, Rhodes S, et al: Validity of the Agency for Healthcare Research and Quality clinical guidelines: How quickly do guidelines become outdated? JAMA 2001;286:1461–1467.
171. Bowman GP: Development and aftercare of clinical guidelines: The balance between rigor and pragmatism. JAMA 2001;286:1509–1511.
172. Gartlehner G, West SL, Lohr KN, et al: Assessing the need to update prevention guidelines: A comparison of two methods. Int J Quality Health Care 2004;16:399–406.
173. Woolf SH: Practice guidelines: A new reality in medicine. III: Impact on patient care. Arch Intern Med 1993;153:2646–2655.
174. Hill MN, Levine DM, Whelton PK: Awareness, use and impact of the 1984 Joint National Committee Report on High Blood Pressure. Am J Public Health 1988;78:1190–1194.
175. Stange KC, Kelly R, Chao J, et al: Physician agreement with the US Preventive Task Services Force recommendations. J Fam Pract 1992;34:409–416.
176. Fowler G, Mant D, Fuller A, Jones L: The "Help Your Patient Stop" initiative: Evaluation of smoking prevalence and dissemination of WHO/UICC guidelines in general practice. Lancet 1989;1(8649):1253–1255.
177. Miles A, Bentley P, Polychronis A, Grey J: Evidence-based medicine: Why all the fuss? This is why. J Eval Clin Pract 1997;3:83–85.
178. Krumholz HM, Radford MJ, Ellerbeck EF, et al: Aspirin for secondary prevention after acute myocardial infarction in the elderly: Prescribed use and outcomes. Ann Intern Med 1996;124:292–298.
179. Krumholz HM, Radford MJ, Wang Y, et al: National use and effectiveness of beta-blockers for the treatment of elderly patients after acute myocardial infarction. National Cooperative Cardiovascular Project. JAMA 1998;280:623–629.
180. Wong JH, Findlay JM, Suarez-Almazor ME: Regional performance of carotid endarterectomy: Appropriateness, outcomes and risk factors for complications. Stroke 1997;28:891–898.
181. Straus SE, McAlister FA: Evidence-based medicine: A commentary on common criticisms. CMAJ 2000;163:837–841.
182. Health Services/Technology Assessment Text: Acute pain management: operative or medical procedures and trauma. Available at www.ncbi.nlm.nih.gov/books/bv.fcgi?rid=hstat6.chapter.8991 (accessed November 1, 2005)
183. Carr DB: The development of national guidelines for pain control: Synopsis and commentary. Eur J Pain 2001;5(Suppl A):91–98.
184. Practice guidelines for acute pain management in the perioperative setting. Available at www.asahq.org/publicationsAndServices/pain.pdf (accessed March 14, 2005).
185. National Health and Medical Research Council (Australia): Acute pain management: Scientific evidence. Available at www.nhmrc.gov.au/publications/_files/cp104.pdf (accessed June 20, 2005).

第 2 部分 术后疼痛与镇痛的科学基础

4 手术对神经内分泌反应、炎症反应和凝血反应的影响

CONOR J. SHIELDS · H. PAUL REDMOND

外科医师和麻醉医师不仅经常协同处理患者疾病所致的后遗症，而且还常需处理患者机体代谢反应所致的生理变化。这种应激反应包括代谢、内分泌、免疫以及血液系统的改变。这些反应使患者能够在不利的环境下生存，并从手术后完全康复。远端脏器合成代谢与分解代谢方面的基本变化都会伴有蛋白质与能量代谢内稳态的改变。尽管这些整合的复杂反应必不可少，但过度反应可能导致机体内环境紊乱，使患者易出现多器官衰竭综合征（multiple organ failure syndrome，MOFS），最终导致死亡[1]。

手术的应激反应可分为几个明显的阶段：Cuthbertson 划分的经典"高潮期"与"低潮期"[1-3]，或 Moore 的 4 期特征（损伤期、转折期、合成代谢期和合成代谢后期）[4]。该反应的时程部分取决于初始创伤的严重程度。

许多刺激因素可引起机体对损伤的生理反应（图 4-1）。手术通常都伴有焦虑、禁食、麻醉药物、疼痛和制动，其中每个因素均轻微增强机体应激反应。组织的分解、体腔的开放以及细胞外液的丢失都可加重机体的应激反应，有时可使反应达到失控的程度；因此，采用微创和腔镜技术可减轻不当的应激反应（表 4-1）[5,6]。

神经内分泌反应

神经传入信号（如疼痛）与中枢神经系统都是神经内分泌反射弧的组成部分，传入 CNS 的信号包括神经信号与内分泌信号两种。伤害性感受器、压力感受器以及化学感受器均可激活交感神经性应激反应，并通过激发逃避反射机制来试图减轻机体的损伤。应激系统的激活可产生针对性的全身性反应，从而提高机体警觉性和认知能力，增加对疼痛的耐受性[7,8]。许多局部炎性介质都能同时激活两大应激反应系统：下丘脑-垂体-肾上腺轴和肾上腺髓质交感神经系统（图 4-2）。这两大应激反应系统对不同种类的刺激信号都可做出反应，包括边缘系统的刺激、昼夜节律变化的刺激以及血液系统的刺激，如来自损伤组织的肿瘤坏死因子-α（tumor necrosis factor-α，TNF-α）、白介素-1（interleukin-1，IL-1）和白介素-6（IL-6）[9]。

下丘脑的控制

疼痛反应是通过脊髓丘脑束以及丘脑后在皮层整合而成，并将信号传递到下丘脑和髓质交感神经中枢，从而激活中枢和区域性神经内分泌反应。虽然疼痛是一种在更高级中枢所呈现的客观性体验，但下丘脑是协调手术创伤自主神经反应的最高级中枢。全麻情况下，痛觉纤维被激活，产生传入信号。硬膜外麻醉和脊麻可减轻这种疼痛反应，但由于急性期蛋白反应主要是由局部分泌的炎性介质所介导，因而往往不受这些麻醉方法的影响[10]。

刺激下丘脑能激活自主神经系统，并影响垂体激素的释放（表 4-2）。这些激素可持续促进下游的靶器官释放一系列的具有生物活性的复合物，如神经垂体

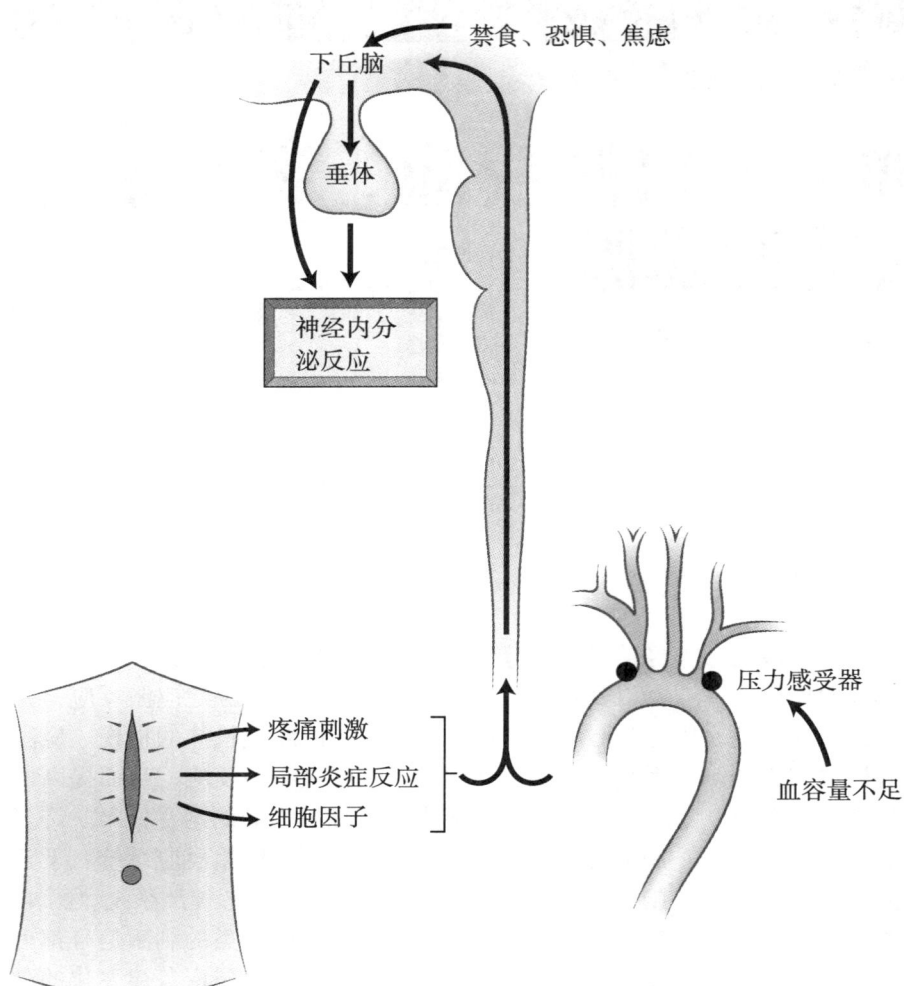

图 4-1 损伤和手术刺激引起的机体代谢反应。创口释放的免疫调节肽类与细胞因子可能加重压力感受器、化学感受器和伤害性感受器引起的代谢反应。

表 4-1	手术所致神经内分泌反应的程度	
手术操作	刺激	神经内分泌反应
腹股沟疝修复 腹腔镜检查 腹腔镜结肠直肠手术	焦虑 恐惧 疼痛 麻醉药物 制动	反应持续 2～5 日 主要是局部炎症反应，伴轻度全身炎症反应
剖腹手术 开放式结肠直肠手术 择期腹主动脉瘤修复术	禁食 细胞外液丢失 侵入体腔 输血 感染	应激反应持续至少 1 周 强烈的、有影响的、确切的炎症反应 循环中碳水化合物、脂肪和蛋白质增加
内脏穿孔剖腹手术 急诊腹主动脉瘤修复术	重度脓毒症 组织坏死 休克	长时间应激反应 前向反馈性炎症反应，并持续激活 蛋白分解代谢占优势
暴发性结肠炎急诊剖腹术	饥饿	可能导致多器官功能衰竭

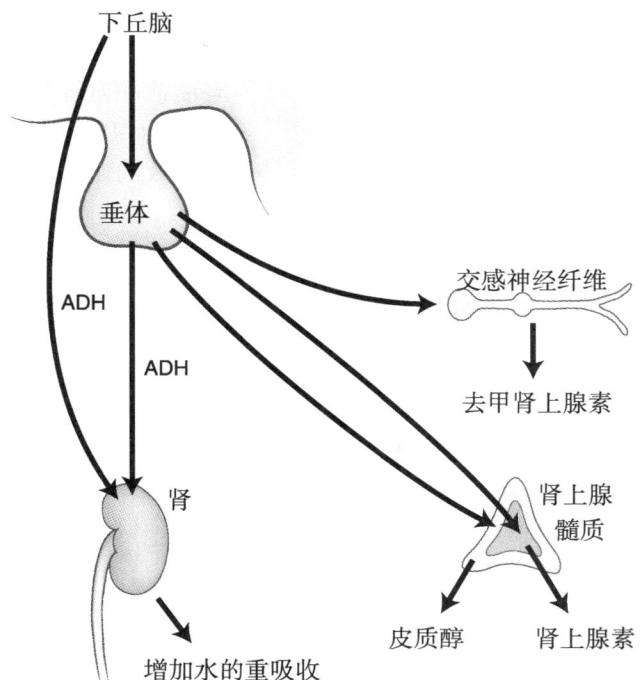

图 4-2 应激系统的传出刺激。下丘脑-垂体-肾上腺轴（图左侧）与肾上腺髓质交感神经系统（图右侧）。下丘脑激活可引起自主神经系统兴奋，通过释放促肾上腺皮质激素释放激素（CRH）和抗利尿激素（ADH），导致水重吸收增加、皮质醇、肾上腺素和去甲肾上腺素释放增加。

释放抗利尿激素（antidiuretic hormone，ADH）、肾上腺髓质释放肾上腺素、交感神经末梢释放去甲肾上腺素。胆碱能系统以及 5-羟色胺能系统的激活可刺激促肾上腺皮质激素释放激素（corticotrophin-releasing hormone，CRH）以及 ADH 的释放，而 CNS 的苯二氮䓬系统和阿片系统可抑制 CRH 和 ADH 的释放[11]。应激系统的激活能导致与疼痛控制相关的下丘脑弓状核以及后脑和脊髓区域中 CRH 介导的阿片类物质和阿片黑皮质素前体（pro-opiomelanocortin，POMC）衍生肽（如 β-内啡呔和脑啡肽）的分泌增加，从而提高机体镇痛反应并减轻对伤害性刺激的交感神经性反应[12]。

垂体激素

生长激素（growth hormone，GH）对维持内环境的稳定起着重要作用，它在夜间以脉冲方式释放；但其在创伤反应中的作用尚不明确。正常情况下，GH 能刺激蛋白质的合成、拮抗胰岛素的作用。在长期病程中，尽管其浓度升高，但其作用并非如上所述[13]。虽然有些报道主张给予外源性 GH，但其功效如何目前仍有争议，某些报道认为其可增加患者死亡率[14]。其他垂体激素在手术创伤反应中的作用似乎并不重要。性激素具有免疫调节的作用，其分泌受 CRH 升高的调节，导致性欲降低和闭经。尽管无活性的甲状腺素（逆三碘甲状腺原氨

表 4-2 激素的变化

来源	激素	作用
下丘脑	促肾上腺皮质激素释放激素（CRH）	促进 ACTH 的释放
	生长激素	作用尚不明了
	抗利尿激素（antidiuretic hormone，ADH）	维持细胞外液容量
		外周与内脏血管收缩
	P 物质	抑制 CRH 分泌
	β-内啡肽	增强镇痛
垂体	促肾上腺皮质激素	增加 ACTH 释放
	促卵泡激素-促黄体激素（FSH-LH）	抑制分泌、抑制性欲、中止月经
	抗利尿激素（ADH）	促进分泌
		维持细胞外液容量
		收缩外周和内脏血管
肾上腺皮质	皮质醇	免疫调节
	醛固酮	增加细胞外液容量
肾上腺髓质	儿茶酚胺	促进分解代谢，代谢亢进
胰腺	胰岛素	胰岛素抵抗情况下促进合成代谢
	胰高血糖素	升高血糖水平，引起损伤后糖生成增加

酸）水平升高，可导致甲状腺功能正常的病态综合征，但应激似乎并不影响促甲状腺激素的水平。

糖皮质激素

CRH 促使腺垂体释放促肾上腺皮质激素（adrenocorticotropic hormone，ACTH），从而引起肾上腺皮质释放糖皮质激素。ACTH 的释放通常呈现昼夜节律性，但手术后 ADH、不同儿茶酚胺、醛固酮和血管紧张素 Ⅱ 以协同方式促使 ACTH 分泌持续升高，其分泌的昼夜节律性丧失[15]。

皮质醇通过肌肉降解提高循环中碳水化合物、游离脂肪酸、三酰甘油和蛋白质的浓度，为创伤组织提供营养环境方面起到重要作用，并导致负氮平衡。由于肝糖原异生增加、胰岛素抵抗和脂质分解增强，使患者糖耐量显著降低。

糖皮质激素的免疫调节作用已十分明确，使其已成为治疗以过度炎性反应为特征的疾病的一项重要措施。其可明显抑制中性粒细胞的不当激活。糖皮质激素的作用部分是通过抑制前炎性细胞因子如 IL-1β 和 IL-6 的基因转录速率，降低其 mRNA 的稳定性[16,17]。其有益的作用还包括抑制受体介导的多形核粒细胞（polymorphonuclear cell，PMN）功能，下调中性粒细胞氧化呼吸暴发的活性和黏附分子的表达，以及抑制 PMN 的活性。其对中性粒细胞-内皮细胞间相互作用的抑制有利于在炎症不当状态时起到保护脏器的作用。

容量调节

维持细胞外液容量及其渗透压是手术和创伤应激反应的基本功能之一。这是通过多种不同激素的共同作用来实现的。血清渗透压升高是 ADH 分泌最常见的刺激因素，而焦虑、疼痛和血容量下降可通过刺激下丘脑而加强肾远曲小管对水分的重吸收。ADH 介导的外周与内脏血管收缩作用可进一步保证有效的灌注。ADH 的增高可持续 1 周以上。ACTH 可刺激肾上腺皮质释放醛固酮，但血管紧张素 Ⅱ 对醛固酮的分泌具有重要的辅助作用。醛固酮作用于远曲小管，以促进氢和钾与钠的交换，结果与 ADH 协同作用来增加细胞外液容量，但可能存在代谢性酸中毒。

细胞外液渗透压的有害变化同样可促进球旁器分泌肾素。局部肌上皮细胞交感神经系统兴奋可刺激肾素的分泌，而 ACTH、ADH 和胰高血糖素可增强该作用。肾素可引起血管紧张素 Ⅰ 的分泌，后者在肺血管经血管紧张素转化酶的作用转化为有活性的血管紧张素 Ⅱ。血管紧张素 Ⅱ 除了能进一步刺激 CRH、ADH 和醛固酮的释放外，其本身也是一种强效的血管收缩剂。

胰岛素

由于严重创伤后出现相对的高血糖和胰岛素抵抗状态，因此人们可能会质疑胰腺分泌的激素（胰岛素）对炎症反应的调节作用。但越来越多的证据充分表明，胰岛素可以促进合成代谢、抑制 TNF-α 的作用，并通过拮抗核因子 κB（nuclear factor B，NFκB）的作用而减少反应性氧族（reactive oxygen species，ROS）的产生，从而达到改善免疫功能的目的[18-20]。研究表明，危重患者采用外源性胰岛素严格控制血糖水平可显著改善患者的预后。这更进一步支持了上述有关胰岛素的特异作用[21]。

心理神经免疫学

目前许多权威人士认同情绪状态和个性特征可能影响免疫反应的观点[22]。传至神经内分泌反射弧靶腺体的信号受到下丘脑的控制，下丘脑对该信号的控制可能受到下丘脑以上刺激的影响。

巴甫洛夫条件反射可抑制动物的免疫应答反应[23]，而医学生在考试时，其自然杀伤细胞活性降低[24]。虽然有人对情绪状态可影响基本生理反应的观点持反对态度，但疼痛感知能力的改变确实可影响机体神经内分泌反应的强度。实际上，神经质是导致胆囊切除术后患者持续性疼痛的一项危险因素，而抑郁或焦虑则不是危险因素[25,26]。

炎症反应

受伤部位产生的传入性冲动传递了局部组织对更多营养物质的需求以及创伤部位及局部环境状态的信息。通过激活急性炎症反应来启动创伤组织的修复可能是由于创伤组织分泌生物活性肽特别是细胞因子所致。活化的巨噬细胞释放的信号分子 TNF-α 能显著增强局部与全身炎症反应。这些炎性介质也可在远端脏

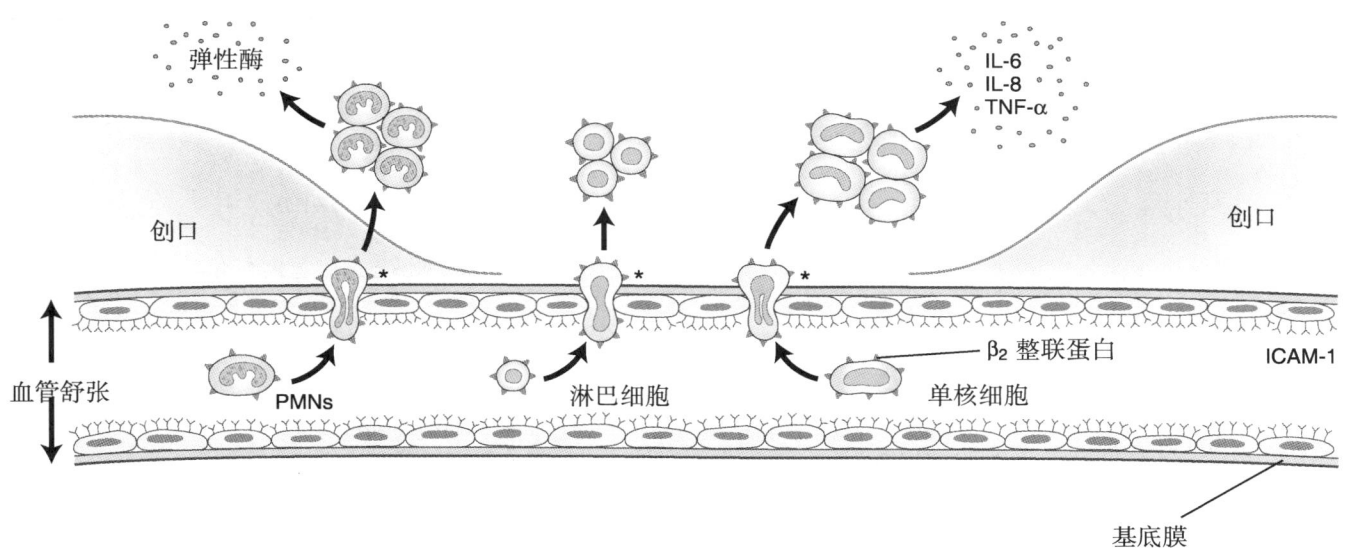

图 4-3 与炎症反应相关的创口。星号（*）表示内皮细胞基底膜通透性增加。局部炎症反应可导致各种免疫活性细胞的趋化作用，伴内皮通透性过高。ICAM-1，细胞间黏附分子 1；IL，白介素；PMN，多形核细胞；TNF-α，肿瘤坏死因子-α。

器发挥促炎作用。因此，从创伤的角度，创伤部位可以被看成一个独立的脏器[27]。局部炎症反应可通过感觉传入纤维引起全身应激而产生急性炎症反应，这种局部炎症反应的后果取决于促炎与抗炎因子之间的复杂相互作用。传入神经元通过分泌促炎或抗炎肽类物质（包括生长抑素和 P 物质）也可影响该后果[28]。

创伤周围血管内皮细胞通透性增加可促进白细胞和其他免疫活性细胞从血管内向创伤部位迁移。创伤部位募集了免疫细胞和辅助细胞，每个细胞都发挥增强促炎信号的作用。最易被募集的细胞是中性粒细胞和巨噬细胞（图 4-3）。

创伤部位激活的肥大细胞可分泌各种免疫活性肽，包括组胺、趋化因子以及蛋白酶。细胞死亡后可释放出细胞内蛋白质如高活力簇信号蛋白 1（high-motility group box protein 1，HMGB1），后者可触发细胞因子、ROS、胞质金属蛋白酶和局部血管扩张剂如一氧化氮（nitric oxide，NO）的进一步释放。炎症部位的疼痛感知至少部分由 NO 所介导[29,30]。虽然大剂量 NO 可增强外周伤害性感受器的敏感性，并诱发疼痛，但能产生低浓度 NO 的化合物，可减轻切口疼痛[29]。

在 ROS 的共同作用下，来自中性粒细胞的弹性蛋白酶可激活胞质金属蛋白酶，引起转化生长因子 β（transforming growth factor-β，TGF-β）的释放，后者具有显著的局部化学募集作用，引起中性粒细胞和巨噬细胞进一步聚集。诱导产生的局部转录因子 NFκB 以及随后表达的多种炎症快速反应基因，使 IL-6、IL-8、TNF-α 以及环氧合酶-2（cyclooxygenase-2，COX-2）的释放达到高峰，从而进一步影响炎性环境（表 4-3）[31]。

随后出现的中性粒细胞在创伤组织中的聚集是补体系统激活以及细胞因子产生，使黏附分子表达激活达顶峰的结果[32]。中性粒细胞暴露于这些内源性炎性介质后可导致 β2 整联蛋白 CD11b/CD18 表达上调，其粘附能力增强。细胞因子引起的炎症反应可引起内皮细胞上细胞间黏附分子-1（intercellular adhesion molecule-1，ICAM-1）和白细胞上 β2 整联蛋白表达上调。这可促进中性粒细胞-内皮细胞间的相互作用，并在一定条件下诱发内皮细胞通透性增高。中性粒细胞旋转是中性粒细胞-内皮细胞紧密粘附达顶峰过程的起始步骤，其中涉及 L-选择素和 P-选择素，两者均由内皮细胞介导（图 4-3）。

肌动蛋白细胞骨架构象改变加上中性粒细胞粘附性变化，可促进中性粒细胞在血管床进一步聚集。激活的中性粒细胞细胞骨架结构由于 F-肌动蛋白的聚合而变得刚性更强，其变形性降低[33]，导致激活的中性粒细胞陷夹在毛细血管内。炎症部位被陷夹的凋亡中性粒细胞的吞噬作用起到了限制中性粒细胞介导组织损伤的作用[34]。这种调节机制的功能障碍是全身炎症反应综合征（systemic inflammatory response syndrome，SIRS）时严重炎症反应增强的主要因素。

细胞内复杂信号转导途径的启动可导致酪氨酸激

表 4-3　创口产生的介质

介质	来源	作用
肿瘤坏死因子-α	巨噬细胞	促炎作用
		促细胞凋亡作用
		产生白介素-1β（IL-1β）
组胺	肥大细胞	血管扩张作用
化学因子	不同来源：巨噬细胞、树突细胞、T 细胞	单核细胞和淋巴细胞趋化作用
IL-1β	巨噬细胞	与 TNF-α 协同增强炎症反应
	内皮细胞	内源性致热源
IL-6	巨噬细胞	介导肝急性期反应蛋白
	T 细胞	同时参与促炎和抗炎反应
IL-8	巨噬细胞	白细胞趋化作用
IL-10	T 细胞	抗炎反应、抑制 TNF-α
IL-12	巨噬细胞	促炎症反应
	树突细胞	辅助 T 淋巴细胞类型 1 的分化
环氧合酶 2（COX-2）	膜磷脂	催化花生四烯酸转变为前列腺素

酶激活所引起的整联蛋白结合亲和力增加，进而引起细胞骨架蛋白再分布[35]。各种蛋白酪氨酸激酶的磷酸化是信号转导中反复出现的反应，包括磷脂酰肌醇-3 激酶（phosphatidylinositol 3-kinase，PI 3-k）[36]、蛋白激酶 C[37]、Src-激酶、有丝分裂原活化蛋白（mitogen-activated protein，MAP）激酶，如 p38 MAP 激酶、细胞外信号相关激酶（extracellular signal-related kinase，ERK）以及 Jun 蛋白 N 端激酶[38]。脂多糖（lipopolysaccharide，LPS）[39]激活的 p38 MAP 激酶通过增强中性粒细胞氧自由基的释放、增强整联蛋白的黏附能力[40]以及调节促炎细胞因子的合成而加强中性粒细胞的免疫活性[41]。

凝血反应

炎症系统和凝血系统是从共同的真核生物祖先中分化产生的高度保守而又密切共生的防御机制。这两种机制联合起来通过防止血管内容量丢失，并抵御微生物的入侵，以维持机体完整。对任何病原微生物的吞噬作用都是由膜结合受体与病原体表面微粒配体相互结合所致[42]。中性粒细胞脱颗粒后释放的蛋白水解酶及产生的 ROS 可杀死病原微生物[43]。这种炎症应答通过以下几个不同途径改变凝血平衡，有利于凝血作用：上调与启动血液凝固与凝血酶产生相关的组织因子、抑制纤溶、在微血管内通过细胞因子介导下下调血管内皮细胞蛋白 C 受体而拮抗抗凝血作用[44,45]。凝血酶以及 TNF-α 也可协同作用来减少血栓调节素（一种蛋白 C 共激活因子）的表达。在炎症反应过度的状态下，血栓调节素的表达减少可能导致临床表现为微血管功能障碍，如低氧、酸中毒以及弥散性血管内凝血。

结论

人类从损伤与手术中恢复的能力提示，伤口愈合是一种人类生存的基本生物学目标。痛觉感受器产生的传入信号是损伤的初始反应之一，最终可导致神经内分泌系统激活，级联性释放下丘脑和垂体激素。从外周看，免疫系统被抗原激活，随后释放具有免疫调节作用的肽类和细胞因子，如 TNF-α、IL-1 和 IL-6，最终导致能量代谢由合成代谢向分解代谢途径的转变。外周感觉神经元起到监测创伤部位环境变化的作用，并通过分泌 P 物质和生长抑素而发挥免疫调制作用。

手术引起的复杂而完整的神经内分泌反应、炎症反应和凝血反应可导致促炎与抗炎作用之间、促凝血倾向与抗凝血倾向之间以及分解代谢与合成代谢之间的平衡丧失。人们已经尝试多种方法来试图打破这种分解代谢占优势的状态，但并无临床效果[46]。危重病患者支持手段和通气治疗的改进使患者总体死亡率略有下降，但这些治疗措施对机体固有的炎症反应过程仍无明显影响[41]。支持治疗，尤其是优化细胞外环境、改善组织氧合以及完善镇痛方法，仍是改善患者预后的首要措施。

(李 杰译 倪 文 邓小明校)

参考文献

1. Boontham P, Chandran P, Rowlands B, Eremin O: Surgical sepsis: Dysregulation of immune function and therapeutic implications. Surgeon 2003;1:187–206.
2. Cuthbertson D: Post-shock metabolic response. Lancet 1942;1:433–437.
3. Sibbald WJ: Shockingly complex: The difficult road to introducing new ideas to critical care. Crit Care 2004;8:419–421.
4. Moore F: Bodily changes in surgical convalescence. 1: The normal sequence-observations and interpretations. Ann Surg 1953;137:289–315.
5. Wu FP, Sietses C, von Blomberg BM, et al: Systemic and peritoneal inflammatory response after laparoscopic or conventional colon resection in cancer patients: A prospective, randomized trial. Dis Colon Rectum 2003;46:147–155.
6. Da Costa ML, Redmond HP, Finnegan N, et al: Laparotomy and laparoscopy differentially accelerate experimental flank tumour growth. Br J Surg 1998;85:1439–1442.
7. Chrousos GP, Gold PW: The concepts of stress and stress system disorders: Overview of physical and behavioral homeostasis. JAMA 1992;267:1244–1252.
8. Chrousos GP: Regulation and dysregulation of the hypothalamic-pituitary-adrenal axis: The corticotropin-releasing hormone perspective. Endocrinol Metab Clin North Am 1992;21:833–858.
9. Johnson JD, O'Connor KA, Watkins LR, Maier SF: The role of IL-1beta in stress-induced sensitization of proinflammatory cytokine and corticosterone responses. Neuroscience 2004;127:569–577.
10. Buyukkocak U, Caglayan O, Oral H, et al: The effects of anesthetic techniques on acute phase response at delivery (anesthesia and acute phase response). Clin Biochem 2003;36:67–70.
11. Grottoli S, Maccagno B, Ramunni J, et al: Alprazolam, a benzodiazepine, does not modify the ACTH and cortisol response to hCRH and AVP, but blunts the cortisol response to ACTH in humans. J Endocrinol Invest 2002;25:420–425.
12. Fukuda Y, Kageyama K, Nigawara T, et al: Effects of corticotropin-releasing hormone (CRH) on the synthesis and secretion of proopiomelanocortin-related peptides in the anterior pituitary: A study using CRH-deficient mice. Neurosci Lett 2004;367:201–204.
13. Shipman J, Guy J, Abumrad NN: Repair of metabolic processes. Crit Care Med 2003;31(Suppl):S512–S517.
14. Takala J, Ruokonen E, Webster NR, et al: Increased mortality associated with growth hormone treatment in critically ill adults. N Engl J Med 1999;341:785–792.
15. Mussi C, Angelini C, Crippa S, et al: Alteration of hypothalamus-pituitary-adrenal glands axis in colorectal cancer patients. Hepatogastroenterology 2003;50(Suppl 2):ccxxviii–ccxxxi.
16. Zitnik RJ, Whiting NL, Elias JA: Glucocorticoid inhibition of interleukin-1-induced interleukin-6 production by human lung fibroblasts: Evidence for transcriptional and post-transcriptional regulatory mechanisms. Am J Respir Cell Mol Biol 1994;10:643–650.
17. Zanker B, Walz G, Wieder KJ, Strom TB: Evidence that glucocorticosteroids block expression of the human interleukin-6 gene by accessory cells. Transplantation 1990;49:183–185.
18. Dandona P, Aljada A, Mohanty P, et al: Insulin inhibits intranuclear nuclear factor kappaB and stimulates IkappaB in mononuclear cells in obese subjects: Evidence for an anti-inflammatory effect? J Clin Endocrinol Metab 2001;86:3257–3265.
19. Satomi N, Sakurai A, Haranaka K: Relationship of hypoglycemia to tumor necrosis factor production and antitumor activity: Role of glucose, insulin, and macrophages. J Natl Cancer Inst 1985;74:1255–1260.
20. Das UN: Is insulin an antiinflammatory molecule? Nutrition 2001;17:409–413.
21. van den Berghe G, Wouters P, Weekers F, et al: Intensive insulin therapy in the critically ill patients. N Engl J Med 2001;345:1359–1367.
22. Carr DJ: Neuroendocrine peptide receptors on cells of the immune system. Chem Immunol 1992;52:84–105.
23. Cohen N, Moynihan JA, Ader R: Pavlovian conditioning of the immune system. Int Arch Allergy Immunol 1994;105:101–106.
24. Malarkey WB, Hall JC, Pearl DK, et al: The influence of academic stress and season on 24-hour concentrations of growth hormone and prolactin. J Clin Endocrinol Metab 1991;73:1089–1092.
25. Borly L, Anderson IB, Bardram L, et al: Preoperative prediction model of outcome after cholecystectomy for symptomatic gallstones. Scand J Gastroenterol 1999;34:1144–1152.
26. Jess P, Jess T, Beck H, Bech P: Neuroticism in relation to recovery and persisting pain after laparoscopic cholecystectomy. Scand J Gastroenterol 1998;33:550–553.
27. Baue AE: Sepsis, systemic inflammatory response syndrome, multiple organ dysfunction syndrome, and multiple organ failure: Are trauma surgeons lumpers or splitters? J Trauma 2003;55:997–998.
28. Coderre TJ, Basbaum AI, Levine JD: Neural control of vascular permeability: Interactions between primary afferents, mast cells, and sympathetic efferents. J Neurophysiol 1989;62:48–58.
29. Prado WA, Schiavon VF, Cunha FQ: Dual effect of local application of nitric oxide donors in a model of incision pain in rats. Eur J Pharmacol 2002;441:57–65.
30. Anbar M, Gratt BM: Role of nitric oxide in the physiopathology of pain. J Pain Symptom Manage 1997;14:225–254.
31. Ardite E, Panes J, Miranda M, et al: Effects of steroid treatment on activation of nuclear factor kappaB in patients with inflammatory bowel disease. Br J Pharmacol 1998;124:431–433.
32. Closa D, Sabater L, Fernandez-Cruz L, et al: Activation of alveolar macrophages in lung injury associated with experimental acute pancreatitis is mediated by the liver. Ann Surg 1999;229:230–236.
33. Skoutelis AT, Kaleridis V, Athanassiou GM, et al: Neutrophil deformability in patients with sepsis, septic shock, and adult respiratory distress syndrome. Crit Care Med 2000;28:2355–2359.
34. Sookhai S, Wang JH, McCourt M, et al: Dopamine induces neutrophil apoptosis through a dopamine D-1 receptor-independent mechanism. Surgery 1999;126:314–322.
35. Yan SR, Berton G: Antibody-induced engagement of beta2 integrins in human neutrophils causes a rapid redistribution of cytoskeletal proteins, Src-family tyrosine kinases, and p72syk that precedes de novo actin polymerization. J Leukoc Biol 1998;64:401–408.
36. Capodici C, Hanft S, Feoktistov M, Pillinger MH: Phosphatidylinositol 3-kinase mediates chemoattractant-stimulated, CD11b/CD18-dependent cell-cell adhesion of human neutrophils: Evidence for an ERK-independent pathway. J Immunol 1998;160:1901–1909.
37. Toker A, Cantley LC: Signalling through the lipid products of phosphoinositide-3-OH kinase. Nature 1997;387(6634):673–676.
38. Scherle PA, Jones EA, Favata MF, et al: Inhibition of MAP kinase kinase prevents cytokine and prostaglandin E2 production in lipopolysaccharide-stimulated monocytes. J Immunol 1998;161:5681–5686.
39. St-Denis A, Chano F, Tremblay P, et al: Protein kinase C-alpha modulates lipopolysaccharide-induced functions in a murine macrophage cell line. J Biol Chem 1998;273:32787–32792.
40. Nick JA, Avdi NJ, Young SK, et al: Common and distinct intracellular signaling pathways in human neutrophils utilized by platelet activating factor and FMLP. J Clin Invest 1997;99:975–986.
41. Denham W, Yang J, Wang H, et al: Inhibition of p38 mitogen activate kinase attenuates the severity of pancreatitis-induced adult respiratory distress syndrome. Crit Care Med 2000;28:2567–2572.
42. Horwitz AH, Williams RE, Liu PS, Nadell R: Bactericidal/permeability-increasing protein inhibits growth of a strain of *Acholeplasma laidlawii* and L forms of the gram-positive bacteria *Staphylococcus aureus* and *Streptococcus pyogenes*. Antimicrob Agents Chemother 1999;43:2314–2316.
43. Krump E, Sanghera JS, Pelech SL, et al: Chemotactic peptide N-formyl-met-leu-phe activation of p38 mitogen-activated protein kinase (MAPK) and MAPK-activated protein kinase-2 in human neutrophils. J Biol Chem 1997;272:937–944.
44. Conway G, Wooley J, Bibring T, LeStourgeon WM: Ribonucleoproteins package 700 nucleotides of pre-mRNA into a repeating array of regular particles. Mol Cell Biol 1988;8:2884–2895.
45. Moore KL, Esmon CT, Esmon NL: Tumor necrosis factor leads to the internalization and degradation of thrombomodulin from the surface of bovine aortic endothelial cells in culture. Blood 1989;73:159–165.
46. Fulkerson WJ, MacIntyre N, Stamler J, Crapo JD: Pathogenesis and treatment of the adult respiratory distress syndrome. Arch Intern Med 1996;156:29–38.

5 术后伤害性疼痛的机制

HENRY FRIZELLE

国际疼痛研究协会对于疼痛的定义是：疼痛是组织损伤或与潜在的组织损伤相关的一种不愉快的躯体感觉和情感经历（表5-1）[1]。伤害性感受是描述疼痛信息传递到中枢神经系统的机制。这种信息最终如何感觉为疼痛尚不明了。通常认为包括以下4个过程：

转导：通过称为伤害性感受器的感觉感受器，将有害性温度、机械性或化学性刺激转化为神经冲动。

传递：将外周转导部位的神经冲动信息传送至大脑和脊髓。

感知：鉴别这些信号为疼痛。

调制：大脑发出的下行性信号改变脊髓中伤害性疼痛信息传递的过程[2,3]。

转导

伤害性感受器是激活阈值较高的感觉感受器，主要感知组织损伤或长期作用于可损伤组织的非伤害性刺激[4]。这些感受器是初级传入神经纤维的游离末梢，遍布在机体外周。伤害性刺激（当刺激持续存在产生损害时，可导致体液和细胞反应，并形成炎症）可激活有髓鞘的A-δ伤害性感受器和无髓鞘的C伤害性感受器。A-δ伤害性感受器对机械性刺激敏感，并以5～25 m/s的速率转导针刺样感觉。C伤害性感受器呈多种模式，传导速度小于2 m/s，传递组织损伤产生的冲动；由于C伤害性感受器呈多种模式，所以它们对温度、化学和机械损伤均可产生反应（图5.1）。

除了直接的伤害，手术创伤可产生神经内分泌炎症反应，导致受损细胞和炎症细胞释放细胞内容物（钾离子、缓激肽、前列腺素）。这可增强损伤部位伤害性感受器的敏感性。结果在损伤部位对疼痛性刺激产生更强的反应（原发性痛觉过敏）。轴突反射将冲动传向脊髓的同时，也将传向伤害性感受器的其余外周分支。这可导致神经肽（P物质、降钙素基因相关肽）的释放，使血管舒张和肥大细胞脱颗粒。肥大细胞脱颗粒后可释放出组胺和血清素[5]。这些促炎症因子可使邻近的A-δ和C伤害性感受器敏感化（继发性痛觉过敏）。正常情况下，许多伤害性感受器（"睡眠感受器"）都不能被激活[6]，只有在病理状态（如炎症）下才激活。

传递

外周末梢产生的神经冲动传递到大脑和脊髓的过程分为几个阶段[7]。感觉神经冲动通过脊髓背角初级传入神经元轴突传导。背根神经节（dorsal root ganglia, DRG）包含A-δ和C伤害性感受器的细胞体。进入脊髓后，伤害性感受器沿Lissauer束上行或下行数个节段后，与脊髓背角Ⅰ、Ⅱ（脊髓灰质）和Ⅴ层中的二级神经元形成突触。在脊髓背角中，伤害性感受器突触传递的主要递质是谷氨酸，主要与急性疼痛感觉相关的受体是α-氨基-3-羟基-5-甲基-异噁唑-4-丙酸（alpha-amino-3-hydroxy-5-methyl-isoxazole-4-propionic acid, AMPA）受体。

二级神经元主要分为两类：特异性伤害性感受

表 5-1	伤害性疼痛的特征		
	内脏痛	表浅感觉痛	深部感觉痛
伤害性感受器定位	内脏器官	皮肤、皮下组织	骨骼、肌肉、肌腱、关节
刺激因素	器官拉伤、炎症、局部缺血	机械性、温度、化学	机械损伤、缺血、炎症
定位	定位不明确	定位准确	弥散或放射状
性质	持续性深部痛或牵涉到皮肤的锐痛	锐痛、灼烧痛、刺痛	钝痛、持续性疼痛、绞痛
症状和体征	恶心、呕吐、出汗、触痛和肌紧张	皮肤触痛、痛觉过敏、感觉过敏	触痛、深部肌肉痉挛
举例	阑尾炎、胰腺炎、消化性溃疡疾病	割伤、擦伤、烧伤	关节炎、肌腱炎

(nociceptive-specific，NS）神经元和"广动力域"(wide dynamic range，WDR）神经元。NS 神经元仅对某种特异类型的伤害性刺激有反应，其感受范围小，并发现其主要位于Ⅰ层。WDR 神经元是非特异性伤害感受器，其对广泛刺激有反应，从轻微的触觉到伤害性刺激。它们的感受范围较广，见于各个层面，但在Ⅴ层尤为集中。二级神经元与广泛的中间神经元形成突触连接，促进或抑制进一步传递（图 5-2）。

中枢性神经疼痛上传通路

有两条主要的上传通路：新脊髓丘脑束和旧脊髓网状丘脑束。针刺样感觉（A-δ 传入）经由新脊髓丘脑束到达中央后回，而由组织损伤导致的疼痛（C 传入）是通过旧脊髓网状丘脑束穿过网状结构到达皮层。在途中，信号的传导需经过丘脑的髓板内核。新脊髓丘脑束是伤害性刺激最重要的传导通路，它位于脊髓前外象限。大多数轴突通过脊髓腹侧白连合交叉到对侧前外象限向上传导，但也有少数轴突在同侧传导。来自远端区域的神经元位置偏外，而近端发出的神经元更集中在中间。脊髓丘脑束神经元分为中间束和侧束投射到丘脑。来自Ⅰ、Ⅱ、Ⅴ层投射到侧丘脑的神经纤维与投射到躯体感觉皮层的神经纤维形成突触连接。因此，这些神经纤维包含疼痛感觉和识别方面的功能。投射到丘脑内侧的神经元来源于较深层的区域（Ⅵ和Ⅹ区）。投射被传送到网状结构、导水管周围灰质（periaqueductal gray matter，PAG）和下丘脑（图 5-3）。

网状结构包含许多与疼痛感觉相关的神经核。巨大细胞性网状核、中缝大核（nucleus raphe magnus，

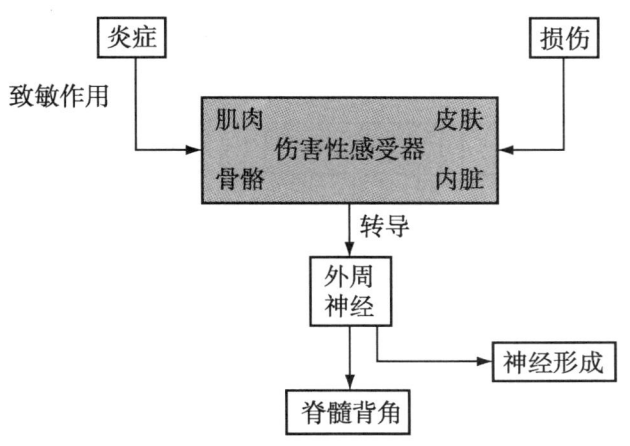

图 5-1 疼痛的外周起源。组织损伤或长时间暴露于无害刺激都可引起伤害性感受器兴奋。炎症可使伤害性感受器致敏，降低其放电阈值。

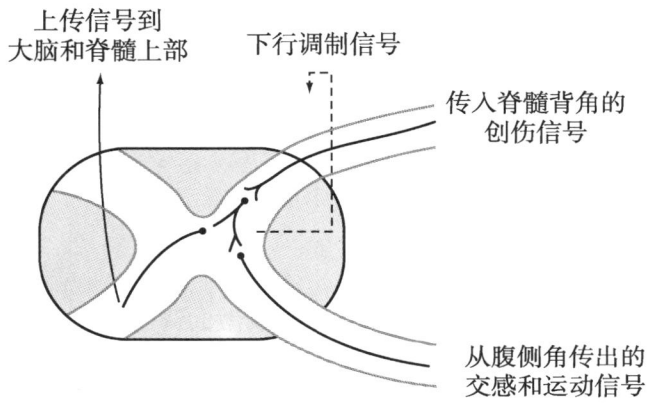

图 5-2 脊髓传导机制简图。图示基本的信号传至背角，其中大多数冲动交叉到对侧，随后沿前部脊髓丘脑束上行。图中也示意同侧反射活性和下行抑制作用。

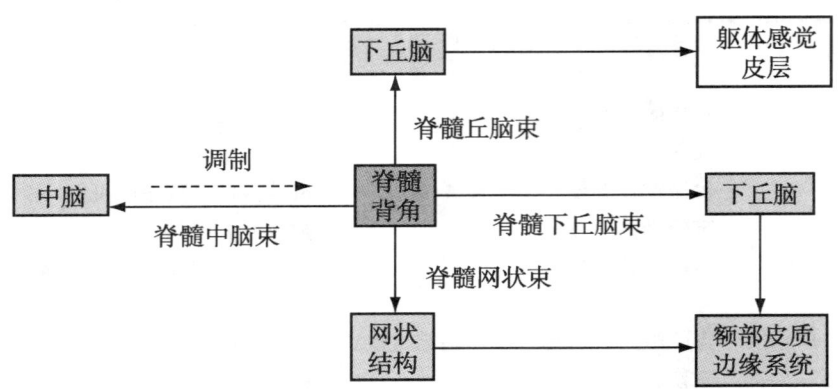

图 5-3 图示伤害性感受冲动从脊髓传导到更高级中枢结构的多种途径。图中显示 4 条主要的投射系统（脊髓丘脑束、脊髓中脑束、脊髓网状束和脊髓下丘脑束）。

NRM）以及 PAG 中的神经元是阿片样物质介导的下行抑制系统的一部分。边缘系统包括下丘脑、海马、杏仁体和扣带回。它与疼痛的行为反应控制有关。额叶皮质控制疼痛性质和记忆。

感知

身体伤害所产生的负面情感（恐惧）和典型的不愉快感受也被称之为疼痛。这与大脑皮质和边缘系统有关。信息从某些背角投射神经元经由丘脑传导到对侧躯体感觉皮层。这种传入映射保留了疼痛位置、强度和性质的信息。其他一些伤害性传入经由丘脑传到边缘系统。它与来自脊髓网状束和脊髓中脑束的传入信息一起共同介导疼痛的情感感受。

疼痛在较高级中枢的整合非常复杂。疼痛识别能力部分具有躯体皮层定位特性，涉及初级和二级感觉皮层。躯体性疼痛的整合在该水平进行，使大脑对疼痛进行定位。情感部分的整合涉及到各种边缘结构，尤其是扣带回皮质。

调制

下行抑制通路

大脑的许多区域与伤害性刺激的调制有关，包括躯体感觉皮层、下丘脑、PAG 和中缝大核。从这些结构发出的神经纤维直接或间接地经由后侧索到达脊髓，投射到Ⅰ层和Ⅴ层。下行系统主要由 3 部分组成：阿片系统、去甲肾上腺素能神经元和 5-羟色胺能神经元。阿片系统与下行性镇痛有关。阿片前体及其相关肽存在于下丘脑、杏仁核、中缝大核和背角。来自蓝斑的去甲肾上腺素能神经元投射到后侧索。来自中缝大核的 5-羟色胺能神经元经后侧索投射到脊髓。

这些通路脊髓门控系统似有影响。虽然 PAG 是阿片类物质介导的下行抑制通路的一部分，但是中缝大核与脊髓之间经由后侧索有直接的联系，其抑制性神经调制作用是由 5-羟色胺所介导的。与这些下行通路有关的其他抑制性神经递质是去甲肾上腺素和 γ-氨基丁酸（gamma-aminobutyric acid，GABA）。抑制性氨基酸（如 GABA）和神经肽（内源性阿片类物质）能与初级传入神经元和背角神经元上的受体相结合，通过突触前和突触后机制抑制伤害性感受的传递[8]。从大脑发出的下行抑制性传入也调制背角伤害性感受的传递。抑制过程是伤害性感受调制系统的一部分，可

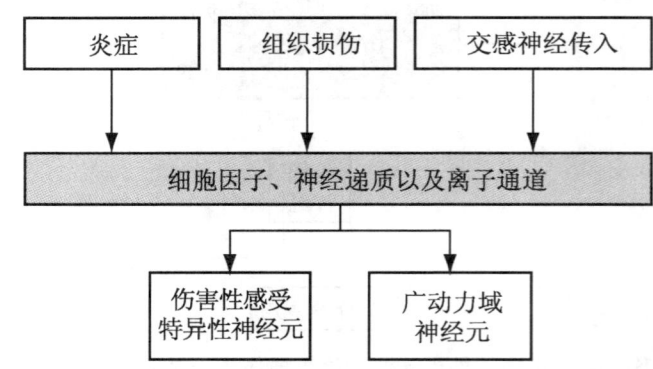

图 5-4 神经末梢致敏现象的简略图示，文中详细介绍细胞因子、神经递质以及离子通道所起的作用。

受器表现为激活阈值降低和放电频率增快[9]。组织损伤后伤害性感受器敏感性增加归咎于以下两种机制之一：缓激肽可能通过与蛋白激酶 C 有关的机制增强热量激活的电流，或前列腺素 E_2 改变离子通道的电压阈值[10]。有力的证据表明，存在与伤害性疼痛冲动传导和传递有关的离子通道翻译后修饰，并同时存在生物物理学致敏性[11]。一般认为，存在于肠道伤害性感受器初级传入神经上的河豚毒素不敏感性钠通道 Na(v) 1.8，是伤害性感受器致敏后兴奋性提高的主要原因[12]。外周致敏在痛觉过敏、异常性疼痛和中枢性致敏中起到重要作用（图 5-4）。

中枢致敏现象是脊髓神经元过度兴奋的一种状态。它使受伤区域周围未受伤害组织中二级痛觉过敏区对无害刺激的反应性增加。对 C 伤害性感受器的反复刺激可引起背角神经元放电频率逐渐增加，称为"wind-up"（图 5-5）[13]。更大量的谷氨酸和 P 物质释放，刺激 AMPA 与神经激肽 I 受体。这可导致正常时无功能的 N-甲基-D-门冬氨酸（N-methyl-d-aspartate，NMDA）受体激活，后者也与谷氨酸作用，引起反应性增强[14]。NMDA 受体的激活可引起 Ca^{2+} 通过离子通道（配体与电压门控通道）内流，导致第二信使 [三磷酸鸟核苷（guanosine triphosphate，GTP）-结合蛋白] 的激活，一氧化氮（nitric oxide，NO）的产生，致癌基因（c-fos）的诱导（图 5-6 和 5-7）。这些第二信使可改变细胞的兴奋性，导致长时程增强作用（long-term potentiation，LTP）。这是一个突触功能用进废退的例子。这种类型的调制作用也发生于伤害性感受传导径路上游。

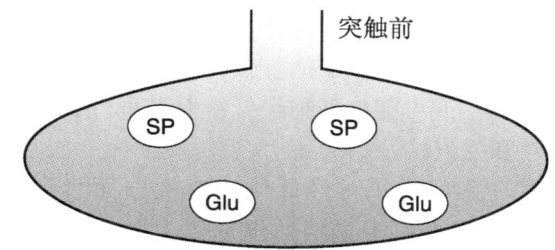
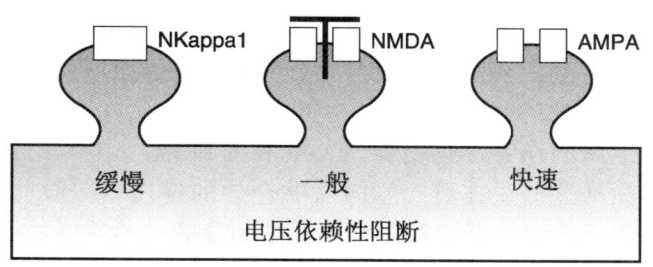

图 5-5 图示称为"wind-up"的背角神经元放电频率增加。从传入神经末梢释放的神经递质激活了缓慢型 NK-1 受体和快速型 AMPA 受体，最后激活第二信使，并启动 NMDA 受体。AMPA，α-氨基-3-羟基-5-甲基噁唑-4-丙酸；Glu，谷氨酸；NMDA，N-甲基-D-门冬氨酸；SP，P 物质。

平衡伤害性感受信号系统。

外周致敏

反复或长时间伤害性刺激和（或）暴露于某些炎症介质中都能使伤害性感受器致敏。致敏的伤害性感

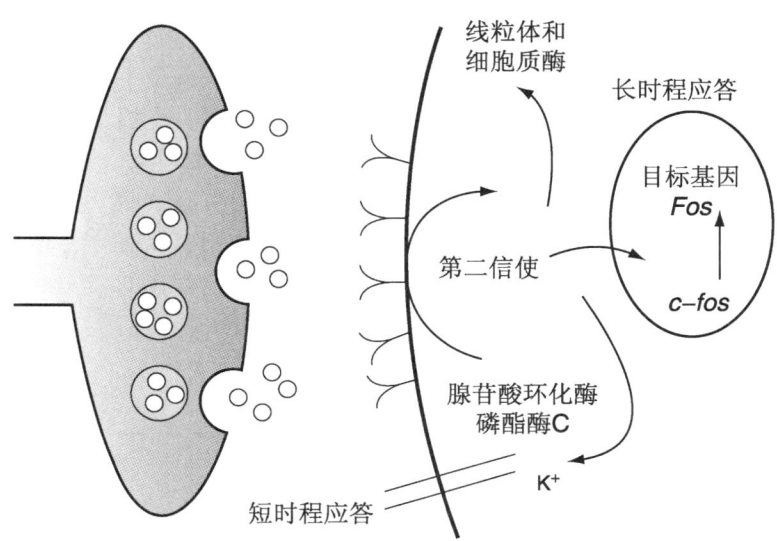

图 5-6 第二信使释放和基因激活。外周神经递质释放可激活突触后受体。第二信使（如 cAMP 和 Ca^{++}）通过减少 K^+ 外流和诱导原癌基因能降低神经元的兴奋性。

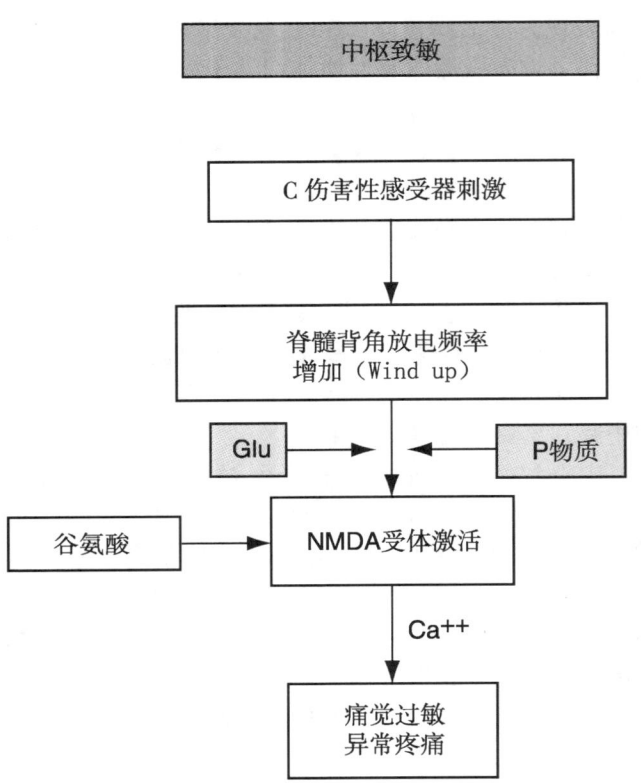

图 5-7 中枢致敏过程的简示图。图示 NMDA 受体、神经递质和钙离子作为第二信使的重要性。Glu，葡萄糖；NMDA，N-甲基-D-门冬氨酸。

中枢致敏的背角发生的另一个变化是反应阈值降低，对阈上刺激的反应在强度和持续时间上都增强，并且背角神经元的感受范围扩大[15]。临床上有很多方式表示这些变化：对伤害性刺激的反应增强（痛觉过敏），正常的无害刺激可产生疼痛反应（异常性疼痛），短暂刺激可产生长时间疼痛（持续疼痛），或者疼痛可能向未受损的组织扩散（牵涉性疼痛）。致敏现象是手术损伤后持续性疼痛和痛觉过敏最常见的原因。受损炎症组织发出的"正常"有害性传入能引起致敏现象，受损神经或神经节发出的"异常"传入也能引起致敏现象。"正常"情况下，致敏作用起到适应作用，以有利于愈合过程中创口的保护。创口愈合后持续存在的致敏现象可能引起慢性疼痛。中枢致敏也可解释为何临床慢性疼痛的治疗要难于急性疼痛。

伤害感受的激动剂与拮抗剂

如上所述，组织损伤、炎症或神经损伤后所产生的许多物质可以改变疼痛的性质，导致痛觉过敏和异常性疼痛。这些化学因子能直接作用于外周神经纤维而产生疼痛，或可能增加神经纤维对各种外源性刺激的敏感性和反应性。

激肽在影响外周神经纤维兴奋性方面起到最重要的作用，因为组织损伤后迅速产生激肽，后者通过作用于外周与中枢神经元而启动一系列互相作用的化学级联反应。缓激肽和血管舒张素（赖氨酰缓激肽）分别是高分子量和低分子量激肽原的产物。它们激活主要的激肽受体 B1 与 B2。主要的药理作用是由 B2 受体激活所产生的。B2 受体存在于大多数组织的伤害性感受器（A-δ 和 C 纤维）中[16]，直接激活这些受体可产生缓激肽介导的疼痛。缓激肽也使这些神经纤维对物理和化学刺激的敏感性增加。这种致敏作用的发生是由于缓激肽与其他炎症介质（如血清素和细胞因子）相互协同作用或通过肥大细胞释放的组胺所致。

B2 受体产生的信号转导是通过数个第二信使系统的激活所产生的，包括膜磷脂酶 C 的配对受体激活和膜磷脂的分裂。结果钠离子通透性增加，导致细胞膜去极化。这种去极化也引起钙离子通透性增加，随后释放感觉神经肽，激活一氧化氮合酶（nitric oxide synthetase，NOS），产生环磷酸鸟苷（cyclic guanosine monophosphate，cGMP）。缓激肽也激活神经节后交感神经纤维，引起类前列腺素和其他炎症介质的释放。B1 受体的数量少于 B2 受体，但是炎症介质（白介素）和生长启动因子可使它们的表达增加。B1 受体在痛觉过敏的产生过程中似乎发挥重要作用，但如何发挥这种作用尚不明了。

神经生长因子（nerve growth factor，NGF）是炎症产生的神经营养物质，它可改变交感神经和感觉神经的兴奋性。炎症期间白介素-1β 和肿瘤坏死因子-α（tumor necrosis factor-α，TNF-α）可刺激 NGF 的产生。NGF 通过介质释放、肥大细胞脱颗粒和 B1 受体增加可诱导伤害性感受器快速间接地致敏。持续较长时间的变化是由于基因调节变化所致。

离子通道的活性

膜离子通道的过度表达能解释为何炎症期间感觉神经元膜兴奋性增加。这些变化能说明炎症产生的痛觉过敏和自发性疼痛。随着认识的深入，发现与伤害性感受有关的各种离子通道数目和作用越来越多。酸敏感性离子通道（acid-sensing ion channel，ASIC）普遍存在于哺乳动物的神经系统中。最近在敲除模型的实验研究证实ASIC与外周伤害性感受有关。尽管明确的机制尚不明了，但目前正在深入研究组织pH值波动的作用[17]。

G蛋白信号系统可能是许多神经递质系统之间的一个共同连接环节。现已证明，G蛋白偶联的内向整流性钾通道（G protein coupled, inwardly rectifying potassium channel，GIRK）是各种神经递质受体与突触传递调节之间的一个共同连接环节。这些受体包括阿片类受体、α-肾上腺素能受体、M胆碱能受体、GABA B受体和大麻素受体；这些受体与突触后GIRK2通道相偶联，可以解释男性大多数抗伤害感受的作用机制[18]。G蛋白信号系统常见于介导伤害性感受的其他离子通道[19]。促炎症反应介质调制离子通道主要是通过G蛋白依赖性途径与cGMP依赖性途径。非阿片肽伤害性感受主要通过结合其自身受体ORL-1来抑制电压依赖性钙电流（ICa）[20]。该受体在结构与功能上与阿片受体类似，同样是G蛋白偶联受体[21]。

阿片受体系统与NMDA受体系统在调节伤害感受中相互作用。如上所述，NMDA受体的激活通过第二信使系统促使兴奋过度现象的出现。在阿片受体亚型中，μ受体和δ受体可能抑制或增强NMDA受体介导的作用，而κ受体则具有抑制作用[22]。在大脑某些区域（丘脑、三叉神经核），NMDA受体的激活为促伤害性感受作用，但在其他脑区（PAG、延髓腹外侧区）NMDA受体的激活为抗伤害性感受作用[23]。

DRG轴突损伤可改变这些神经元中钠离子通道的表达。SNS/PN3和NaN钠通道基因下调，而以前静息性III型钠通道基因上调。该过程可改变DRG神经元电生理特性，结果发生自发性放电或以不恰当高频方式放电。目前正在探讨这种基因表达改变与开发镇痛药之间的关联[24]。

结论

近年来，人们对术后伤害性疼痛机制的认识有了很大提高。对相关的大量神经递质与受体研究提示存在镇痛药治疗的许多可能靶点。但是，存在大量潜在的治疗靶位点，加上神经系统能改变这种靶点，这就意味着单一镇痛药可能无效。

（张庆兵译　范晓华　邓小明校）

参考文献

1. Merskey H, Bogduk N (eds): Classification of Chronic Pain: Descriptions of Chronic Pain Syndromes and Definitions of Pain Terms, 2nd ed. Seattle, IASP Press, 1994.
2. Besson JM, Chaouch A: Peripheral and spinal mechanisms of nociception. Physiol Rev 1987;67:67–186.
3. Pasero C, Paice JA, McCaffery M: Basic mechanisms underlying the causes and effects of pain. In McCaffery M, Pasero C (eds): Pain Clinic Manual, 2nd ed. St Louis, Mosby Inc, 1999, pp 15–34.
4. Merskey H, Bogduk N: Classification of Chronic Pain: Descriptions of Chronic Pain Syndromes and Definitions of Pain Terms, 2nd ed. Seattle, IASP Press, 1994.
5. Song SO, Carr DB: Pain and Memory. Pain: Clinical Updates 1999;VII:1.
6. Siddal PJ, Cousins MJ: Spinal pain mechanisms. Spine 1997;22:98–104.
7. Willis WD, Westlund KN: Neuroanatomy of the pain system and of the pathways that modulate pain. J Clin Neurophysiol 1997;14:2–31.
8. Terman GW, Bonica JJ: Spinal mechanisms and their modulation. In Loeser JD, Butler SH, Chapman CR, Turk DC (eds): Bonica's Management of Pain, 3rd ed. Baltimore, Lippincott Williams & Wilkins, 2001, pp 73–152.
9. Woolf CJ: Recent advances in the pathophysiology of acute pain. Br J Anaesth 1989;63:139–146.
10. Cesare P, McNaughton P: Peripheral pain mechanisms. Curr Opin Neurobiol 1997;7:493–499.
11. Bhave G, Gereau RW 4th: Posttranslational mechanisms of peripheral sensitization. J Neurobiol 2004;61:88–106.
12. Cervero F, Laird JM: Role of ion channels in mechanisms controlling gastrointestinal pain pathways. Curr Opin Pharmacol 2003;3:608–612.
13. Woolf CJ: Evidence for a central component of post-injury pain hypersensitivity. Nature 1983;306:686–688.
14. Eide PK: Wind up and the NMDA receptor complex from a clinical perspective. Eur J Pain 2000;4:5–17.
15. Dickenson AH: Central acute pain mechanisms. Ann Med 1995;27:223–227.
16. Steranka LR, Manning D, DeHaas CJ, et al: Bradykinin as a pain mediator: Receptors are localized to sensory neurons and antagonists have analgesic actions. Proc Natl Acad Sci U S A 1988;85:3245–3249.
17. Krishtal O: The ASICs: Signalling molecules? Modulators? Trends Neurosci 2003;26:477–483.
18. Blednov YA, Stoffel M, Alva H, Harris RA: A pervasive mechanism for analgesia: Activation of GIRK2 channels. Proc Natl Acad Sci U S A 2003;100:277–282.
19. Liu L, Yang T, Bruno MJ, et al: Voltage-gated ion channels in nociceptors: Modulation by cGMP. J Neurophysiol 2004;92:2323–2332.
20. Yeon KY, Sim MY, Choi SY, et al: Molecular mechanisms underlying calcium current modulation by nociceptin. Neuroreport 2004;15:2205–2209.
21. New DC, Wong YH: The ORL1 receptor: Molecular pharmacology and signalling systems. Neurosignals 2002;11:197–212.
22. Riedel W, Neeck G: Nociception, pain and antinociception: Current concepts. Z Rheumatol 2001;60:404–415.
23. Fundytus ME: Glutamate receptors and nociception: Implications for the drug treatment of pain. CNS Drugs 2001;15:29–58.
24. Waxman SG: The molecular pathophysiology of pain: Abnormal expression of sodium channel genes and its contributions to hyperexcitability of primary sensory neurons. Pain 1999;(Suppl 6):S133–S140.

6 术后神经性疼痛的机制

RICHARD M. TALBOT · CONNAIL R. McCRORY

典型的神经性疼痛是由于神经系统任何部分包括外周神经、背根神经节（dorsal root ganglion，DRG）、背根或中枢神经系统（central nervous system，CNS）受到损伤所致的疼痛（图 6-1 和图 6-2）。鉴于所有的术后患者都会发生伤害性疼痛，即使是经历很小的外科手术后也不例外，神经性疼痛会被混杂在各种原因所致的综合性疼痛中，从而可能更难于诊断和治疗。神经性疼痛可能转变为慢性疼痛，因此诊治神经性疼痛具有特别重要的意义。目前研究重点在于手术后慢性疼痛的患病率。据估计，约 20% 的患者出现术后慢性疼痛[1]。术后急性疼痛控制差是术后慢性疼痛的最主要原因[2,3]。然而，目前并不明确术后神经性疼痛的患病率和最佳治疗方案。其中的原因很多，包括难以从已接受阿片类药物治疗的患者中采集详细病史；而且缺乏研究证实手术作为一种炎性反应的过程，可诱发神经性疼痛或加重术前已有神经性疼痛患者的疼痛程度。

本章探讨手术炎性反应与神经性疼痛之间的相互作用，讨论手术对已有神经性疼痛的影响，并提出诊断和治疗术后神经性疼痛的循证结论。

定义

国际疼痛研究协会（International Association for the Study of Pain, ISAP）已将神经性疼痛定义为"神经系统原发性损害或功能障碍启动或引起的疼痛"[4]。它是神经结构和（或）功能改变所致，涉及中枢或外周神经损害。

发病率

据估计美国有 800 万，英国有 50 万患者患有神经性疼痛[5]。目前尚无前瞻性资料明确术后单纯神经性疼痛的发病率。但是，有研究显示某些手术后常伴有神经性疼痛，如胸廓切开术和乳房切除术。

病因学

患者需手术治疗的创伤事件可能是神经损伤以及其后神经性疼痛的主要原因。旁注 6-1 列出了神经性疼痛综合征的病因。术后神经性疼痛可能由手术、麻醉或非手术性创伤引起。表中列出与神经性疼痛综合征发生相关的因素；这些因素可能会促使术后神经性疼痛的发生或（术前）已有的神经性疼痛加重。

机制

神经性疼痛是由外周或中枢神经系统的创伤或者病变所致。

疼痛发生的机制如下[6-11]（从图 6-3 到图 6-6）：
- 伤害感受
- 外周致敏
- 表型转换和异位兴奋性
- 中枢致敏

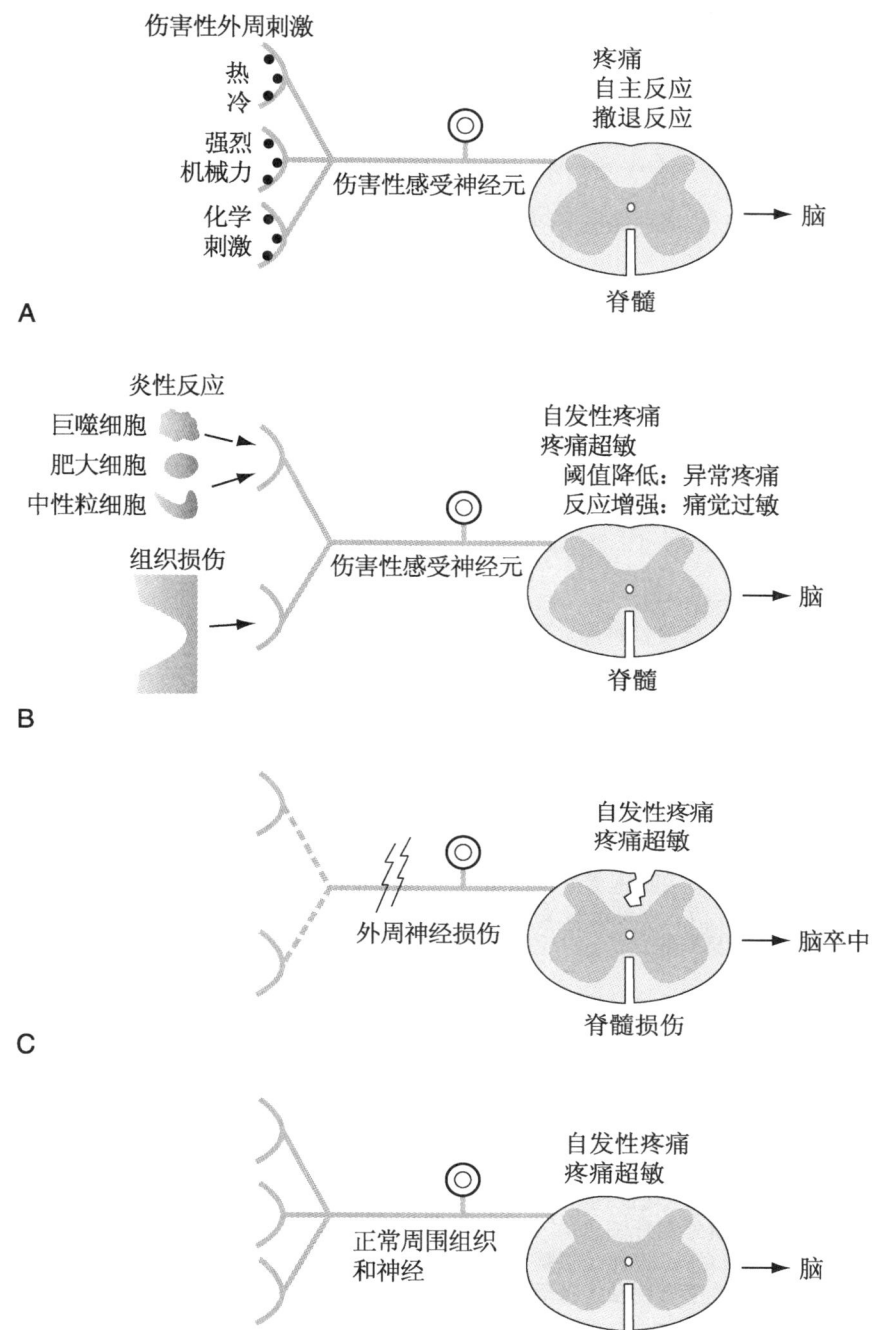

图 6-1 疼痛的 4 种主要类型。A. 伤害感受性疼痛；B. 炎症性疼痛；C. 神经性疼痛；D. 功能性疼痛。(Modified from Woolf CJ: Pain: Moving from symptom control toward mechanism-specific pharmacologic management. Ann Intern Med 2004;140:441-451.)

- 神经免疫系统的调理
- 易化增强
- 结构重组
- 抑制减弱（脱抑制）
- 神经损伤时其他蛋白的表达

任何一种疼痛状态的发生机制都是非特异的。所有的术后疼痛，包括术后神经性疼痛，都是由各种机制共同产生的（表 6-1）。

神经性疼痛的病因学、发生机制和临床特征之间的关系很复杂（图 6-3）。

神经损伤引起的外周神经性疼痛可表现为自发性疼痛（刺激非依赖性疼痛）或者对刺激产生超敏性疼

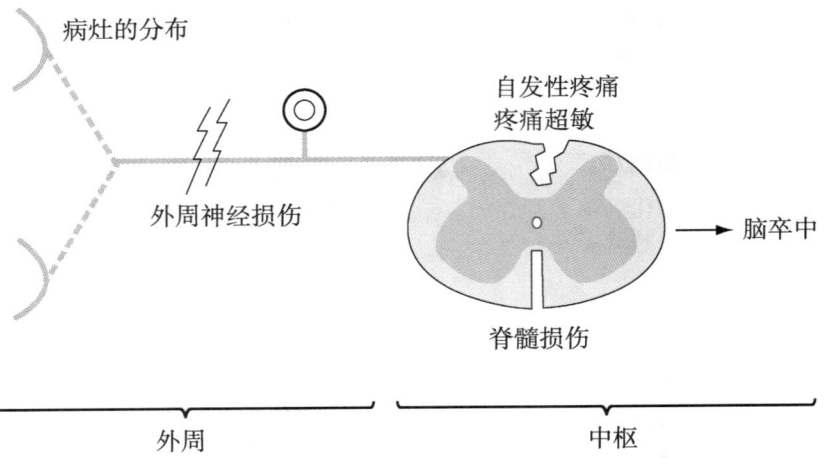

图 6-2 神经性疼痛损害的分布。(Modified from Woolf CJ: Pain: Moving from symptom control toward mechanism-specific pharmacologic management. Ann Intern Med 2004;140:441-451.)

痛（刺激诱发的疼痛）（图 6-4）[11]。

伤害性感受

伤害性感受是对有害性刺激的感觉，它是由于刺激激活伤感受器的外周末梢所致。所谓伤害性感受器是指"优先对伤害性刺激或者长时间存在会产生伤害的刺激敏感的受体"[4]。伤害性感受包括转导、传导和感知三部分。

传递离子的通道一般是钠通道或者非选择性阳离子通道。这些通道并非由电压门控，而是受温度、化学配体和机械力所控制。感觉神经元上表达的许多电压门控钠离子通道中只有两种与伤害性感受器有关，即$Na_v1.8$ 和 $Na_v1.9$[12,13]。

旁注 6-1　神经疼痛综合征的病因学

外周神经损伤
手术创伤
- 截肢术后
- 拉钩损伤
- 神经结扎
- 挤压或牵拉伤

麻醉创伤
- 导致直接和间接神经损伤的区域麻醉／镇痛技术并发症

非手术创伤
- 神经卡压
- 腕管综合征
- 跗管综合征
- 肘管综合征
- 桡骨综合征
- 感觉异常性股痛（股外侧皮神经）
- 胸廓出口综合征

代谢性疾病
- 糖尿病
- 甲状腺功能减退
- 尿毒症性神经病
- 淀粉样变性病
- 多发性骨髓瘤
- 卟啉病（遗传性与获得性）
- Wilson 病
- 血色素沉着症

缺血性损害
- 外周血管疾病
- 中枢神经系统梗死

营养性
- 脚气病（硫胺素缺乏）
- 酒精中毒（多种维生素缺乏）
- 糙皮病（烟酸缺乏）

血管受压
- 异常动脉环：在某些三叉神经痛呈现为神经慢性损伤

恶性肿瘤
- 直接肿瘤挤压
- 化疗药物毒性作用：顺铂、长春新碱、紫杉醇
- 放射治疗后纤维化：慢性神经压迫和缺血
- 相关的代谢紊乱
- 类肿瘤性效应：感觉运动神经病
  - 与癌肿相关（非特异性）
  - 与异常蛋白血症相关（如多发性骨髓瘤）
  - 亚急性感觉神经元病变（最常见小细胞瘤）

中毒性
- 异烟肼（维生素 B6 拮抗剂）
- 金
- 铊
- 砷
- 氰化物
- 铅

感染性
- 获得性免疫缺陷综合征
- 疱疹后神经痛
- 急性炎性多发性神经病（Guillain-Barré 综合征）
- Lyme 病

自身免疫性疾病
- 多发性动脉炎
- 系统性红斑狼疮

遗传性（罕见）
- Fabry 病

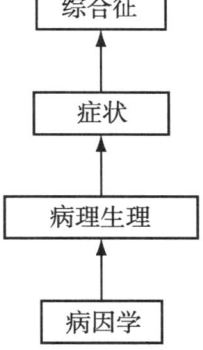

图 6-3　神经性疼痛的病因、发病机制和症状。(Modified from Woolf CJ, Mannion RJ: Neuropathic pain: Aetiology, symptoms, mechanisms and management. Lancet 1999;353:1959-1964.)

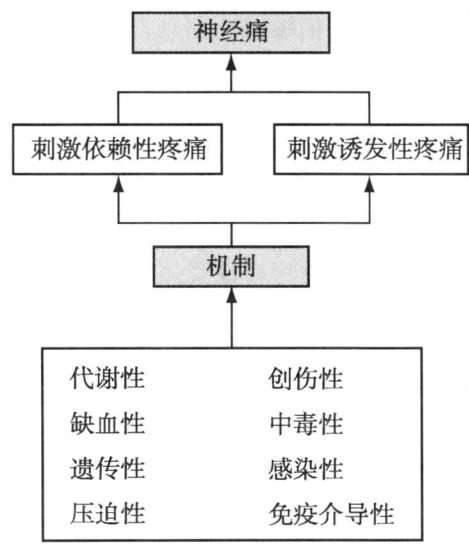

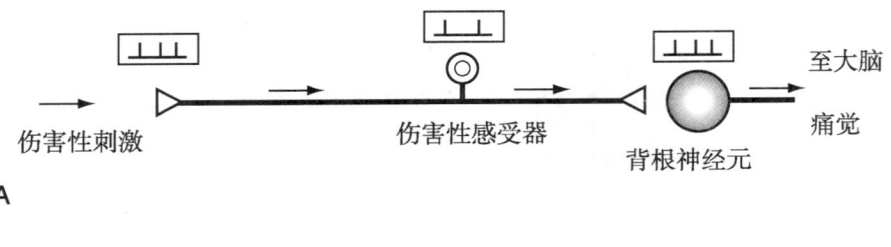
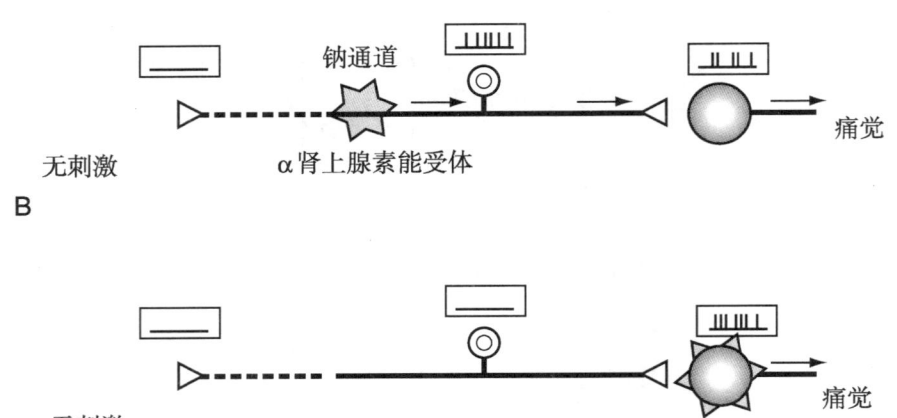

图 6-4 神经损伤后自发性疼痛的机制。A. 正常感觉功能；B. 神经损伤后沿轴突自发性放电的感觉功能；C. 神经损伤后脊髓背角神经元自发性放电的感觉功能。(Modified from Woolf CJ, Mannion RJ: Neuropathic pain: Aetiology, symptoms, mechanisms and management. Lancet 1999;353:1959-1964.)

外周致敏

不论是损伤后还是手术后的疼痛超敏基本均由中枢与外周致敏所致。

组织损伤和随后的炎症反应可导致细胞内容物如钾离子和 ATP 酶（adenosine triphosphatase，ATPase）释放到细胞外间隙，导致被募集来的炎性细胞生物合成各种细胞因子、化学因子和生长因子[14]。这些因子可激活或者使伤害感受器敏感。所谓外周致敏是指伤害感受器末梢敏感性和兴奋性的增强。外周致敏可导致局限于炎症区域的疼痛敏感性增强。

有关这些激活因子的一个例子就是 ATP 酶及其对配体门控的 P2X$_3$ 嘌呤伤害感受器受体的激活，该受体可检出组织损伤的快速型伤害感受器[15]。

致敏因子如前列腺素 E2 可与表达在伤害感受器末梢膜表面的特异性受体结合，并与细胞内激酶相偶联。前列腺素 E2 可激活腺苷酸环化酶（cAMP），使 cAMP 水平升高。后者可激活 cAMP 依赖性蛋白激酶 A。不论是由末梢内微粒体释放的钙，还是由膜通道进入的钙，都可以激活钙离子依赖性蛋白激酶 C[15]。细胞内激酶如蛋白激酶 A 和蛋白激酶 C，可使许多蛋白中的丝氨酸和苏氨酸残基磷酸化。磷酸化可改变蛋白质结构（翻译后的改变），从而改变受体与离子通道的活性及其激活阈值。例如，热敏感传感器瞬时受体电位 V1 通道（transient receptor potential V1 channel，TRPV1）磷酸化后，从 42℃降低到接近正常体温时，其激活阈值也降低[16]，从而使得被阳光灼伤患者在温水洗浴时也会出现灼伤痛。有一些受体是结构组成的，如缓激肽 B2 受体。它可以被缓激肽激活和敏化[17]。另外一些受体则是炎症或者损伤后诱发的，如缓激肽 B1 受体。

肿瘤坏死因子-α（tumor necrosis factor-α，TNF-α）和白介素-1β（interleukin-1，IL-1β）可以在炎症反应发生数小时内诱导出环氧合酶-2（COX-2）[18]。因此，非甾体类抗炎药（nonsteroidal anti-inflammatory drug，NSAID）或者 COX-2 选择性药物对慢性 COX-2 酶表达的情况具有快速镇痛作用，如类风湿性关节炎；但在急性情况下则无此作用，如伤害性疼痛和急性炎症反应性疼痛。可能同时存在一些敏感化因子（前列腺素 E2、神经生长因子和缓激肽），所以仅阻止一种因子的产生并不能排除外周致敏。这些过多的敏感化因子使 COX-2 抑制剂等镇痛药的作用受限。

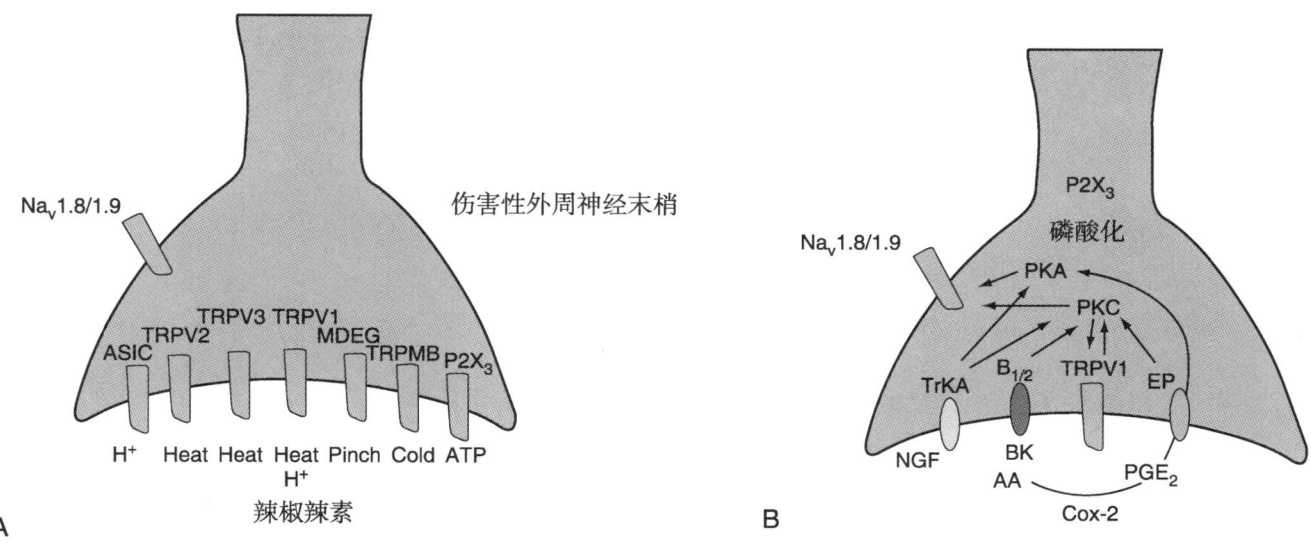
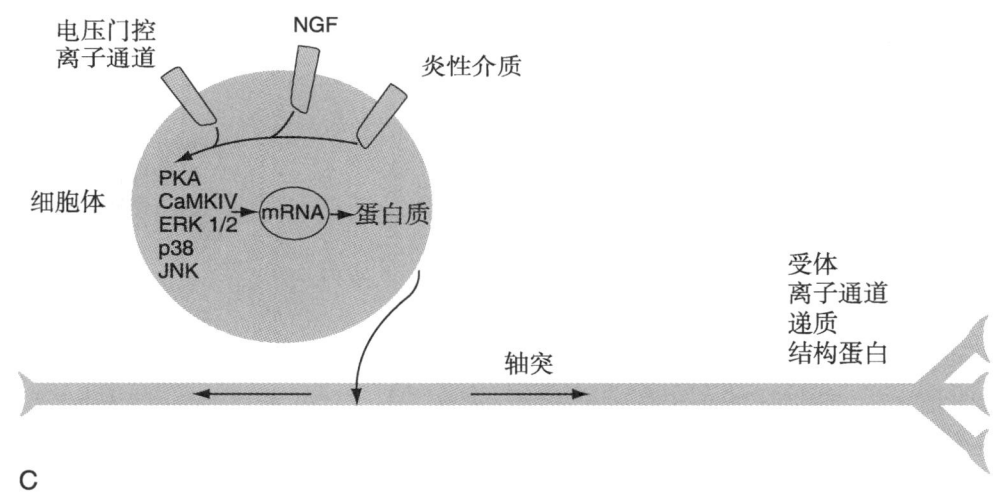

图6-5 初级感觉神经元在疼痛中的作用。A. 一个伤害性感受器神经元外周末梢。图中标出了对温度、机械力和化学刺激能产生反应的离子通道。感觉神经元的接受能力以转导离子通道来表达。B. 在组织损伤和炎症期间释放出炎症介质 PGE_2、缓激肽（BK）和神经生长因子（NGF）。这些介质可激活细胞内激酶，后者磷酸化转导离子通道，降低其阈值或者提高钠通道兴奋性。C. 炎症介质、活性物质和生长因子可激活感觉神经元胞内信号转导级联反应。调制基因表达的转录因子受这些级联反应的控制。这可导致基因表达水平的改变，引起受体、离子通道和其他功能蛋白水平的变化。基因表达的改变可引起蛋白质的变化，这可能导致神经元表型的改变。AA，花生四烯酸；ASIC，酸敏感性离子通道；ATP，三磷酸腺苷；$B_{1/2}$，缓激肽 B_1 和 B_2 受体；BK，缓激肽；CaMKⅣ，钙调激酶Ⅳ；COX-2，环氧合酶-2；DRG，背根神经节；EP，前列腺素 E 受体；ERK，胞外信号调节激酶；JNK，jun 激酶；MDEG，哺乳动物退化蛋白；mRNA，信使 RNA；$Na_V1.8/1.9$，电压门控的钠离子通道 1.8/1.9；NGF，神经生长因子；PKA，蛋白激酶 A；$P2X_3$，配体门控的 ATP 嘌呤伤害性受体；PKC，蛋白激酶 C；TRP，瞬时型感受器电压受体。（From Woolf CH: Pain: Moving from symptom control toward mechanism-specific pharmacologic management. Ann Intern Med 2004;140;441-451.）

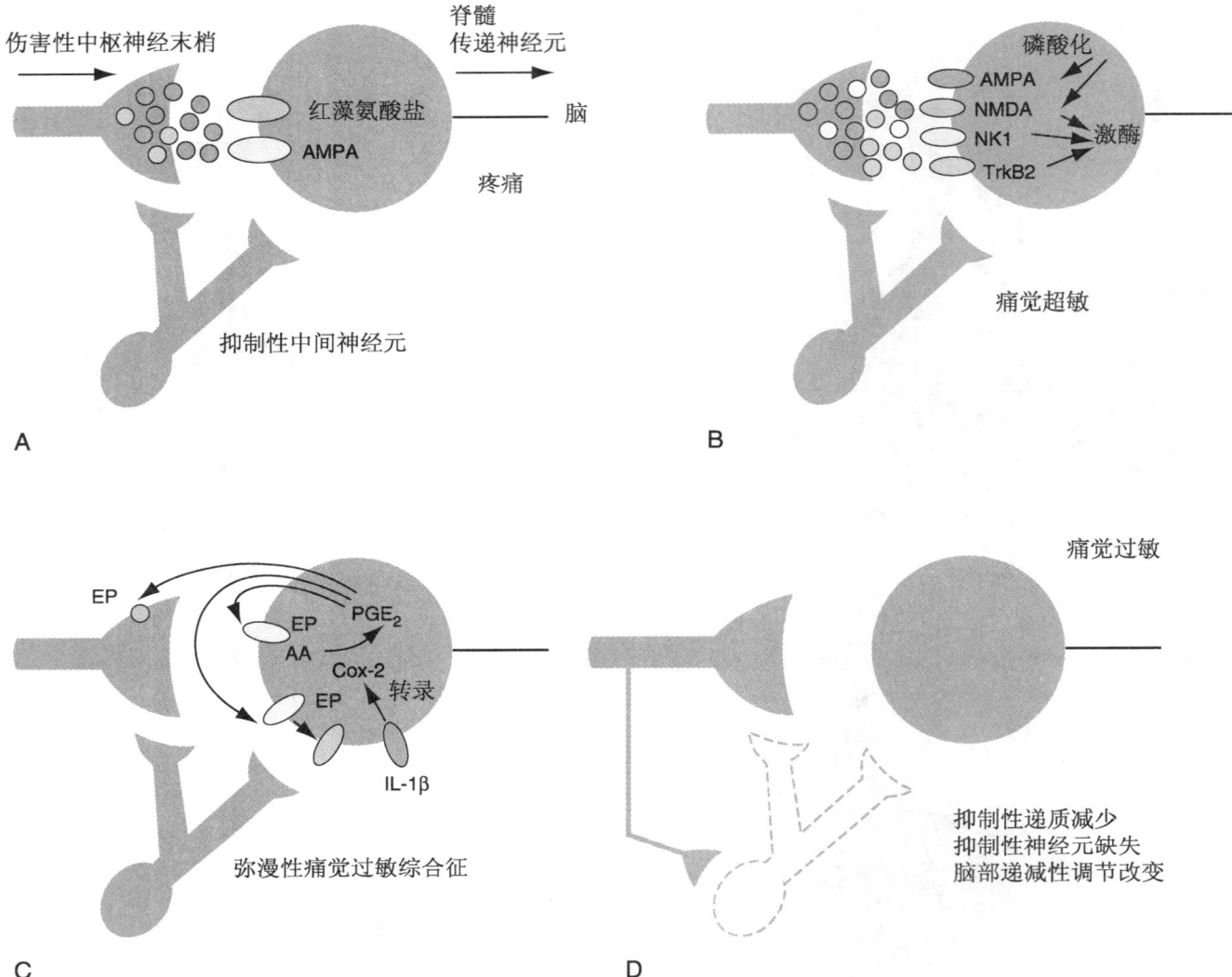

图6-6 脊髓背角神经元在疼痛中的作用。A．伤害性传递。B．中枢致敏的急性期。C．中枢致敏的后期。一些基因表达的改变被活化，并且局限于区域效应，如强啡肽；但其他一些基因表达的改变呈广泛性，并且导致全脑功能改变，如外周炎症后中枢神经元环氧合酶-2的诱导。D．脱抑制。AA，花生四烯酸；AMPA，α-氨基-3-羟基-5-甲基-4-异噁唑丙酸；EP，前列腺素E受体；IL-1β，白介素-1β；NK1，神经激肽-1；NMDA，N-甲基-D-天（门）冬氨酸；PGE_2，前列腺素 E_2；TrkB2，酪氨酸激酶B2。(From Woolf CH: Pain: Moving from symptom control toward mechanism-specific pharmacologic management. Ann Intern Med 2004;140;441-451.)

表6-1 与疼痛状态相关的疼痛机制

	伤害感受	外周敏感	表型改变	中枢敏感	异位兴奋	结构重组	抑制下降
伤害感受性疼痛	●	●		●			
炎症性疼痛		●		●			
神经性疼痛		●	●	●	●	●	●
功能性疼痛				●		●	

Adapted from text in Woolf CJ: Pain: Moving from symptom control toward mechanism-specific pharmacologic management. Ann Intern Med 2004;140: 441-451.

表型转换与异位兴奋性

外周神经损伤后，数百条基因上调或者下调[19,20]。最初，炎性介质、NGF和其他一些因子和配体可与受体和离子通道相结合，激活感觉神经元细胞内转导级联反应。这些转导级联反应控制着调制基因表达的转录因子。基因表达的改变可导致受体、离子通道和其他一些功能蛋白水平的变化，从而引起神经元兴奋性、转导和递质特性的改变，从而导致神经元表型的改变。

如在正常情况下，C类纤维表达神经调质脑源性神经营养因子和P物质。但在外周神经损伤后，A类纤维也开始表达同样的神经调质[21,22]。这提示A类纤维可能会诱发正常情况下只有C类纤维才有的中枢致敏[23]。

再举一个例子，外周炎性反应后，伤害感受器外周末梢中热敏感性TRPV1通道水平增加，从而增加外周的热敏感性[24]，改变突触调节因子、P物质和脑源性神经营养因子的水平[25]，放大向脊髓的中枢传入信号。这种修饰作用是炎症组织中NGF产生增加所致。这种外周NGF被转运到背根神经节感觉神经元的胞体上。在这里，它激活了细胞内信号途径。这些途径包括NGF诱导的p38丝裂原激活的蛋白激酶的激活，这可增加外周炎症反应后一级感觉神经元中TRPV1的表达和外周转运，从而可加剧热痛觉过敏[24]。

外周轴突损伤后，随着DRG上$\alpha_2\delta$钙通道亚基增加，μ阿片样受体数量下调，提示对吗啡敏感性显著下降，而对加巴喷丁敏感性增强[26]。神经损伤后，钾与钠离子通道的表达和分布发生改变，使膜兴奋性增加，引起自发性异位兴奋性。这是自发性神经性疼痛的主要促发因素[27]。

中枢致敏

中枢致敏是用于描述在脊髓背角躯体感觉神经元中建立的一种更强突触效应的术语。通常发生在外周强烈的伤害性刺激之后，如手术切口；但是，炎症期间伤害感受器敏感化或神经损伤后感觉神经元产生的自发性异位活性也可能诱发中枢致敏。早在20年前就有人提出中枢致敏的概念[28,29]。中枢致敏在急性术后疼痛、创伤后疼痛以及神经性疼痛发展过程中起主要作用[11,30-34]。

中枢致敏存在两种形式[34]。第一种（急性期）为活性依赖性形式，其响应伤害感受器的传入活性，这种传入活性可通过磷酸化和电压变化来调节突触传递；或者响应配体门控离子通道受体；这种中枢致敏可在数秒钟内被诱发，并持续数分钟。第二种（晚期）为转录依赖形式，它需数小时才能被诱导出来[9,35]，并且持续时间长于初始刺激时间。其中枢致敏的机制类似于外周致敏，包括细胞内激酶的激活、蛋白的磷酸化以及基因诱导。

伤害感受器中枢末梢释放的递质可引起脊髓背角活性增强，导致受体特性改变（密度、阈值、动力学、分布和活性）。这是中枢致敏的早期活性依赖形式。在活性依赖的中枢致敏中发挥主要作用的是谷氨酸激活的N-甲基-D-门冬氨酸（N-methyl-d-aspartate，NMDA）受体[36]。中枢致敏期间NMDA受体的磷酸化可增加其从细胞内库存中向突触膜的分布。去除具有阻滞NMDA通道作用的Mg^{2+}以及通道开放时间较长可引起该受体对谷氨酸的反应增强，兴奋性升高[9,37]。这种兴奋性升高提示原阈值下水平时即可激活（异常性疼痛）、正常刺激水平时反应加剧（痛觉过敏）以及可能传播至非损伤区域（次级痛觉过敏）。

现已证实，竞争性NMDA受体拮抗剂氯胺酮可减轻中枢致敏早期相以及随后的疼痛超敏[31,36]，并且在慢性神经性疼痛治疗中起到一定作用[38]。寻找其他NMDA受体拮抗剂的努力也取得了一些效果。例如抗病毒和抗帕金森病药物金刚烷胺可作为一种非竞争性NMDA受体拮抗剂，减轻癌症患者手术性和神经性疼痛[39]。NMDA受体广泛分布于整个神经系统中，而且治疗指数低下，所以限制了这类药物的临床应用。

中枢致敏晚期形式，即转录依赖性形式，与转录因子激活以及转录和基因表达变化有关。突触介导的细胞内转导途径的激活或体液信号可能引发这种形式的中枢致敏。基因表达的早期变化局限于接受受损组织传入的神经系统部分。例如，内源性阿片肽强啡肽受到分裂素激活的蛋白激酶（mitogen-activated protein kinases，MAPK）的调节[40]。而MAPK为基因的体液型激活，具有更广泛的作用。

晚期形式的重要例子是外周局部组织损伤后数小时在中枢神经系统许多区域都有COX-2的表达。炎性细胞释放入循环的体液细胞因子可刺激脑血管内皮细胞产生IL-1β，IL-1β进入脑脊液并与神经元表达的IL-1β受体结合，最终产生COX-2[41]。随后产生的前列腺素 E2 具有突触前与突触后效应，从而发挥多种广泛的作用。

这些研究结果的临床意义在于，不论是外周诱导还是中枢诱导的 COX-2，都可作为治疗疼痛的靶点。除了通过区域麻醉/镇痛技术来减少感觉向中枢神经系统的传入外，还须用选择性 COX-2 抑制剂来抑制体液介导的中枢 COX-2 的生成[6]。

神经免疫系统的调理

越来越多的证据表明免疫系统在神经病和神经性疼痛中发挥一定的作用[42]。据估计，临床 50% 的神经性疼痛患者与外周神经的感染或炎症有关，而与神经创伤无关[43]。有人综述了免疫系统在疼痛中的作用[44]，总结如下：

- 疼痛性神经病变与神经创伤和炎症有关
- 抗体对外周神经的攻击可引起疼痛性神经病变
- 对外周血管的免疫攻击可引起疼痛性神经病变
- DRG 和背根上的免疫作用可引起疼痛

创伤和炎性神经性疼痛动物模型的研究表明，在外周神经水平起关键作用的免疫细胞是从体循环募集到受累区域的中性粒细胞和巨噬细胞，以及诸多的局部细胞。正常情况下外周神经内可见成纤维细胞、内皮细胞、Schwann 细胞、肥大细胞、巨噬细胞和树突细胞[45]。释放的促炎性细胞因子 NO 和活性氧簇可杀死入侵的病原体，但是也直接提高神经兴奋性，破坏髓鞘，改变血-神经屏障[46]。免疫反应不会局限于外周，在脊髓也发生免疫反应，表现为胶质细胞的激活[47]。

抗体介导的对神经的攻击包括两种完全不同的类型。第一种，抗体攻击神经细胞膜，改变离子通道的功能；第二种，IgM、IgG1 和 IgG3 抗体激活补体级联反应。补体级联反应的激活可导致血-神经屏障的破坏，巨噬细胞和中性粒细胞募集进入神经，Schwann 细胞功能遭破坏，膜攻击复合体形成并对神经产生损伤，促进抗体结合位点的巨噬细胞破坏[48]。一般认为这些抗体具有"分子拟态"能力，因为产生的抗体能识别病毒、细胞和肿瘤细胞外表面的片段（"抗原决定簇"），但是也可能攻击正常神经表面与这些抗原形状类似的区域[49]。原发性或医源性神经创伤都可使外周神经的蛋白暴露出来[50]，也可能产生这些抗体。最后，抗体也有可能直接针对已侵入神经的病原体。至少

70% 的吉兰-巴雷综合征患者有神经性疼痛[51,52]。

对外周血管的免疫攻击引起的疼痛性神经病变称为血管性神经病变[53]。通常情况下对血管的攻击呈全身弥漫性。一般认为，血管损伤、血管内凝血和坏死引起的缺血可引起这种病变[54]。

DRG 的感觉神经元胞体周围有许多免疫细胞，而这些神经元能释放出兴奋性氨基酸和 L-精氨酸，后者是神经元 NO 合成的底物。此外，外周神经损伤可激活卫星细胞，使其在 DRG 神经元周围释放出促炎细胞因子和各种生长因子[42]。免疫源性物质如促炎性细胞因子可能通过激活受体引起疼痛，也有可能通过直接作用兴奋感觉神经纤维和脊髓神经根[55]。

术后应激反应与神经免疫调理之间可能存在联系。

易化增强

大脑对脊髓感觉过程的下行性抑制与易化作用尚不明了。长期以来，人们都认为炎症和外周神经损伤后可激活或者增强易化控制作用[56]。动物实验的研究表明了易被 5-HT$_3$ 拮抗剂（如昂丹司琼）所阻滞的延髓脊髓下行易化通道的存在，并且证实拮抗 5-HT$_3$ 受体可减轻伤害性感受引起的行为与电活动指标[57,58]。已有报道对神经性疼痛患者和纤维肌痛患者使用 5-HT$_3$ 受体拮抗剂后具有镇痛效果[59-62]。

结构重组

来自外周的感受伤害性传入纤维以高度有序的方式终止于背角。动物实验证明，外周损伤后在脊髓背角中枢低阈值传入末梢萌生至正常由伤害性感受器末梢占据的区域[63]。如果在人类也能证实存在这种结构重组现象，那将有助于解释一些非反应性神经性疼痛情况。

抑制减弱（脱抑制）

突触前与突触后抑制共同将到来的感觉传入精细地调节到一个有限而短暂的恰当反应水平。脊髓抑制性神经元可释放抑制性神经递质甘氨酸和 γ-氨基丁酸（gamma-aminobutyric acid，GABA）。研究显示，外周神经损伤可导致 GABA 能抑制作用选择性缺失[64]，而给予 GABA 受体激动剂可减轻神经性疼痛[65]。因此推

测抑制减弱（脱抑制）可促进神经性疼痛患者疼痛超敏反应的发生。

神经损伤时其他蛋白的表达

磷脂酰肌醇蛋白聚糖-1（glypican-1）是广泛表达于发育期与成熟期神经系统以及培养的 Schwann 细胞中的一种蛋白。磷脂酰肌醇蛋白聚糖-1 可以作为许多配体的共受体，包括裂缝轴突向导蛋白。Bloechlinger 等的一项研究表明，在 DRG 神经元中含蛋白多糖的磷脂酰肌醇蛋白聚糖-1 表达以生长依赖性方式与损伤诱导方式被调节[66]；外周损伤时这种变化持续 1 个月以上，而中枢切断后持续的时间较短。成熟 DRG 中裂缝-1、robo 2 和磷脂酰肌醇蛋白聚糖-1 的存在表明这些分子能组成一种功能性复合物。当磷脂酰肌醇蛋白-1 出现在细胞表面时，该复合物可能调节成熟神经系统轴突的生长。一般认为，robo 蛋白可以形成一种受体复合体，使神经元对裂缝蛋白的活动、导向轴突的生长与定向产生反应。

小结

随着更多蛋白质的发现以及对各种不同炎症级联反应、免疫过程和基因表达之间复杂相互作用的更多了解，人们正逐步深入地认识疼痛的发生机制。蛋白质的表达、分布和修饰既可同时，也可先后发生，这就是理解并成功治疗各种临床疼痛情况的困难所在。

麻醉医师的作用

麻醉医师在神经性疼痛治疗中的作用包括以下几个步骤：
- 识别患者可能的风险；
- 评估患者术前疼痛；
- 实施预先干预策略；
- 做出诊断。

诊断

通过以下方法可能为神经性疼痛做出诊断：
- 病史和体格检查
- 临床诊断

尽管一些辅助检查可能有助于诊断，但对于神经性疼痛并无特异性检查结果。

病史

病史应该反映患者自发性疼痛、刀刺样疼痛或烧灼样疼痛以及诱发性疼痛方面的信息（图 6-3）。

以下是神经性疼痛的症状[4]：
- 感觉迟钝：一种不愉快的异常感觉，呈自发性或诱发性。
- 异常性疼痛：由一种正常情况下不会诱发疼痛的刺激而引发的疼痛。
- 痛觉减退：对有害刺激的敏感性降低。
- 痛觉增敏：对正常的疼痛刺激反应性增强。
- 感觉减退：对刺激的敏感性降低，除外特异感觉。
- 感觉过敏：对刺激的敏感性增强，除外特异感觉。
- 痛觉过敏：以对刺激的反应增强为特征的一种痛觉综合征，特别是反复刺激以及阈值升高。

体格检查

可能也有局部神经缺陷：无力或局部自主神经改变（出汗、血管舒缩功能不稳）以及营养性变化（皮肤、皮下组织或毛发和指甲）。

有时应用的辅助检查包括电诊断研究（肌电图和神经传导速率有助于确定神经系统损伤的存在）和热像图（偶尔用于确定自主神经功能障碍）。在评价复杂性区域疼痛综合征（complex regional pain syndrome，CRPS）或者交感介导性疼痛的可能病例时，人们一直主张观察静息或诱发性催汗不对称性[定量催汗轴突反射（quantitative sudomotor axon reflex，QSART)]、对全身滴注 α-肾上腺素拮抗剂的反应、止血带缺血试验、激光多普勒表皮血流测定以及经皮氧分压差测定。

不论这些试验多么有意义，但作为一个临床诊断，最主要的是对所有试验结果做出仔细的解释，以避免盲从试验结果和误诊。磁共振成像与神经传导研究相结合能够辨别损害的特殊位置，这可能揭示手术中神经损伤的原因。

预防措施

麻醉医师在预防神经性疼痛中的作用包括以下几点：

1. 风险评估（旁注 6-2 和表 6-2）。

2. 最优化地治疗糖尿病[67]、甲状腺疾病、维生素缺乏和其他可能易发生神经功能障碍和神经病变的疾病。
3. 避免医源性神经损伤。

下面列出了围手术期神经损伤的机制，它们可能单独发生或数种机制联合发生[68,69]：

- 针、缝线、器械造成的直接创伤和神经内注射。
- 注射神经毒性物质或者局部麻醉药的直接神经毒性作用，后者呈浓度和剂量依赖性。
- 由于手术操作和围手术期体位所致的机械性牵拉和压迫，或血肿压迫。血肿可由先天性以及更特殊地由于获得性凝血异常所致（如给予抗凝药和预防深静脉血栓形成的药物）。
- 由于压迫或者长时间严重低血压影响血供而导致的缺血。

穿行距离长的神经易受牵拉性损伤，经过或者邻近骨性突起的神经易受压迫性损伤。美国麻醉医师学会（American Society of Anesthesiologists，ASA）索赔终审项目（www.asaclosedclaims.org）是一个鉴别有关麻醉失误、损伤模式和预防措施方面最终医疗事故判决而进行的深入调查项目。"失误"指导致医疗事故索赔的所有情况，而不仅是感觉丧失。该项目研究的 4 183 例有 16% 为麻醉相关性神经损伤。这些投诉发生率从高至低依次为：尺神经（28%）、臂丛（20%）、腰骶神经根（16%）和脊髓（13%）[70]。全身麻醉、中枢神经系统阻滞以及区域麻醉/镇痛均可能导致神经损伤[71,72]。

神经损伤存在以下 3 种类型：

- 神经失用性损伤发生于鞘膜受损而轴突完好时，这可导致神经功能丧失，是麻醉中最常见的类型。尽管恢复需要数周到数月，但预后良好。
- 轴突断裂伤发生于轴突断裂而神经鞘膜完好。随着轴突以每日 1 mm 的速度再生，其功能可能逐渐恢复。
- 神经断裂伤发生于神经完全离断时，此时轴突、鞘膜和结缔组织均断裂。这种神经损伤通常不会恢复，患者可能出现慢性神经性疼痛。

症状在 1 天内出现，但也可能 2~3 周都不会出现。损伤的严重性决定了症状的程度和持续时间[69]。

预防措施包括尽可能在患者清醒时实施区域麻醉/镇痛技术，使用神经刺激器而不是引出异感，以更好地了解解剖结构。最重要的预防措施是确保患者处于适当的体位，以避免神经和神经丛的牵拉和压迫。

公认的术后神经性疼痛状况

开胸术后疼痛

开胸术后疼痛综合征的发生率约为 50%[73]。综述 6 项研究共 878 例患者的报道表明，47% 的患者有开

旁注 6-2	发生术后神经性疼痛的特殊原因

术前神经性疼痛
老年人
女性
工作状态（从业者与失业者比较）
糖尿病
酗酒
尿毒症
获得性免疫缺陷综合征或者其他免疫功能低下
恶性肿瘤，如骨肉瘤
新辅助化疗/放疗
纤维肌痛
创伤
药物或毒物：疼痛性多发性神经病（异烟肼、金、醚醇硝唑、呋喃妥因、长春新碱、顺铂、紫杉醇、砷、氰化物、铊）
营养性特异性维生素缺乏（如烟酸、B_{12}、B_6）
抑郁症

表 6.2	慢性疼痛的预测因子
术前因素	疼痛，中度到重度，持续超过 1 个月
	反复手术
	心理易感性
	工人的赔偿金
术中因素	有神经损伤风险的手术径路
术后因素	疼痛（急性，中度到重度）
	放疗区域
	神经毒性化疗
	抑郁症
	心理易感性
	神经过敏症
	焦虑症

Adapted from Perkins FM, Kehlet H: Chronic pain as an outcome of surgery: A review of predictive factors. Anesthesiology 2000;93: 1123-1133.

胸术后疼痛综合征[3]。其病因可能取决于神经损伤，后者表现为胸壁切开术后疼痛程度增加[74]，并且与腹壁浅反射丧失相关的开胸术后疼痛综合征发生率较高[75,76]。肿瘤复发可能对上述数据分布的差异起一定作用[74]。两项研究表明，前路开胸手术患者肋间神经功能障碍和开胸术后疼痛综合征的发生率低于后外侧路开胸术；然而，这两项研究的样本量小，并且没有把慢性术后疼痛作为一个主要观察指标[76,77]。尽管术后疼痛强度已被认为是开胸术后疼痛综合征的一项预测指标，但其他一些研究已经注意到术前疼痛，而并没有把这种术前疼痛作为一项独立的危险因素[78]。

2004年的一篇综述报道可视胸腔镜手术（video-assisted thoracic surgery，VATS）具有更好的疗效，并且并发症相当于治疗气胸的开胸术和微创手术[79]。这种治疗方法还有住院时间更短以及镇痛药用量更少的优点。

与单独术后硬膜外镇痛相比，联合术中与术后硬膜外镇痛可将6个月时疼痛的发生率从67%降到33%[80]。

乳房切除术后痛

乳房切除术后疼痛是指妇女在乳房肿块切除术或者乳房切除术后的一种慢性神经性疼痛综合征。乳腺癌手术后1年疼痛发生率约50%。27%的乳腺癌幸存者有慢性术后乳房疼痛[81]。乳房手术后的妇女可能有胸壁痛、乳房痛或瘢痕痛（11%~57%）、乳房幻觉痛（13%~24%）以及手臂或肩痛（12%~51%）[3]。术后神经性疼痛可能在瘢痕周围，并可能放射到腋窝。

一项前瞻性研究并没有发现术前乳房疼痛是一项预测因子，这与以往研究结果不同[82-84]；术前焦虑和抑郁更为常见，尽管没有统计学意义[83]。手术类型与范围可能影响疼痛的发生率。例如，腋窝切除的范围与手臂疼痛的发生率和症状相关[85,86]，乳房切除加假体植入术术后疼痛的发生率（53%）高于单纯乳房切除术（31%）[87]。

已证实急性术后疼痛的程度和所需镇痛药物的剂量是预测持续性乳房疼痛和同侧手臂疼痛的最佳指标。此外，术后辅助性放疗和化疗是乳房和手臂慢性神经性疼痛的危险因素[88,89]。

乳房手术后大多数疼痛是由于神经损伤所致[89-92]。据报道，48%~84%腋窝切除术妇女出现肋间臂丛神经分布区域感觉改变；感觉变化的妇女中有25%~50%有肋间臂神经痛[93,94]。

腹股沟疝修补术后疼痛

腹股沟疝修补术后慢性疼痛的发病率在0%~37%，总体发生率为11.5%[3]。一项研究证实，开放性腹股沟疝修补术后患者有30%出现慢性疼痛（疼痛持续时间超过3个月）[95]。其中46%为神经性疼痛。研究认为与慢性疼痛相关的危险因素包括年轻、门诊手术、存在术前疼痛以及复发性疝手术。

术后1周和4周时腹股沟疝术后疼痛的程度可预测1年时的疼痛[96]。推测神经损伤是这种术后神经性疼痛综合征的主要因素[97-99]。

至今尚无确凿证据证实，麻醉或手术疝修补技术在腹股沟疝修复术后神经性疼痛中起到任何重要作用[100]。

幻觉痛和残肢痛

幻觉痛的经典描述是指发生在肢体截断术后的幻肢痛，但是幻觉痛一词是指身体任何部分截去后出现的疼痛；这种疼痛在乳房切除术后和拔牙后都会出现。通常认为幻觉痛是一种去传入性疼痛。去传入性疼痛定义为"由于传入到中枢神经系统的感觉丧失而产生的疼痛，可见于臂丛神经撕脱或者其他外周神经损伤时，或者由于中枢神经系统病变所致"[4]。人们一直认为中枢致敏是去传入性疼痛的主要病理生理机制。据报道幻肢痛的发病率为30%~81%；66%的幻觉痛患者有残肢痛，而无幻觉痛患者中有50%有残肢痛，这提示残肢痛的发病率超过60%[3]。

并非所有的流行病学调查都能够将幻觉痛从非疼痛性幻觉和残肢痛中区别出来。幻觉包括外感受性感觉（触觉、温觉、压力感觉、瘙痒和疼痛）、本体感觉（位置感觉、长度与体积感觉）和运动感觉（主动性与自发性运动感觉）。尽管症状可能发生在去神经支配后的任何时间，但幻觉痛和幻觉一般在神经损伤后很快出现。幻肢痛疼痛发作的发生率和发生频率在截肢术后第1年内呈逐渐降低趋势[101,102]，但约50%的长期幻觉痛患者并不出现疼痛强度减弱[103]。

已有文献表明幻觉痛的先兆有截肢术前痛和持续残肢痛（急性和慢性）[103-105]，非疼痛性幻觉与幻觉痛之间存在相关性。化疗与幻觉痛的发生率较高有关[105]。传统认为幻觉痛的预测因子包括高龄、近端截肢术、上肢损伤、急性截肢和原有精神异常；然而近期研究并没有证实这些因素为预测因子[106]。一篇关于幻肢痛的综述列举了在幻肢痛的发生过程中可能起一定作用的其他内源性和外源性因素（表6-3）[107]。

残肢痛最有可能与损伤神经末端神经瘤的形成有关，因此一般被认为是一种外周神经性疼痛。其典型发作延迟数月出现，并且其发病率低于幻觉痛。值得注意的是，许多截肢术后患者同时存在残肢痛与幻觉痛。

少数研究关注围手术期硬膜外持续给药与残肢痛和幻觉痛的发生率。研究证实，术前开始硬膜外镇痛（联合布比卡因、可乐定和二乙酰吗啡）可有效地减少截肢术后的幻觉痛[108]；然而，随后的一项研究并没有证实该结论[109]。这两项研究的样本量都较小。

也有人研究了神经鞘膜内滴注局麻药，以确定持续性滴注盐酸布比卡因是否可减少截肢术后缓解疼痛所需的麻醉药用量，以及是否可影响幻觉痛的发病率。一项研究证实了这种方法有效[110]，但另一项研究显示该方法并不能防止下肢截肢术后患者残肢或幻肢痛[111]。一项研究探讨了手术前通过硬膜外留置导管滴注局麻药进行围手术期硬膜外阻滞（开始于截肢术前24 h）的效果，并与硬膜外麻醉相比较，结果表明前者预防幻觉痛方面并无优势，但可更好地缓解手术后早期残肢痛[112]。这些研究的样本量也很小。

表6-3	可能调制幻觉痛体验的因素
内部因素	遗传倾向
	焦虑/情绪应激
	注意/精神涣散
	排尿/排便
	其他疾病（脑出血，椎间盘脱出）
外部因素	天气改变
	残肢接触
	假体的使用
	脊髓麻醉
	机能恢复
	治疗

Adapted from Nikolajsen L, Jensen TS: Phantom limb pain. Br J Anaesth 2001;87:107-116.

胆囊切除术后痛

胆囊切除术后常见慢性腹痛（3%～56%），即所谓的胆囊切除术后综合征[3]。除腹痛外，还有许多其他表现，可能存在多种原因。原因包括术后腹壁切口痛、Oddi括约肌功能障碍引起的疼痛、胆管结石引起的疼痛、除了胆结石外术前未能诊断出来的疾病引起的疼痛，以及其他术前因素，如心理脆弱、女性、术前长期忍受症状[113-118]。值得注意的是，有典型胆石病症状的病史与慢性疼痛危险性降低相关[119-121]。腹腔镜胆囊切除术与开腹式胆囊切除术后腹痛的远期结局方面似乎并无差异[122,123]。

目前认识到腹腔镜胆囊切除术后入口位点疼痛可能严重。一项前瞻性随机研究比较了双入口与四入口腹腔镜胆囊切除术在总体疼痛评分、镇痛需求、住院时间以及患者对手术和瘢痕方面满意评分。结果显示，双入口腹腔镜胆囊切除术造成的入口位点疼痛较少，但是其他方面的结果相近[124]。

胆囊切除术后综合征的前瞻性研究并没有将神经性疼痛和瘢痕疼痛区别于其他原因导致的慢性内脏痛和症状。

术后复杂性区域疼痛综合征

复杂性区域疼痛综合征（complex regional pain syndrome, CRPS）是用于描述损伤后疼痛和血管舒缩不稳定的一种综合征，典型的以外周初始伤害性事件开始，它并不局限于单支神经分布上，并且与初始事件不成比例[125,126]。它可分为两种类型（旁注6-3和表6-4）。

CRPS Ⅰ型或Ⅱ型患者根据其对交感阻滞或干涉的反应[127]，可以具有交感依赖性疼痛或者非交感依赖性疼痛。患者可能具有其中一类表现，或者常见同时具有两类表现[128]。

CRPS并非一种罕见的术后并发症。其发病率因手术类型与部位、环境以及患者评估时期而异。人们已经注意到CRPS的发病率在术后前3个月内下降，在6个月时稳定[129]。对140例CRPS患者的回顾性研究表明有16.4%是由手术所致[130]。大多数CRPS病例发生在矫形外科手术后，提示两者间存在因果关系，因为既往已有研究报道所有创伤病例中有5%患者出现CRPS[131]。

旁注 6-3	复杂性区域疼痛综合征（Complex Regional Pain Syndrome，CRPSs）Ⅰ型与Ⅱ型

Ⅰ型 CRPS（以前称为交感反射性营养不良）是由一个初始的有害事件所致。

Ⅱ型 CRPS（以前称为灼痛）是由神经损伤所致。

Ⅰ型与Ⅱ型均具有如下特征：

- 发生自发性疼痛或者异常性疼痛/痛觉过敏，并且不限于单支外周神经分布的区域（并且对于 CRPS Ⅰ型，其疼痛的程度与诱发事件不成比例）。
- 自诱发事件以来，疼痛区域存在或者一直在水肿、皮肤血流异常或异常出汗增多等现象。
- 因为存在解释该疼痛或者功能障碍程度的疾病而排除 CRPS 的诊断。

表 6-4　复杂性区域疼痛综合征（CRPS）与矫形外科手术操作

矫形外科手术操作	CRPS 估计发生率（%）
膝关节镜手术	2.3～4
腕管手术	2.1～5
踝部手术	13.6
全膝关节成形术	0.8～13
腕骨骨折	7～37
Dupuytren 挛缩而行筋膜切除术	4.5～40

Data from Reuben SS: Preventing the development of complex regional pain syndrome after surgery. Anesthesiology. 2004;101:1215-1224.

一篇关于防止 CRPS 发生的综述显示，干预 CRPS 的措施包括手术时机、区域麻醉技术、超前多模式镇痛和药理学疗法[132]。

手术时机

由于缺少循证医学研究，对有 CRPS 病史的患者最佳手术时机尚不明了。一种观点认为，CPRS 发病期进行手术可能导致患者 CRPS 病情加重[133,134]。因此，如果可能的话，手术应该推迟到 CRPS 症状得到很好控制之后[135]。

研究已证实，术前疼痛是各种手术后慢性疼痛的一项先兆[3]。因此，将评价术前疼痛程度作为术后可能严重疼痛的一个标志将很有价值[129]。

区域麻醉技术

已有个案报道，以往有 CRPS 病史的患者接受手术实施全身麻醉后可复发 CRPS，而实施区域麻醉后则不会复发[136,137]。一项前瞻性研究观察了 17 例既往行下肢截除术患者接受 23 次脊髓麻醉的影响，结果只有 1 例患者出现了临床明显的幻肢痛，持续仅数分钟[138]。已报道可能降低术后 CRPS 发病率的技术有星状神经节阻滞、区域静脉内麻醉和硬膜外麻醉。

星状神经节阻滞　并非所有上肢区域麻醉技术都可导致交感神经阻滞。一项回顾性研究证实，围术期星状神经节阻滞可降低 CRPS 的发生[139]。但是，至今尚无研究证实这种降低见于无 CRPS 病史的患者。

区域静脉内麻醉　与星状神经节阻滞相比，区域静脉内麻醉技术要求较低，并发症发生率也较低。前瞻性随机对照临床研究中用于检查交感反射性神经营养不良中疼痛缓解有效性的药物包括胍乙啶[140-144]、利血平[141,142]、氟哌利多[145]、阿托品[146]、溴苄铵[147]和酮色林[148]。这些临床研究的主要结果建议总结如下[143,149,150]：①确定区域静脉内麻醉时溴苄铵和酮色林的有效镇痛作用有限；②结果一致证实区域静脉内麻醉时胍乙啶和利血平并无镇痛效果；③证明区域静脉内麻醉中使用氟哌利多和阿托品无效的数据有限[132]。一项研究和一篇综述都主张使用静脉内利多卡因和 α_2-肾上腺素激动剂可乐定（1μg/kg）作为治疗急性术后痛和上肢 CRPS 症状的一种有效方法[151-153]。

硬膜外麻醉　病例报道推荐下肢远端 CRPS 患者手术时选择硬膜外麻醉作为麻醉方法[136,137,154]。由于缺乏前瞻性研究，因此并不明确最佳时机、治疗时程、安全性、有效性以及恰当的联合镇痛方法（可能时）。在这些药物治疗方案中，可乐定有可能起到关键性作用[155]。

超前多模式镇痛

CRPS 的可能病理生理机制提示外周伤害性感受可导致中枢致敏。镇痛技术的目标在于降低中枢致敏。这种伤害性传入不仅来自于切口（超前镇痛），也可来自于整个手术后时期（预防性镇痛）[156,157]。一般建议联合使用不同作用机制的镇痛药进行多模式镇痛[158]。研究已经证实这种方法有效[159-161]。

药理学疗法

围手术期可使用各种药物来降低术后 CRPS 的发病率。有假设认为，组织损伤时产生了过多的毒性氧自由基，使机体对组织损伤的炎症反应过强，从而诱发 CRPS。因此研究了自由基清除剂。已经研究了二甲基亚砜[162,163]、甘露醇[164]、N-乙酰半胱氨酸[163]、肉碱[165]和维生素 C[166,167]治疗 CRPS 的作用。迄今为止，只有维生素 C 通过前瞻性随机安慰剂对照双盲研究，以评价其作为一种自由基清除剂减少 CRPS 发病的有效性[166]。值得注意的是，该研究包括通过非手术保守治疗的腕部骨折患者；结果表明，维生素 C 可显著降低 1 年时 CRPS 的发病率。最近一项前瞻性非随机研究也证明维生素 C 用于手术治疗腕部骨折（患处钢针固定）的患者具有这种益处[167]。

其他经过研究的药物疗法有降钙素和酮色林疗法。降钙素是由甲状腺产生的一种多肽激素，可调节血钙浓度和骨钙代谢。随着在中枢神经系统降钙素结合位点的发现，有人就提出其抗伤害性感受的作用[168]。作用的可能机制包括钙离子流动、儿茶酚胺能和 5-羟色胺能机制、蛋白磷酸化、β-内啡肽产生、环氧合酶抑制和组胺干扰等[168,169]。随后的研究量化并证实了降钙素基因相关肽在 CRPS 患者中的重要作用[170]。还需要进行大样本随机前瞻性研究来确定围手术期使用降钙素降低高危矫形手术后 CRPS 发病率和复发率的有效性[132]。

酮色林是 5-羟色胺 II 型受体的拮抗剂，可能具有镇痛作用，因此对 CRPS 患者有利[143,148]。

术后神经性疼痛的治疗

一旦确诊术后神经性疼痛，就要采取与慢性神经性疼痛相同的治疗原则。表 6-5 列出所用的各种治疗方法，但神经性疼痛的最佳治疗方案尚未确定。抗癫痫药、三环类抗抑郁药和阿片类镇痛药是药理学治疗的基础。神经性疼痛治疗困难，有时对治疗或干预毫无反应。鉴于患者对药物的反应不同，药物使用的剂量和副作用也有所不同，本章列出的药物及其用药方案仅供指导（表 6-6 至表 6-8；旁注 6-4）。一些常用于治疗神经性疼痛的药物，其初期的作用并不是治疗神经性疼痛。用于治疗神经性疼痛的药物包括普瑞巴林、加巴喷丁和辣椒素。

抗癫痫药

抗癫痫药对神经性疼痛具有镇痛作用（见表 6-6）。这些药物的作用机制不同，因此用一种药物失败，并不能排除其他抗癫痫药可能有效。

普瑞巴林在结构上与加巴喷丁相关，但前者与 $\alpha_2\delta$ 亚基蛋白的亲和力远远大于后者。这种亚基蛋白与在神经性疼痛中起作用的电压门控钙通道有关[171,171]。普瑞巴林对这些钙通道具有调制作用，可减少神经递质释

表 6-5　神经性疼痛的治疗选择

治疗方案	举例
直接针对病因的手术治疗	外周神经解压术（如腕管松解） 神经根解压术（如椎间盘切除术）
全身性药物治疗	三环类抗抑郁药（如阿米替林） 抗癫痫药（如加巴喷丁、普瑞巴林） 抗交感药物（如胍乙啶、酚妥拉明） 阿片类药物（如羟考酮、吗啡） 钠通道阻断剂（如利多卡因、美西律） NMDA 拮抗剂（如氯胺酮）
区域药物治疗	表面用药（如辣椒素、利多卡因） 外周： 　传导阻滞 　类固醇注射 　交感神经切除术 椎管： 　传导阻滞 　类固醇注射 　交感阻滞 　阿片类药物
电刺激	经皮神经刺激 直接外周神经刺激 脊髓刺激 深部脑刺激
功能性治疗	理疗 职业疗法
行为修饰/心理疗法	生物反馈 松弛技术
毁坏神经系统技术	外周神经松解 外周神经切除 通过化学与手术方法实施神经根切除术 脊髓丘脑外侧束切断术 脑损伤立体定向治疗

Adapted from Panlilio LM, Tella P, Raja SN: Neuropathic pain: Outcome studies on the role of nerve blocks. In Prithvi RJ (ed): Textbook of Regional Anesthesia. Philadelphia, Churchill Livingstone 2002, p 972.

表6-6　用于治疗神经性疼痛的抗癫痫药

药物	静脉剂量	口服剂量	全身副作用	神经毒副作用	罕见副作用
卡马西平	不适用	从2~3mg/(kg·d)起，每5日增加1次剂量，直到10mg/(kg·d)；由于肝自身诱导作用，2~3月后可能需要进一步增加剂量到15~20mg/(kg·d)；最大用量1.6 g/d	恶心、呕吐、腹泻、低钠血症、皮疹、瘙痒	困倦、头晕、视力模糊或复视、嗜睡、头痛	粒细胞缺乏症、Stevens-Johnson综合征、再生障碍性贫血、肝衰竭、皮炎/皮疹、血清病、胰腺炎
加巴喷丁	不适用	第1日300 mg；第2日300 mg，每日2次；第3日300 mg，每日3次；必要时可增至1800 mg/d，分3次服用；建议肾功能不全患者使用较低剂量	未知	嗜睡、头晕、共济失调	未知
拉莫三嗪	不适用	对于使用酶诱导性抗癫痫药物的患者：25 mg，每日2次；必要时每1~2周增加5 mg，直到适当剂量。对于服用丙戊酸盐的患者：隔日服用25 mg；必要时每2周增加25~50mg，直到最大剂量300~500mg/d	皮疹、恶心	头昏、嗜睡	Stevens-Johnson综合征、超敏反应
奥卡西平	不适用	以300~600 mg/d，分2~3次服用开始，1周内每日可增加600 mg，直至总量达900~3000 mg/d，分2~3次服用。	恶心、皮疹、低钠血症	镇静、头痛、头晕、眩晕、共济失调、复视	未知
苯妥英	15mg/kg（不大于50mg/min）：剂量以苯妥英当量表示。癫痫持续状态：以100~150mg/min的速度给予15~20mg/kg。非急症负荷量：静脉注射或肌肉注射10~20mg/kg。维持剂量：每日4~6mg/kg	9~12 h以上分3次口服15 mg/kg；维持剂量5 mg/(kg·d)	牙龈肥大、体毛增加、皮疹、淋巴结病	谵妄、言语不清、复视、共济失调、神经病变（长期服用）	粒细胞缺乏症、再生障碍性贫血、Stevens-Johnson综合征、肝衰竭、皮炎/皮疹、血清病

药物	剂量			副作用		进一步说明
噻加宾	4 mg, 每日1次；对成年人, 1周内增加4~8 mg/d, 直到出现临床反应, 或达56 mg/d, 分次服用	不适用		头晕、无力、嗜睡、恶心、神经质、震颤、精神不集中、腹痛	未知	
托吡酯	50 mg/d, 应用1周；然后1周内以50 mg 的递增速度增加剂量, 直到有效剂量	不适用		疲劳、神经质、精神不集中、厌食、谵安、抑郁、语言障碍、焦虑、情绪异常、震颤	体重减轻、肾结石、感觉异常	急性近视和青光眼少汗与体温过高主要发生于儿童
丙戊酸盐	作为辅助治疗, 推荐每日总量 200 mg, 每日2次	15 mg/(kg·d), 分2~4次服用；必要时可每周以5~10 mg/(kg·d) 的速度增大剂量	以 20 mg/min 速度滴注60 min 以上, 必要时最大剂量可达 2500 mg/d, 分2~4次 快速滴注: 5~10 min 以上可滴注总量达 15mg/kg[1.5~3 mg/(kg·min)]	体重增加、恶心、呕吐、毛发脱落、易擦伤	震颤	粒细胞缺乏症、Stevens-Johnson综合征、再生障碍性贫血、肝炎、皮疹、血清病、胰腺炎

Modified from Bajwa ZH, Sami N, Ho CC: Antiepileptic drugs in the treatment of neuropathic pain. In UpToDate February 17, 2004. Available at www.uptodate.com/

表 6-7　用于治疗神经性疼痛的三环类抗抑郁药

药物	剂量	作用机制	副作用	进一步说明
阿米替林	10~150 mg/d	去甲肾上腺素和5-羟色胺重吸收抑制剂	抗胆碱能作用、镇静、直立性低血压	以下患者慎用：青光眼；服用单胺氧化酶抑制剂（MAOI）者（5-羟色胺综合征患者）；不能耐受抗胆碱能或镇静副作用者
去甲替林（阿米替林的活性代谢物）	25 mg, 3~4次/日 最大量：150 mg/d	去甲肾上腺素和5-羟色胺重吸收抑制剂	抗胆碱能作用、镇静、直立性低血压	副作用少于阿米替林；心血管疾病患者慎用
米帕明	25mg, 3次/日；可增至150 mg/d	去甲肾上腺素和5-羟色胺重吸收抑制剂	抗胆碱能作用、镇静、直立性低血压、震颤	以下患者慎用：青光眼；服用单胺氧化酶抑制剂（MAOI）者（5-羟色胺综合征患者）；不耐受抗胆碱能或镇静副作用者
地帕明（米帕明的活性代谢产物）	100~200 mg/d	去甲肾上腺素和5-羟色胺重吸收抑制剂	抗胆碱能作用、镇静、震颤	抗胆碱能副作用发生率最低的药物之一

From Namaka M, Gramlich CR, Ruhlen D, et al: A treatment algorithm for neuropathic pain. Clin Ther 2004;26:951-979.

6 术后神经性疼痛的机制

表6-8 用于治疗神经性疼痛的阿片类镇痛剂

药名	剂量	作用机制	副作用	进一步说明
吗啡	个体差异	μ阿片样受体激动剂	躯体依赖、呼吸抑制、恶心、呕吐、镇静	金标准
美沙酮	5~10 mg，每4~8 h；长期使用时，使用间隔时间不宜短于12 h	下行传导径路中的μ阿片样受体激动剂	同吗啡	可用于应用吗啡后疼痛加剧或兴奋的患者
曲马多	50~100 mg，必要时每4~6 h重复，口服或肌注，可缓慢滴注（2~3 min以上）	弱阿片样受体激动剂，去甲肾上腺素重吸收抑制剂，促进5-羟色胺释放	躯体依赖、胃痛、头晕、困倦、皮疹、恶心	有报道发生癫痫（一般在快速静脉给药后）
芬太尼	表面贴用：每小时25~300 μg，持续72h 糖浆：初始剂量200 μg，15 min以上；必要时在第一次剂量后15 min可重复一次剂量；对每次疼痛发作使用不超过两个剂量单位； 每日最大4个剂量单位	μ阿片样受体激动剂	副作用与吗啡相同 贴敷局部反应，如皮疹、红斑、瘙痒	如果发热，由于吸收可能增加，宜监测患者 给药部位外部暴露也有可能增加药物吸收 作用时间长
丁丙诺啡	表面贴用：35~70 μg/h，持续72 h 舌下：200~400 μg/(6~8h)	部分激动μ阿片样受体并且解离缓慢，从而导致镇痛作用延长	副作用与吗啡相同 贴敷局部反应，如皮疹、红斑、瘙痒、延迟性局部变态反应伴重度炎症反应 丁丙诺啡具有阿片样激动剂的特性，可能会对其他戒断症状依赖的患者引起戒断症状；纳洛酮只能部分逆转其作用	如果发热，由于吸收可能增加、副作用增加，宜监测患者 给药部位外部热暴露也有可能增加药物吸收 作用时间长 与苯二氮䓬类药物合用时可发生严重呼吸抑制
羟考酮	口服：必要时5 mg/(4~6h)；每日最大量一般为400 mg 静脉内：必要时1~10 mg/4h 皮下：必要时5 mg/4h	阿片样受体激动剂	副作用与吗啡相同	避免用于哮喘症患者

Adapted from Namaka M, Gramlich CR, Ruhlen D, et al: A treatment algorithm for neuropathic pain. Clin Ther 2004;26:951-979; further data from British National Formulary 48, September 2004. London, British National Association and Pharmaceutical Society of Great Britain. www.bnf.org.

旁注 6-4	用于治疗神经性疼痛的表面用药

利多卡因凝胶和 5% 利多卡因贴膏
0.025% 和 0.075% 辣椒素乳膏
乙醚 / 阿司匹林

放；研究显示其对神经性疼痛具有镇痛作用[173,174]。

三环类抗抑郁药

三环类抗抑郁药（tricyclic antidepressant，TCA）在神经性疼痛患者中具有镇痛作用[175-180]，这种镇痛作用可能与其抗抑郁作用没有直接关系，并且可能存在剂量-反应关系[181,182]。TCA 影响去甲肾上腺素和 5-羟色胺的释放与重吸收，从而增强了下行性 5-羟色胺能和去甲肾上腺素能系统的抑制作用与抗伤害感受作用（见表 6-7）[183-185]。

阿片类镇痛药

已有研究表明，阿片类镇痛药（吗啡、美沙酮、曲马多、芬太尼、丁丙诺啡和羟考酮）在神经性疼痛中具有镇痛作用（见表 6-8）[186-195]。阿片类物质与阿片样受体结合，在 NMDA 受体上呈非竞争性拮抗作用，包括对伤害感受神经元上钙通道的作用[196,197]。

表面药物

研究显示，利多卡因贴膏可有效治疗疱疹后神经性疼痛[198,199]；并且进一步研究提示该药还可用于治疗其他神经性疼痛状态[200,201]。一篇表面使用辣椒素的综述认为，对于其他治疗无反应的患者，联合或单独应用该药可能有效[202]。研究表明，表面用阿司匹林/乙醚混合物对急性疱疹和疱疹后神经性疼痛有效（旁注 6-4）[203-205]。

术后神经性疼痛的可能治疗方案

以下是可用于治疗术后神经性疼痛的药物或联合用药：

- 三环类：阿米替林
- 普瑞巴林
- 羟考酮和三环类
- 全身麻醉中使用氯胺酮
- 曲马多
- 局部麻醉
- 超前镇痛：该概念很吸引人，但尚无有力证据支持。

总结

术后神经性疼痛可能会被漏诊。4 例肿瘤患者中就有 1 例存在神经性疼痛，而其中大量的病例可能是由于医源性神经损伤所致[206]。其病理生理机制尚不完全明了，因此仍不能确定最佳的治疗方案。一般建议对术前神经性疼痛实施最佳治疗，并对新诊断出来的术后神经性疼痛患者进行早期干预。

（刘 佳译 包 睿 邓小明校）

参考文献

1. Davies HT, Crombie IK, Macrae WA, Rogers KM: Pain clinic patients in northern Britain. Pain Clin 1992;5:129–135.
2. Carr DB, Goudas LC: Acute pain. Lancet 1999;353:2051–2058.
3. Perkins FM, Kehlet H: Chronic pain as an outcome of surgery: A review of predictive factors. Anesthesiology 2000;93:1123–1133.
4. Merskey H, Bogduk N (eds): Classification of Chronic Pain, 2nd ed. IASP Task Force on Taxonomy. Seattle, IASP Press, 1994. See also IASP website: www.iasp-pain.org/terms-p.html/
5. Melton L: Taking a shot at neuropathic pain. Lancet Neurol 2003;2:719.
6. Woolf CJ. Pain: Moving from symptom control toward mechanism-specific pharmacologic management. Ann Intern Med 2004;140:441–451.
7. Scholz J, Woolf CJ: Can we conquer pain? Nat Neurosci 2002;5(Suppl):1062–1067.
8. Julius D, Basbaum AI: Molecular mechanisms of nociception. Nature 2001;413: 203–210.
9. Woolf CJ, Salter MW: Neuronal plasticity: Increasing the gain in pain. Science 2000;288:1765–1769.
10. Mogil JS, Yu L, Basbaum AI: Pain genes? Natural variation and transgenic mutants. Ann Rev Neurosci 2000;23:777–811.
11. Woolf CJ, Mannion RJ: Neuropathic pain: Aetiology, symptoms, mechanisms and management. Lancet 1999;353:1959–1964.
12. Waxman SG, Wood JN: Sodium channels from mechanisms to medicines? Brain Res Bull 1999;50:309–310.
13. Amaya F, Decosterd I, Samad TA, et al: Diversity of expression of the sensory neuron-specific TTX-resistant voltage-gated sodium ion channels SNS and SNS2. Mol Cell Neurosci 2000;15:331–342.
14. Levine JD, Reichling DB: Peripheral mechanisms of inflammatory pain. In Wall PD, Melzack R (eds): Textbook of Pain, 4th ed. Edinburgh, Churchill Livingstone, 1999, pp 59–84.
15. McCleskey EW, Gold MS: Ion channels of nociception. Annu Rev Physiol 1999;61:835–856.
16. Numazaki M, Tominaga T, Toyooka H, Tominaga M: Direct phosphorylation of capsaicin receptor VR1 by protein kinase Cepsilon and identification of two target serine residues. J Biol Chem 2002;15:13375–13378.
17. Walker K, Perkins M, Dray A: Kinins and kinin receptors in the nervous system. Neurochem Int 1995;26:1–16.
18. Vane JR, Bakhle YS, Botting RM: Cyclooxygenases 1 and 2. Annu Rev Pharmacol Toxicol 1998;38:97–120.

19. Costigan M, Befort K, Karchewski L, et al: Replicate high-density rat genome oligonucleotide microarrays reveal hundreds of regulated genes in the dorsal root ganglion after peripheral nerve injury. BMC Neurosci 2002;3:16.
20. Xiao HS, Huang QH, Zhang FX, et al: Identification of gene expression profile of dorsal root ganglion in the rat peripheral axotomy model of neuropathic pain. Proc Natl Acad Sci U S A 2002;99:8360–8365.
21. Noguchi K, Kawai Y, Fukuoka T, et al: Substance P induced by peripheral nerve injury in primary afferent sensory neurons and its effect on dorsal column nucleus neurons. J Neurosci 1995;15:7633–7643.
22. Fukuoka T, Kondo E, Dai Y, et al: Brain-derived neurotrophic factor increases in the uninjured dorsal root ganglion neurons in selective spinal nerve ligation model. J Neurosci 2001;21:4891–4900.
23. Decosterd I, Allchorne A, Woolf CJ: Progressive tactile hypersensitivity after a peripheral nerve crush: Non-noxious mechanical stimulus-induced neuropathic pain. Pain 2002;100:155–162.
24. Ji RR, Samad TA, Jin SX, et al: p38 MAPK activation by NGF in primary sensory neurons after inflammation increases TRPV1 levels and maintains heat hyperalgesia. Neuron 2002;36:57–68.
25. Mannion RJ, Costigan M, Decosterd I, et al: Neurotrophins: Peripherally and centrally acting modulators of tactile stimulus-induced inflammatory pain hypersensitivity. Proc Natl Acad Sci U S A 1999;96:9385–9390.
26. Luo ZD, Chaplan SR, Higuera ES, et al: Upregulation of dorsal root ganglion (alpha)2(delta) calcium channel subunit and its correlation with allodynia in spinal nerve-injured rats. J Neurosci 2001;21:1868–1875.
27. Liu CN, Devor M, Waxman SG, Kocsis JD: Subthreshold oscillations induced by spinal nerve injury in dissociated muscle and cutaneous afferents of mouse DRG. J Neurophysiol 2002;87:2009–2017.
28. Woolf CJ: Evidence for a central component of post-injury pain hypersensitivity. Nature 1983;306:686–688.
29. Woolf CJ, Wall PD: Relative effectiveness of C primary afferent fibers of different origins in evoking a prolonged facilitation of the flexor reflex in the rat. J Neurosci 1986;6:1433–1442.
30. Eliav E, Teich S, Benoliel R, et al: Large myelinated nerve fiber hypersensitivity in oral malignancy. Oral Surg Oral Med Oral Pathol Oral Radiol Endod 2002;94:45–50.
31. Stubhaug A, Breivik H, Eide PK, et al: Mapping of punctuate hyperalgesia around a surgical incision demonstrates that ketamine is a powerful suppressor of central sensitization to pain following surgery. Acta Anaesthesiol Scand 1997;41:1124–1132.
32. Campbell JN, Raja SN, Meyer RA, Mackinnon SE: Myelinated afferents signal the hyperalgesia associated with nerve injury. Pain 1988;32:89–94.
33. Koltzenburg M, Scadding J: Neuropathic pain. Curr Opin Neurol 2001;14:641–647.
34. Woolf CJ: Dissecting out mechanisms responsible for peripheral neuropathic pain: Implications for diagnosis and therapy. Life Sci 2004;74:2605–2610.
35. Ji RR, Kohno T, Moore KA, Woolf CJ: Central sensitization and LTP: Do pain and memory share similar mechanisms? Trends Neurosci 2003;26:696–705.
36. South SM, Kohno T, Kaspar BK, et al: A conditional deletion of the NR1 subunit of the NMDA receptor in adult spinal cord dorsal horn reduces NMDA currents and injury-induced pain. J Neurosci 2003;23:5031–5040.
37. Ji RR, Woolf CJ: Neuronal plasticity and signal transduction in nociceptive neurons: Implications for the initiation and maintenance of pathological pain. Neurobiol Dis 2001;8:1–10.
38. Felsby S, Nielsen J, Arendt-Nielsen L, Jensen TS: NMDA receptor blockade in chronic neuropathic pain: A comparison of ketamine and magnesium chloride. Pain 1996;64:283–291.
39. Pud D, Eisenberg E, Spitzer A, et al: The NMDA receptor antagonist amantadine reduces surgical neuropathic pain in cancer patients: A double blind, randomized, placebo controlled trial. Pain 1998;75:349–354.
40. Ji RR, Befort K, Brenner GJ, Woolf CJ: ERK MAP kinase activation in superficial spinal cord neurons induces prodynorphin and NK-1 upregulation and contributes to persistent inflammatory pain hypersensitivity. J Neurosci 2002;22:478–485.
41. Samad TA, Moore KA, Sapirstein A, et al: Interleukin-1beta-mediated induction of Cox-2 in the CNS contributes to inflammatory pain
42. Watkins LR, Maier SF: Beyond neurons: Evidence that immune cells and glial cells contribute to pathological pain states. Physiol Rev 2002;82:981–1011.
43. Said G, Hontebeyrie-Joskowicz M: Nerve lesions induced by macrophage activation. Res Immunol 1992;143:589–599.
44. Watkins LR, Maier SF: Neuropathic pain: The immune connection. Pain: Clin Updates 2004;12:1.
45. Olsson Y: Microenvironment of the peripheral nervous system under normal and pathological conditions. Crit Rev Neurobiol 1990;5:265–311.
46. Stoll G, Jander S, Myers RR: Degeneration and regeneration of the peripheral nervous system: From Augustus Waller's observations to neuroinflammation. J Peripher Nerv Syst 2002;7:13–27.
47. Watkins LR, Milligan ED, Maier SF: Glial activation: A driving force for pathological pain. Trends Neurosci 2001;24:450–455.
48. Koski CL: Mechanisms of Schwann cell damage in inflammatory neuropathy. J Infect Dis 1997;176:S169–S172.
49. Quarles RH, Weiss MD: Autoantibodies associated with peripheral neuropathy. Muscle Nerve 1999;22:800–822.
50. Koski CL: Humoral mechanisms in immune neuropathies. Neurol Clin 1992;10:629–649.
51. Moulin DE, Hagen N, Feasby TE, et al: Pain in Guillain-Barré syndrome. Neurology 1997;48:328–331.
52. Nguyen DK, Agenarioti-Belanger S, Vanasse M: Pain and the Guillain-Barré syndrome in children under 6 years old. J Paediatr 1999;134:773–776.
53. Hawke SH, Davies L, Pamphlett R, et al: Vasculitic neuropathy: A clinical and pathological study. Brain 1991;114:2175–2190.
54. Heuss D, Probst-Cousin S, Kayser C, Neundorfer B: Cell death in vasculitic neuropathy. Muscle Nerve 2000;23:999–1004.
55. Sorkin LS, Xiao WH, Wagner R, Myers RR: Tumour necrosis factor-alpha induces ectopic activity in nociceptive primary afferent fibres. Neuroscience 1997;81:255–262.
56. Porreca F, Ossipov MH, Gebhart GF: Chronic pain and medullary descending facilitation. Trends Neurosci 2002;25:319–325.
57. Suzuki R, Morcuende S, Webber M, et al: Superficial NK1-expressing neurons control spinal excitability through activation of descending pathways. Nat Neurosci 2002;5:1319–1326.
58. Zeitz KP, Guy N, Malmberg AB, et al: The 5-HT3 subtype of serotonin receptor contributes to nociceptive processing via a novel subset of myelinated and unmyelinated nociceptors. J Neurosci 2002;22:1010–1019.
59. McCleane GJ, Suzuki R, Dickenson AH: Does a single intravenous injection of the 5HT3 receptor antagonist ondansetron have an analgesic effect in neuropathic pain? A double-blinded, placebo-controlled cross-over study. Anesth Analg 2003;97:1474–1478.
60. Farber L, Stratz TH, Bruckle W, et al; German Fibromyalgia Study Group: Short-term treatment of primary fibromyalgia with the 5-HT3-receptor antagonist tropisetron: Results of a randomized, double-blind, placebo-controlled multicenter trial in 418 patients. Int J Clin Pharmacol Res 2001;21:1–13.
61. Haus U, Varga B, Stratz T, et al: Oral treatment of fibromyalgia with tropisetron given over 28 days: Influence on functional and vegetative symptoms, psychometric parameters and pain. Scand J Rheumatol Suppl 2000;113:55–58.
62. Stratz T, Farber L, Varga B, et al: Fibromyalgia treatment with intravenous tropisetron administration. Drugs Exp Clin Res 2001;27:113–118.
63. Woolf CJ, Shortland P, Coggeshall RE: Peripheral nerve injury triggers central sprouting of myelinated afferents. Nature 1992;355:75–78.
64. Moore KA, Kohno T, Karchewski LA, et al: Partial peripheral nerve injury promotes a selective loss of GABAergic inhibition in the superficial dorsal horn of the spinal cord. J Neurosci 2002;22:6724–6731.
65. Hwang JH, Yaksh TL: The effect of spinal GABA receptor agonists on tactile allodynia in a surgically-induced neuropathic pain model in the rat. Pain 1997;70:15–22.
66. Bloechlinger S, Karchewski LA, Woolf CJ: Dynamic changes in glypican-1 expression in dorsal root ganglion neurons after peripheral and central axonal injury. Eur J Neurosci 2004;19:1119–1132.
67. The effect of intensive diabetes therapy on the development and progression of neuropathy. The Diabetes Control and Complications Trial Research Group. Ann Intern Med 1995;122:561–568.
68. Werrett G: Nerve injuries. In Allman KG, Wilson IH (eds): Oxford Handbook of Clinical Anaesthesia. Oxford, Oxford University Press, 2001,

69. Sawyer RJ, Richmond MN, Hickey JD, Jarrratt JA: Peripheral nerve injuries associated with anaesthesia. Anaesthesia 2000;55:980–991.
70. Cheney FW, Domino KB, Caplan RA, Posner KL: Nerve injury associated with anesthesia: A closed claims analysis. Anesthesiology 1999;90:1062–1069.
71. Ben-David B: Complications of regional anesthesia: An overview. Anesthesiol Clin North Am 2002;20:665–667.
72. Borgeat A, Ekatodramis G: Nerve injury associated with regional anesthesia. Curr Top Med Chem 2001;1:199–203.
73. Katz J, Jackson M, Kavanagh BP, Sandler AN: Acute pain after thoracic surgery predicts long-term post-thoracotomy pain. Clin J Pain 1996;12:50–55.
74. Keller SM, Carp NZ, Levy MN, Rosen SM: Chronic post thoracotomy pain. J Cardiovasc Surg 1994;35(Suppl 1):161–164.
75. Benedetti F, Vighetti S, Ricco C, et al: Neurophysiologic assessment of nerve impairment in posterolateral and muscle-sparing thoracotomy. J Thorac Cardiovasc Surg 1998;115:841–847.
76. Benedetti F, Amanzio M, Casadio C, et al: Postoperative pain and superficial abdominal reflexes after posterolateral thoracotomy. Ann Thorac Surg 1997;64:207–210.
77. Nomori H, Horio H, Fuyuno G, Kobayashi R: Non-serratus-sparing antero-axillary thoracotomy with disconnection of anterior rib cartilage: Improvement in postoperative pulmonary function and pain in comparison to posterolateral thoracotomy. Chest 1997;111:572–576.
78. Perttunen K, Tasmuth T, Kalso E: Chronic pain after thoracic surgery: A follow-up study. Acta Anaesthesiol Scand 1999;43:563–567.
79. Sedrakyan A, van der Meulen J, Lewsey J, Treasure T: Video assisted thoracic surgery for treatment of pneumothorax and lung resections: Systematic review of randomised clinical trials. BMJ 2004;329(7473):1008.
80. Obata H, Saito S, Fujita N, et al: Epidural block with mepivacaine before surgery reduces long-term post-thoracotomy pain. Can J Anaesth 1999;46:1127–1132.
81. Carpenter JS, Andrykowki MA, Sloan P, et al: Postmastectomy/postlumpectomy pain in breast cancer survivors. J Clin Epidemiol 1998;51:1285–1292.
82. Kroner K, Krebs B, Skov J, Jorgensen HS: Immediate and long-term phantom breast syndrome after mastectomy: Incidence, clinical characteristics and relationship to pre-mastectomy breast pain. Pain 1989;36:327–334.
83. Tasmuth T, Estlanderb AM, Kalso E: Effect of present pain and mood on the memory of past postoperative pain in women treated surgically for breast cancer. Pain 1996;68:343–347.
84. Tasmuth T, von Smitten K, Kalso E: Pain and other symptoms during the first year after radical and conservative surgery for breast cancer. Br J Cancer 1996;74:2024–2031.
85. Maunsell E, Brisson J, Deschenes L: Arm problems and psychological distress after surgery for breast cancer. Can J Surg 1993;36:315–320.
86. Keramopoulos A, Tsionou C, Minaretzis D, et al: Arm morbidity following treatment of breast cancer with total axillary dissection: A multivariate approach. Oncology 1993;50:445–449.
87. Wallace MS, Wallace AM, Lee J, Dobke MK: Pain after breast surgery: A survey of 282 women. Pain 1996;66:195–205.
88. Tasmuth T, Kataja M, Blomqvist C, et al: Treatment-related factors predisposing to chronic pain in patients with breast cancer—a multivariate approach. Acta Oncol 1997;36:625–630.
89. Tasmuth T, von Smitten K, Hietanen P, et al: Pain and other symptoms after different treatment modalities of breast cancer. Ann Oncol 1995;6:453–459.
90. Watson CP, Evans RJ, Watt VR: The post-mastectomy pain syndrome and the effect of topical capsaicin. Pain 1989;38:177–186.
91. Killer HE, Hess K: Natural history of radiation-induced brachial plexopathy compared with surgically treated patients. J Neurol. 1990;237:247–250.
92. Vecht CJ, Van de Brand HJ, Wajer OJ: Post-axillary dissection pain in breast cancer due to a lesion of the intercostobrachial nerve. Pain 1989;38:171–176.
93. Abdullah TI, Iddon J, Barr L, et al: Prospective randomized controlled trial of preservation of the intercostobrachial nerve during axillary node clearance for breast cancer. Br J Surg 1998;85:1443–1445.
94. Bratschi HU, Haller U: [Significance of the intercostobrachial nerve in axillary lymph node excision] Geburtshilfe Frauenheilkd 1990;50:
95. Poobalan AS, Bruce J, King PM, et al: Chronic pain and quality of life following open inguinal hernia repair. Br J Surg 2001;88:1122–1126.
96. Callesen T, Bech K, Kehlet H: Prospective study of chronic pain after groin hernia repair. Br J Surg 1999;86:1528–1531.
97. Seid AS, Amos E: Entrapment neuropathy in laparoscopic herniorrhaphy. Surg Endosc 1994;8:1050–1053.
98. Starling JR, Harms BA: Diagnosis and treatment of genitofemoral and ilioinguinal neuralgia. World J Surg 1989;13:586–591.
99. Heise CP, Starling JR: Mesh inguinodynia: A new clinical syndrome after inguinal herniorrhaphy? J Am Coll Surg 1998;187:514–518.
100. Callesen T: Inguinal hernia repair: Anaesthesia, pain and convalescence. Dan Med Bull 2003;50:203–218.
101. Krane EJ, Heller LB: The prevalence of phantom sensation and pain in pediatric amputees. J Pain Symptom Manage 1995;10:21–29.
102. Jensen TS, Krebs B, Nielsen J, Rasmussen P: Immediate and long-term phantom limb pain in amputees: Incidence, clinical characteristics and relationship to pre-amputation limb pain. Pain 1985;21:267–278.
103. Sherman RA, Sherman CJ, Parker L: Chronic phantom and stump pain among American veterans: Results of a survey. Pain 1984;18:83–95.
104. Nikolajsen L, Ilkjaer S, Kroner K, et al: The influence of preamputation pain on postamputation stump and phantom pain. Pain 1997;72:393–405.
105. Smith J, Thompson JM: Phantom limb pain and chemotherapy in pediatric amputees. Mayo Clin Proc 1995;70:357–364.
106. Portenoy RK: Neuropathic pain. In Kanner R (ed): Pain Management Secrets, 2nd ed. Philadelphia, Hanley & Belfus, 2003, pp 147–170.
107. Nikolajsen L, Jensen TS: Phantom limb pain. Br J Anaesth 2001;87:107–116.
108. Jahangiri M, Jayatunga AP, Bradley JW, Dark CH: Prevention of phantom pain after major lower limb amputation by epidural infusion of diamorphine, clonidine and bupivacaine. Ann R Coll Surg Engl 1994;76:324–326.
109. Nikolajsen L, Ilkjaer S, Christensen JH, et al: Randomised trial of epidural bupivacaine and morphine in prevention of stump and phantom pain in lower-limb amputation. Lancet 1997;350:1353–1357.
110. Fisher A, Meller Y: Continuous postoperative regional analgesia by nerve sheath block for amputation surgery—a pilot study. Anesth Analg 1991;72:300–303.
111. Pinzur MS, Garla PG, Pluth T, Vrbos L: Continuous postoperative infusion of a regional anesthetic after an amputation of the lower extremity: A randomized clinical trial. J Bone Joint Surg Am 1996;78:1501–1505.
112. Lambert AW, Dashfield AK, Cosgrove C, et al: Randomized prospective study comparing preoperative epidural and intraoperative perineural analgesia for the prevention of postoperative stump and phantom limb pain following major amputation. Reg Anesth Pain Med 2001;26:316–321.
113. Jorgensen T, Teglbjerg JS, Wille-Jorgensen P, et al: Persisting pain after cholecystectomy. A prospective investigation. Scand J Gastroenterol 1991;26:124–128.
114. Jess P, Jess T, Beck H, Bech P: Neuroticism in relation to recovery and persisting pain after laparoscopic cholecystectomy. Scand J Gastroenterol 1998;33:550–553.
115. Borly L, Anderson IB, Bardram L, et al: Preoperative prediction model of outcome after cholecystectomy for symptomatic gallstones. Scand J Gastroenterol 1999;34:1144–1152.
116. Middelfart HV, Kristensen JU, Laursen CN, et al: Pain and dyspepsia after elective and acute cholecystectomy. Scand J Gastroenterol 1998;33:10–14.
117. Bates T, Ebbs SR, Harrison M, A'Hern RP: Influence of cholecystectomy on symptoms. Br J Surg 1991;78:964–967.
118. Stefaniak T, Vingerhoets A, Babinska D, et al: Psychological factors influencing results of cholecystectomy. Scand J Gastroenterol 2004;39:127–132.
119. Fenster LF, Lonborg R, Thirlby RC, Traverso LW: What symptoms does cholecystectomy cure? Insights from an outcomes measurement project and review of the literature. Am J Surg 1995;169:533–538.
120. Gilliland TM, Traverso LW: Modern standards for comparison of cholecystectomy with alternative treatments for symptomatic cholelithiasis with emphasis on long-term relief of symptoms. Surg

121. Gui GP, Cheruvu CV, West N, et al: Is cholecystectomy effective treatment for symptomatic gallstones? Clinical outcome after long-term follow-up. Ann R Coll Surg Engl 1998;80:25–32.
122. Vander Velpen GC, Shimi SM, Cuschieri A: Outcome after cholecystectomy for symptomatic gall stone disease and effect of surgical access: Laparoscopic v open approach. Gut 1993;34:1448–1451.
123. Ros A, Nilsson E: Abdominal pain and patient overall and cosmetic satisfaction one year after cholecystectomy: Outcome of a randomized trial comparing laparoscopic and minilaparotomy cholecystectomy. Scand J Gastroenterol 2004;39:773–777.
124. Poon CM, Chan KW, Lee DW, et al: Two-port versus four-port laparoscopic cholecystectomy. Surg Endosc 2003;17:1624–1627.
125. Stanton-Hicks M, Janig W, Hassenbusch S, et al: Reflex sympathetic dystrophy: Changing concepts and taxonomy. Pain 1995;63:127–133.
126. Benzon HT: Taxonomy: Definitions of pain terms and chronic pain syndromes. In Eds; Benzon HT, Raja SN, Borsook D, et al (eds): Essentials of Pain Medicine and Regional Anesthesia. Philadelphia, Churchill Livingstone, 1999, pp 10–11.
127. Roberts WJ: A hypothesis on the physiological basis for causalgia and related pains. Pain 1986;24:297–311.
128. Boas RA: Sympathetic nerve blocks: In search of a role. Reg Anesth Pain Med 1998;23:292–305.
129. Harden RN, Bruehl S, Stanos S, et al: Prospective examination of pain-related and psychological predictors of CRPS-like phenomena following total knee arthroplasty: A preliminary study. Pain 2003;106:393–400.
130. Pak TJ, Martin GM, Magness JL, Kavanaugh GJ: Reflex sympathetic dystrophy: Review of 140 cases. Minn Med 1970;53:507–512.
131. Bonica JJ: Causalgia and other reflex sympathetic dystrophies. In Bonica JJ, Liebeskind JC, Albe-Fressard D, et al (eds): Advances in Pain Research and Therapy, vol 3. New York, Raven Press, 1979, pp 141–166.
132. Reuben SS: Preventing the development of complex regional pain syndrome after surgery. Anesthesiology 2004;101:1215–1224.
133. Katz MM, Hungerford DS: Reflex sympathetic dystrophy affecting the knee. J Bone Joint Surg Br 1987;69:797–803.
134. Veldman PH, Goris RJ: Surgery on extremities with reflex sympathetic dystrophy. Unfallchirurg 1995;98:45–48.
135. Katz MM, Hungerford DS, Krackow KA, Lennox DW: Reflex sympathetic dystrophy as a cause of poor results after total knee arthroplasty. J Arthroplasty 1986;1:117–124.
136. Rocco AG: Sympathetically maintained pain may be rekindled by surgery under general anesthesia. Anesthesiology 1993;79:865.
137. Viel EJ, Pelissier J, Eledjam JJ: Sympathetically maintained pain after surgery may be prevented by regional anesthesia. Anesthesiology 1994;81:265–266.
138. Tessler MJ, Kleiman SJ: Spinal anaesthesia for patients with previous lower limb amputations. Anaesthesia 1994;49:439–441.
139. Reuben SS, Rosenthal EA, Steinberg RB: Surgery on the affected upper extremity of patients with a history of complex regional pain syndrome: A retrospective study of 100 patients. J Hand Surg [Am] 2000;25:1147–1151.
140. Glynn CJ, Basedow RW, Walsh JA: Pain relief following post-ganglionic sympathetic blockade with I.V. guanethidine. Br J Anaesth 1981;53:1297–1302.
141. Rocco AG, Kaul AF, Reisman RM, et al: A comparison of regional intravenous guanethidine and reserpine in reflex sympathetic dystrophy: A controlled, randomized, double-blind crossover study. Clin J Pain 1989;5:205–209.
142. Blanchard J, Ramamurthy S, Walsh N, et al: Intravenous regional sympatholysis: A double-blind comparison of guanethidine, reserpine, and normal saline. J Pain Symptom Manage 1990;5:357–361.
143. Jadad AR, Carroll D, Glynn CJ, McQuay HJ: Intravenous regional sympathetic blockade for pain relief in reflex sympathetic dystrophy: A systematic review and a randomized, double-blind crossover study. J Pain Symptom Manage 1995;10:13–20.
144. Ramamurthy S, Hoffman J: Intravenous regional guanethidine in the treatment of reflex sympathetic dystrophy/causalgia: A randomized, double-blind study. Guanethidine Study Group. Anesth Analg 1995;81:718–723.
145. Kettler RE, Abram SE: Intravenous regional droperidol in the management of reflex sympathetic dystrophy: A double-blind, placebo-controlled, crossover study. Anesthesiology 1988;69:933–936.
146. Glynn CJ, Stannard C, Collins PA, Casale R: The role of peripheral sudomotor blockade in the treatment of patients with sympathetically
147. Hord AH, Rooks MD, Stephens BO, et al: Intravenous regional bretylium and lidocaine for treatment of reflex sympathetic dystrophy: A randomized, double-blind study. Anesth Analg 1992;74:818–821.
148. Hanna MH, Peat SJ: Ketanserin in reflex sympathetic dystrophy: A double-blind placebo controlled cross-over trial. Pain 1989;38:145–150.
149. Kingery WS: A critical review of controlled clinical trials for peripheral neuropathic pain and complex regional pain syndromes. Pain 1997;73:123–139.
150. Perez RS, Kwakkel G, Zuurmond WW, de Lange JJ: Treatment of reflex sympathetic dystrophy (CRPS type 1): A research synthesis of 21 randomized clinical trials. J Pain Symptom Manage 2001;21:511–526.
151. Reuben SS, Steinberg RB, Klatt JL, Klatt ML: Intravenous regional anesthesia using lidocaine and clonidine. Anesthesiology 1999;91:654–658.
152. Reuben SS, Steinberg RB, Madabhushi L, Rosenthal E: Intravenous regional clonidine in the management of sympathetically maintained pain. Anesthesiology 1998;89:527–530.
153. Reuben SS, Rosenthal EA, Steinberg RB, et al: Surgery on the affected upper extremity of patients with a history of complex regional pain syndrome: The use of intravenous regional anesthesia with clonidine. J Clin Anesth 2004;16:517–522.
154. Cramer G, Young BM, Schwarzentraub P, et al: Preemptive analgesia in elective surgery in patients with complex regional pain syndrome: A case report. J Foot Ankle Surg 2000;39:387–391.
155. Rauck RL, Eisenach JC, Jackson K, et al: Epidural clonidine treatment for refractory reflex sympathetic dystrophy. Anesthesiology 1993;79:1163–1169.
156. Kissin I: Preemptive analgesia: Terminology and clinical relevance. Anesth Analg 1994;79:809–810.
157. Katz J: Pre-emptive analgesia: evidence, current status and future directions. Eur J Anaesthesiol Suppl 1995;10:8–13.
158. Kehlet H, Dahl JB: The value of "multimodal" or "balanced analgesia" in postoperative pain treatment. Anesth Analg 1993;77:1048–1056.
159. Gatt CJ Jr, Parker RD, Tetzlaff JE, et al: Preemptive analgesia: Its role and efficacy in anterior cruciate ligament reconstruction. Am J Sports Med 1998;26:524–529.
160. Reuben SS, Sklar J: Pain management in patients who undergo outpatient arthroscopic surgery of the knee. J Bone Joint Surg Am 2000;82:1754–1766.
161. Reuben SS, Makari-Judson G, Lurie SD: Evaluation of efficacy of the perioperative administration of venlafaxine XR in the prevention of postmastectomy pain syndrome. J Pain Symptom Manage 2004;27:133–139.
162. Zuurmond WW, Langendijk PN, Bezemer PD, et al: Treatment of acute reflex sympathetic dystrophy with DMSO 50% in a fatty cream. Acta Anaesthesiol Scand 1996;40:364–367.
163. Perez RS, Zuurmond WW, Bezemer PD, et al: The treatment of complex regional pain syndrome type I with free radical scavengers: A randomized controlled study. Pain 2003;102:297–307.
164. Zyluk A: The reasons for poor response to treatment of posttraumatic reflex sympathetic dystrophy. Acta Orthop Belg 1998;64:309–313.
165. De Grandis D, Minardi C: Acetyl-L-carnitine (levacecarnine) in the treatment of diabetic neuropathy: A long-term, randomised, double-blind, placebo-controlled study. Drugs R D 2002;3:223–231.
166. Zollinger PE, Tuinebreijer WE, Kreis RW, Breederveld RS: Effect of vitamin C on frequency of reflex sympathetic dystrophy in wrist fractures: A randomised trial. Lancet 1999;354:2025–2028.
167. Cazeneuve JF, Leborgne JM, Kermad K, Hassan Y: [Vitamin C and prevention of reflex sympathetic dystrophy following surgical management of distal radius fractures.] Acta Orthop Belg 2002;68:481–484.
168. Braga PC: Calcitonin and its antinociceptive activity: Animal and human investigations 1975-1992. Agents Actions 1994;41:121–131.
169. Yoshimura M: Analgesic mechanism of calcitonin. J Bone Miner Metab 2000;18:230–233.
170. Birklein F, Schmelz M, Schifter S, Weber M: The important role of neuropeptides in complex regional pain syndrome. Neurology 2001;57:2179–2184.
171. Jones DL, Sorkin LS: Systemic gabapentin and S(+)-3-isobutyl-gamma-aminobutyric acid block secondary hyperalgesia. Brain Res 1998;810:93–99.
172. Field MJ, Hughes J, Singh L: Further evidence for the role of the alpha(2)delta subunit of voltage dependent calcium channels in models

173. Fink K, Dooley DJ, Meder WP, et al: Inhibition of neuronal Ca(2+) influx by gabapentin and pregabalin in the human neocortex. Neuropharmacology 2002;42:229–236.
174. Lesser H, Sharma U, LaMoreaux L, Poole RM: Pregabalin relieves symptoms of painful diabetic neuropathy: A randomized controlled trial. Neurology 2004;63:2104–2110.
175. Watson CP, Evans RJ, Reed K, et al: Amitriptyline versus placebo in postherpetic neuralgia. Neurology 1982;32:671–673.
176. Bowsher D: Acute herpes zoster and postherpetic neuralgia: Effects of acyclovir and outcome of treatment with amitriptyline. Br J Gen Pract 1992;42:244–246.
177. Kvinesdal B, Molin J, Froland A, Gram LF: Imipramine treatment of painful diabetic neuropathy. JAMA 1984;251:1727–1730.
178. Max MB, Lynch SA, Muir J, et al: Effects of desipramine, amitriptyline, and fluoxetine on pain in diabetic neuropathy. N Engl J Med 1992;326:1250–1256.
179. Watson CP, Vernich L, Chipman M, Reed K: Nortriptyline versus amitriptyline in postherpetic neuralgia: A randomized trial. Neurology 1998;51:1166–1171.
180. Sawynok J, Esser MJ, Reid AR: Antidepressants as analgesics: An overview of central and peripheral mechanisms of action. J Psychiatry Neurosci 2001;26:21–29.
181. Max MB, Culnane M, Schafer SC, et al: Amitriptyline relieves diabetic neuropathy pain in patients with normal or depressed mood. Neurology 1987;37:589–596.
182. Sindrup SH, Gram LF, Skjold T, et al: Concentration-response relationship in imipramine treatment of diabetic neuropathy symptoms. Clin Pharmacol Ther 1990;47:509–515.
183. Botney M, Fields HL: Amitriptyline potentiates morphine analgesia by a direct action on the central nervous system. Ann Neurol 1983;13:160–164.
184. Ansuategui M, Naharro L, Feria M: Noradrenergic and opioidergic influences on the antinociceptive effect of clomipramine in the formalin test in rats. Psychopharmacology 1989;98:93–96.
185. McCleane G: Pharmacological strategies in relieving neuropathic pain. Expert Opin Pharmacother 2004;5:1299–1312.
186. Rowbotham MC, Twilling L, Davies PS, et al: Oral opioid therapy for chronic peripheral and central neuropathic pain. N Engl J Med 2003;348:1223–1232.
187. Kalman S, Osterberg A, Sorensen J, et al: Morphine responsiveness in a group of well-defined multiple sclerosis patients: A study with i.v. morphine. Eur J Pain 2002;6:69–80.
188. Raja SN, Haythornthwaite JA, Pappagallo M, et al: Opioids versus antidepressants in postherpetic neuralgia: A randomized, placebo-controlled trial. Neurology 2002;59:1015–1021.
189. Gimbel JS, Richards P, Portenoy RK: Controlled-release oxycodone for pain in diabetic neuropathy: A randomized controlled trial. Neurology 2003;60:927–934.
190. Duhmke RM, Cornblath DD, Hollingshead JR: Tramadol for neuropathic pain. Cochrane Database Syst Rev 2004;(2):CD003726.
191. Kouya PF, Hao JX, Xu XJ: Buprenorphine alleviates neuropathic pain-like behaviors in rats after spinal cord and peripheral nerve injury. Eur J Pharmacol 2002;450:49–53.
192. Watson CP, Moulin D, Watt-Watson J, et al: Controlled-release oxycodone relieves neuropathic pain: A randomized controlled trial in painful diabetic neuropathy. Pain 2003;105:71–78.
193. Zhao C, Tall JM, Meyer RA, Raja SN: Antiallodynic effects of systemic and intrathecal morphine in the spared nerve injury model of neuropathic pain in rats. Anesthesiology 2004;100:905–911.
194. Sartain JB, Mitchell SJ: Successful use of oral methadone after failure of intravenous morphine and ketamine. Anaesth Intensive Care 2002;30:487–489.
195. Mancini I, Lossignol DA, Body JJ: Opioid switch to oral methadone in cancer pain. Curr Opin Oncol 2000;12:308–313.
196. Yamakura T, Sakimura K, Shimoji K: Direct inhibition of the N-methyl-D-aspartate receptor channel by high concentrations of opioids. Anesthesiology 1999;91:1053–1063.
197. McDowell TS: Fentanyl decreases Ca^{2+} currents in a population of capsaicin-responsive sensory neurons. Anesthesiology 2003;98:223–231.
198. Galer BS, Rowbotham MC, Perander J, Friedman E: Topical lidocaine patch relieves postherpetic neuralgia more effectively than a vehicle topical patch: Results of an enriched enrollment study. Pain 1999;80:533–538.
199. Davies PS, Galer BS: Review of lidocaine patch 5% studies in the treatment of postherpetic neuralgia. Drugs 2004;64:937–947.
200. Galer BS, Jensen MP, Ma T, et al: The lidocaine patch 5% effectively treats all neuropathic pain qualities: Results of a randomized, double-blind, vehicle-controlled, 3-week efficacy study with use of the neuropathic pain scale. Clin J Pain 2002;18:297–301.
201. Argoff CE, Galer BS, Jensen MP, et al: Effectiveness of the lidocaine patch 5% on pain qualities in three chronic pain states: Assessment with the Neuropathic Pain Scale. Curr Med Res Opin. 2004;20(Suppl 2):21–28.
202. Mason L, Moore RA, Derry S, et al: Systematic review of topical capsaicin for the treatment of chronic pain. BMJ 2004;328(7446):991.
203. Bareggi SR, Pirola R, De Benedittis G: Skin and plasma levels of acetylsalicylic acid: A comparison between topical aspirin/diethyl ether mixture and oral aspirin in acute herpes zoster and postherpetic neuralgia. Eur J Clin Pharmacol 1998;54:231–235.
204. De Benedittis G, Lorenzetti A: Topical aspirin/diethyl ether mixture versus indomethacin and diclofenac/diethyl ether mixtures for acute herpetic neuralgia and postherpetic neuralgia: A double-blind crossover placebo-controlled study. Pain 1996;65:45–51.
205. De Benedittis G, Besana F, Lorenzetti A: A new topical treatment for acute herpetic neuralgia and post-herpetic neuralgia: The aspirin/diethyl ether mixture. An open-label study plus a double-blind controlled clinical trial. Pain 1992;48:383–390.
206. Marchettini P, Formaglio F, Lacerenza M: Iatrogenic painful neuropathic complications of surgery in cancer. Acta Anaesthesiol Scand 2001;45:1090–1094.

7 术后疼痛：遗传学和基因组学

ULRIKE M. STAMER · FRANK STÜBER

人类基因组计划揭示了几乎完整的基因组序列资料，这些资料为进一步研究基因组变异对疼痛状态下伤害性感受的敏感性和易感性以及对疼痛药物疗法反应性的影响提供了基础。目前正在研究与疼痛感觉、疼痛过程和疼痛治疗相关的基因，如阿片受体、运载体以及药物治疗的其他靶点。而且，已经建议将筛选药物代谢酶表达变异作为一种可能的诊断工具，以改善患者的治疗效果。代谢酶基因多态性变异表达可能是药物不良反应的主要因素，可能影响住院时间和总的治疗费用。

遗传学基础

孟德尔于1866年发表了"遗传定律"，并且用豌豆实验证明亲代将遗传性的不同元素传给子代。特殊表现是由存在不同形式的基因或等位基因所决定的，看得见的特征就是所谓的显型，比如花的颜色和哺乳动物的肤色。黑色和白色老鼠同一基因有不同的等位基因，这取决于所遗传亲代等位基因的优势关系。

但是，并不是所有的特征都按照孟德尔法则遗传。许多遗传因素均可调节复杂性疾病，如糖尿病、高血压病、冠状动脉疾病、精神分裂症和偏头痛。不同的遗传特征常以很小的信息性标记出现，如基因碱基序列的个体差异。而有一些却以高度信息性标记的形式出现，这是一些遗传疾病（即Huntington舞蹈症、囊性纤维病）的主要原因。基因组变异可以为单个碱基变异或单核苷酸多态性（single-nucleotide polymorphism，SNP），以插入/缺失变异形式，或者更复杂的较长序列DNA和大量等位基因编码变异的形式出现。这些复杂变异组成微随体、小卫星序列和不定数串列重复区（图7-1）。等位基因是指整个功能性基因的不同复制编码，因为基因复制编码可能与蛋白质表达水平密切相关，所以其是基因分型的目靶。

这些基因变异称为基因多态性或突变，这就是为何在基因组某一位点的DNA序列中存在不同个体的原因。多态性是指种群中等位基因频率高于1%的变异，而突变是指等位基因频率低于1%的变异。

已经进行了很多有关实验性疼痛状况下的研究工作，如近亲交配的鼠种或基因敲除或转基因小鼠对急性和慢性疼痛的行为反应[1,2]。相反，在人类很难进行机械学研究，并且动物实验结果往往不适用于人类。

遗传学和基因组学

基因组时代提出了一种新医学，其着重于预测医学，而不是预防或治疗医学[3]。其主要探寻易使个体发生某种疾病或防止个体发生疾病如慢性疼痛的基因变异，并且将使疾病的治疗个体化和人性化。如在开胸术、乳房切除术、四肢截肢等手术后，哪位患者是发生慢性疼痛综合征的危险个体？哪位患者在术后疼痛治疗中需要极大剂量阿片类药物，而且将对术后

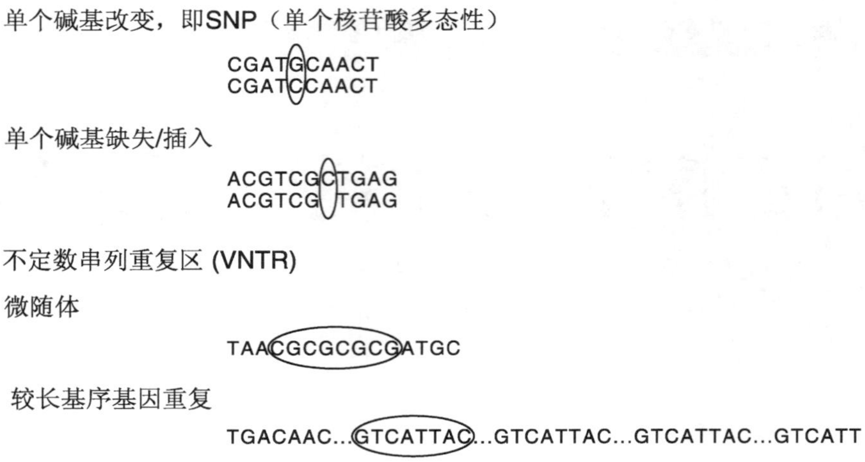

单个碱基改变，即SNP（单个核苷酸多态性）
CGATGCAACT
CGATCCAACT
单个碱基缺失/插入
ACGTCGCTGAG
ACGTCG TGAG
不定数串列重复区 (VNTR)
微随体
TAACGCGCGCGATGC
较长基序基因重复
TGACAAC...GTCATTAC...GTCATTAC...GTCATTAC...GTCATT

图 7–1 基因组变异

疼痛治疗的标准方案反应差？2004 年开始的流行病学研究检查了候选基因变异体和神经性疼痛之间潜在的相关性[4]。文献筛选了相关的 200 个可能基因。在以往发表的研究基础上，有 20 个基因可能影响神经性疼痛。科学界正期待第一个大型遗传流行病学试验的结果。

严重和持续性疼痛的个体差异曾归因于损伤的严重性，患者的年龄、人格特征、社会背景、情绪和心理因素、经济状况，以及其他的环境影响。疼痛过程的分子介质，例如炎性介质（5–羟色胺、组胺、缓激肽、细胞因子），第二信使、受体以及内源性神经递质正在研究中，希望这些研究能为将来个体化疼痛处理揭示新的策略。

药物疗法有时使临床医师不得不面对意想不到的治疗无效或者出现的严重不良反应。这种情形对某些患者而言可能会危及生命。一项对 39 项前瞻性研究的荟萃分析估计严重不良药物反应（adverse drug reaction，ADR）的总体发生率是 6.7%。严重事件是指那些需要住院治疗或导致永久性残疾或死亡的事件[5]。

ADR 的发生与发病率、死亡率和实际医疗费用相关。ADR 的潜在危险因素或治疗失败的原因包括患者年龄、性别、合并疾病、给药方法、器官功能（特别是肝肾功能）和饮食习惯以及吸烟和饮酒嗜好等某些生活方式因素（图 7–2）。而且，基因变量能改变药物的药代动力学和药效动力学，因此诱发 ADR 或者降低药效。DNA 序列的变更可以影响机体对药物的敏感性及其代谢途径的调节。在不同个体，镇痛药的效应部位也不一样。受体多态性、离子通道、药物载体以及药物治疗的其他目标等已广泛认可，而且解释了与镇痛药和复合镇痛药相对应的变化。其他混杂变量是疼痛强度、疼痛类型或疼痛综合征（腹部手术与骨科手术后急性术后疼痛比较，慢性良性疼痛与癌性疼痛比较，内脏疼痛与神经性疼痛比较等）和环境影响以

非药理学效应
安慰剂效应
社会影响
其他环境影响
心理应对策略
年龄
生理学改变
性别
器官功能
遗传背景：
药物代谢敏感性
药代动力学
药效动力学
反应性
合并疾病
联合用药
营养饮食

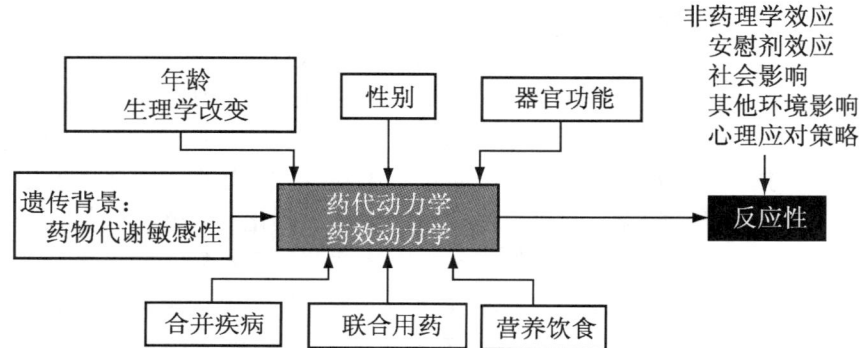

图 7–2 决定某种药物 / 镇痛药反应的变量

及心理方面。

药物基因学描述了基因决定药物代谢的不同。这些基因变异可以导致 ADR、药物的毒性或一种药物治疗失败。德国儿科医师 Friedrich Vogel 认识到药物代谢受遗传影响，1958 年他首次引入了这一概念。药物基因学概念是一更新、更广泛的概念，其涉及分子生物学和相关技术取得的新进展。我们现在认为基因组学包括基因动态结构、转录子、编码子和蛋白质组等，而不是仅仅关注于单个碱基的改变。药物基因学包括药物作用的所有方面，包含药物吸收、分布、代谢、排泄和靶受体亲和力。而且，这一概念也指在不断增加基因知识的基础上新药理学因子的发展和发现。现已经认识到药物遗传学/药物基因组学可能会改善多种药物治疗的临床结果，而且代表了基因组时代重要的生物医学进步。

药物代谢的基因学

药物效应的变化可能是由基因多态性所致。这些多态现象可以发生于药物摄取、运转、效应分子（比如受体或离子通道）、代谢和排泄等各个系统。扩展的药理学效应、ADR、毒性、药物前体缺乏、有效剂量的增减以及药物与药物之间更强的相互作用都可能是基因变异的潜在作用[6]。

药物代谢包括两个步骤。代谢 I 相，底物的功能性分子群通过氧化、氧合、还原和水解等改变，从而在药物分子中产生特殊功能组。它们通过 II 相酶（如 N-乙酰转移酶，尿苷二磷酸葡萄糖苷酸转移酶，谷胱甘肽-S 转移酶）催化而作为葡糖糖醛酸、硫酸盐或谷胱甘肽连接位点。细胞色素 P450 基因族（cytochrome P450 gene family，CYP）在 I 相代谢中起重要作用，其代谢内源性和外源性物质。在所有生物体内都存在这些酶。在十多亿年的种群发展中，其产生了许多亚群。作为适应过程中的一部分，由于环境影响和选择压力，各物种和亚群都形成了新的 CYP 基因。

细胞色素 P450 2D6

多态性细胞色素 P450 酶是很多药物的代谢酶

表 7-1	通过特异性细胞色素 P450 异构体 CYP2C9、CYP2C19 和 CYP_2D_6* 代谢的药物		
同功酶	代谢的药物	药物：举例	酶活性改变情况下的不良反应
CYP2C9	华法林		出血
	苯妥英		共济失调
	NSAID	布洛芬、双氯芬酸、萘普生、美洛昔康、塞来昔布	胃肠道出血
	口服降血糖药	甲苯磺丁脲、格列吡嗪	低血糖
	血管紧张素 II 阻滞剂	氯沙坦、厄贝沙坦	无资料
CYP2C19	质子泵抑制剂	奥美拉唑、泮托拉唑	无资料
	抗癫痫药	地西泮、苯妥英	镇静
CYP2D6	抗抑郁药	阿米替林、氯米帕明、地昔帕明、丙米嗪、帕罗西汀	镇静、心脏毒性
	β 受体阻断剂	美托洛尔、噻吗洛尔	过量
	抗心律失常药	普罗帕酮、美西律、氟卡尼、阿义马林	心律失常
	抗精神病药	氟哌啶醇	帕金森综合征
	5-羟色胺拮抗剂	昂丹司琼、托烷司琼	恶心、呕吐
	止吐药	甲氧氯普胺	无资料
	镇痛药	可待因、曲马多、羟考酮、右美沙芬	无痛或减轻疼痛
	苯丙胺	摇头丸	无资料；毒性？

*For more detailed information, see http://medicine.iupi.edu/flockart

（表 7-1）而且在催化活性方面存在很大的个体差异。关键碱基改变或缺失导致信使 RNA（mRNA）和蛋白质有缺陷，从而引起代谢能力的改变。

CYP2D6 是细胞色素 P450 系统中一种高度多态性的同工酶。CYP2D6 存在 50 多种不同变异，因此在人群中存在广泛的代谢谱[7,8]。在基因命名网站有所有已知细胞色素等位基因的详细目录[9]。

个别显示正常酶活性的酶称为泛代谢者（extensive metabolizer，Em）。相反，酶活性下降或缺乏酶则为乏代谢者（poor metabolizer，PM），其在 2D6 基因位点存在单个碱基改变或缺失。PM 呈现两个无活性等位基因，其主要特点是使一些常用药物不能羟化，如 β 受体阻断剂、抗心律失常药、抗抑郁药、神经镇静药以及镇痛药等（见表 7-1）。

药物代谢功能的遗传变异性具有重要的临床意义，因为大约 10% 的白种人具有无功能的等位基因常染色体隐形遗传特性[7,10]。CYP2D6 基因的复制和多复制与某些药物的超速代谢相关。"超速代谢者"（ultrarapid metabolizer，Um）酶活性显著增高，导致底物低于治疗的血药浓度。4%～5% 的白种人是 Um。然而其他种族的患者有不同的概率。携带多重 CYP2D6 基因拷贝最多的个体是埃塞俄比亚人和沙特阿拉伯人，总数分别达 21% 和 25%（见表 7-2）。

不同人种和种族背景人群中不同概率的基因变异使得治疗策略需修改。白种人中 CYP2D6*4 等位基因存在高概率（等位基因概率 20%），占 CYP2D64 等位基因突变的 75% 以上，而中国人群中这种基因突变几乎不存在（见表 7-2）。

可待因

可待因是一种没有镇痛效果的药物前体。它主要是通过糖脂化作用而消除，经 O-脱甲基作用转变为吗啡以及 N-脱甲基作用转变为去甲可待因，是次要消除途径。可待因经 O-脱甲基作用产生活性代谢产物吗啡依赖于 CYP2D6 活性[11]，CYP2D6 活性与 PM 相对缺乏有关。

可待因广泛用于治疗手术后疼痛，特别是儿科患者。与美国和英国相反，可待因在德国并不用作常规单一镇痛药。然而，可待因是许多药物的成分（如对乙酰氨基酚加可待因），而且广泛应用于急性和慢性疼痛治疗。一些研究已经证实，在 PM 患者中可待因镇痛效果相对缺乏[10,12]。Williams 等人研究了可待因对行增殖腺扁桃体切除术儿童的止痛效果[13,14]。吗啡血浆浓度非常低，并且与代谢表型有关，同时在 2 例 PM 患者和某些有代谢能力下降的杂合子患者中没有检测到吗啡或其代谢产物 [吗啡-6-葡萄糖苷酸（morphine-6-glucuronide，M6G）或吗啡-3-葡萄糖苷酸（morphine-3-glucuronide，M3G）]。在临床实践中，可待因效果存在很大个体差异，其对大约 10% 白种患者基本无效或完全无效[13,15]。

曲马多

曲马多是一种合成的阿片类药物，研究表明其止痛效果很少伴有呼吸抑制作用和出现耐药性、成瘾性和药物滥用的情况。此消旋混合物是通过它的两种对映体：（+）-曲马多、（-）-曲马多及其代谢产物的协同作用从而发挥止痛作用。肝细胞色素 P450 将曲马

表 7-2	不同人种变异体 CYP2D6 等位基因根据等位基因频率的分布				
等位基因变异体	酶功能	高加索人	亚洲人	非洲黑人	衣索比亚人、沙特阿拉伯人
*2×N	基因复制：酶活性增加	1～5	0～2	2	10～16
*4	剪接缺陷：钝化酶	12～21	1	2	1～4
*5	删除：没有酶	2～7	6	4	1～3
*10	不稳定酶	1～2	51	6	3～9
*17	减少底物亲和力	0	无数据	34	3～9

From Ingelman-Sundberg M, Oscarson M, McLellan RA: Polymorphic human cytochrome P450 enzymes: An opportunity for individualized drug treatment. Trends Pharmacol Sci 1999;20:342-349.

多代谢为 11-去甲基化复合物，其中主要为 M1（O-去甲基曲马多）且具有镇痛作用。已经证实（+）-O-去甲基曲马多和 μ-阿片类受体有亲和力，而且比原始复合物大约强 200 倍。因此，其是主要的阿片受体介导的止痛作用，而（+）-曲马多和（-）-曲马多抑制神经递质 5-羟色胺和去甲肾上腺素的重摄取[16,17]。O-去甲基化形成 M1 需要 CYP2D6。

药物遗传学可以解释患者术后对疼痛治疗药物的某些不同反应[18]。一项对腹部手术患者恢复期的前瞻性临床研究证实 CYP2D6 基因型影响曲马多镇痛效果。在此研究中，有 300 例患者给予术后患者自控镇痛方法（patient-controlled analgesia，PCA）镇痛。分析有 CYP2D6 突变 PM 患者的基因型。Em 和 PM 人口统计学和外科相关因素均相似。PM 的曲马多负荷量、相继曲马多消耗量以及补充剂量比有一种以上野生型等位基因的患者更多。PM 组中的无效比例比 EM 组更高。由此说明，术后给予曲马多治疗的 PM 患者比 EM 患者出现的疼痛更多。

5-羟色胺-3-受体拮抗剂

所有手术患者中约 30% 发生术后恶心和呕吐（postoperative nausea and vomiting，PONV）。挥发性麻醉药和阿片类药物（用于麻醉技术的一部分或用于术后疼痛治疗）是发生 PONV 的主要病因。5-羟色胺-3（serotonin-3，5HT₃）受体拮抗剂最初用于预防化疗导致的恶心呕吐，现在也广泛应用于 PONV 的预防和治疗。Kaiser 等人已经证实托烷司琼和昂丹司琼预防癌症患者恶心呕吐的效用取决于患者活性 CYP2D6 基因编码[19]。在对健康韩国人受试者的托烷司琼药代动力学研究发现，血药水平与特定的基因型相关，Ums 患者的血清浓度最低[20]。随后对术后患者的试验结果证实具有 CYP2D6 等位基因多功能复制的个体和 UM 状态的患者昂丹司琼无效的发生率更高[21]。这些结果说明，给予 5HT₃ 拮抗剂托烷司琼和昂丹司琼止吐治疗的疗效取决于患者 CYP2D6 酶活性，Um 患者的反应性较低。

药物相互作用

基因多态性也可以影响药物相互作用。酶活性抑制或诱导是各种药理学效应变化的可能因素。特定酶活性抑制剂产生药理学上确定的乏代谢者，如胺碘酮、甲氧氯普胺、氟哌啶醇、塞来昔布和其他一些药物（旁注 7-1）可抑制 CYP2D6。通过同时给予 CYP2D6 底物美托洛尔提高血浆药物浓度证实，连续 7 d，给予 2×200 mg/d 塞来考昔或连续 6 d 给予胺碘酮 1.2 g/d 可抑制 CYP2D6[22,23]。因代谢下降，β 受体阻断剂的血药浓度平均增加 2 倍。个别患者的这一药物相互作用取决于 CYP2D6 的基因型[23]。

因此，如果患者长期服用塞来考昔、西咪替丁、雷尼替丁等，给予可待因和曲马多行术后镇痛是不明智的（见旁注 7-1）。

阿片受体

阿片类药物是严重急性和慢性疼痛患者药物治疗的主要药物。阿片受体基因克隆已经引发了有关控制阿片受体表达的基因定子的讨论。诸如细胞因子等转录因子能够调节这些基因。转录后事件包括剪接改变和 mRNA 稳定性和翻译有效性的改变。而且，这些受体显示的多态区域可以影响结合位点的表达和功能。

现今对 μ-阿片受体的一些多态现象和突变已有描述。T802C（S268P）等位基因变异对脱敏作用以及 μ-阿片受体的 G 蛋白偶联均有影响[24]。人类 μ-阿片受体功能缺失可影响机体阿片物质调节行为或药物成瘾性[25]。

μ-阿片受体外显子 1 中 A118G 多态现象导致 40 位点天冬酰胺转换成天冬氨酸，并显示可使吗啡的主要活性代谢物 M6G 的瞳孔收缩效应下降[26]。携带两个

旁注 7-1	CYP2D6 抑制剂*
胺碘酮	
西咪替丁、雷尼替丁	
塞来昔布	
可乐定	
可卡因	
帕罗西汀	
普罗帕酮	
美沙酮	
组胺 H1 受体拮抗剂	
氟西汀（百忧解）	
氟哌啶醇	

*不断升级版见网上在线：http://medicine.iupi.edu/flockart/

G118等位基因受试者比只携带一个基因拷贝和携带两个野生型等位基因的受试者具有较低的M6G效应。

这一结果已在有关2例行吗啡癌痛控制治疗的病例报道中得到证实[27]。M6G经肾清除，肾功能衰竭患者出现蓄积。与在位点118突变的患者相比，只有野生型受体的患者出现如镇静、嗜睡和警戒性下降等中枢神经系统副作用。已证实M6G蓄积是出现阿片类药物毒性的危险因素，特别是在吗啡治疗期间出现中枢神经系统副作用。因此，假设118G基因型可防止M6G相关的阿片类药物毒性[27]。

Klepstad等将μ-阿片受体基因型与恶性疾病所致疼痛患者的阿片类药物需要量相关联[28]。与那些杂合子等位基因患者（n=17）或纯合子野生型等位基因患者（n=78）相比，纯合子118G等位基因患者（n=4）需要更大剂量的吗啡才能控制疼痛。但是，此研究中样本量较小，目前需要更大样本的研究证实这些结果并排除一些可能的"机会性"结果[4,29]。

μ-阿片受体多态现象和药物耐受、药物滥用的发生和疼痛治疗中阿片类药物效应之间存在潜在的相关性。迄今为止，研究结果并不一致，这可能是由于种群不同和所研究的患者数目不同。目前的研究注重于分析更多的单倍体（单个染色体在紧密连接位点上的等位基因复合物）及基因型-表现型的联系[30]。

μ阿片受体的选择性剪接

对芬太尼、氢吗啡酮、羟考酮和美沙酮等阿片类药物相对于吗啡的镇痛效能已有很好的描述。然而，这些标准转换率均为平均值，而个体反应可能完全不同，需要量可能更低或者更高。一名患者如需增加吗啡剂量，则提示出现耐药性或者出现吗啡依赖性副作用，此时通常会更换其他阿片类药物，如氢吗啡酮、羟考酮或美沙酮。这种阿片类药物的更换常常证实，与预期的那些药物相关功效相比，更小剂量即已足够。在高耐药性患者中常常观察到不完全的交叉耐药现象。好像对不同μ-阿片类药物相对敏感性不同。

同时，有证据表明μ-阿片受体存在多种亚型。已经确定在细胞羟基末端存在很多基因剪接变异[31]。它们都包含同样的前3个外显子。但是μ-阿片受体-1（MOR-1）的外显子4被更多的外显子复合替代。这些剪接改变导致细胞内3'末端序列不同，从而影响受体的功效和运输[32]。这种剪接变异的区域性分布是唯一的，剪接机制似乎是细胞和局部所特有的[33,34]。最终，必须阐明阿片受体亚型的药理学功能，剪接变异与患者中阿片类药物不同反应以及临床发现的不完全交叉耐药现象之间的联系仍需阐证。

非阿片类镇痛药

非阿片类镇痛药广泛用于治疗小手术后急性疼痛或联合应用阿片类药物用于大手术后疼痛治疗。它们是多模式疼痛治疗中必不可少的一部分，因为作用机制不同的镇痛药联合应用可以增加治疗效果而且减少不良反应，如阿片类药物引起的恶心呕吐和呼吸抑制。

很多调查研究证实基因对非阿片类镇痛药效果有明确影响。在动物模型里，特殊物种（鼠类）似乎对非甾体类抗炎药（NSAID）或对乙酰氨基酚尤为敏感，而其他物种却对这些药物有一定程度的耐药性[1,35]。推测可能人类也存在类似的非阿片类药物效应差别。

双氯芬酸、布洛芬、萘普生和吡罗昔康等NSAID药物由CYP2C9代谢。已经证实这种细胞色素的多态现象与酶活性的缺乏相关。1%~3%的白种人为PM。CYP2C9的多态现象可能在NSAID的镇痛效果和毒性方面起到重要作用。与野生型基因型CYP2C9*1/*1携带者相比，CYP2C9*3纯合子携带者口服塞来昔布后清除率下降2倍多，CYP2C9*3等位基因杂合子携带者的清除率则介于两者之间[36]。Tang等人报道在两例CYP2C9*1/*3和一例*3/*3受试者中[37]，在单一口服剂量后，塞来昔布血药浓度增加了2.2倍[按照2~24 h曲线下面积（AUC）计算][36]。在CYP2D9*3杂合子和纯合子携带者中检测到羧化-塞来昔布和羟化-塞来昔布的浓度降低，这一结果说明CYP2C9多态性位点影响塞来昔布药代动力学参数[38]。由于环氧合酶-2抑制剂在血液和组织中广泛蓄积，CYP2D9*3等位基因纯合子携带者大大延长了塞来昔布体内潴留时间。这种差异是否与药物效能更强或更高的不良反应发病率及不良反应严重性（如肾损伤和其他剂量依赖性的不良结果）相关，仍有待进一步研究。

布洛芬药代动力学和布洛芬介导的对环氧合酶1和2的抑制明显受CYP2D9基因型影响。在两名CYP2C9*3等位基因携带者中，外消旋布洛芬和S-布洛芬清除率下降。S-布洛芬清除率下降伴有更强的药效学活性，这对接受这种 NSAID 药物治疗的患者身上可能有重要临床意义。

右美沙芬，是 N-甲基-D-天冬氨酸（N-methyl-d-aspartate，NMDA）拮抗剂，是一种很好的抗抑郁药，作为联合镇痛药常规应用于慢性疼痛治疗，其是 CYP2D6 的作用底物。至于曲米帕明，其生物利用度和全身清除率则明显依赖于 CYP2D6 基因型。CYP2D6 PM 患者生物利用度高和全身清除率低可导致机体内曲米帕明过高，增加药物不良反应风险。另一方面，CYP2D6 基因复制体携带者对三环类抗抑郁药的超速代谢可导致血药浓度不足，从而增加对治疗反应差的可能[39]。在其他抗抑郁药和抗精神药中也发现类似结果。基因引起的血药浓度不同使得剂量需适当调整[40]。

性别差异

有关实验性疼痛和慢性疼痛的人类研究表明女性疼痛发病率高于男性[41,42]。尚无随机试验验证急性术后疼痛的性别特异性。在肘关节交叉韧带重建术后[43]和一项包括各种手术的队列研究发现女性疼痛更剧烈[44]。而且，队列研究中女性每公斤体重需要多给予 30% 的吗啡才能获得同等水平的镇痛效果[44]。

尤其是 κ-受体介导的镇痛似乎存在男女性别差异。纳布啡和喷他佐辛等 κ-激动药对女性能产生显著的镇痛效果，而对男性则无镇痛效果[45,46]。Mogil 等[47]证实小鼠体内黑皮质素-1 受体（melanocortin-1 receptor，MC1R）调节 κ-阿片受体诱导敏感性，但只见于雌性小鼠。在人类，MC1R 基因的两种突变体等位基因与浅色皮肤和红毛发有关。喷他佐辛镇痛对这一基因型女性比对男性更有效。其他一些结果表明，红发人对热疼痛更敏感，而对皮下给予利多卡因镇痛有抵抗。另外，红发女性需增加 19% 的地氟烷才能抑制伤害性电刺激的反应活动[48,49]。

其他相关基因

其他一些可能与疼痛感觉、调节和治疗有关的相关基因仍在研究中。儿茶酚-O 位-甲基转移酶（catechol-O-methyltransferase，COMT）基因很有可能是一相关基因，其参与儿茶酚胺类物质代谢，因此可能是多巴胺和肾上腺素、去甲肾上腺素等神经递质的关键调节基因。*val 158met* 多态性可使 COMT 活性降低 3~4 倍。Zubieta 等将这一多态性与疼痛反应改变相联系[50]。通过正电子发射断层扫描显示放射性标记的卡芬太尼与阿片受体的结合减少，由此说明纯合子甲基 158 基因类型个体的局部 μ-阿片类系统对疼痛的应答下降。另外，有报道蛋氨酸纯合子疼痛敏感性和疼痛的情感分级更高。

除了代谢酶、大麻素、NMDA、多巴胺和 5-羟色胺-肾上腺素能受体、离子通道、白介素、内源性阿片类物质和其他物质是疼痛和疼痛治疗的特异标靶[4]。转运蛋白的基因编码在决定特定部位药物浓度中起着重要作用，如中枢神经系统和突触间隙。P-糖蛋白是相关基因，其在血脑屏障、5-羟色胺和多巴胺转运蛋白表达，在突触间隙调节这些神经递质的重摄取。

结论

疼痛领域的研究已经开始阐明影响疼痛机制和感受的基因变异，以及疼痛信号传递和脊髓对疼痛的处理等。已经很好地确立了临床前期动物模型，但是新型镇痛药的治疗效能还在研究中。由于更快、更好的基因分型技术的发展，已经确定的基因编码药物代谢酶、药物载体以及受体基因的多态性数量正在迅速增加。在很多病例中，这些基因因素对某一个别药物的药代动力学和药效动力学均有很大影响，特别是在治疗指数窄的情况下。将来，临床医师可根据基因型推荐特定的药物剂量。

因为个体差异和人种差异均可能很高，这需要尖端的吞吐量高的技术用于基因分析和大量者样本。用于床旁或临床或诊所来诊断患者的药物敏感性的遗传药理学 DNA 芯片已经在研究中。这些发展将使得患者治疗更加个体化，从而有望减少疼痛药物治疗的不良药物反应，并增强疗效。

（周 懿译 万小健 邓小明校）

参考文献

1. Mogil JS, Wilson SG, Bon K, et al: Heritability of nociception I: Responses of 11 inbred mouse strains on 12 measures of nociception. Pain 1999;80:67–82.
2. Seitzer Z, Wu T, Max MB, Diehl SR: Mapping a gene for neuropathic pain-related behaviour following peripheral neurectomy in the mouse. Pain 2000;93:101–106.
3. Dausset J: Journal of Biomedicine and Biotechnology [editorial]. J Biomed Biotechnol 2001;1:1-2.
4. Belfer I, Wu T, Kingman A, et al: Candidate gene studies of human pain mechanisms. Anesthesiology 2004;100:1562–1572.
5. Lazarou J, Pomeranz BH, Corey PN: Incidence of adverse drug reactions in hospitalized patients: A meta-analysis of prospective studies. JAMA 1998;279:1200–1205.
6. Tsai YJ, Hoyme HE: Pharmacogenomics: The future of drug therapy. Clin Genet 2002;62:257–264.
7. Daly AK, Brockmoller J, Broly F, et al: Nomenclature for human CYP2D6 alleles. Pharmacogenetics 1996;6:193–201.
8. Marez D, Legrand M, Sabbagh N, et al: Polymorphism of the cytochrome P450 CYP2D6 gene in a European population: Characterization of 48 mutations and 53 alleles, their frequencies and evolution. Pharmacogenetics 1997;7:193–202.
9. Human Cytochrome P450 (CYP) Allele Nomenclature Committee: Home page. Available at http://www.imm.ki.se/CYPalleles/
10. Sachse C, Brockmoller J, Bauer S, Roots I: Cytochrome P450 2D6 variants in a Caucasian population: Allele frequencies and phenotypic consequences. Am J Hum Genet 1997;60:284–295.
11. Poulsen L, Brosen K, Arendt-Nielsen L, et al: Codeine and morphine in extensive and poor metabolizers of sparteine: Pharmacokinetics, analgesic effect and side effects. Eur J Clin Pharmacol 1996;51:289–295.
12. Eckhardt K, Li S, Ammon S, et al: Same incidence of adverse drug events after codeine administration irrespective of the genetically determined differences in morphine formation. Pain 1998;76:27–33.
13. Williams DG, Hatch DJ, Howard RF: Codeine phosphate in paediatric medicine. Br J Anaesth 2001;86:413–421.
14. Williams DG, Patel A, Howard RF: Pharmacogenetics of codeine metabolism in an urban population of children and its implications for analgesic reliability. Br J Anaesth 2002;89:839–845.
15. Fagerlund TH, Braaten Ø: No pain relief from codeine…? An introduction to pharmacogenomics. Acta Anaesthesiol Scand 2001;68:140–149.
16. Raffa RB, Friderichs E, Reimann W, et al: Complementary and synergistic antinociceptive interaction between the enantiomers of tramadol. J Pharmacol Exp Ther 1993;267:331–340.
17. Poulsen L, Arendt-Nielsen L, Brosen K, Sindrup SH: The hypoalgesic effect of tramadol in relation to CYP2D6. Clin Pharmacol Ther 1996;60:636–644.
18. Stamer UM, Lehnen K, Höthker F, et al: Impact of CYP2D6 genotype on postoperative tramadol analgesia. Pain 2003;105:231–238.
19. Kaiser R, Sezer O, Papies A, et al: Patient-tailored antiemetic treatment with 5-hydroxytryptamine type 3 receptor antagonists according to cytochrome P-450 2D6 genotypes. J Clin Oncol 2002;20:2805–2811.
20. Kim M-K, Cho J-Y, Lim H-S, et al: Effect of the CYP2D6 genotype on the pharmacogenetics of tropisetron in healthy Korean subjects. Eur J Clin Pharmacol 2003;9:111–116.
21. Candiotti KA, Birnbach DJ, Lubarsky DA, et al: The impact of pharmacogenomics on postoperative nausea and vomiting: Do CYP2D6 allele copy number and polymorphisms affect the success or failure of ondansetron prophylaxis? Anesthesiology 2005;102:543–549.
22. Werner U, Werner D, Rau T, et al: Celecoxib inhibits metabolism of cytochrome P450 2D6 substrate metoprolol in humans. Clin Pharmacol Ther 2003;74:130–137.
23. Werner D, Wuttke H, Fromm MF, et al: Effect of amiodarone on the plasma levels of metoprolol. Am J Cardiol 2004;94:1319–1321.
24. Koch T, Kroslak T, Averbeck M, et al: Allelic variation S268P of the human mu-opioid receptor affects both desensitization and G protein coupling. Mol Pharmacol 2000;58:328–334.
25. Befort K, Filliol D, Decaillot FM, et al: A single nucleotide polymorphic mutation in the human mu-opioid receptor severely impairs receptor signaling. J Biol Chem 2001;276:3130–3137.
26. Lötsch J, Skarke C, Grosch S, et al: The polymorphism A118G of the human mu-opioid receptor gene decreases the pupil constrictory effect of morphine-6-glucuronide but not that of morphine. Pharmacogenetics 2002;12:3–9.
27. Lötsch J, Zimmermann M, Darimont J, et al: Does the A118G polymorphism at the mu-opioid receptor gene protect against morphine-6-glucuronide toxicity? Anesthesiology 2002;97:814–819.
28. Klepstad P, Rakvag TT, Kaasa S, et al: The 118 A→G polymorphism in the human micro-opioid receptor gene may increase morphine requirements in patients with pain caused by malignant disease. Acta Anaesthesiol Scand 2004;48:1232–1239.
29. Eisenach JC: Fishing for genes: Practical ways to study polymorphisms for pain. Anesthesiology 2004;100:1343–1344.
30. Hoehe MR, Kopke K, Wendel B, et al: Sequence variability and candidate gene analysis in complex disease: Association of mu-opioid receptor gene variation with substance dependence. Hum Mol Genet 2000;9:2895–2908.
31. Pasternak GW, Pan YX: Alternative splicing of mu-opioid receptors. In Mogil JS (ed): The Genetics of Pain. Seattle, IASP Press, 2004, pp 85–103.
32. Koch T, Schulz S, Pfeiffer M, et al: C-terminal splice variants of the mouse mu-opioid receptor differ in morphine-induced internalization and receptor resensitization. J Biol Chem 2001;276:31408–31414.
33. Abbadie C, Pan YX, Pasternak GW: Differential distribution in rat brain of mu opioid receptor carboxy terminal splice variants MOR-1C-like and MOR-1-like immunoreactivity: Evidence for region-specific processing. J Comp Neurol 2000;419:244–256.
34. Abbadie C, Pasternak GW, Aicher SA: Presynaptic localization of the carboxy-terminus epitopes of the mu opioid receptor splice variants MOR-1C and MOR-1D in the superficial laminae of the rat spinal cord. Neuroscience 2001;106:833–842.
35. Pick CG, Cheng J, Paul D, Pasternak G: Genetic influences in opioid analgesic sensitivity in mice. Brain Res 1991;556:295–298.
36. Kirchheiner J, Störmer E, Meisel C, et al: Influence of CYP2C9 genetic polymorphisms on pharmacokinetics of celecoxib and its metabolites. Pharmacogenetics. 2003;13:473–480.
37. Tang C, Shou M, Rushmore TH, et al: In-vitro metabolism of celecoxib, a cyclooxygenase-2 inhibitor, by allelic variant forms of human liver microsomal cytochrome P450 2C9: Correlation with CYP2C9 genotype and in-vivo pharmacokinetics. Pharmacogenetics 2001;11:223–235.
38. Kirchheiner J, Meineke I, Freytag G, et al: Enantiospecific effects of cytochrome P450 2C9 amino acid variants on ibuprofen pharmacokinetics and on the inhibition of cyclooxygenases 1 and 2. Clin Pharmacol Ther 2002;72:62–75.
39. Kirchheiner J, Sasse J, Meineke I, et al: Trimipramine pharmacogenetics after intravenous and oral administration in carriers of CYP2D6 genotypes predicting poor, extensive and ultrahigh activity. Pharmacogenetics 2004;13:721–728.
40. Kirchheiner J, Nickchen K, Bauer M, et al: Pharmacogenetics of antidepressants and antipsychotics: The contribution of allelic variations to the phenotype of drug response. Mol Psychiatry 2004;9:442–473.
41. Unruh AM: Gender variations in clinical pain experience. Pain 1996;65:23–67.
42. Riley J, Robinson MG, Wise EA, et al: Sex differences in the perception of noxious experimental stimuli: A meta-analysis. Pain 1998;74:180–187.
43. Taenzer AH, Clark C, Curry CS: Gender affects report of pain and function after arthroscopic anterior cruciate ligament reconstruction. Anesthesiology 2000;53:670–675.
44. Cepeda MS, Carr DB: Women experience more pain and require more morphine than men to achieve a similar degree of analgesia. Anesth Analg 2003;97:1464–1468.
45. Gear RW, Miaskowski C, Gordon NC, et al: Kappa-opioids produce significantly greater analgesia in women than in men. Nat Med 1996;2:1248–1250.
46. Gear RW, Miaskowski C, Gordon NC, et al: The kappa opioid nalbuphine produces gender- and dose-dependent analgesia and antianalgesia in patients with postoperative pain. Pain 1999;83:339–345.
47. Mogil JS, Wilson SG, Chesler EJ, et al: The melanocortin-1 receptor gene mediates female-specific mechanisms of analgesia in mice and humans. Proc Natl Acad Sci USA 2003;100:4867–4872.
48. Liem EB, Lin CM, Suleman MI, et al: Anesthetic requirement is increased in redheads. Anesthesiology 2004;101:279–283.
49. Liem EB, Joiner TV, Tsueda K, Sessler DI: Increased sensitivity to thermal pain and reduced subcutaneous lidocaine efficacy in redheads. Anesthesiology 2005;102:509–514.
50. Zubieta JK, Heitzeg MM, Smith YR, et al: COMT val158met genotype affects mu-opioid neurotransmitter responses to a pain stressor. Science 2003;299(5610):1240–1243.

8 术后疼痛处理与患者结局

CHRISTOPHER L. WU · ROBERT W. HURLEY

近几十年来，我们对伤害性感受的神经生物学、术后疼痛的急性与慢性有害影响以及术后疼痛各种治疗方法的认识有了成倍的提高。这些认识的进步也同时提高了人们对术后疼痛治疗的认识，这体现在美国医疗保健质量与研究机构提出了美国急性疼痛处理实践指南以及专家委员会提出的急性疼痛处理临床实践指南[1-3]。另外，美国医院认证的医疗保健机构认证联合委员会（Joint Commission on Accreditation of Healthcare Organizations，JCAHO）也执行新的疼痛处理标准[4]。最后，术后疼痛治疗的进步已经使术后镇痛的实施达到最佳水平。

尽管传统上一直以主要并发症的发病率和死亡率来判断治疗结果，但通常还要结合一些非传统的判断指标，如患者满意度、生活质量以及康复质量。然而，尚不明了术后疼痛本身能否真正影响患者结局。当然，术后疼痛对患者生理与心理有诸多害处，最终可能导致患者发病率和死亡率升高。动物与人体的研究均提示，控制术后疼痛可能降低其中的一些有害作用，从而改善患者术后结局。此外，不同镇痛方案在不同水平发挥镇痛作用，可能对患者结局产生不同影响。最后，术后疼痛治疗的组织实施（如"急性疼痛治疗"）也可能影响患者的结局。

术后疼痛的急性与慢性后果

要理解术后疼痛及其治疗如何最大限度地影响患者结局，就需要全面了解术后疼痛对机体的急性和慢性影响，包括对伤害性感受的神经生物学的了解。术后疼痛对患者传统性与非传统性治疗结果均能产生广泛的有害性急性与慢性影响。

急性作用

手术所造成的创伤可引起各种病理生理反应，而伤害性感受传入可能加重这些反应，且可能增加患者疼痛的发病率和死亡率。局部炎症及全身介质所介导的神经内分泌应激反应部分是由于伤害性感觉信息传递到中枢神经系统（central nervous system，CNS）所致。这种神经内分泌应激反应本质上是一种分解代谢亢进的高代谢状态，代谢和氧耗水平增加，导致水钠潴留以及血液葡萄糖、游离脂肪酸、酮体和乳酸升高。这种神经内分泌应激反应可能影响身体其他器官系统和区域。患者可能存在血液高凝（包括纤溶抑制、血小板反应性增高以及血浆黏滞性增加）[5]、术后免疫抑制[6]及伤口愈合差[7]。

未予控制的术后疼痛主要通过激活交感神经系统可能导致发病率或死亡率增加。交感神经激活可增加心肌氧耗或通过冠状血管收缩而减少心肌氧供，可能增加心肌缺血和心肌梗死的发生[8]。未被控制的术后疼痛可引起交感传出兴奋增加，也可能进一步减弱胃肠功能，延缓其恢复。此外，术后疼痛还能引起一些有害的神经反射活动而损害术后呼吸系统的功能，尤其是上腹部手术和胸部手术[9]，同时亦抑制胃肠功能[10,11]。

慢性作用

术后出现慢性疼痛可能是由于术后对疼痛控制不理想所致[12,13]。尽管这种因果关系并不明确，但是研究提示术后疼痛由急性向慢性转变比以前想像的要早得多[14]。某些手术后发生慢性疼痛较常见，包括截肢术（高达83%）、胸廓切开术（高达67%）、胸骨切开术（27%）、乳房手术（高达57%）及胆囊手术（高达56%）[12-15]。胸腔手术、疝修补术、截肢术、乳房手术及胆囊手术术后急性疼痛的严重程度可能是发生慢性疼痛的重要预测因子[15-22]。此外，控制术后疼痛的严重程度可能改善患者的远期结局[23-25]。

疼痛通路及伤害性感受的神经生物学

由于控制术后疼痛对于术后出现慢性疼痛可能具有重要意义，因此了解伤害性感受的神经生物学有助于我们理解各种传导通路的重要性，以及它们在急性疼痛向慢性疼痛转化中的作用。术后组织损伤可引起炎性介质释放，从而激活外周伤害性感受器。直径小的A-δ和C纤维可将伤害性信息传递到脊髓背角。神经传递由数量众多的肽类和氨基酸类物质来执行，包括P物质、降钙素、促生长激素、肠多肽以及生长激素等。这些神经递质可激活脊髓次级投射神经元，这些神经元具有各种各样的受体，其中一些可促进伤害性疼痛的传递。这些受体包括兴奋性氨基酸受体如NMDA受体、AMPA/KA受体、mGluR以及P物质（SP）与神经激肽（NK-1）受体。

脊髓背角是伤害性感受整合的重要部位之一，因为它同时接受来自外周伤害性感受器和下行调理部位的传入信息。外周伤害性刺激不断传入可引起脊髓或中枢敏化，表现为伤害性感受器激活阈值降低，激活后放电频率增高，基础或自发性放电频率增快[14]。虽然目前尚不明确各种神经递质在伤害性感受过程中的确切作用，但某些受体（如NMDA）似乎对急性损伤后发生慢性疼痛更为重要[26]。浅表和深部背角突触前后均能发现NMDA受体，它们可增加伤害性疼痛信息的传递[27]。因此，就目前对伤害性感受神经生物学的认识，手术损伤引起的外周持续性伤害性传入可使中枢敏化并导致慢性疼痛。减轻或防止中枢敏化和术后疼痛可降低术后慢性疼痛的发生率[28,29]。

超前镇痛

应用抗伤害性治疗来防止或减弱术后中枢敏化及兴奋性增高（如超前镇痛）对患者术后恢复可能具有短期（如术后疼痛减轻）和长期（如慢性疼痛减少）的双重作用（图8-1）。虽然实验研究表明超前镇痛可有效减少术后疼痛，但是临床试验结果尚有争议[30-33]。超前镇痛临床意义存在争论的原因之一就是超前镇痛的确切定义尚未确定。人们提出了数种定义，大体分为"狭义"（即术中）和"广义"（即围手术期）两类[30]。狭义超前镇痛的定义主要集中在镇痛介入的时间（即切皮前或切皮后），但是没有涉及这种镇痛治疗失效后术后疼痛可能会引起中枢敏化的问题。因此，这种狭义的定义可能是导致不同临床研究中难以测定超前镇痛作用的原因。

广义定义说明了超前镇痛其他方面的作用（即介入的强度与持续时间），其可能与治疗切口与炎性损伤的临床相关性更强，后两者对中枢敏化的启动与维持具有重要作用（图8-2）。因此，镇痛干预本身的确切时机可能不如其防止中枢敏化的作用重要。已经应用各种药物与技术来研究这个问题，但仍未得到一个有

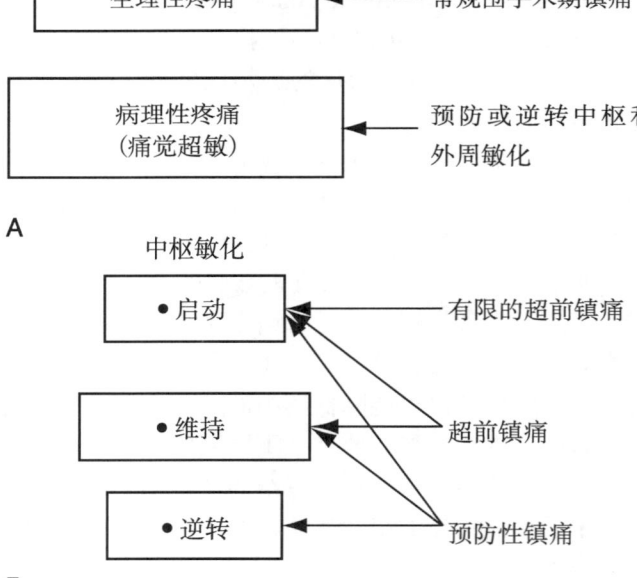

图8-1 中枢敏化和术后疼痛。A. 术后疼痛治疗：与常规围手术期镇痛方法相比较，超前镇痛只着眼于病理性疼痛的预防。B. 采用不同方法以排除中枢敏化对术后疼痛的促进作用。(From Kissin I: Preemptive analgesia. Anesthesiology 2000; 93:1138-1143.)

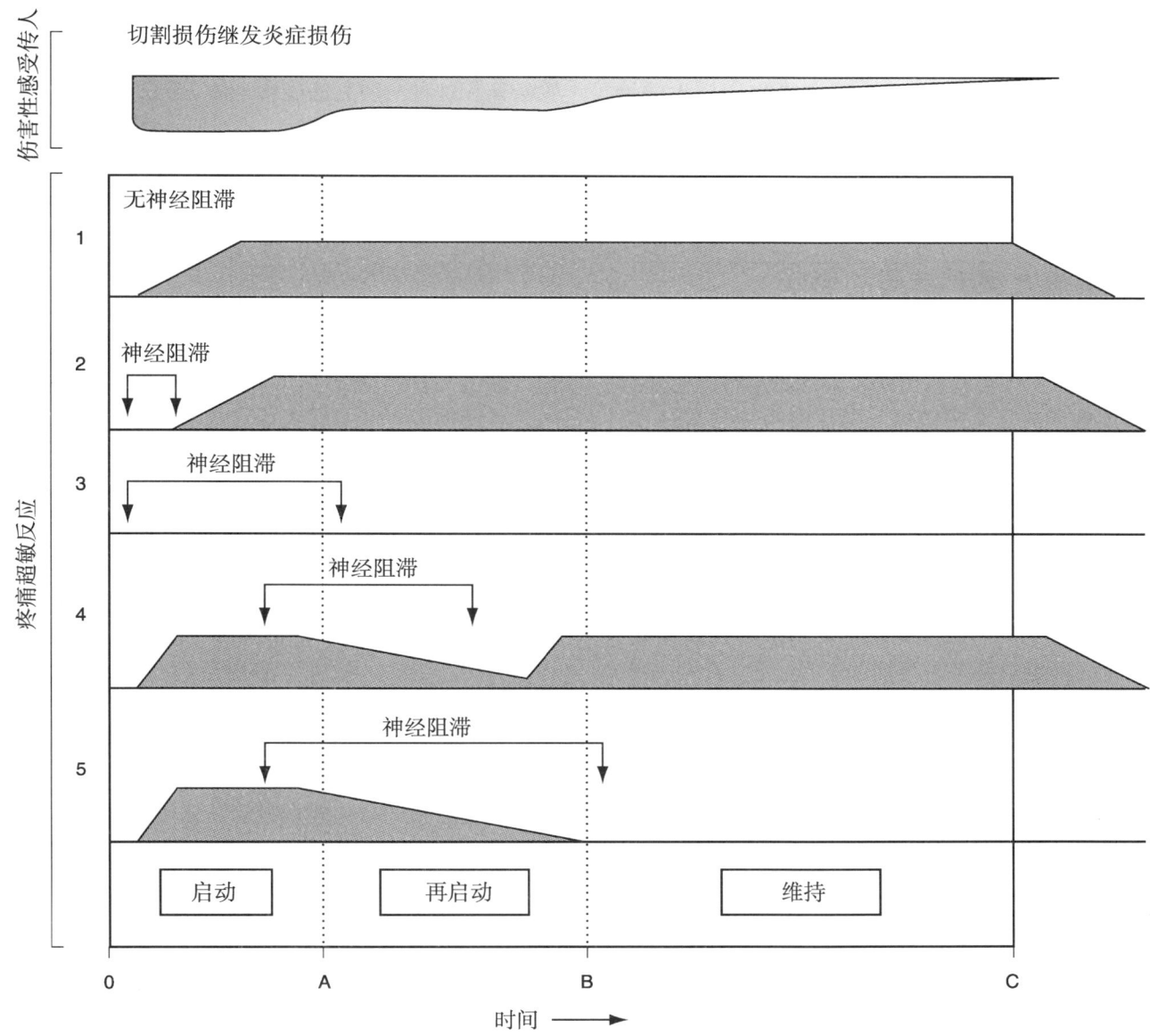

图 8-2 该模型阐明神经阻滞下疼痛超敏先占效应和逆转所必需的假设条件。图示顶端显示切割损伤、炎症损伤或者两者同时存在引起的伤害性感受传入,条带宽度表示传入的强度。图示底部显示不同神经阻滞条件下对伤害性传入可能产生的变化的5种疼痛超敏反应:已经建立疼痛超敏时给予神经阻滞:①没有;②较短时间;③持续较长时间;④损伤前阻滞但较短;⑤损伤前阻滞但持续时间较长。时间A指该时间以后伤害性传入不能启动疼痛超敏,但是强度足够再次启动(如果神经阻滞前已经建立疼痛超敏);时间B指该时间以后指伤害性传入不能再次启动疼痛超敏,但是能维持疼痛超敏性(到时间C终止)。能够启动并维持中枢敏化的伤害性传入持续时间决定了可能先占效应的效力。如果阻滞一直持续到传入衰减至不能触发中枢超敏化的水平时,先占效应可能具有临床意义(见于变量2、3)。中枢超敏的逆转取决于两个因素:持续中枢敏化以及能启动、再次启动并维持(分别与传入强度下降水平相一致)疼痛超敏的持续传入冲动。阻滞作用应该持续到中枢敏化衰减,并且传入强度低于可能有效地再次启动中枢超敏的水平(变量5)。由于再次启动中枢超敏的传入强度低于其启动中枢超敏的强度,因此成功逆转疼痛超敏(允许较大的输入衰减)的神经阻滞作用时间应该长于先占效应时间(允许较强的传入衰减)。(From Kissin I: Preemptive analgesia. Anesthesiology 2000;93:1138-1143; modified from Kissin I, Lee SS, Bradley EL Jr: Effect of prolonged nerve block on inflammatory hyperalgesia in rats: Prevention of late hyperalgesia. Anesthesiology 1998;88:224-232.)

关超前镇痛的确切临床结论[33]。然而，采用超前镇痛广义定义的临床试验结果表明，这种模式是一种临床相关现象，只有当术中完全阻断有害刺激，并将这种阻断作用延续到术后，才可取得临床最大的治疗效果[34]。因此，应用超前镇痛来防止中枢敏化，尤其是综合应用多种强效的镇痛措施（见后述），可能会减轻术后急性与慢性疼痛[12,28]。

不同镇痛方案对结局的影响

尽管有很多镇痛方法可用于治疗术后疼痛，但只有某些特殊方法才可改善围手术期患者结局。这里讨论的最常见方法是全身镇痛（阿片类药物与NSAID）与区域镇痛（椎管内阻滞与外周神经阻滞）技术。每种镇痛技术或药物对患者结局的影响可能与多种因素有关，包括所提供的镇痛水平、围手术期伤害刺激影响是否减弱以及有无副作用。此外，某种特殊技术或药物（如硬膜外镇痛）对不同患者结局的影响可能也有所不同。尽管某些镇痛方法显然有利于患者结局，但是临床医师也必须考虑可能的不良事件，其中某些副作用虽然罕见，但却可能是致命性的，所以对每例患者均应选择合适的镇痛方法。

全身镇痛

数种全身性镇痛药可用于治疗术后疼痛，但是最常用的两种药物是阿片类药物和NSAID。这两类药物均可口服或静脉给药，但是后者更常用于术后不能耐受口服药物的患者。这些药物能提供良好的术后镇痛作用。然而，仅用于全身性给药时，这些药物可能不足以减轻围手术期病理生理反应，以改善传统意义上的患者结局。

全身应用阿片类药物

尽管阿片类药物用于治疗术后疼痛可能有效，但其在镇痛中的作用常受限于诸如易出现耐受，以及恶心、呕吐、镇静和呼吸抑制等典型副作用的出现[35]。阿片类药物可经皮下、肌内或皮肤给药，但是最有效的给药途径是静脉内给药，尤其病人自控静脉给药（intravenous patient-controlled anesthesia，IV-PCA）方式。经皮给予芬太尼已经用于处理急性疼痛[36]，然而芬太尼经皮持续稳定释放的给药模式在急性疼痛治疗中不易调节给药剂量。新近也有PCA经皮芬太尼电子给药装置用于急性疼痛的报道[37,38]。

全身性阿片类药物的最佳给药途径是通过PCA装置给药。这种给药方法能够个体化用药，满足术后阿片类药物需求量在个体间存在的巨大差异，并最大限度地减少患者个体间药效动力学和药代动力学差异的影响。通过PCA装置给予阿片类药物的镇痛效果一般优于其他"按需"给药方法（肌内、皮下）。经皮PCA给予阿片类药物所产生的镇痛作用与IV-PCA相似[38]。

全身应用阿片类药物对患者结局的影响 与其他镇痛方法相比，全身性阿片类药物在改善患者术后结局方面似乎并无优越性。尚无确切证据提示全身应用阿片类药物可降低术后患者死亡率。但是，患者的结局因全身阿片类药物给药方法的不同而异。PCA装置（无论静脉内或经皮）是各种全身性使用阿片类药物方法中的"金标准"。

与传统"按需"给药方式（一般为肌内或皮下）相比，IV-PCA不仅可提供更好的术后镇痛效果，而且可提高患者满意度，降低肺部并发症的风险[39,40]。对15项随机试验（"按需"肌内给药与IV-PCA相比）进行的荟萃分析结果显示，IV-PCA的镇痛效果明显较优，但是死亡率或发病率并无显著下降[40]。随后的一项定量系统回顾（对IV-PCA与非IV-PCA全身给予阿片类药物进行比较）显示，使用IV-PCA的患者肺部并发症的风险较低（图8-3）[39]。

与传统"按需"镇痛方案相比，IV-PCA也可能改善患者自我评价的结果，如患者满意度，尽管这种结果的评价极为复杂。与其他方法如"按需"肌内或皮下给予阿片类药物相比，患者更易接受IV-PCA[39-41]。患者对IV-PCA满意度较高的原因尚不明了，但可能与其镇痛效果较好、可自控给药以及避免向护理人员主诉疼痛或索要镇痛药有关[41-44]。尽管各种镇痛技术的副作用发生率不同可能影响患者满意度，但是IV-PCA所引起的阿片类药物相关副作用的发生率与肌内、皮下或经皮给药镇痛并无明显差异[38]。

非甾体类抗炎药

NSAID包括阿司匹林和对乙酰氨基酚，通过抑制环氧合酶和前列腺素的合成而发挥镇痛作用，这两者都是外周与中枢敏化的重要介质。NSAID对轻中度术后疼痛具有良好的镇痛作用，是阿片类药物治疗中重

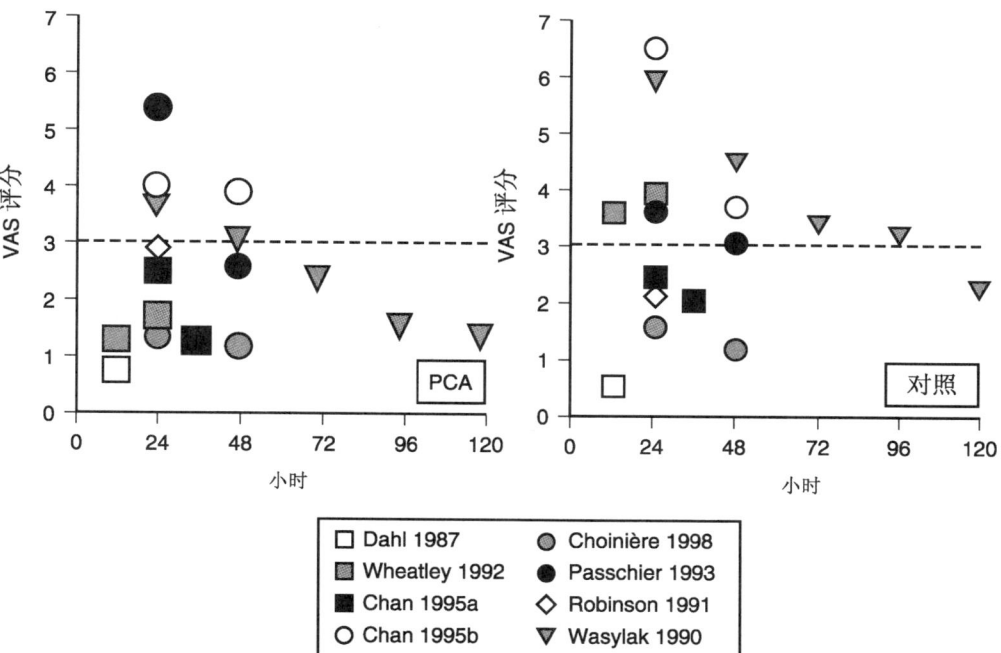

图8-3 患者自控镇痛（PCA）（左）和对照（右）的疼痛强度评分。数据来自于8项吗啡试验所报道的视觉模拟评分（VAS）疼痛强度。记号大小与试验样本大小成比例。图中虚线表示中度疼痛。(From Walder B, Schafer M, Henzi I, Tramer MR: Efficacy and safety of patient-controlled opioid analgesia for acute postoperative pain: A quantitative systematic review. Acta Anaesthesiol Scand 2001;45:795-804.)

度术后疼痛的有效辅助药物。随着特异性环氧合酶抑制剂（如环氧合酶2抑制剂）的问世，人们一般认为口服或肠道外给予NSAID是多模式镇痛方案的组成部分，因为其镇痛机制不同于阿片类药物和局部麻醉药。

对患者结局的影响 与阿片类药物一样，与其他镇痛药物相比，NSAID本身对死亡率或发病率无显著影响。然而，NSAID可能改善镇痛效果和患者的自我评价（如患者满意度），这部分是由于可减少患者对阿片类药物的需求，从而减少阿片类药物的副作用以及促进患者恢复[46-48]。当作为全身阿片类药物的辅助用药时，NSAID可改善术后镇痛效果，且可减少对阿片类药物的需求达50%。后一种作用可能减少阿片类药物相关副作用，促进胃肠功能恢复，减少呼吸抑制，提高患者满意度。然而，并非所有研究都认为同时使用NSAID能减少阿片类药物相关副作用[49-51]。

区域镇痛与外周镇痛

各种椎管内（主要是硬膜外）及外周镇痛技术可有效地治疗术后疼痛。硬膜外及外周镇痛方法，尤其是应用以局部麻醉药为主的镇痛配方时，所产生的镇痛效果优于全身使用阿片类药物[52,53]。与全身应用阿片类药物镇痛不同的是，区域镇痛技术可能对患者的生理功能有利，包括可能减少手术的围手术期伤害作用，从而改善患者结局，包括使常见并发症的发病率下降。具体如何采用区域镇痛技术（如导管位置、局部麻醉药与阿片类药物镇痛方案、镇痛持续时间）将影响患者结局的改善程度。

椎管内阿片类药物

椎管内应用阿片类药物为主的镇痛方法，可以采取单次或持续给药的方式，可有效地控制术后疼痛。根据阿片类药物的亲脂性可将椎管内阿片类药物进行分类，亲脂性药物（如芬太尼、舒芬太尼）较疏脂性/亲水性药物（如吗啡、氢吗啡酮）起效快，但作用时间较短。总体上说，与静脉持续给药方式相比，持续硬膜外给予亲脂性阿片类药物的优点最少，但是持续硬膜外给予亲水性阿片类药物的镇痛效果优于传统上"按需"静脉内给予阿片类药物[55,56]。硬膜外持续给予阿片类药物的镇痛效果可能优于间断单次给药，且前者副作用较少[57,58]。

椎管内阿片类药物对患者结局的影响 椎管内应用阿片类药物可能减弱围手术期病理生理反应（如神经内分泌应激反应），这种作用一般并不见于全身应用常规临床剂量的阿片类药物时，因此可能影响围手术期患者结局。尽管椎管内应用阿片类药物所产生的镇痛作用优于全身应用阿片类药物，但是椎管内给予阿片类药物一般只能部分减弱围手术期病理生理反应。椎管内应用阿片类药物可调节围手术期应激反应，但是减轻程度不如应用以局部麻醉药为主的硬膜外镇痛方法[59]。这种部分而不是完全地抑制围手术期病理生理反应的作用可能是由于椎管内阿片类药物允许伤害性信息中枢神经系统中的传递,因此不能完全阻止神经内分泌应激反应。所以,椎管内应用阿片类药物对患者结局的影响可能不如应用以局部麻醉药为主的硬膜外镇痛方案。

即使椎管内应用阿片类药物只能部分减弱围手术期病理生理反应,但是一些研究表明,椎管内应用阿片类药物尤其是硬膜外吗啡的患者术后结局可优于全身应用阿片类药物(表 8-1)[60-67]。随机研究表明,围手术期硬膜外吗啡患者的心血管和肺部并发症少于全身应用阿片类药物患者[61,62,64-67]。数项随机试验的荟萃分析结果证实,与全身应用阿片类药物相比,硬膜外使用吗啡可降低术后肺不张的发生率[68]。因此,围手术期椎管内应用阿片类药物在某些情况下可能改善患者结局。最后,椎管内所应用阿片类药物的某些副作用可能影响患者结局[69]。例如,椎管内应用阿片类药物可导致剂量依赖性恶心与呕吐的发生[71,72],单次剂量后发生率为20%~50%,持续给药可达到45%~80%[73]。此外,60%椎管内给予阿片类药物的患者可能发生瘙痒,而硬膜外给予局部麻醉药或全身使用阿片类药物的患者只有15%~18%出现瘙痒[39,74,75]。

以局部麻醉药为主的硬膜外镇痛

以局部麻醉药为主的硬膜外镇痛(一般应用小量亲脂性阿片类药物)是治疗术后疼痛的一种有效方法[76]。以局部麻醉药为主的硬膜外镇痛方法所产生的镇痛效果优于全身应用阿片类药物(图 8-4)[53]。硬膜外镇痛可以采用持续给药方式或患者自控硬膜外镇痛方式(patient-controlled epidural analgesia,PCEA)。与 IV-PCA 一样,PCEA 能满足术后镇痛的个体化用药需求,在几个方面可能优于持续性硬膜外给药(如药物需求量较少,患者满意度较高,镇痛效果较好),是一种安全有效的术后镇痛方法[80,81]。总之,PCEA 的镇痛效果和患者满意度均优于 IV-PCA[82,83]。硬膜外局部麻醉药可引起一些副作用,可能影响患者某些结局。例如,局部麻醉药可能引起低血压(发生率为 0.7%~3%)[54,80,84],或可能导致下肢运动阻滞(2%~3%)[54,80]。

硬膜外镇痛对患者结局的影响 以局部麻醉药为主的硬膜外镇痛配方能减弱或甚至完全抑制围手术期

表 8-1 硬膜外吗啡与全身应用阿片类药物术后镇痛的结局研究

研究	研究人群(例数)	试验设计	发病率(EA vs SYST)	死亡率(EA vs SYST)
Park et al (2001)[60]	ABD (1021)	RCT	22% vs 37%*	综合资料
Tsui et al (1997)[61]	ABD-THOR (578)	RCT	EA 改善肺部(EA:13% vs 25%;$P=0.002$)和 CV(EA:21% vs 43%;$P<0.001$)结果以及 LOS(EA:22±20 vs 30±37;$P=0.005$)	EA:8% vs 14%;$P=0.038$
Mojor et al (1996)[62]	ABD (65)	OBS	EA 改善 CV($P=0.002$)和肺($P=0.019$)结果以及 ICU 中 LOS($P=0.024$)	无报道
Liu et al (1995)[63]	ABD (54)	RCT	硬膜外与全身阿片类药物对 GI 恢复无差异	无报道
Beattie et al (1993)[64]	Mixed (55)	RCT	EA 改善 CV 缺血(EA:17.2% vs 50%;$P<0.01$)和快速型心律失常(EA:20.7% vs 50%;$P<0.05$)	无报道
Her et al (1990)[65]	ABD (49)	OBS	EA 改善机械通气需求($P=0.002$)、呼吸衰竭($P=0.018$)和 ICU 中 LOS(EA:2.7d vs 3.8d;$P=0.003$)	无报道
Hasenbos et al (1987)[66]	THOR (129)	RCT	EA 改善肺部并发症(EA:12.1% vs 38%)	无报道
Rawal et al (1984)[67]	ABD	RCT	EA 改善肺部并发症(EA:13% vs 40%)、GI GIal ce(EA:56.7±3.1h vs 75.1±3.1h;$P<0.05$)和 LOS(EA:7±0.5d vs 9±0.6d;$P<0.05$)	无报道

*所显示的资料来自显示总体无差异的(主动脉瘤修复手术)研究的亚组患者。发病率和死亡率综合资料。
ABD,腹部手术;CV,心血管;EA,硬膜外麻醉;GI,胃肠;ICU,加强医疗病房;LOS,住院时间;OBS,观察;RCT,随机对照试验;SYST,

病理生理反应。结果，这些患者的发病率与死亡率可能低于全身使用阿片类药物镇痛的患者[10,11,68,85,86]。此外，相比于全身应用阿片类药物，硬膜外镇痛效果更优，可能改善患者结局。研究已提示，术中应用局部麻醉药可降低患者死亡率；对随机试验的一项荟萃分析[区域麻醉随机试验共同观察（Collaborative Overview of Randomised Trials of Regional Anaesthesia，CORTRA）荟萃分析：包括9559例对象的141项试验]结果证实，椎管内麻醉与镇痛可将30日死亡率降低约30%（图8-5）[86]。

与某些情况下全身甚或椎管内应用阿片类药物相比，以局部麻醉药为主的硬膜外镇痛可降低术后凝血系统以及胃肠、肺和心脏并发症的发生率（图8-6）[10,11,86]。以局部麻醉药为主的胸部硬膜外镇痛可抑制交感神经冲动传出，减少阿片类药物应用总量，减轻胃肠道的脊髓反射性抑制作用[10,87]，从而促进胃肠动力的恢复。随机对照试验（randomized controlled trial，RCT）表明，以局部麻醉药为主的术后胸部硬膜外镇痛可使患者胃肠功能恢复时间以及达到出院标准的时间均早于全身应用阿片类药物镇痛的患者[63,82,88]。此外，接受硬膜外局部麻醉药的患者，腹部手术后胃肠动力恢复也早于接受硬膜外阿片类药物的患者[63,89,90]。尚无资料显示，胸部硬膜外局部麻醉药镇痛是否可引起肠吻合口裂开[91]。

以局部麻醉药为主的硬膜外镇痛方案还可通过维护患者术后肺功能、提供更佳镇痛效果、减弱脊髓对膈肌功能的反射性抑制作用[10]，从而降低胸腹部手术高危患者术后肺部并发症的发生率[68,85]。对约50项RCT的荟萃分析以及一项大型RCT证实，以局部麻醉药为主的胸部硬膜外镇痛患者的肺部感染和并发症发生率均低于硬膜外或全身应用阿片类药物的患者（图8-7）。对15项试验1178例冠状动脉旁路移植患

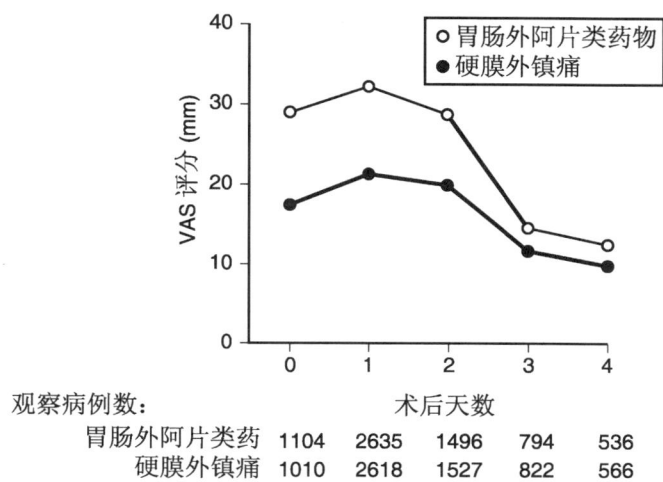

图8-4 胃肠外阿片类药物和硬膜外镇痛用于控制术后疼痛的比较。术后前4天硬膜外镇痛效果显著优于胃肠外阿片类药物。VAS，视觉模拟评分。(From Block BM, Liu SS, Rowlingson AJ, et al: Efficacy of postoperative epidural analgesia: A meta-analysis. JAMA 2003;290:2455-2463.)

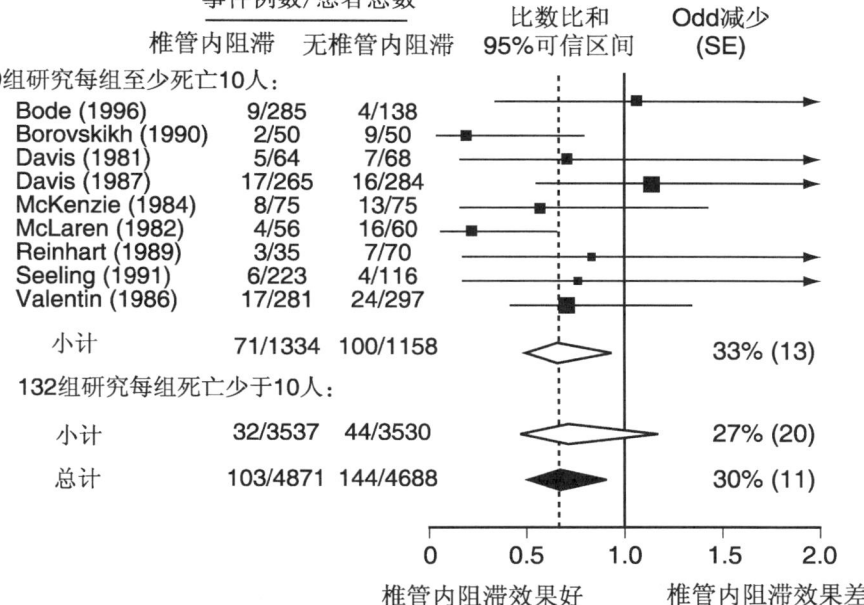

图8-5 椎管内阻滞对术后30天内死亡率的影响。菱形显示综合试验结果比数比的95%可信区间。纵轴表示总体结果。SE，抽样误差。(From Rodgers A, Walker N, Schug S, et al: Reduction of postoperative mortality and morbidity with epidural or spinal anaesthesia: Results from overview of randomised trials. BMJ 2000;321:1493.)

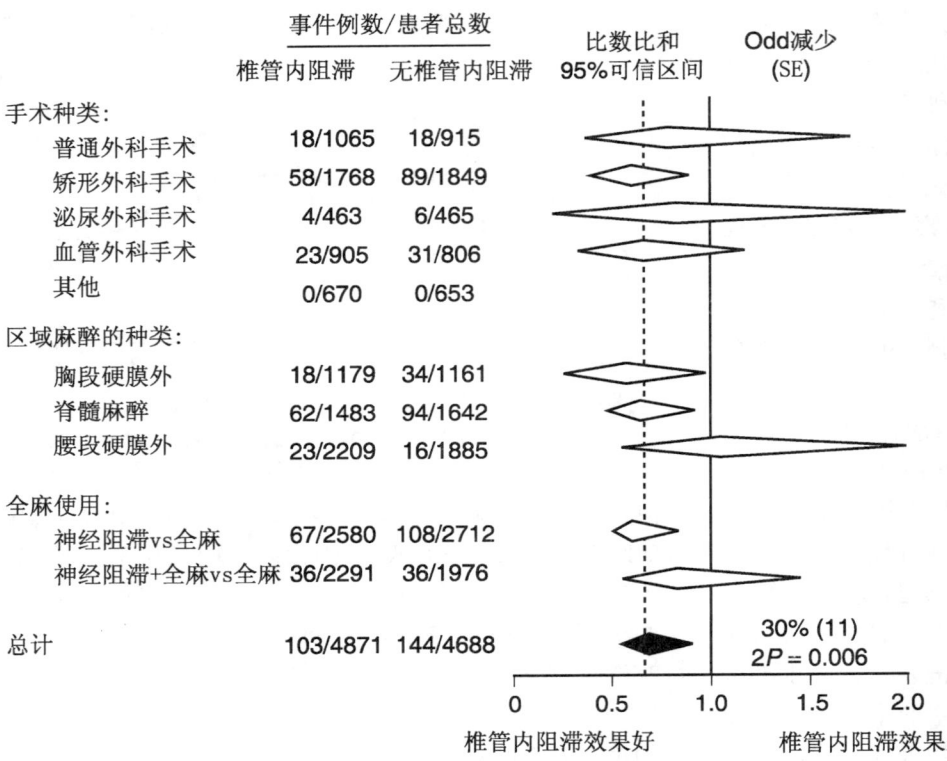

图 8-6 椎管内阻滞对术后并发症的影响。菱形表示综合试验结果比数比的 95% 可信区间。纵轴表示总体综合结果。(From Rodgers A, Walker N, Schug S, et al: Reduction of postoperative mortality and morbidity with epidural or spinal anaesthesia: Results from overview of randomised trials. BMJ 2000;16:321.)

者的荟萃分析结果表明，胸部硬膜外镇痛可明显降低心律失常风险[比数比（OR）0.52]和肺部并发症发生率（OR 0.41），并使拔管时间提前 4.5h[92]（图 8-8）。

此外，术中硬膜外麻醉和腰麻可能降低围手术期患者的高凝状态，如深静脉血栓形成（deep venous thrombosis，DVT）、肺动脉栓塞以及血管移植失败。CORTRA 荟萃分析中进一步分析了术中椎管内麻醉对围手术期发病率的影响；作者注意到，椎管内麻醉和镇痛可将 DVT 发生率降低 44%，肺栓塞发生率降低 55%（图 8-6）[86]。一项较早的荟萃分析也表明，与全身麻醉相比，术中椎管内麻醉可使 DVT 发生率降低

31%[93]；全身麻醉下发生 DVT 的发病率高出约 4 倍。一项关于下肢择期血管重建手术患者的 RCT 中，随机接受围手术期硬膜外麻醉/镇痛的患者血管需再次搭桥或需行栓子切除术的几率要低于接受全身麻醉的患者。另外一项关于下肢血管再通术患者的 RCT 表明，麻醉方案中包含硬膜外麻醉-镇痛的患者血栓形成（外周动脉移植冠状动脉或深静脉血栓形成）的发生率较低[95]。围手术期应用硬膜外麻醉可能通过增加血流量和减弱围手术期应激反应来降低高凝事件的发生率。然而，应该注意的是，许多较早期的试验并没有同时预防性应用抗凝药物；因此，目前尚不明了围手术期

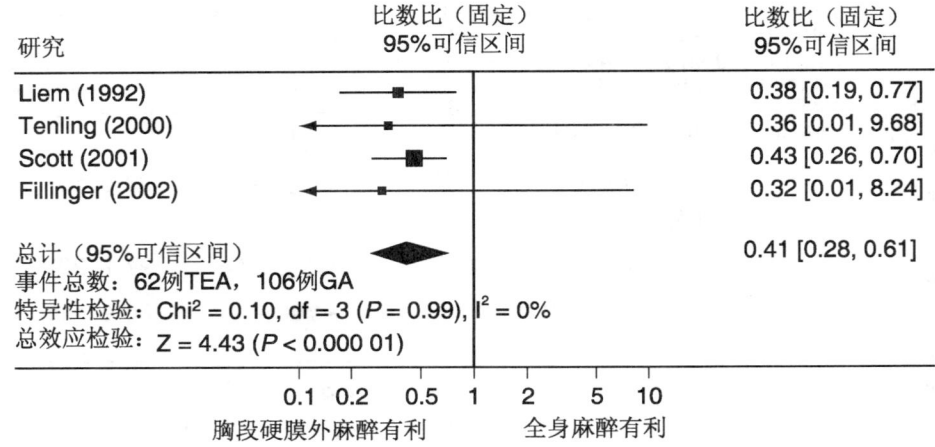

图 8-7 围手术期硬膜外镇痛对冠脉旁路移植患者肺部并发症发生率的影响。菱形表示试验结果比数比的 95% 可信区间。GA，全麻；OR，比数比；TEA，胸段硬膜外麻醉。(Data from Liu SS, Block BM, Wu CL: Effects of perioperative central neuraxial analgesia on outcome after coronary artery bypass surgery: A meta-analysis. Anesthesiology 2004;101:153-161.)

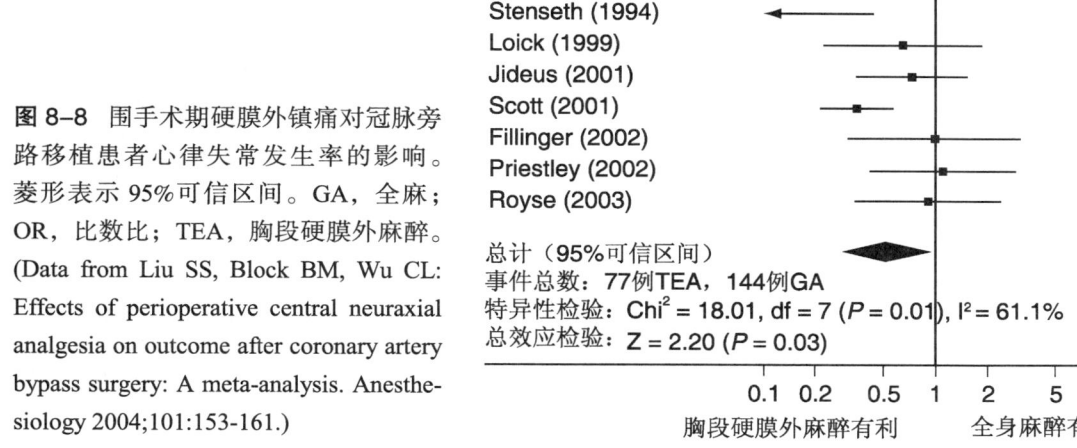

图 8-8 围手术期硬膜外镇痛对冠脉旁路移植患者心律失常发生率的影响。菱形表示 95%可信区间。GA,全麻;OR,比数比;TEA,胸段硬膜外麻醉。(Data from Liu SS, Block BM, Wu CL: Effects of perioperative central neuraxial analgesia on outcome after coronary artery bypass surgery: A meta-analysis. Anesthesiology 2004;101:153-161.)

硬膜外麻醉镇痛除了具有预防性抗凝作用外,还具有哪些其他优点。

最后,经胸段而不是腰段硬膜外导管给予以局部麻醉药为主的镇痛配方可能降低术后心肌梗死的发生率(图 8-9)[96]。这种作用的机制尚不明了,但可能与减轻应激反应和高凝状态、术后镇痛效果完善以及冠脉血流改善有关[5,97]。试验数据还表明,以局部麻醉药为主的胸部硬膜外镇痛具有一些生理优点:包括减少心肌梗死面积、削弱交感神经兴奋介导的冠脉收缩作用以及改善缺血区域的冠脉血流量[98-100]。显然,"导管-切口平面一致"的硬膜外镇痛的优势最明显,即硬膜外导管置管位置与切口位置相对应,这样所需药物较少,药物副作用发生率较低[80,101-103]。与硬膜外"导管-切口平面不一致"的硬膜外镇痛相比,硬膜外"导管-切口平面一致"可使胃肠功能恢复较早,心肌梗死发生率较低[103,104,96],镇痛效果较好[105,106]。

尽管以局部麻醉药为主的硬膜外方法在降低术后胃肠、肺以及可能心脏的发病率方面具有明显优势,但是硬膜外镇痛对术后凝血功能、认知功能障碍以及免疫功能的影响尚不确定。RCT 提示,术中区域阻滞麻醉可降低高凝状态相关事件(如 DVT)的发生率。然而,术后硬膜外镇痛在降低高凝状态相关事件发生率方面的优势尚不明了。最后,以局部麻醉药为主的硬膜外方法可改善患者的自我评估指标,包括患者满意度以及生活质量,这可能一定程度上反映以局部麻醉药为主的硬膜外方法镇痛效果优于全身应用阿片类药物。

外周区域镇痛

外周区域镇痛有多种技术(如臂丛、腰丛、股神经、坐骨-腘神经);可单次给药,主要用于术中麻醉,或辅助用于术后镇痛,或通过导管持续给予局麻药。应用外周区域镇痛技术不论是单次注射或持续给药,其镇痛效果均优于全身应用阿片类药物[111-113],甚至可改善患者结局[23,110,114,115]。应用以局部麻醉药为主单次注射阻断外周神经的镇痛效果较好,可改善结局,如阿片类药物相关副作用较少,这可能与阿片类药物用量减少有关,且患者满意度较高[111-115]。与全身应用阿片类药物相比,持续或患者自控给药的外周神经阻滞用于术后镇痛所产生的镇痛效果较好,阿片类药物相关的副作用较少,且患者满意度较高[110,116,117]。尽管外周神经阻滞的镇痛效果较好,并且可能具有有利的生理影响,但尚无大样本随机试验证实这种技术具有降低手术患者围手术期死亡率或并发症发病率的效果。

多模式镇痛

术后镇痛本身可能并不足以减少围手术期并发症的发病率和死亡率;然而,患者恢复期应用多模式镇痛方法进行完善的术后镇痛,可对患者结局产生最有利的影响[118,119]。这种多模式措施涉及了患者治疗的诸多方面,包括控制患者疼痛以有利于其尽早活动、早期肠道营养、患者教育以及通过以局部麻醉药为主的区域镇痛技术[120]与其他镇痛药物相结合的方法(多模式镇

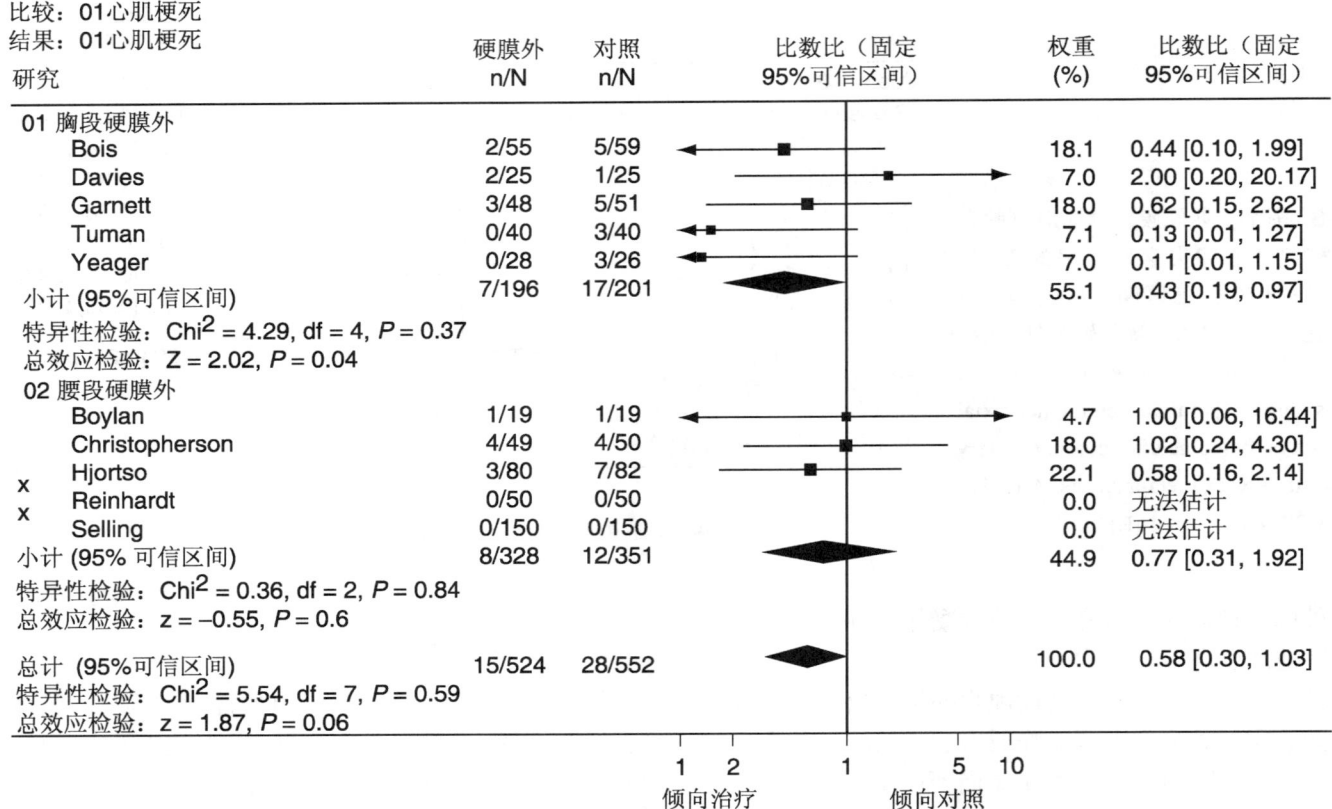

图 8-9 术后硬膜外镇痛对术后心肌梗死的影响。注意：只有胸段而不是腰段硬膜外镇痛可减少术后心肌梗死发生率。菱形表示 95% 可信区间。(From Beattie WS, Badner NH, Choi P: Epidural analgesia reduces postoperative myocardial infarction: A meta-analysis. Anesth Analg 2001;93:853-858.)

痛）来减弱围手术期应激反应，以促使患者恢复[46]。以局部麻醉药为主的硬膜外或外周神经镇痛技术的镇痛效果完善，有利于改善患者生理功能，是多模式镇痛方法的重要组成部分。

一些研究结果提示，多模式镇痛方法可控制术后病理生理反应，促进患者恢复，并缩短住院时间[118]。数项研究表明，接受多模式镇痛的胸部或腹部手术患者的应激反应较少而全身一般情况良好，拔管时间提前，疼痛评分较低，肠道功能恢复较快，达到离开加强医疗病房标准的时间较早[121-124]。一份研究显示，接受多模式"快通道"康复患者的总体并发症，尤其是心肺并发症，发生率明显低于常规治疗患者，尽管两组再次入院率无明显差异[124]。围手术期发病率显著下降可能是由于常规临床治疗中应用了标准化多模式治疗方法（如液体限制和硬膜外镇痛）[125]。

术后疼痛服务

自从 1988 年首次描述以麻醉学为基础的急性疼痛服务以来[126]，逐渐发展了许多围手术期疼痛处理模式，通常称为"急性疼痛服务"[127]。尽管有数种急性疼痛服务模式，但是资料提示所有围手术期疼痛服务会影响围手术期患者的结局，如疼痛评分、患者满意度，可能还包括患者发病率，特别是应用硬膜外镇痛时[11,128-131]。许多情况下，应用急性疼痛服务可能降低术后疼痛评分，某些患者严重疼痛评分可降低 50% 以上[129,132]。随着以护士为主的急性疼痛服务的介入，这些疼痛评分有所下降[133,134]。此外，一些研究显示，急性疼痛服务的应用可改善患者满意度，减少麻醉药相关的副作用，如恶心、镇静、瘙痒和呼吸抑制[128,131]，但这些结论尚无定论[132]。急性镇痛服务最大的作用之一是建立或协调多模式康复计划（"快通道"手术、临床通径），因为：①术后死亡率和发病率很可能取决于许多因素（如患者教育程度、镇痛质量、已有的术后康复计划）；②疼痛缓解本身不可能显著改善术后患者结局[132]。

小结

术后疼痛对围手术期患者结局可能产生不良影响。术后疼痛的控制，尤其是通过应用可提供完善镇痛、对患者生理有利的镇痛方法，可以减轻围手术期病理生理反应；而这种镇痛手段作为患者恢复中多模式方法的一部分可能有利于患者术后结局。某些镇痛技术如以局部麻醉药为主的硬膜外镇痛可减轻围手术期病理生理反应，患者发病率降低，某些试验中死亡率也下降。然而，必须认识到，如何使用这些技术可能比技术本身更为重要。如"硬膜外镇痛"并不单纯是一项总称；该技术有各种方法，如镇痛药物的选择与剂量、导管放置的位置、围手术期镇痛作用开始与持续时间等，均可不同程度地影响患者结局。未来的研究目标应该是比较不同镇痛方法与技术对患者结局（如满意度、生活质量和恢复质量）的影响。

（晨　光　张　瑛译　陈　辉　邓小明校）

参考文献

1. Carr DB, Jacox AK, Chapman RC, et al: Clinical Practice Guideline: Acute Pain Management: Operative or Medical Procedures and Trauma. Rockville, Md, Agency for Health Care Policy and Research, 1992.
2. American Society of Anesthesiologists: Practice guidelines for acute pain management in the perioperative setting: A report by the American Society of Anesthesiologists task force on pain management, acute pain section. Anesthesiology 1995;82:1071–1081.
3. American Pain Society Quality of Care Committee: Quality improvement guidelines for the treatment of acute pain and cancer pain. JAMA 1995;274:1874–1880.
4. Phillips DM: JCAHO pain management standards are unveiled. JAMA 2000;284:428–429.
5. Rosenfeld BA: Benefits of regional anesthesia on thromboembolic complications following surgery. Reg Anesth 1996;21(Suppl):9–12.
6. Desborough JP: The stress response to trauma and surgery. Br J Anaesth 2000;85:109–117.
7. Pomposelli JJ, Baxter JK 3rd, Babineau TJ, et al: Early postoperative glucose control predicts nosocomial infection rate in diabetic patients. JPEN J Parenter Enteral Nutr 1998;22:77–81.
8. Warltier DC, Pagel PS, Kersten JR: Approaches to the prevention of perioperative myocardial ischemia. Anesthesiology 2000;92:253–259.
9. Fratacci MD, Kimball WR, Wain JC, et al: Diaphragmatic shortening after thoracic surgery in humans: Effects of mechanical ventilation and thoracic epidural anesthesia. Anesthesiology 1993;79:654–665.
10. Liu S, Carpenter RL, Neal JM: Epidural anesthesia and analgesia: Their role in postoperative outcome. Anesthesiology 1995;82:1474–1506.
11. Wu CL, Fleisher LA: Outcomes research in regional anesthesia and analgesia. Anesth Analg 2000;91:1232–1242.
12. Perkins FM, Kehlet H: Chronic pain as an outcome of surgery: A review of predictive factors. Anesthesiology 2000;93:1123–1233.
13. Macrae WA: Chronic pain after surgery. Br J Anaesth 2001;87:88–98.
14. Carr DB, Goudas LC: Acute pain. Lancet 1999;353:2051–2058.
15. Kalso E, Mennander S, Tasmuth T, et al: Chronic post-sternotomy pain. Acta Anaesthesiol Scand 2001;45:935–939.
16. Katz J, Jackson M, Kavanagh BP, et al: Acute pain after thoracic surgery
17. Kalso E, Perttunen K, Kaasinen S: Pain after thoracic surgery. Acta Anaesthesiol Scand 1992;36:96–100.
18. Ochroch EA, Gottschalk A, Augostides J, et al: Long-term pain and activity during recovery from major thoracotomy using thoracic epidural analgesia. Anesthesiology 2002;97:1234–1244.
19. Callesen T, Bech K, Kehlet H: Prospective study of chronic pain after groin hernia repair. Br J Surg 1999;86:1528–1531.
20. Tasmuth T, Kataja M, Blomqvist C, et al: Treatment-related factors predisposing to chronic pain in patients with breast cancer—a multivariate approach. Acta Oncol 1997;36:625–630.
21. Fisher A, Meller Y: Continuous postoperative regional analgesia by nerve sheath block for amputation—a pilot study. Anesth Analg 1991;72:300–303.
22. Borly L, Anderson IB, Bardram L, et al: Preoperative prediction model of outcome after cholecystectomy for symptomatic gallstones. Scand J Gastroenterol 1999;34:1144–1152.
23. Capdevila X, Barthelet Y, Biboulet P, et al: Effects of perioperative analgesic technique on the surgical outcome and duration of rehabilitation after major knee surgery. Anesthesiology 1999;91:8–15.
24. Gottschalk A, Smith DS, Jobes DR, et al: Preemptive epidural analgesia and recovery from radical prostatectomy: A randomized controlled trial. JAMA 1998;279:1076–1082.
25. Carli F, Mayo N, Klubien K, et al: Epidural analgesia enhances functional exercise capacity and health-related quality of life after colonic surgery: Results of a randomized trial. Anesthesiology 2002;97:540–549.
26. Wu CL, Garry MG, Zollo RA, et al: Gene therapy for the management of pain. Part II: Molecular targets. Anesthesiology 2001;95:216–240.
27. Liu H, Wang H, Sheng M, et al: Evidence for presynaptic N-methyl-D-aspartate autoreceptors in the spinal cord dorsal horn. Proc Natl Acad Sci U S A 1994;91:8383–8387.
28. Obata H, Saito S, Fujita N, et al: Epidural block with mepivacaine before surgery reduces long-term post-thoracotomy pain. Can J Anaesth 1999;46:1127–1132.
29. Schug SA, Burrell R, Payne J, et al: Pre-emptive epidural analgesia may prevent phantom limb pain. Reg Anesth 1995;20:256.
30. Kissin I: Preemptive analgesia. Anesthesiology 2000;93:1138–1143.
31. Kissin I: Preemptive analgesia: Why its effect is not always obvious. Anesthesiology 1996;84:1015–1019.
32. Woolf CJ, Chong MS: Preemptive analgesia—treating postoperative pain by preventing the establishment of central sensitization. Anesth Analg 1993;77:362–379.
33. Moiniche S, Kehlet H, Dahl JB: A qualitative and quantitative systematic review of preemptive analgesia for postoperative pain: The role of timing of analgesia. Anesthesiology 2002;96:725–741.
34. Kissin I, Lee SS, Bradley EL Jr: Effect of prolonged nerve block on inflammatory hyperalgesia in rats: Prevention of late hyperalgesia. Anesthesiology 1998;88:224–232.
35. Taylor DA, Fleming WW: Unifying perspectives of the mechanisms underlying the development of tolerance and physical dependence to opioids. J Pharmacol Exp Ther 2001;297:11–18.
36. Lehmann LJ, DeSio JM, Radvany T, et al: Transdermal fentanyl in postoperative pain. Reg Anesth 1997;22:24–28.
37. Chelly JE, Grass J, Houseman TW, et al: The safety and efficacy of a fentanyl patient-controlled transdermal system for acute postoperative analgesia: A multicenter, placebo-controlled trial. Anesth Analg 2004;98:427–433.
38. Viscusi ER, Reynolds L, Chung F, et al: Patient-controlled transdermal fentanyl hydrochloride vs intravenous morphine pump for postoperative pain: A randomized controlled trial. JAMA 2004;291:1333–1341.
39. Walder B, Schafer M, Henzi I, et al: Efficacy and safety of patient-controlled opioid analgesia for acute postoperative pain: A quantitative systematic review. Acta Anaesthesiol Scand 2001;45:795–804.
40. Ballantyne JC, Carr DB, Chalmers TC, et al: Postoperative patient-controlled analgesia: Meta-analyses of initial randomized control trials. J Clin Anesth 1993;5:182–193.
41. Thomas V, Heath M, Rose D, et al: Psychological characteristics and the effectiveness of patient-controlled analgesia. Br J Anaesth 1995;74:271–276.
42. Pellino TA, Ward SE: Perceived control mediates the relationship between pain severity and patient satisfaction. J Pain Symptom Manage 1998;15:110–116.
43. Chumbley GM, Hall GM, Salmon P: Why do patients feel positive about

44. Jamison RN, Taft K, O'Hara JP, et al: Psychosocial and pharmacologic predictors of satisfaction with intravenous patient-controlled analgesia. Anesth Analg 1993;77:121–125.
45. Morgan PJ, Halpern S, Lam-McCulloch J: Comparison of maternal satisfaction between epidural and spinal anesthesia for elective Cesarean section. Can J Anaesth 2000;47:956–961.
46. Jin F, Chung F: Multimodal analgesia for postoperative pain control. J Clin Anesth 2001;13:524–539.
47. Crews JC: Multimodal pain management strategies for office-based and ambulatory procedures. JAMA 2002;288:629–632.
48. White PF: The role of non-opioid analgesic techniques in the management of pain after ambulatory surgery. Anesth Analg 2002;94:577–585.
49. Ballantyne JC: Use of nonsteroidal antiinflammatory drugs for acute pain management. Problems in Anesthesia 1998;10:23–36.
50. Grass JA, Sakima NT, Valley M, et al: Assessment of ketorolac as an adjuvant to fentanyl patient-controlled epidural analgesia after radical retropubic prostatectomy. Anesthesiology 1993;78:642–648.
51. Schug SA, Sidebotham DA, McGuinnety M, et al: Acetaminophen as an adjunct to morphine by patient-controlled analgesia in the management of acute postoperative pain. Anesth Analg 1998;87:368–372.
52. Dolin SJ, Cashman JN, Bland JM: Effectiveness of acute postoperative pain management. I: Evidence from published data. Br J Anaesth 2002;89:409–423.
53. Block BM, Liu SS, Rowlingson AJ, et al: Efficacy of postoperative epidural analgesia: A meta-analysis. JAMA 2003;290:2455–2463.
54. Wheatley RG, Schug SA, Watson D: Safety and efficacy of postoperative epidural analgesia. Br J Anaesth 2001;87:47–61.
55. Loper KA, Ready LB: Epidural morphine after anterior cruciate ligament repair: A comparison with patient-controlled intravenous morphine. Anesth Analg 1989;68:350–352.
56. Malviya S, Pandit UA, Merkel S, et al: A comparison of continuous epidural infusion and intermittent intravenous bolus doses of morphine in children undergoing selective dorsal rhizotomy. Reg Anesth Pain Med 1999;24:438–443.
57. de Leon-Casasola OA, Lema MJ: Postoperative epidural opioid analgesia: What are the choices? Anesth Analg 1996;83:867–875.
58. Rauck RL, Raj PP, Knarr DC, et al: Comparison of the efficacy of epidural morphine given by intermittent injection or continuous infusion for the management of postoperative pain. Reg Anesth 1994;19:316–324.
59. Gourlay GK, Kowalski SR, Plummer JL, et al: Fentanyl blood concentration-analgesic response relationship in the treatment of postoperative pain. Anesth Analg 1988;67:329–337.
60. Park WY, Thompson JS, Lee KK: Effect of epidural anesthesia and analgesia on perioperative outcome: A randomized, controlled Veterans Affairs cooperative study. Ann Surg 2001;234:560–569.
61. Tsui SL, Law S, Fok M, et al: Postoperative analgesia reduces mortality and morbidity after esophagectomy. Am J Surg 1997;173:472–478.
62. Major CP Jr, Greer MS, Russell WL, Roe SM: Postoperative pulmonary complications and morbidity after abdominal aneurysmectomy: A comparison of postoperative epidural versus parenteral opioid analgesia. Am Surg 1996;62:45–51.
63. Liu SS, Carpenter RL, Mackey DC, et al: Effects of perioperative analgesic technique on rate of recovery after colon surgery. Anesthesiology 1995;83:757–765.
64. Beattie WS, Buckley DN, Forrest JB: Epidural morphine reduces the risk of postoperative myocardial ischaemia in patients with cardiac risk factors. Can J Anaesth 1993;40:532–541.
65. Her C, Kizelshteyn G, Walker V, et al: Combined epidural and general anesthesia for abdominal aortic surgery. J Cardiothorac Anesth 1990;4:552–557.
66. Hasenbos M, van Egmond J, Gielen M, Crul JF: Post-operative analgesia by high thoracic epidural versus intramuscular nicomorphine after thoracotomy. Part III: The effects of peri- and post-operative analgesia on morbidity. Acta Anaesthesiol Scand 1987;31:608–615.
67. Rawal N, Sjostrand U, Christoffersson E, et al: Comparison of intramuscular and epidural morphine for postoperative analgesia in the grossly obese: Influence on postoperative ambulation and pulmonary function. Anesth Analg 1984;63:583–592.
68. Ballantyne JC, Carr DB, deFerranti S, et al: The comparative effects of postoperative analgesic therapies on pulmonary outcome: Cumulative meta-analyses of randomized, controlled trials. Anesth Analg 1998;86:
69. Wu CL, Richman JM: Postoperative pain and quality of recovery. Curr Opin Anesthesiol 2004;17:455–460.
70. Bailey PL, Rhondeau S, Schafer PG, et al: Dose-response pharmacology of intrathecal morphine in human volunteers. Anesthesiology 1993;79:49–59.
71. Kirson LE, Goldman JM, Slover RB: Low-dose intrathecal morphine for postoperative pain control in patients undergoing transurethral resection of the prostate. Anesthesiology 1989;71:192–195.
72. Chaney MA: Side effects of intrathecal and epidural opioids. Can J Anaesth 1995;42:891–903.
73. Gedney JA, Liu EH: Side-effects of epidural infusions of opioid bupivacaine mixtures. Anaesthesia 1998;53:1148–1155.
74. Kjellberg F, Tramer MR: Pharmacological control of opioid-induced pruritus: A quantitative systematic review of randomized trials. Eur J Anaesthesiol 2001;18:346–357.
75. Bucklin BA, Chestnut DH, Hawkins JL: Intrathecal opioids versus epidural local anesthetics for labor analgesia: A meta-analysis. Reg Anesth Pain Med 2002;27:23–30.
76. Grass JA: Epidural analgesia. Problems in Anesthesia 1998;10:45–67.
77. Ferrante FM, Lu L, Jamison SB, et al: Patient-controlled epidural analgesia: Demand dosing. Anesth Analg 1991;73:547–552.
78. Lubenow TR, Tanck EN, Hopkins EM, et al: Comparison of patient-assisted epidural analgesia with continuous-infusion epidural analgesia for postoperative patients. Reg Anesth 1994;19:206–211.
79. Gambling DR, McMorland GH, Yu P, et al: Comparison of patient-controlled epidural analgesia and conventional intermittent "top-up" injections during labor. Anesth Analg 1990;70:256–261.
80. Liu SS, Allen HW, Olsson GL: Patient-controlled epidural analgesia with bupivacaine and fentanyl on hospital wards: Prospective experience with 1,030 surgical patients. Anesthesiology 1998;88:688–695.
81. Wigfull J, Welchew E: Survey of 1057 patients receiving postoperative patient-controlled epidural analgesia. Anaesthesia 2001;56:70–75.
82. Mann C, Pouzeratte Y, Boccara G, et al: Comparison of intravenous or epidural patient-controlled analgesia in the elderly after major abdominal surgery. Anesthesiology 2000;92:433–441.
83. Blake DW, Stainsby GV, Bjorksten AR, et al: Patient-controlled epidural versus intravenous pethidine to supplement epidural bupivacaine after abdominal aortic surgery. Anaesth Intensive Care 1998;26:630–635.
84. de Leon-Casasola OA, Parker B, Lema MJ, et al: Postoperative epidural bupivacaine-morphine therapy: Experience with 4,227 surgical cancer patients. Anesthesiology 1994;81:368–375.
85. Rigg JR, Jamrozik K, Myles PS, et al: Epidural anaesthesia and analgesia and outcome of major surgery: A randomised trial. Lancet 2002;359:1276–1282.
86. Rodgers A, Walker N, Schug S, et al: Reduction of postoperative mortality and morbidity with epidural or spinal anaesthesia: Results from overview of randomised trials. BMJ 2000;321:1493–1496.
87. Rimback G, Cassuto J, Wallin G, et al: Inhibition of peritonitis by amide local anesthetics. Anesthesiology 1988;69:881–886.
88. Jayr C, Thomas H, Rey A, et al: Postoperative pulmonary complications: Epidural analgesia using bupivacaine and opioids versus parenteral opioids. Anesthesiology 1993;78:666–676.
89. Scheinin B, Asantila R, Orko R: The effect of bupivacaine and morphine on pain and bowel function after colonic surgery. Acta Anaesthesiol Scand 1987;31:161–164.
90. Thoren T, Sundberg A, Wattwil M, et al: Effects of epidural bupivacaine and epidural morphine on bowel function and pain after hysterectomy. Acta Anaesthesiol Scand 1989;33:181–185.
91. Holte K, Kehlet H: Epidural analgesia and risk of anastomotic leakage. Reg Anesth Pain Med 2001;26:111–117.
92. Liu SS, Block BM, Wu CL: Effects of perioperative central neuraxial analgesia on outcome after coronary artery bypass surgery: A meta-analysis. Anesthesiology 2004;101:153–161.
93. Sorenson RM, Pace NL: Anesthetic techniques during surgical repair of femoral neck fractures: A meta-analysis. Anesthesiology 1992;77:1095–1104.
94. Christopherson R, Beattie C, Frank SM, et al: Perioperative morbidity in patients randomized to epidural or general anesthesia for lower extremity vascular surgery. Anesthesiology 1993;79:422–434.
95. Tuman KJ, McCarthy RJ, March RJ, et al: Effects of epidural anesthesia and analgesia on coagulation and outcome after major vascular surgery.

96. Beattie WS, Badner NH, Choi P: Epidural analgesia reduces postoperative myocardial infarction: A meta-analysis. Anesth Analg 2001; 93:853–858.
97. Veering BT, Cousins MJ: Cardiovascular and pulmonary effects of epidural anaesthesia. Anaesth Intensive Care 2000;28:620–635.
98. Davis RF, DeBoer LW, Maroko PR: Thoracic epidural anesthesia reduces myocardial infarct size after coronary artery occlusion in dogs. Anesth Analg 1986;65:711–717.
99. Rolf N, Van de Velde M, Wouters PF, et al: Thoracic epidural anesthesia improves functional recovery from myocardial stunning in conscious dogs. Anesth Analg 1996;83:935–940.
100. Kock M, Blomberg S, Emanuelsson H, et al: Thoracic epidural anesthesia improves global and regional left ventricular function during stress-induced myocardial ischemia in patients with coronary artery disease. Anesth Analg 1990;71:625–630.
101. Magnusdottir H, Kirno K, Ricksten SE, et al: High thoracic epidural analgesia does not inhibit sympathetic nerve activity in the lower extremities. Anesthesiology 1999;91:1299–1304.
102. Chisakuta AM, George KA, Hawthorne CT: Postoperative epidural infusion of a mixture of bupivacaine 0.2% with fentanyl for upper abdominal surgery: A comparison of thoracic and lumbar routes. Anaesthesia 1995;50:72–75.
103. Hodgson PS, Liu SS: Thoracic epidural anaesthesia and analgesia for abdominal surgery: Effects on gastrointestinal function and perfusion. Balliere's Clini Anesthesiol 1999;13:9–22.
104. Scott AM, Starling JR, Ruscher AE, et al: Thoracic versus lumbar epidural anesthesia's effect on pain control and ileus resolution after restorative proctocolectomy. Surgery 1996;120:688–695.
105. Broekema AA, Gielen MJ, Hennis PJ: Postoperative analgesia with continuous epidural sufentanil and bupivacaine: A prospective study in 614 patients. Anesth Analg 1996;82:754–759.
106. Kahn L, Baxter FJ, Dauphin A, et al: A comparison of thoracic and lumbar epidural techniques for post-thoracoabdominal esophagectomy analgesia. Can J Anaesth 1999;46:415–422.
107. Wu CL, Hsu W, Richman JM, Raja SN: Postoperative cognitive function as an outcome of regional anesthesia and analgesia. Reg Anesth Pain Med 2004;29:257–268.
108. de Leon-Casasola OA: Immunomodulation and epidural anesthesia and analgesia. Reg Anesth 1996;21(Suppl):24–25.
109. Dalldorf PG, Perkins FM, Totterman S, et al: Deep venous thrombosis following total hip arthroplasty: Effects of prolonged postoperative epidural anesthesia. J Arthroplasty 1994;9:611–616.
110. Wu CL, Naqibuddin M, Fleisher LA: Measurement of patient satisfaction as an outcome of regional anesthesia and analgesia. Reg Anesth Pain Med 2001;26:196–208.
111. Allen HW, Liu SS, Ware PD, et al: Peripheral nerve blocks improve analgesia after total knee replacement surgery. Anesth Analg 1998; 87:93–97.
112. Mulroy MF, Larkin KL, Batra MS, et al: Femoral nerve block with 0.25% or 0.5% bupivacaine improves postoperative analgesia following outpatient arthroscopic anterior cruciate ligament repair. Reg Anesth Pain Med 2001;26:24–29.
113. Allen JG, Denny NM, Oakman N: Postoperative analgesia following total knee arthroplasty: A study comparing spinal anesthesia and combined sciatic femoral 3-in-1 block. Reg Anesth Pain Med 1998;23:142–146.
114. Wang H, Boctor B, Verner J: The effect of single-injection femoral nerve block on rehabilitation and length of hospital stay after total knee replacement. Reg Anesth Pain Med 2002;27:139–144.
115. Stevens RD, Van Gessel E, Flory N, et al: Lumbar plexus block reduces pain and blood loss associated with total hip arthroplasty. Anesthesiology 2000;93:115–121.
116. Borgeat A, Schappi B, Biasca N, et al: Patient-controlled analgesia after major shoulder surgery: Patient-controlled interscalene analgesia versus patient-controlled analgesia. Anesthesiology 1997;87:1343–1347.
117. Singelyn FJ, Deyaert M, Joris D, et al: Effects of intravenous patient-controlled analgesia with morphine, continuous epidural analgesia, and continuous three-in-one block on postoperative pain and knee rehabilitation after unilateral total knee arthroplasty. Anesth Analg 1998;87:88–92.
118. Kehlet H, Wilmore DW: Multimodal strategies to improve surgical outcome. Am J Surg 2002;183:630–641.
119. Kehlet H: Multimodal approach to control postoperative pathophysiology and rehabilitation. Br J Anaesth 1997;78:606–617.
120. Kehlet H, Holte K: Effect of postoperative analgesia on surgical outcome. Br J Anaesth 2001;87:62–72.
121. Barratt SM, Smith RC, Kee AJ, et al: Multimodal analgesia and intravenous nutrition preserves total body protein following major upper gastrointestinal surgery. Reg Anesth Pain Med 2002;27:15–22.
122. Brodner G, Pogatzki E, Van Aken H, et al: A multimodal approach to control postoperative pathophysiology and rehabilitation in patients undergoing abdominothoracic esophagectomy. Anesth Analg 1998;86:228–234.
123. Brodner G, Van Aken H, Hertle L, et al: Multimodal perioperative management—combining thoracic epidural analgesia, forced mobilization, and oral nutrition—reduces hormonal and metabolic stress and improves convalescence after major urologic surgery. Anesth Analg 2001;92:1594–1600.
124. Basse L, Thorbol JE, Lossl K, Kehlet H: Colonic surgery with accelerated rehabilitation or conventional care. Dis Colon Rectum 2004;47: 271–277.
125. Neal JM, Wilcox RT, Allen HW, Low DE: Near-total esophagectomy: The influence of standardized multimodal management and intraoperative fluid restriction. Reg Anesth Pain Med 2003;28:328–334.
126. Ready LB, Oden R, Chadwick HS, et al: Development of an anesthesiology-based postoperative pain management service. Anesthesiology 1988;68:100–106.
127. Rawal N: 10 years of acute pain services—achievements and challenges. Reg Anesth Pain Med 1999;24:68–73.
128. Brodner G, Mertes N, Buerkle H, et al: Acute pain management: Analysis, implications and consequences after prospective experience with 6349 surgical patients. Eur J Anaesthesiol 2000;17:566–575.
129. Bardiau FM, Braeckman MM, Seidel L, et al: Effectiveness of an acute pain service inception in a general hospital. J Clin Anesth 1999; 11:583–589.
130. Sartain JB, Barry JJ: The impact of an acute pain service on postoperative pain management. Anaesth Intensive Care 1999;27: 375–380.
131. Miaskowski C, Crews J, Ready LB, et al: Anesthesia-based pain services improve the quality of postoperative pain management. Pain 1999; 80:23–29.
132. Werner MU, Soholm L, Rotboll-Nielsen P, Kehlet H: Does an acute pain service improve postoperative outcome? Anesth Analg 2002; 95:1361–1372.
133. Stadler M, Schlander M, Braeckman M, et al: A cost-utility and cost-effectiveness analysis of an acute pain service. J Clin Anesth 2004;16:159–167.
134. Bardiau FM, Taviaux NF, Albert A, et al: An intervention study to enhance postoperative pain management. Anesth Analg 2003;96: 179–185.

9 阿片类药物的异化效应（痛觉过敏和耐受）及其对术后镇痛的影响

OLIVER H. G. WILDER-SMITH

现已明确，神经系统并非通过某个独立通道（hard-wired）对传入性伤害刺激进行处理。通过最近十几年对疼痛的研究发现，伤害性感受（对有害刺激的处理）会放大随后发生的伤害性感觉[1]，这种过程称为"伤害性神经可塑性"。外科手术所致的中枢性敏化导致痛觉过敏和疼痛加剧即为一典型例证[2]。显然，用于麻醉和镇痛的药物凭其特性可调节伤害性传入并影响随后的伤害性疼痛的处理。因此，给予阿片类药物可通过提高痛阈抑制伤害性传入，还可以抑制外科手术伤害性传入所致的中枢性敏化[2]。

最近发现，阿片类药物在治疗疼痛时有不良的影响。使用该类药物能导致神经可塑性发生异化，表现为药物耐受和痛觉过敏[6]，其他相关表现还有肌痉挛、癫痫发作和恶心呕吐。显然，这些表现对患者术后康复不利。外科手术后不期望出现痛觉过敏有两个原因，首先，在术后早期出现痛觉过敏会导致术后疼痛加剧，从而导致患者应激加剧，并发症增多，住院治疗时间延长[7-9]；其次，手术后痛觉过敏过于强烈或持续时间过长可能会导致疼痛的"慢性化"，这是因为外科手术后慢性疼痛的形成与神经损害（导致痛觉超敏的原因）和术后发生持续、强烈的急性痛（痛觉过敏的症状）有关[10,11]。另外，还由于大家已逐渐承认，异常持久的中枢致敏是导致疼痛"慢性化"的重要原因[1,12]。

本文旨在：①简要概述阿片类物质产生痛觉过敏（opioid-induced hyperalgesia，OIH）和药物耐受的机制；②总结关于OIH和药物耐受的动物实验证据；③通过自愿受试者和临床研究提供OIH和药物耐受存在的证据；④提出临床针对阿片类药物所致药物耐受和OIH可能的解决方法。

定义

本文中阿片类药物导致的痛觉过敏（OIH）定义为痛阈低于基础值，它被认为是机体积极适应或敏感化的一种现象。药物耐受指在疼痛状态稳定的情况下，需要更多药物才能达到相同镇痛效果，它被认为是机体消极适应或脱敏感化的一种现象。本文需强调的是：临床上阿片类药物导致的耐受可能是由于机体对药物的敏感性丧失，也可能是由于疼痛的敏感性增加如痛觉过敏所致（后文讨论）。

阿片致痛觉过敏的机制

即使是单次应用，阿片类药物与μ受体(MOR)结合后对疼痛处理均有抑制和兴奋作用[6]。因此，MOR结合后同时启动了负反馈（抑制，耐受）环路和正反馈（兴奋，超敏）环路。

负反馈环路的机制可能为：
- 下调MOR的分布数量。该理论并未得到广泛认可[6]。
- 与抑制性G蛋白解偶联后使得MOR脱敏，导致相关钾离子通道反应性降低[13,14]。
- 增强神经元细胞表面MOR胞吞作用。瑞芬太尼尤其可能通过这个机制发挥作用[3]。
- 长期使用阿片类药物可对脊髓产生神经毒性。这可能是一种潜在的不可逆改变，包括神经元发生可塑性变化以及通过 NMDA 受体、NO 和多聚二磷酸腺苷合成酶 (PARS) 介导的凋亡[17]。

正反馈环路的机制可能为：

● 通过蛋白激酶 Cγ（PKCγ）磷酸化和激活 NMDA 受体[6]。众所周知，NMDA 激动剂是伤害前递质。这种机制提供了一个正反馈环路——其效果类似于细胞内钙增加导致的长时程增强效应，并进一步刺激 PKCγ 的产生[18]。NMDA 受体的涉入意味着伤害性传入后 OIH 和中枢性敏化之间存在确切的交叉感知 "cross-talk"。激活 NMDA 受体后，通过钙-钙调素调节可产生 NO。NO 不仅可调节 μ 阿片受体（MOR）的表达[19]，还可能激活神经胶质细胞。目前认为神经胶质细胞与中枢敏化的产生有密切的联系[20-23]。

● 通过增加蛋白激酶 A（PKA），增强 G 蛋白偶联的 MOR 的兴奋性[16]。MOR 可处于抑制状态 (Gi/Go 偶联) 或兴奋 (Gs 偶联) 状态[16]。

● 释放脊髓伤害前递质如强啡肽。长时间使用阿片药物可导致脊髓过度产生强啡肽，从而产生疼痛过敏，并使阿片类药物丧失镇痛效应[24-26]。

● 延髓头端腹内侧群(RVM)的下行易化。RVM 内的细胞网络可对脊髓伤害性神经传入进行抑制和兴奋性调控[27-30]。目前认为，伤害性传入可被"开放"型细胞 (On-cells) 易化，而被"关闭"型细胞抑制。这些细胞均与 MOR 相联系；突触的活性呈一种平衡，MOR 的活化使该平衡向"开放"型细胞偏移，则表现为痛觉过敏。

● 其他 OIH 的可能机制：兴奋性代谢物质（如吗啡-3-葡糖苷酸）可能通过抗甘氨酸能机制起作用[31、32]。

与 OIH 形成相关的机制总结于旁注 9-1。

阿片类药物诱导疼痛过敏的证据

动物数据

动物实验现已证实的确存在 OIH 现象。2000 年，Celerier 等[33]证实，给大鼠注射 4 次芬太尼（间隔 15 分钟，剂量为 20～100μg/kg）后，存在剂量依赖性的疼痛过敏，且可持续 5d 以上（图 9-1）。其他研究亦显示相同的效果[33-38]。Laulin 等[37]报道了一个重要现象，他们发现上述实验中的这种 OIH 现象可降低以后吗啡的镇痛效果，10d 后应用纳洛酮仍可诱发出 OIH

（图 9-2）。该组实验中使用海洛因的其他研究表明 OIH 具有长时程性，即：使用海洛因超过 12d 以上导致的 OIH，停用海洛因 2 周后才能消除[35]。而当 OIH 消除一周后，再次单次、小剂量应用海洛因（整个研究开始时间已 >1 月），将产生典型的长时程 OIH（复燃）（图 9-3）[35]。连续 12d 给大鼠使用海洛因，停用 2 个月后使用纳洛酮仍可能诱导出 OIH[35]。海洛因诱导的痛觉过敏在 1 个月后重复出现，这种现象表明痛觉过敏具有一定的稳定性（即每一循环基线上的曲线下面积）。在持续每日予以海洛因 0.2mg/kg 12d 后，比较第 1d 和第 13d 大鼠的痛觉过敏状态，很明显诱导痛觉过敏的基线已向痛觉过敏方向偏移（图 9-4），此可解释阿片耐受现象[35]。基于角叉菜胶诱导以及手术诱导出的伤害性感受进行的动物实验证据表明，OIH 和伤害性感受诱导的痛觉过敏（NIH）相互作用，会产生更强、更广泛的痛觉过敏（图 9-5）[39,40]。

总之，研究已充分表明啮齿类动物中的 OIH 现象：

● 是确切可靠可诱导的现象
● 至少为阿片耐受现象提供了部分解释
● 可能为剂量依赖
● 可长时间影响以后的阿片镇痛效果
● 长时间后仍可诱发出来或复燃
● 机体状态呈长时间持续改变并可影响感觉处理
● 可能与 NIH 有协同作用

人类数据

有关人类 OIH 和耐受现象的证据比动物更加有限。然而，许多关于 OIH 的综述（包括其临床相关性）已发表[6,41-43]，甚至在正式研究该现象之前，已有个案报道了 OIH 的存在[44-46]。在临床文献中，人类 OIH 存在的最早证据来自于对阿片类药物成瘾者的研究，结果清楚地表明，其痛阈比正常人低，并且他们

旁注 9-1　与 OIH 形成相关的机制

中枢性谷氨酸能系统：NMDA 受体
脊髓释放强啡肽
下行/脊髓上易化：延脑头端腹内侧的"开放"细胞与"关闭"细胞
兴奋性 Gs 偶联的 μ 阿片受体：表达增加/效能作用
抗甘氨酸能机制
代谢产物（吗啡-3-葡糖苷酸）

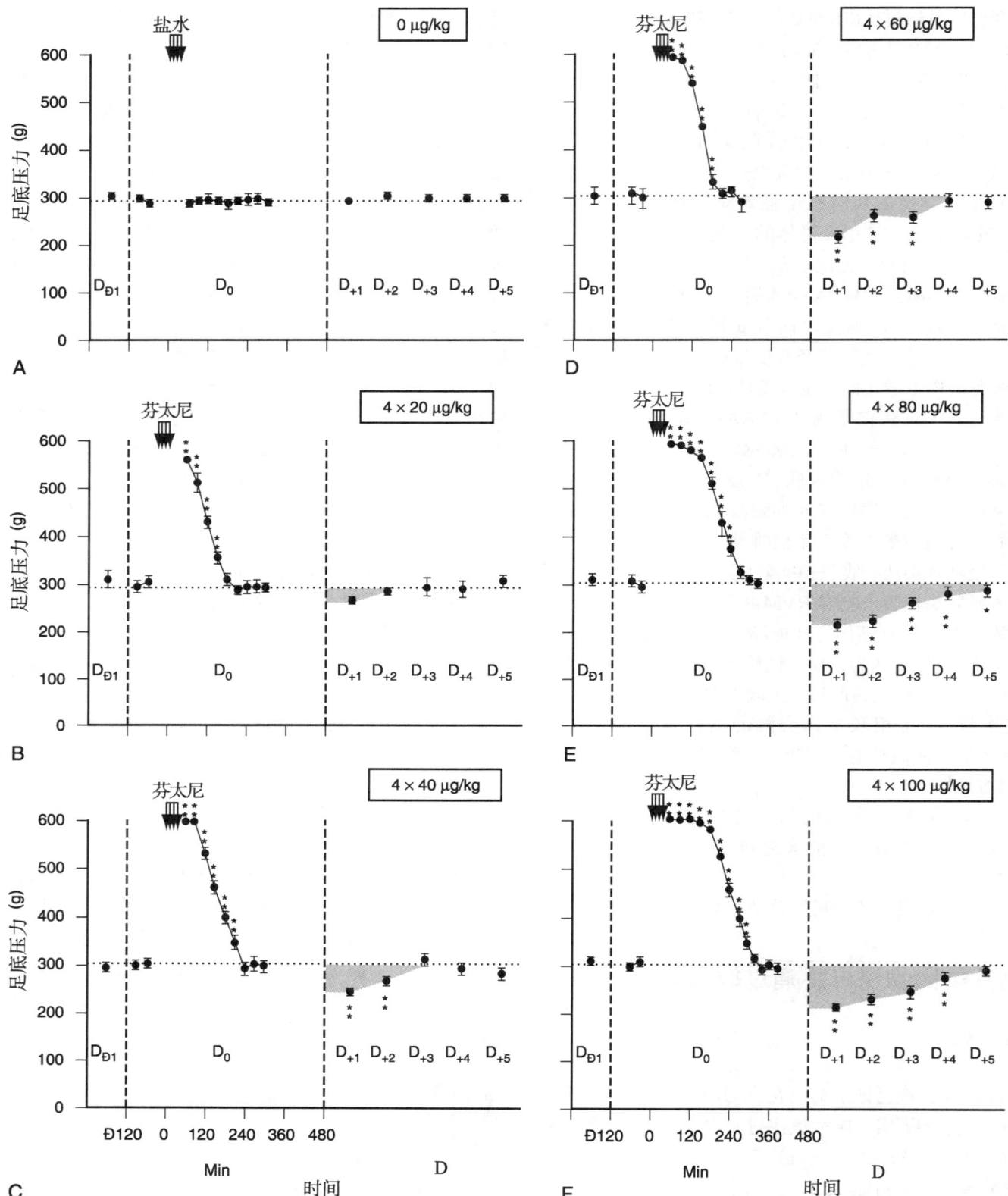

图 9-1 A–F，芬太尼对痛觉过敏大鼠的短期剂量依赖性。通过使大鼠发出叫声的足底刺激强度（克）来鉴定疼痛敏感性。数值由平均数±SEM 来表示。圆圈连线显示痛阈变化过程。星号代表与基线阈值相比有统计学意义，$^*P<0.05$；$^{**}P<0.01$。D，天；Min，分钟。(From Celerier E, Rivat C, Jun Y, et al: Long-lasting hyperalgesia induced by fentanyl in rats: Preventive effect of ketamine. Anesthesiology 2000; 92: 465-472.)

9 阿片类药物的异化效应（痛觉过敏和耐受）及其对术后镇痛的影响

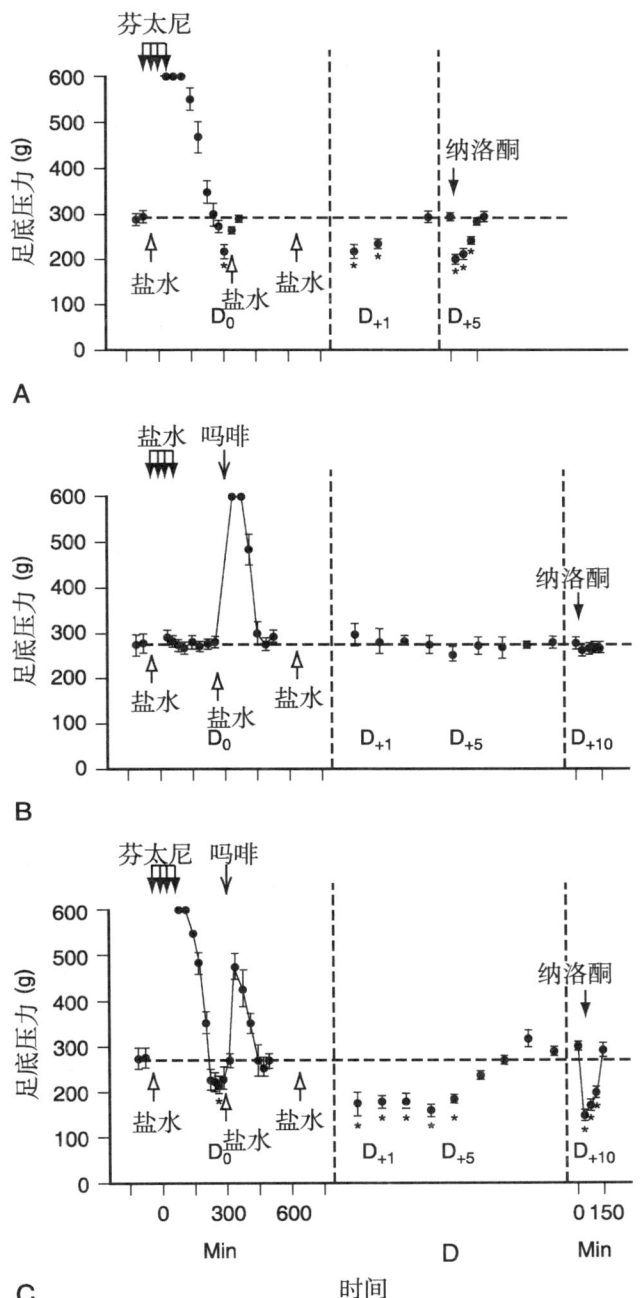

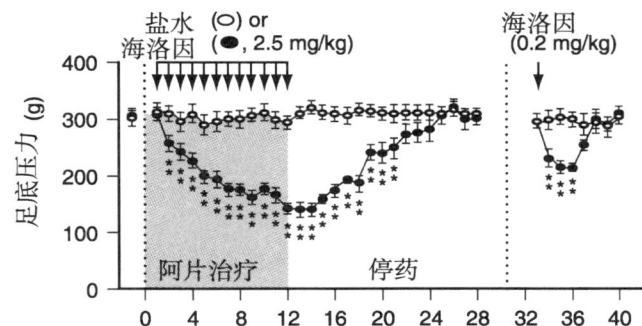

图 9-3 海洛因（每天 2.5 mg/kg，连续 12 天）对大鼠痛觉敏感性的长期效应。通过使大鼠发出叫声的足底刺激强度（g）来鉴定疼痛敏感性。记录到长期和累计的阿片类药物能够产生痛觉过敏，并且这种现象可以被单次、小剂量注射海洛因复燃。圆圈连线显示痛阈变化过程。星号代表与基线阈值相比有统计学意义，$^*P<0.05$；$^{**}P<0.01$。(From Celerier E, Laulin JP, Corcuff JB, et al: Progressive enhancement of delayed hyperalgesia induced by repeated heroin administration: A sensitization process. J Neurosci 2001;21:4074-4080.)

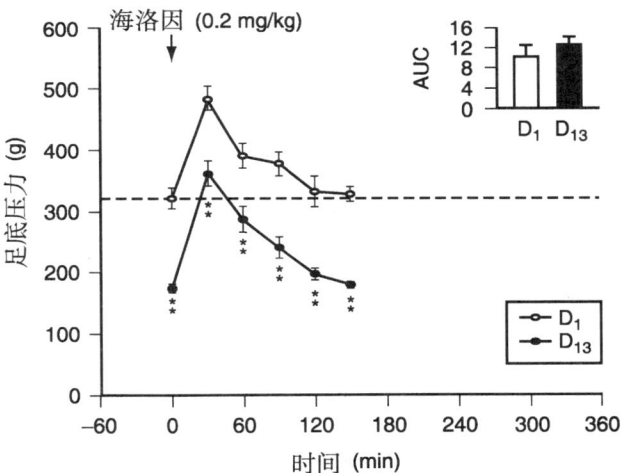

图 9-2 A-C，中期给予芬太尼（皮下给予 4~60μg）产生的疼痛敏感性和给予吗啡（皮下注射 5 mg/kg）产生的痛觉缺失。通过使大鼠发出叫声的足底刺激强度（克）来鉴定疼痛敏感性。C 图记录阿片类药物产生的长时程痛觉过敏，盐酸纳洛酮使用后可以使阿片致痛敏性持续 10 天。圆圈连线显示痛阈变化过程。星号代表与基线阈值相比有统计学意义，$^*P<0.05$；$^{**}P<0.01$。D，天；Min，分钟。(From Laulin JP, Maurette P, Corcuff JB, et al: The role of ketamine in preventing fentanyl-induced hyperalgesia and subsequent acute morphine tolerance. Anesth Analg 2002; 94:1263-1269.)

图 9-4 分别于皮下注射 0.2 mg/kg 海洛因（连续 12 天）之前和之后给予 2.5 mg/kg 海洛因，比较两者产生的痛觉敏感性，如图中 D_1 和 D_{13} 所示。通过使大鼠发出叫声的足底刺激强度（克）来鉴定疼痛敏感性。记录曲线下面积来表明 D_1 和 D_{13} 产生的镇痛效应。因此，曲线下面积的缩减就代表镇痛作用（相当于耐药性）强弱的变化。圆圈连线显示痛阈变化过程。星号代表与基线阈值相比有统计学意义，$^*P<0.05$；$^{**}P<0.01$。D，天；Min，分钟。(From Celerier E, Laulin JP, Corcuff JB, et al: Progressive enhancement of delayed hyperalgesia induced by repeated heroin administration: A sensitization process. J Neurosci 2001;21:4074-4080.)

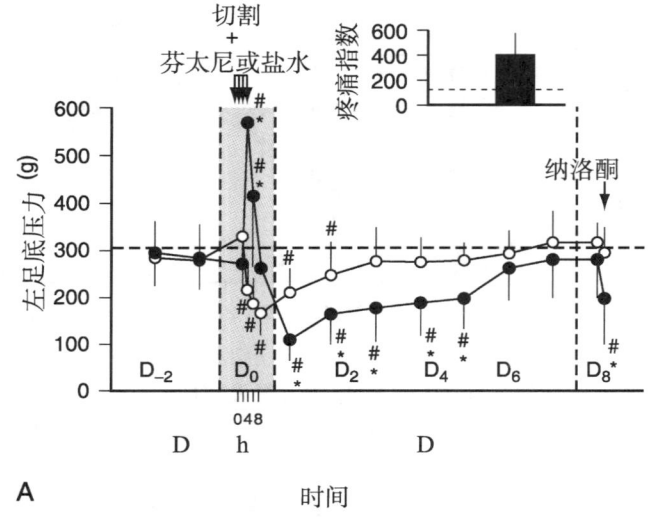

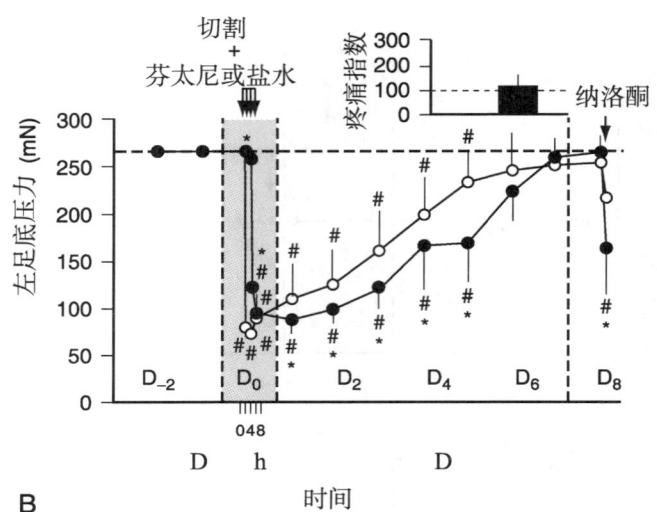

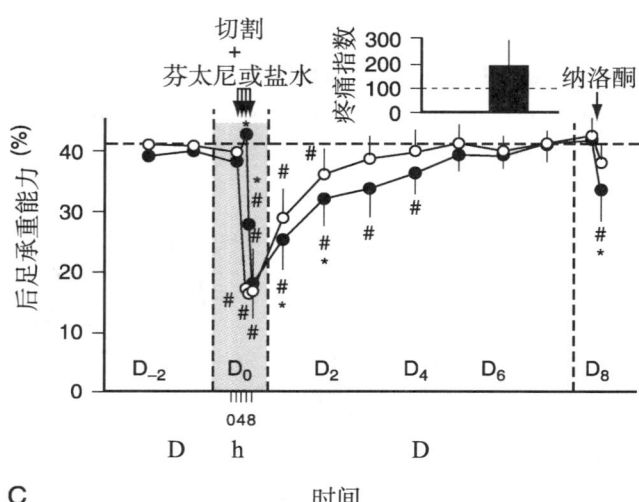

图 9-5 芬太尼对大鼠左足切割痛的协同效应：机械痛敏（A），触诱发痛（B）和承重能力的变化（C）。在 D_0 时，氟烷麻醉，切开大鼠的后足皮肤。皮下（SC）间隔 15 分钟给予 4 个剂量的芬太尼（100μg/kg）或含盐注射液，总剂量为 400μg/kg（n＝12）。外科手术施行完后第 2 次给予芬太尼。三种疼痛参数分别在手术前 D_{-2}、D_1、D_0 以及手术当天（D_0）的术后 2、4、6 小时评价，之后每天评价一次直到术后第 8 天。实验结束（D_8），所有老鼠注射纳洛酮（1 mg/kg SC），这 3 种疼痛参数在 5 分钟后测量。插图表示术后每天 3 种疼痛指数——机械痛敏（A）、异常触痛（B）和承重能力（C）的变化。疼痛参数值和疼痛指数用 $\bar{x}\pm SD$ 来表达。空心圆表示给予生理盐水注射的大鼠，实心圆表示给予芬太尼的老鼠；#，Dunnett 检验，与 D_0 基础值比较 $P<0.05$；*，Dunnett 检验，两组相比 $P<0.05$；†，疼痛指数的比较用 Mann-Whitney 检验，$P<0.05$。(From Richebe P, Rivat C, Laulin JP, et al: Ketamine improves the management of exaggerated postoperative pain observed in perioperative fentanyl-treated rats. Anesthesiology 2005;102:421-428.)

对阿片类药物的镇痛效果更差（图 9-6）[47]。进一步（间接）的研究来自于志愿者，使用瑞芬太尼输注，并定期测量压痛阈值。研究结果表明，瑞芬太尼以 0.1μg/(kg·min) 的速度输注 90min 后，镇痛作用降低，在输注瑞芬太尼 240min 后，压痛阈值与最初的基数值已无差别（图 9-7）[3]。

已有为数不多的安慰剂对照和前瞻性试验开始正式研究 OIH，研究对象为志愿者[5,48,49]。所有这些研究中，一些正式定量感觉实验（对一确定的感觉刺激所产生的疼痛强度）已被用来量化痛觉过敏程度，因为仅凭疼痛报告不足以证明存在痛觉过敏。所引用的 3 项研究显示：以临床常用剂量短期（长达 30min）输注瑞芬太尼停用后均发生了痛觉过敏[5,48,49]。其中一项用压力痛阈作为痛觉过敏最终指标的研究证明，停用瑞芬太尼后不但存在痛觉过敏，而且在输注瑞芬太尼期间其镇痛作用就已减弱（耐受性）（图 9-8）[49]。

迄今为止，只有一项安慰剂对照的前瞻性研究证实了手术后存在 OIH，该研究已发表[50]。虽然上述志愿者参与的这些研究在临床工作中的重要性或相关性不大，但仍可为人类存在 OIH 提供证据。

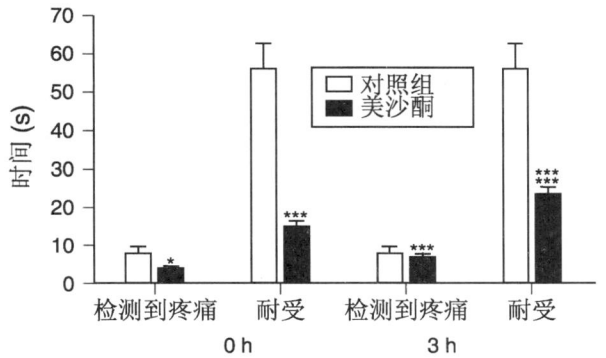

图9-6 美沙酮持续给药患者和正常对照组在冷加压试验中疼痛耐受和检测到疼痛的时间。在给予患者美沙酮30分钟前测量1次，3小时后测量第2次。数值由平均值±SEM表示。星号表示有统计学意义。*，表示0时美沙酮组与对照组检测到疼痛的时间相比 $P<0.05$。***，表示0时美沙酮组与对照组产生耐受的时间相比 $P<0.001$；3小时对照组与美沙酮产生耐受的时间相比 $P<0.001$。0和3小时之间美沙酮组检测到疼痛的时间和耐受性相比 $P<0.001$。(From Doverty M, White JM, Somogyi AA, et al: Hyperalgesic responses in methadone maintenance patients. Pain 2001;90:91-96.)

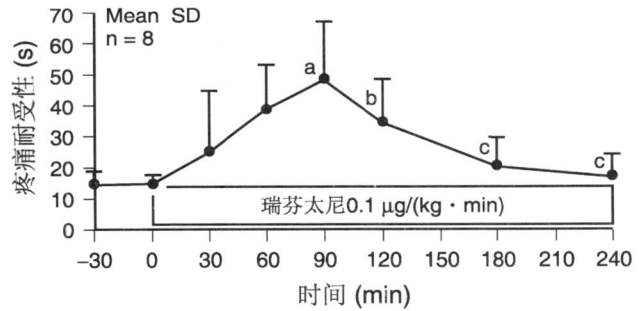

图9-7 持续给予 $0.1\mu g/(kg\cdot min)$ 剂量瑞芬太尼的志愿者对冷加压实验的疼痛耐受性。a，与0时比，$P<0.0001$；b，与90 min 时比，$P<0.05$；c，与90 min 时比，$P<0.0001$。(From Vinik HR, Kissin I: Rapid development of tolerance to analgesia during remifentanil infusion in humans. Anesth Analg 1998;86:1307-1311.)

对阿片类药物诱导疼痛过敏进行调节的证据

动物资料

大量理论依据认为，OIH 的发生与兴奋性氨基酸受体系统的激活密切相关，例如 NMDA 受体与 OIH

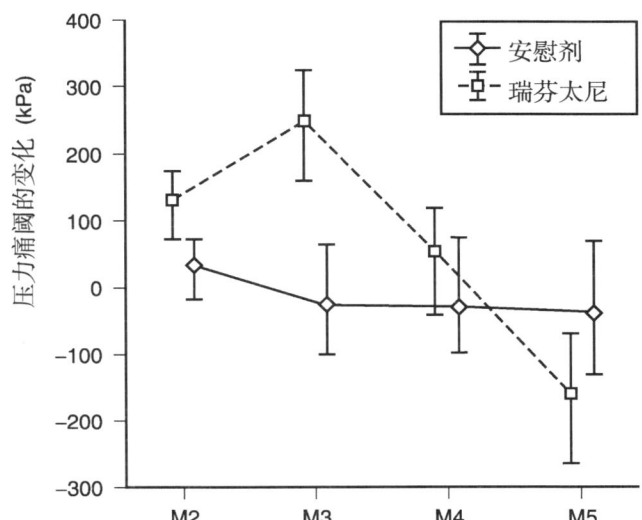

图9-8 给予瑞芬太尼或安慰剂（生理盐水）后压力痛阈 (kPa) 的变化（与基础值比较）。在第2个检测时间点 (M2)，瑞芬太尼的血药浓度为 $1\mu g/ml$, M3 时为 $2\mu g/ml$, M4 时为 $1\mu g/kg$。M5 为最后给药10分钟后检测的数值。数值用95%可信区间表示。(Modified from Luginbuhl M, Gerber A, Schnider TW, et al: Modulation of remifentanil-induced analgesia, hyperalgesia, and tolerance by small-dose ketamine in humans. Anesth Analg 2003;96:726-732.)

和药物耐受相关。因此，多数关于 OIH 和药物耐受的动物实验研究都把焦点集中于应用 NMDA 受体阻滞剂来预防或治疗 OIH 及药物耐受。有研究表明，给予氯胺酮可非竞争性地阻滞 NMDA 受体，从而降低大鼠对阿片类药物的耐受[51]。另外几项研究证实，使用氯胺酮[33,37]或 MK-801[34,35]阻滞 NMDA 受体可有效预防大鼠 OIH 的发生。因此，在使用芬太尼前，给予单次剂量的氯胺酮可减轻继发的痛觉过敏，并能增强吗啡镇痛效果，且重复给药效果更佳[37]（图9-9）。同样，在长期应用海洛因之前，给予重复剂量的 MK-801，不但可以预防 OIH，并可抑制由阿片类药物或阿片拮抗剂所致的 OIH 复燃（图9-10）[35]。尤为重要的是，通过氯胺酮阻断 NMDA 受体可降低 OIH 和 NIH 的协同作用（图9-11）[39,40]。

总之，动物研究已充分证明，在应用阿片类药物之前，使用氯胺酮阻断 NMDA 受体可有效抑制随后继发的 OIH，还可预防远期 OIH 的诱发和复燃。这些效应于长期和短期内都可观察到。若 NMDA 受体阻滞剂继续以超过初次使用的剂量使用，则效果更加明显。但目前尚无确切证据表明 NMDA 受体阻滞剂将会作为

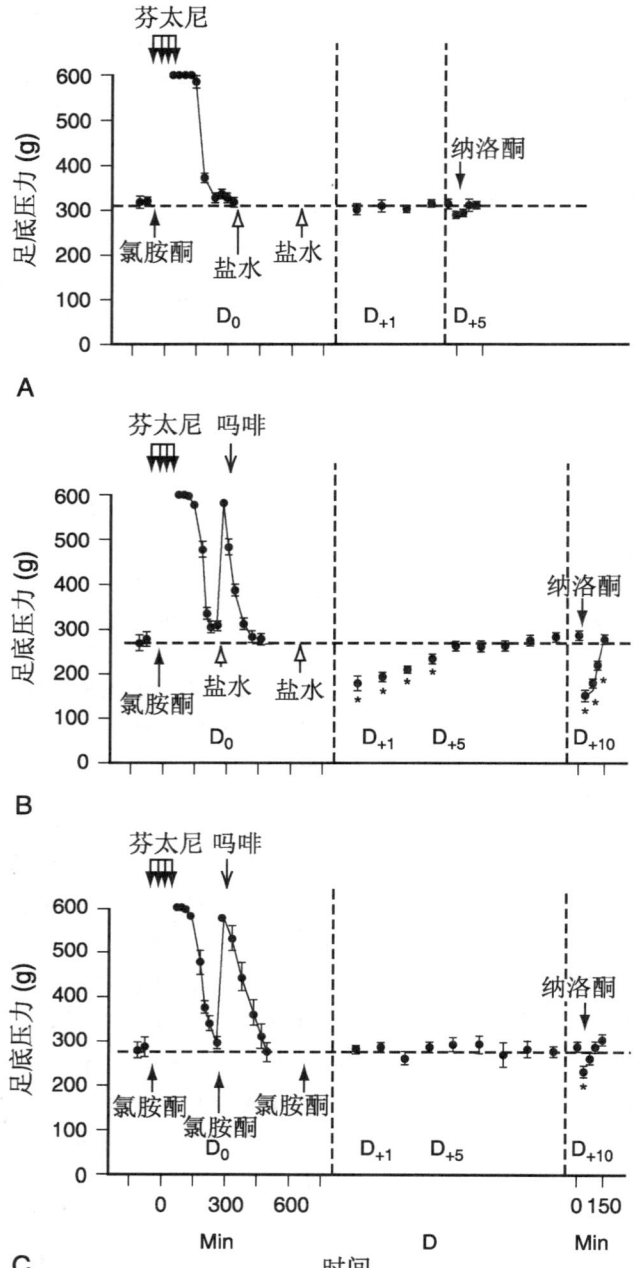

图 9-9 A 到 C，在给予大鼠芬太尼（4× 60μg/kg，皮下）前，单次或持续给予氯胺酮（皮下 10 mg/kg）对疼痛敏感性及吗啡（5 mg/kg SC）镇痛作用的影响。通过使大鼠发出叫声的足底刺激强度（g）来鉴定疼痛敏感性。数值由平均数±SEM 表示。星号表示有统计学意义。D，天；Min，分钟。(From Laulin JP, Maurette P, Corcuff JB, et al: The role of ketamine in preventing fentanyl-induced hyperalgesia and subsequent acute morphine tolerance. Anesth Analg 2002; 94: 1263-1269.)

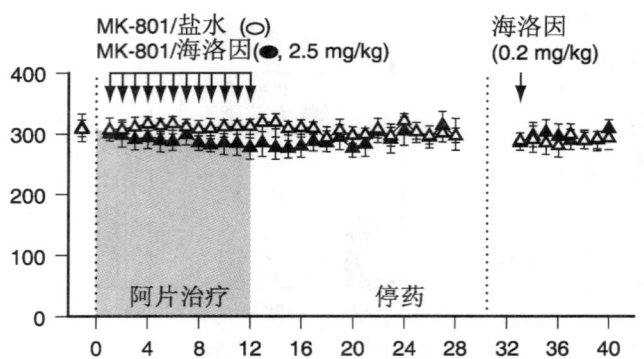

图 9-10 每次在给予海洛因 30 分钟前皮下给予 0.15 mg/kg MK-801，不但可以预防持续 12 天给予海洛因导致的阿片类药物诱发的疼痛过敏，并且可阻断此后给予小剂量海洛因发生疼痛过敏复燃现象。通过使大鼠发出叫声的足底刺激强度（g）来鉴定疼痛敏感性。数值由平均数±SEM 表示。与图 9-4 比较。(From Celerier E, Laulin JP, Corcuff JB, et al: Progressive enhancement of delayed hyperalgesia induced by repeated heroin administration:A sensitization process. J Neurosci 2001; 21:4074-4080.)

治疗措施而应用于临床（与预防性使用相反）。在手术创伤情况下，最有可能的结果是，必须证实 NMDA 受体阻滞剂可以抑制 OIH 和 NIH 之间的协同作用。

人类资料

已证实 NMDA 受体阻滞剂对手术患者的术后疼痛及阿片类药物消耗量有影响，NMDA 受体阻滞剂对 OIH 和药物耐受具有积极的效应[52-56]。人类预防性应用 NMDA 阻滞剂来防治 OIH 的效果到底如何，目前仅有 3 项[5,48,49]正式的志愿者参与的安慰剂对照的前瞻性研究。Koppert 等[5,48]进行的两项研究中，采用经皮刺激诱发和维持的痛觉过敏模型，结果证实，与单独应用瑞芬太尼相比，在瑞芬太尼输注前应用氯胺酮可以防止痛觉过敏区域的增加（图 9-12）。有趣的是，这些研究中有一组证明，虽然氯胺酮对感觉的客观测定（疼痛超敏区域）有较大影响，但 α2 受体激动剂可乐定对主观性疼痛体验有更大影响，提示不同药对 OIH 有不同的效果（图 9-13）[5]。Luginbuhl 等[49]使用压痛阈值进行了第 3 项研究，未能证实氯胺酮的显著效果，可能与芬太尼输注时间过短，加之血浆氯胺酮浓度过低有关。最近的一项研究证实：在腹部大手术后应用氯胺酮对治疗瑞芬太尼诱导的痛觉过敏有效[50]。

9 阿片类药物的异化效应（痛觉过敏和耐受）及其对术后镇痛的影响

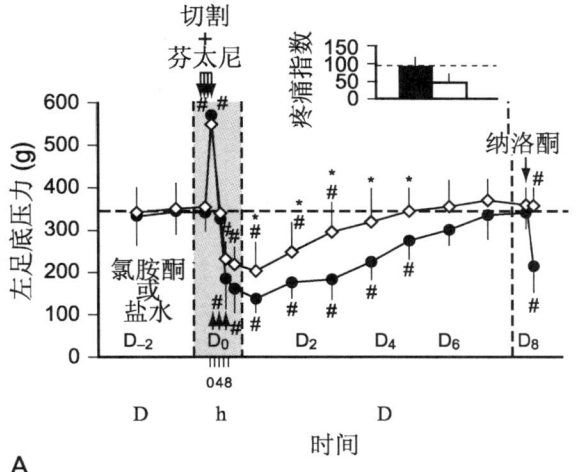

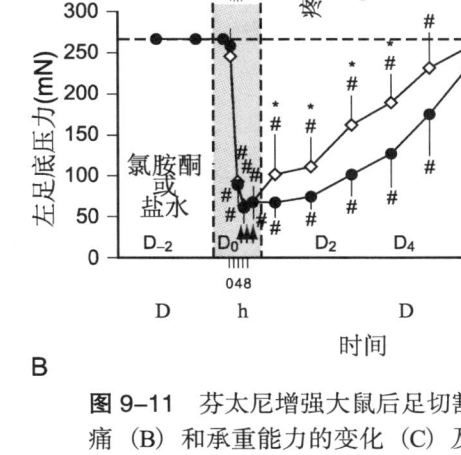

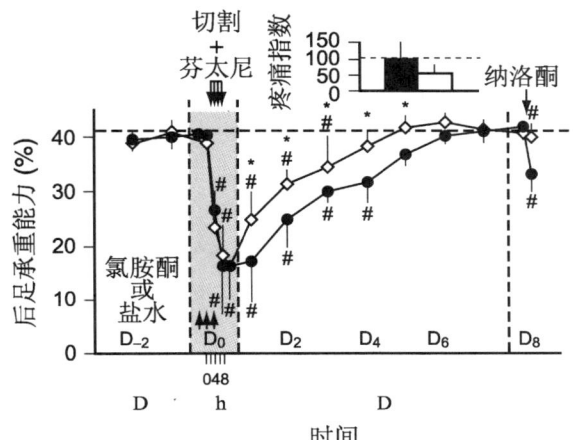

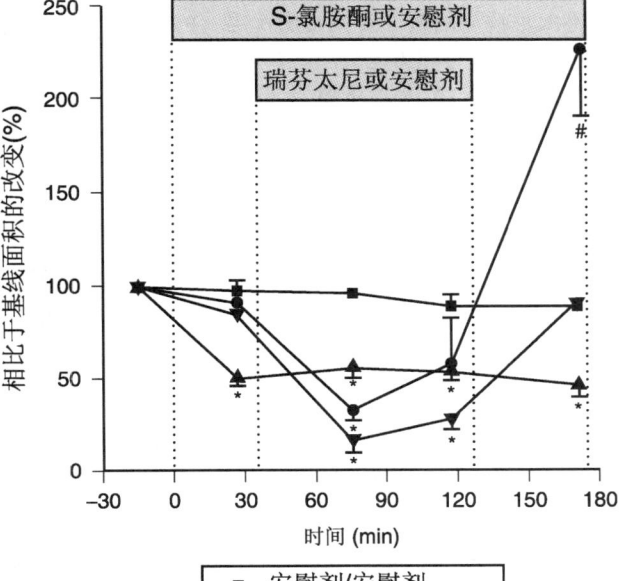

图 9-11 芬太尼增强大鼠后足切割诱发的机械痛敏（A）、触诱发痛（B）和承重能力的变化（C）及氯胺酮对芬太尼这一作用的影响。在 D_0 时通过氟烷麻醉切开大鼠后足底皮肤，皮下（SC）间隔 15 分钟给予 4 次芬太尼（100μg/kg）或含盐注射液，总量为 400μg/kg（n=12）。外科手术结束后给予第二次芬太尼。三次皮下注射氯胺酮（3×10 mg/kg；n=12）或生理盐水（n=12）。首剂芬太尼在外科手术之前 30 分钟给予，随后每 5 小时注射一次。在术前 D_{-2}、D_{-1} 和 D_0 时间点、术后 2、4、6 和 10 小时及随后的 8 天用 3 个参数评价疼痛程度；实验结束时（D_8），所有大鼠均注射纳洛酮（1 mg/kg，SC），这 3 种疼痛参数在 5 分钟后测量。插图表示手术切割后每天机械痛敏（A）、触诱发痛（B）和承重能力（C）三种疼痛指数的变化。疼痛参数值和疼痛指数用均值±SD 来表达。空心圆表示给予生理盐水的大鼠，实心圆表示给予氯胺酮或芬太尼的大鼠；Dunnett 检验，与 D_0 基础值比较 $P<0.05$；*，Dunnett 检验，两组之间相比 $P<0.05$；†，疼痛指数的比较用 Mann-Whitney 检验，$P<0.05$。(From Richebe P, Rivat C, Laulin JP, et al: Ketamine improves the management of exaggerated postoperative pain observed in perioperative fentanyl-treated rats. Anesthesiology 2005;102:421-428.)

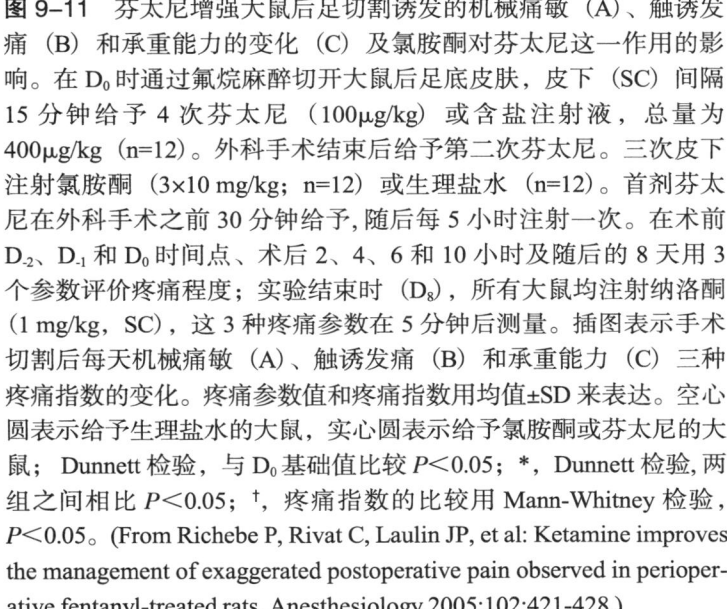

图 9-12 注射 NMDA 受体阻断剂 S-氯胺酮。阿片类激动剂瑞芬太尼、S-氯胺酮和瑞芬太尼混合剂能有效地缩小机械痛敏 50%～75%（*）。但是一旦停止给药（#），机械痛敏的范围将超过单独预给予瑞芬太尼 130%。同时给予 S-氯胺酮将会消除单独给予瑞芬太尼导致的痛觉过敏。在整个实验过程中，生理盐水对照组机械痛敏的区间范围没有发生改变（双因素重复检验，方差分析，与所有对照组相比 $P<0.01$）。数值由平均数± SD 表示。(From Angst MS, Koppert W, Pahl I, et al: Short-term infusion of the mu-opioid agonist remifentanil in humans causes hyperalgesia during withdrawal. Pain 2003;106:49-57.)

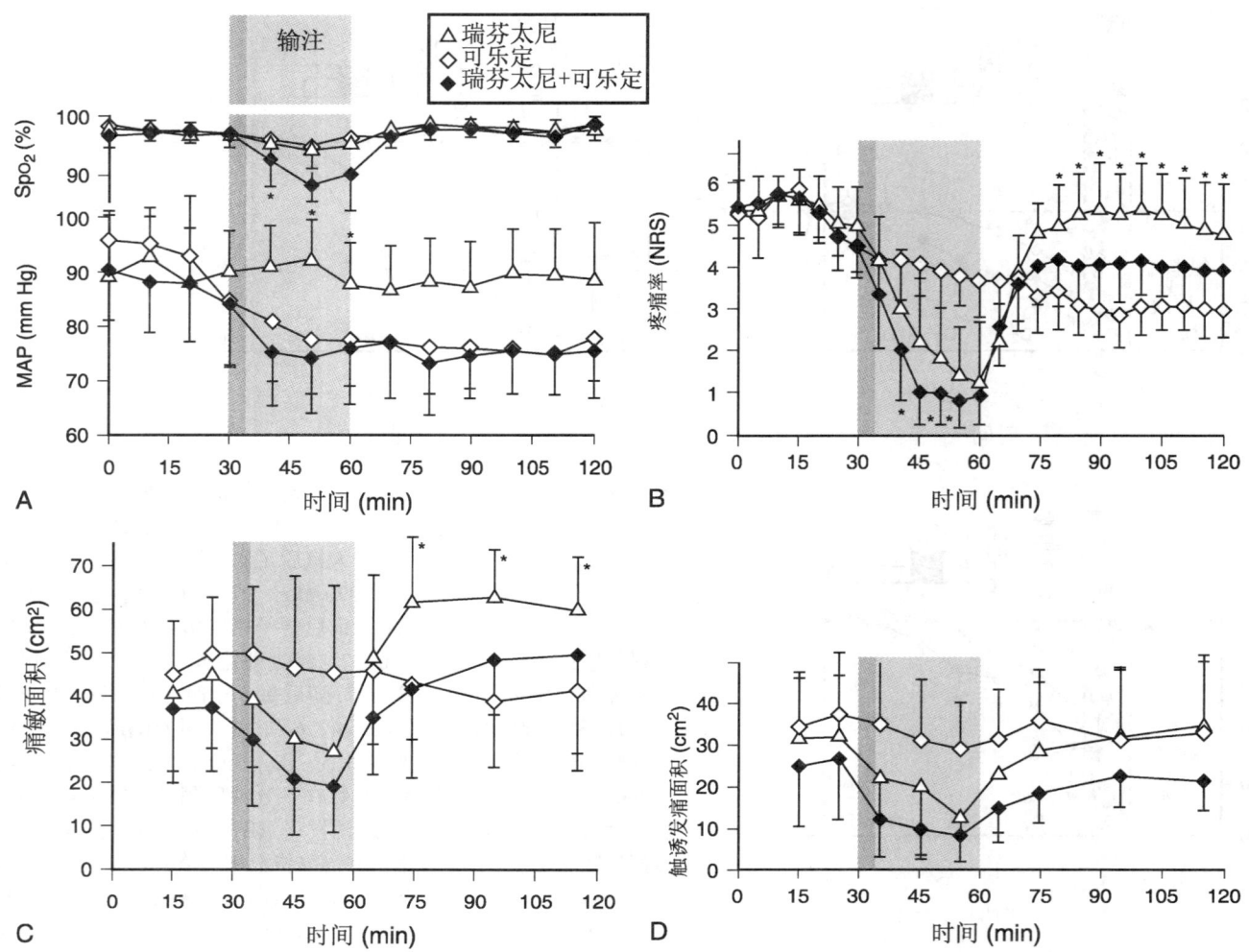

图 9-13 A.在实验期间氧饱和度（SpO$_2$）和平均动脉压（MAP）的时间曲线。同时给予可乐定[给予瑞芬太尼 0.1μg/（kg·min）之前注射 2μg/kg，5 分钟以上）以缩短瑞芬太尼镇痛起效时间，减少瑞芬太尼诱导的输注后抗镇痛作用（$P<0.001$，方差分析）(B)；机械刺激痛敏（方差分析 $P<0.001$）(C)；触诱发痛区域未受影响（D)（每组方差分析，P 值无差异）。数据用平均数±SD（n=13）表示。*，与经 Bonferroni 公式校正过的数据比较，$P<0.05$。NRS，数字评定量表。(From Koppert W, Sittl R, Scheuber K, et al: Differential modulation of remifentanil-induced analgesia and postinfusion hyperalgesia by S-ketamine and clonidine in humans. Anesthesiology 2003;99:152-159.)

目前，在人类通过氯胺酮阻断 NMDA 受体来防止 OIH 的研究尚有限，但被认为是有前景的。显然，确定这种效果的临床真实性和重要性有待更进一步的研究。

总结和结论

目前已有令人信服的动物研究证实了 OIH 和药物耐受的机制。这些研究提示潜在的状态改变可能是长期的，并且影响之后应用的阿片类药物的镇痛效果，甚至在相当长的时间后，应用某种作用于阿片受体的药物后，仍会诱发或导致该现象复燃。在人类中的研究虽然不多，但亦提示了 OIH 和药物耐受的真实存在，其本质与动物实验结果是一致的。目前尚需更深入的研究来确定手术后这种现象的临床相关性。

与有关阿片类药物和 NMDA 受体的关系的理论推测一致，动物试验亦提示 NMDA 受体阻滞剂氯胺酮或 MK-801 可有效抑制 OIH 和药物耐受的形成。尽管动物试验令人信服，但人类研究尚局限于少量的志愿者和临床研究。因此，尚需在人类中进行进一步的研究来验证初始研究的结论，从而确定其临床相关性及意义。

本章开始就已指出，手术后的痛觉过敏是大家都不希望看到的。无论是长期和短期的痛觉过敏，都会严重影响结局。已有的研究显示，目前使用的镇痛方式可能会引起甚至恶化我们正试图避免的临床状况，这让我们感到困惑，因此迫切需要引起大家的关注。显然，该课题目前需要精心设计且与临床密切相关的研究。

这里提出的研究结论将如何影响临床医生的日常实践？手术后痛觉过敏的处理对改善术后疼痛可能是非常关键的。关于 OIH 及其 NMDA 受体阻滞剂的调节作用，目前尚缺乏公认的、特异性、权威性、高水准的临床证据。但已有具备强烈建议性的支持性证据存在，另外，有关小剂量氯胺酮对术后镇痛的积极作用已获得了令人信服的高水准的证据支持[51,54-56]，该证据可使每一位临床医师在日常实践中会考虑到这一概念存在的可能性，直至有权威性结论出现为止。

（杨宇光　毛燕飞译　卞金俊　熊源长校）

参考文献

1. Woolf CJ, Salter MW: Neuronal plasticity: Increasing the gain in pain. Science 2000;288:1765–1769.
2. Wilder-Smith OH, Tassonyi E, Crul BJ, Arendt-Nielsen L: Quantitative sensory testing and human surgery: Effects of analgesic management on postoperative neuroplasticity. Anesthesiology 2003;98:1214–1222.
3. Vinik HR, Kissin I: Rapid development of tolerance to analgesia during remifentanil infusion in humans. Anesth Analg 1998;86:1307–1311.
4. Leung A, Wallace MS, Ridgeway B, Yaksh T: Concentration-effect relationship of intravenous alfentanil and ketamine on peripheral neurosensory thresholds, allodynia and hyperalgesia of neuropathic pain. Pain 2001;91:177–187.
5. Koppert W, Sittl R, Scheuber K, et al: Differential modulation of remifentanil-induced analgesia and postinfusion hyperalgesia by S-ketamine and clonidine in humans. Anesthesiology 2003;99:152–159.
6. Simonnet G, Rivat C: Opioid-induced hyperalgesia: Abnormal or normal pain? Neuroreport 2003;14:1–7.
7. Kehlet H: Postoperative pain relief—what is the issue? Br J Anaesth 1994;72:375–378.
8. Carli F, Mayo N, Klubien K, et al: Epidural analgesia enhances functional exercise capacity and health-related quality of life after colonic surgery: Results of a randomized trial. Anesthesiology 2002;97:540–549.
9. Rodgers A, Walker N, Schug S, et al: Reduction of postoperative mortality and morbidity with epidural or spinal anaesthesia: Results from overview of randomised trials. BMJ 2000;321:1493.
10. Macrae WA: Chronic pain after surgery. Br J Anaesth 2001;87:88–98.
11. Perkins FM, Kehlet H: Chronic pain as an outcome of surgery: A review of predictive factors. Anesthesiology 2000;93:1123–1133.
12. Coderre TJ, Katz J, Vaccarino AL, Melzack R: Contribution of central neuroplasticity to pathological pain: Review of clinical and experimental evidence. Pain 1993;52:259–285.
13. Christie MJ, Williams JT, North RA: Mechanisms of tolerance to opiates in locus coeruleus neurons. NIDA Res Monogr 1987;78:158–168.
14. Christie MJ, Williams JT, North RA: Cellular mechanisms of opioid tolerance: Studies in single brain neurons. Mol Pharmacol 1987;32:633–638.
15. Whistler JL, Chuang HH, Chu P, et al: Functional dissociation of mu opioid receptor signaling and endocytosis: Implications for the biology of opiate tolerance and addiction. Neuron 1999;23:737–746.
16. Crain SM, Shen KF: Antagonists of excitatory opioid receptor functions enhance morphine's analgesic potency and attenuate opioid tolerance/dependence liability. Pain 2000;84:121–131.
17. Mao J, Mayer DJ: Spinal cord neuroplasticity following repeated opioid exposure and its relation to pathological pain. Ann N Y Acad Sci 2001;933:175–184.
18. Aanonsen LM, Wilcox GL: Nociceptive action of excitatory amino acids in the mouse: Effects of spinally administered opioids, phencyclidine and sigma agonists. J Pharmacol Exp Ther 1987;243:9–19.
19. Cadet P, Mantione K, Bilfinger TV, Stefano GB: Real-time RT-PCR measurement of the modulation of Mu opiate receptor expression by nitric oxide in human mononuclear cells. Med Sci Monit 2001;7:1123–1128.
20. Watkins LR, Milligan ED, Maier SF: Glial activation: A driving force for pathological pain. Trends Neurosci 2001;24:450–455.
21. Watkins LR, Milligan ED, Maier SF: Glial proinflammatory cytokines mediate exaggerated pain states: Implications for clinical pain. Adv Exp Med Biol 2003;521:1–21.
22. DeLeo JA, Tanga FY, Tawfik VL: Neuroimmune activation and neuroinflammation in chronic pain and opioid tolerance/hyperalgesia. Neuroscientist 2004;10:40–52.
23. Wieseler-Frank J, Maier SF, Watkins LR: Immune-to-brain communication dynamically modulates pain: Physiological and pathological consequences. Brain Behav Immun 2005;19:104–111.
24. Vanderah TW, Ossipov MH, Lai J, et al: Mechanisms of opioid-induced pain and antinociceptive tolerance: Descending facilitation and spinal dynorphin. Pain 2001;92:5–9.
25. Gardell LR, Wang R, Burgess SE, et al: Sustained morphine exposure induces a spinal dynorphin-dependent enhancement of excitatory transmitter release from primary afferent fibers. J Neurosci 2002;22:6747–6755.
26. Ossipov MH, Lai J, Vanderah TW, Porreca F: Induction of pain facilitation by sustained opioid exposure: Relationship to opioid antinociceptive tolerance. Life Sci 2003;73:783–800.
27. Fields HL, Vanegas H, Hentall ID, Zorman G: Evidence that disinhibition of brain stem neurones contributes to morphine analgesia. Nature 1983;306:684–686.
28. Schnell C, Ulucan C, Ellrich J: Atypical on-, off- and neutral cells in the rostral ventromedial medulla oblongata in rat. Exp Brain Res 2002;145:64–75.
29. McGaraughty S, Reinis S, Tsoukatos J: Two distinct unit activity responses to morphine in the rostral ventromedial medulla of awake rats. Brain Res 1993;604:331–333.
30. Heinricher MM, Neubert MJ: Neural basis for the hyperalgesic action of cholecystokinin in the rostral ventromedial medulla. J Neurophysiol 2004;92:1982–1989.
31. Yaksh TL, Harty GJ: Pharmacology of the allodynia in rats evoked by high dose intrathecal morphine. J Pharmacol Exp Ther 1988;244:501–507.
32. Smith MT: Neuroexcitatory effects of morphine and hydromorphone: Evidence implicating the 3-glucuronide metabolites. Clin Exp Pharmacol Physiol 2000;27:524–528.
33. Celerier E, Rivat C, Jun Y, et al: Long-lasting hyperalgesia induced by fentanyl in rats: Preventive effect of ketamine. Anesthesiology 2000;92:465–472.
34. Celerier E, Laulin J, Larcher A, et al: Evidence for opiate-activated NMDA processes masking opiate analgesia in rats. Brain Res 1999;847:18–25.
35. Celerier E, Laulin JP, Corcuff JB, et al: Progressive enhancement of delayed hyperalgesia induced by repeated heroin administration: A sensitization process. J Neurosci 2001;21:4074–4080.
36. Laulin JP, Celerier E, Larcher A, et al: Opiate tolerance to daily heroin administration: An apparent phenomenon associated with enhanced pain sensitivity. Neuroscience 1999;89:631–636.
37. Laulin JP, Maurette P, Corcuff JB, et al: The role of ketamine in preventing fentanyl-induced hyperalgesia and subsequent acute morphine tolerance. Anesth Analg 2002;94:1263–1269.
38. Laulin JP, Larcher A, Celerier E, et al: Long-lasting increased pain sensitivity in rat following exposure to heroin for the first time. Eur J Neurosci 1998;10:782–785.
39. Rivat C, Laulin JP, Corcuff JB, et al: Fentanyl enhancement of carrageenan-induced long-lasting hyperalgesia in rats: Prevention by the N-methyl-D-aspartate receptor antagonist ketamine. Anesthesiology 2002;96:381–391.
40. Richebe P, Rivat C, Laulin JP, et al: Ketamine improves the management of exaggerated postoperative pain observed in perioperative fentanyl-treated rats. Anesthesiology 2005;102:421–428.
41. Koppert W: [Opioid-induced hyperalgesia. Pathophysiology and clinical relevance.] Anaesthesist 2004;53:455–466.
42. Mao J: Opioid-induced abnormal pain sensitivity: Implications in clinical opioid therapy. Pain 2002;100:213–217.
43. Mercadante S, Ferrera P, Villari P, Arcuri E: Hyperalgesia: An emerging

44. Twycross R: Paradoxical pain. BMJ 1993;306:793.
45. Hanks GW, O'Neill WM, Fallon MT: Paradoxical pain. BMJ 1993;306:793.
46. Bowsher D: Paradoxical pain. BMJ 1993;306:473–474.
47. Doverty M, White JM, Somogyi AA, et al: Hyperalgesic responses in methadone maintenance patients. Pain 2001;90:91–96.
48. Angst MS, Koppert W, Pahl I, et al: Short-term infusion of the mu-opioid agonist remifentanil in humans causes hyperalgesia during withdrawal. Pain 2003;106:49–57.
49. Luginbuhl M, Gerber A, Schnider TW, et al: Modulation of remifentanil-induced analgesia, hyperalgesia, and tolerance by small-dose ketamine in humans. Anesth Analg 2003;96:726–732.
50. Joly V, Richebe P, Guignard B, et al: Remifentanil-induced postoperative hyperalgesia and its prevention with small-dose ketamine. Anesthesiology 2005;103:147–155.
51. Kissin I, Bright CA, Bradley EL Jr: The effect of ketamine on opioid-induced acute tolerance: Can it explain reduction of opioid consumption with ketamine-opioid analgesic combinations? Anesth Analg 2000;91:1483–1488.
52. Schmid RL, Sandler AN, Katz J: Use and efficacy of low-dose ketamine in the management of acute postoperative pain: A review of current techniques and outcomes. Pain 1999;82:111–125.
53. De Kock M, Lavand'homme P, Waterloos H: 'Balanced analgesia' in the perioperative period: Is there a place for ketamine? Pain 2001;92:373–380.
54. McCartney CJ, Sinha A, Katz J: A qualitative systematic review of the role of N-methyl-D-aspartate receptor antagonists in preventive analgesia. Anesth Analg 2004;98:1385–1400.
55. Raith K, Hochhaus G: Drugs used in the treatment of opioid tolerance and physical dependence: A review. Int J Clin Pharmacol Ther 2004;42:191–203.
56. Subramaniam K, Subramaniam B, Steinbrook RA: Ketamine as adjuvant analgesic to opioids: A quantitative and qualitative systematic review. Anesth Analg 2004;99:482–495.

第3部分 术后疼痛管理

10 疼痛管理目标的制定

PETER G. MOORE

人性化治疗的基本原则

近年来，疼痛误诊和治疗上的缺陷相当普遍，这个问题已经引起了立法者、州、联邦管理机构以及医疗保健机构的关注[1-5]。为此，卫生保健组织和机构制定了新的规则和标准，即把疼痛治疗作为首要治疗目的[4,6,7]。

在建立国家级治疗程序时，卫生保健组织联合委员会（Joint Commission on Accreditation of Healthcare Organizations，JCAHO）主席Dennis S. O'Leary教授说："不能缓解的疼痛在生理上和心理上对患者都有巨大影响。"联合委员会认为，有效的疼痛治疗是良好治疗的重要组成部分。他还说："研究工作清楚地表明了不能缓解的疼痛会延缓患者康复的速度，增加患者和家属的负担，并增加卫生保健体系的费用[8]。"

术后疼痛的定义是指与手术相关的组织损伤所引起的急性疼痛。虽然手术及其伴发损伤会引起急性痛，但这可能不是引起术后疼痛的唯一原因。许多疼痛是由于长时间手术制动以及局部受压所致。此外，很多患者术前还忍受着慢性疼痛的折磨，这种疼痛是潜在疾病或损伤引起的——如一些退行性或恶性疾病可能在术后产生剧烈疼痛。

术后疼痛治疗的基本原则是建立在这样一个理念基础上的，即解除疼痛是人类的基本权利，疼痛是可以治愈的，疼痛治疗能促进患者康复[9]。该原则否定了疼痛是组织损伤和手术后不可避免的结果这一说法。术后疼痛治疗的目的就是止痛和促进康复。JCAHO在为医疗保健机构制定治疗目标时建立了新的基本原则（表10-1），要求医疗机构和医护人员肯定患者进行疼痛治疗的权利[8]。

JCAHO标准首先提出患者有权利对疼痛进行合适的评估和治疗。其基本观点就是疼痛治疗不是一种辅助治疗措施，而是整个疾病治疗中的基本的不可分割的一部分。疼痛治疗人性化原则的基本原理源于以下3方面：

- 患者的基本权利——尽管外科手术会造成身体

表10-1　JCAHO推荐的疼痛治疗原则

权利和伦理	承认患者有恰当的疼痛评估和疼痛治疗的权利
疼痛评估	对每个患者都进行评估，如果有疼痛，记录疼痛的性质和程度，便于再次评估及随访
患者护理	建立便于有效止痛药物处方和发放的政策和操作流程
患者教育	对患者及其家属进行有效疼痛管理培训
后继治疗	为出院患者制定疼痛治疗计划
提高止痛质量和医疗机构的性能	确保所有医务人员有资格进行疼痛评估和疼痛治疗，并对新医务人员进行疼痛评估和治疗的能力培训

Adapted from Joint Commission on Accreditation of Healthcare Organizations: Joint Commission focuses on pain management. Aug 3, 1999. Available at www.jcaho.org/news+room/health+care+issues/jcaho+focus+on+pain+management.htm

的损伤，但必须让患者脱离或减轻疼痛。
- 患者的知情同意权——患者有权知道他（她）所接受的治疗情况。
- 人人平等的治疗权——确立以患者需要为基础的治疗标准。

基于上述基本原理，我们认识到患者有权利知道他们的病情、了解各项治疗措施包括治疗可能引起的风险以及在手术期间的治疗计划等。这些必须告之患者，使其同意并参与治疗计划。

患者术前培训证据

尽管最近关注的焦点问题仍集中在疼痛未及时治疗上，但不恰当的疼痛治疗也需要注意。有证据表明手术患者虽然在术后进行了疼痛治疗，却有近50%的患者疼痛治疗可能并不恰当，这些患者中重度疼痛的发生率达25%~40%[10-12]。此结果和以前的研究相比已有很大进步。既往曾有报道称中至重度疼痛的发生率为87%，并且药物延迟治疗的比率占到了41%[13]。术后疼痛仍是一个基本问题的原因在于患者总认为疼痛是外科手术的必然并发症，因而常常被忽略[12]。

未控制的疼痛或控制不佳的疼痛，即使偶尔发作一次——尽管时间短暂，也可能会很大程度地影响患者对治疗的看法。但在对患者的调查过程中，这种影响往往被忽视[14-16]。

单凭患者的自我感觉并不能有效地测量疼痛治疗的效果。只有使用疼痛评估系统及一些特定检查来了解患者的疼痛经历，才能正确评定疼痛治疗的有效性[15,17-22]。

对患者进行术前培训的优点包括缓解患者的焦虑、恐惧、担心，以及让他们了解止痛是术后治疗的目的之一[23-40]。疼痛治疗过程中，来自患者的障碍主要包括文化和语言上的障碍、自身或亲属朋友的相关经历以及担心药物成瘾等[17,25,37,41-45]。通过对患者的教育和个别辅导可以改变患者的态度，克服这些障碍[40,45-47]。有充分的证据表明，通过专业医师或护士对患者进行积极的术前教育，能在术后疼痛治疗中取得更佳结局[26,34,35,48-63]。

对先前已存在疼痛的术前疼痛治疗证据

据估计，大多数择期手术患者术前存在中到重度的慢性疼痛[24,25,31,49,64,65]。退行性关节病行关节成形术的患者术前都存在严重疼痛，对他们积极进行术前疼痛治疗能显著改善术后疼痛治疗的效果并有助于患者的康复[20,24,26,27,34,35,39,49,54,64-75]。2004年9月罗非考昔撤离市场使环氧合酶-2（cyclooxygenase-2，COX-2）类镇痛药引起了特别关注[76-86]。因为这是一个突发事件，所以手术期间停用COX-2类药物所带来的影响尚不清楚[87,88]。

超前镇痛证据

超前镇痛的概念是建立在实验研究基础之上的，即术前镇痛可以阻断或者减少伤害性刺激诱发的神经生理和神经递质的变化，从而减轻术后疼痛的强烈程度。换言之，超前镇痛抑制了"wind-up"现象[89-91]。从大量动物模型中得到的动物研究结果尚可，但超前镇痛在临床上的结果却不尽相同。虽然在术后早期单独或联合使用氯胺酮[92-94]、神经阻滞[89,92,95-97]、局部止痛[98-100]、非甾体类抗炎药（nonsteroidal anti-inflammatory drug，NSAID）[101-117]以及非口服阿片类等药物对早期疼痛有不同的疗效[94,98-100,103,105,108-111,114-119]，但对于慢性术后疼痛综合征的治疗效果却欠佳，甚至无效[92,97-99,112,118,120,121]。

联合疼痛治疗证据

大量临床研究有力地证明了术后疼痛是个多因素问题，需要联合治疗[67,99,110,117,122-131]。联合治疗较单项治疗更能改善外科手术结局。联合治疗术后措施包括作用于不同部位的各种药物治疗以及治疗急性疼痛的各种支持性和辅助性治疗措施，几项结局性研究对此提供了坚实的证据[132-135]。

"急性疼痛治疗小组"证据

建立公共疼痛服务机构或"急性疼痛治疗小组"主要是为了改善住院患者的疼痛治疗[136-142]。虽然一些研究质疑急性疼痛治疗小组的效能，但他们已经最大程度地证明了自身的价值[50,143-145]。然而，建立急性疼痛治疗小组以及发挥其效能仍然面临着巨大的挑战[144,146-150]，其中最主要的障碍在于运行成本，因为这项服务收费低廉[147,148]。急性疼痛治疗小组的功能除了有益于患者外，还能够降低医院成本（包括改善手术结局、促进患者康复以及提前出院）[145]。

建立疼痛标准改善患者护理的证据

针对住院患者疼痛治疗的不足，在2000年，作为美国建立质量标准的主要机构，JCAHO提出了疼痛治疗的国家性目标和标准[2]。这个提议的提出基于这样一个基本观念，即有效的疼痛治疗能改善患者护理[143]。但在2003—2004年发表的一些调查表明，虽然疼痛治疗已经有了很大程度的改善，但仍有大量患者在住院治疗时承受了中到重度的疼痛[12,50,146,149-151]。普遍的观点认为，现在住院患者的疼痛治疗已经有了提高，在疼痛管理标准提高之前，更多的工作应该放在对患者和医护人员的教育上[12,152-154]。JCAHO提出的原则就是要让所有参加围术期治疗的医务人员明白，缓解疼痛和痛苦是疾病治疗不可质疑的目的，即疼痛治疗不是辅助治疗，而是疾病整体治疗的一部分[155-157]。

推荐

以患者为中心的多种治疗模式

作为外科治疗的一部分，术后疼痛治疗的主要目标是预防和（或）减轻患者的疼痛和痛苦。术中疼痛管理必须根据患者的需要进行个体化治疗，使患者潜在的疾病或手术创伤带来的疼痛和痛苦得到缓解，以加快患者恢复（甚至恢复到正常功能）。

一个多模式疼痛治疗计划的制定应该考虑到各种可能引起伤害性刺激和潜在疼痛的发生机制以及先前存在的疼痛情况，除此以外，还要考虑到可能影响患者痛觉、汇报疼痛状况意愿和放大疼痛可能的心理因素，如恐惧、焦虑和误解等。

制度的实施

有效的术后疼痛治疗需要一个明确的疼痛治疗制度来保障，所有参与治疗的医务人员必须把缓解患者疼痛作为患者手术治疗和康复过程中的首要目的来对待。制度能强制性地规定整个治疗过程的标准，并让所有医护工作者学习和执行这些标准，确保所有患者都能得到恰当的疼痛评估和治疗。疼痛治疗制度的建立和对医务工作者的教育必须在多学科疼痛治疗工作小组的指导下进行，包括疼痛专科医师、麻醉医师、外科医师、临床专科护士、药剂师以及制度制订人员、教育人员和密切监督和实施质量控制的人员（图10-1）。

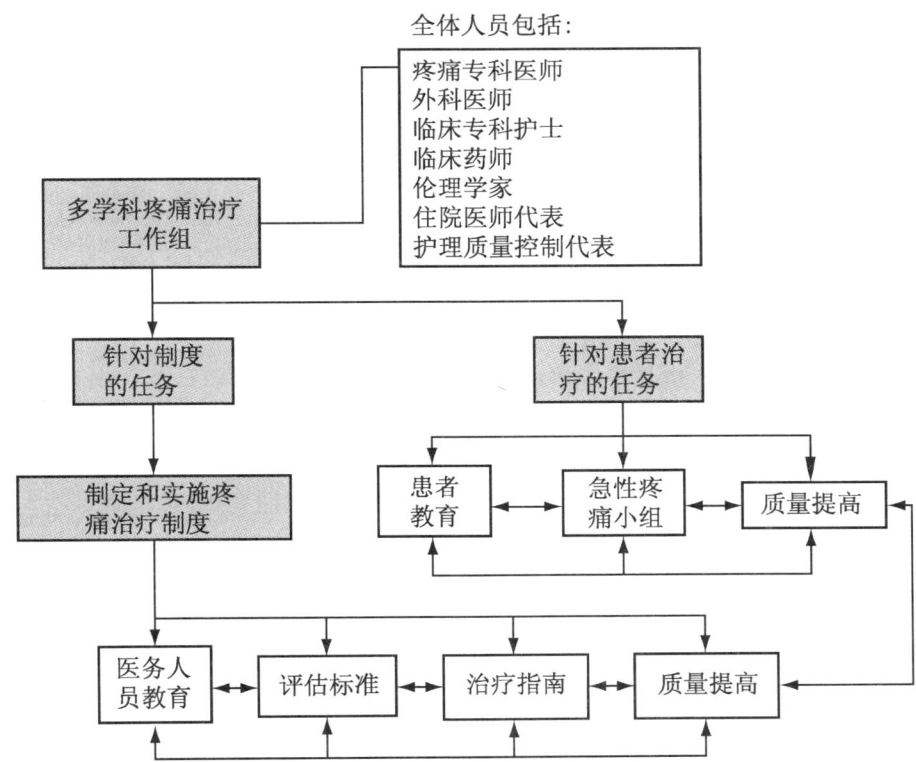

图10-1 疼痛治疗制度以及急性疼痛治疗流程。

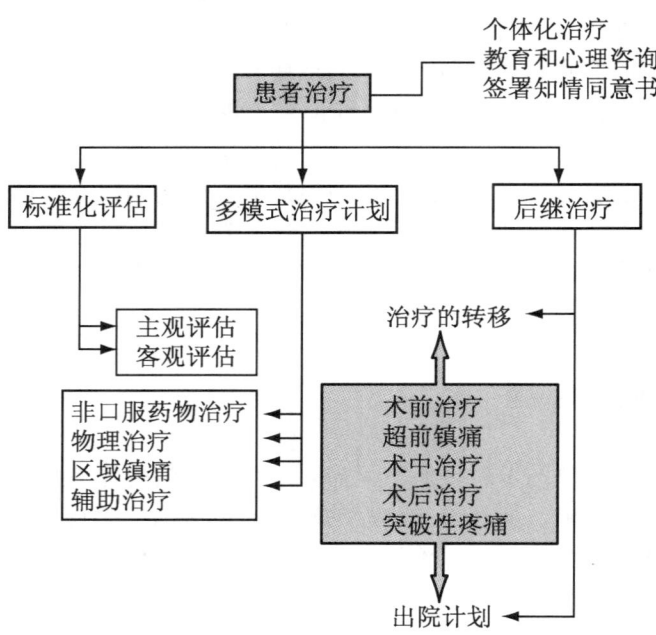

图 10-2 外科手术后的整体疼痛治疗流程。

建立急性疼痛治疗小组是患者治疗过程中的关键步骤，他们可以和患者诊疗小组进行协商，指导和协调疼痛治疗计划（图 10-2）。考虑到患者住院期间有效疼痛治疗的重要性以及患者住院期间要进行多次交接，急性疼痛治疗小组的一个工作中心就是确保患者住院和出院后疼痛治疗的连续性。对病人手术期间各个不同阶段（术前、术中和术前）间的有效管理和过渡缺乏系统性，是导致疼痛治疗有效性低的主要原因，无论疼痛测量方法和治疗水平如何皆如此。

全国性议程

关于疼痛治疗的全国性议程必须从学校和其他培训机构的教育开始。疼痛治疗必须是护理和医学院教育课程的一部分，也是毕业培训计划的一部分。此外，医学、护理继续教育以及换发证程序必须保证有资格且有执照的医师保持对当前疼痛治疗实践的能力。即使有了这些非常重要的步骤，加强疼痛治疗的知识性和系统性还需要一个观念的转变，即止痛药物的基本作用——疼痛是可以治愈的，只要存在疼痛就应该治疗。最近的事件表明，即使医师不能尽职治疗疼痛，立法机构和检查机构会强制要求。

（葛建云　毛燕飞译　杜健儿　熊源长校）

参考文献

1. Thomson H: A new law to improve pain management and end-of-life care: Learning how to treat patients in pain and near death must become a priority. West J Med 2001;174:161–162.
2. Phillips DM: JCAHO pain management standards are unveiled. Joint Commission on Accreditation of Healthcare Organizations. JAMA 2000; 284:428–429.
3. Acello B: Meeting JCAHO standards for pain control. Nursing 2000; 30:52–54.
4. Practice guidelines for acute pain management in the perioperative setting. A report by the American Society of Anesthesiologists Task Force on Pain Management, Acute Pain Section. Anesthesiology 1995;82:1071–1081.
5. Rich BA: Physicians' legal duty to relieve suffering. West J Med 2001; 175:151–152.
6. National Pharmaceutical Council, Inc: Pain: Current understanding of assessment, management, and treatments. Dec 1, 2001. Available at www.jcaho.org/news+room/health+care+issues/pain_mono_+npc.pdf
7. Practice guidelines for postanesthetic care: A report by the American Society of Anesthesiologists Task Force on Postanesthetic Care. Anesthesiology 2002;96:742–752.
8. Joint Commission on Accreditation of Healthcare Organizations: Joint Commission focuses on pain management. Aug 3, 1999. Available at www.jcaho.org/news+room/health+care+issues/jcaho+focus+on+pain+management.htm
9. Cousins MJ, Brennan F, Carr DB: Pain relief: A universal human right. Pain 2004;112:1–4.
10. Dolin SJ, Cashman JN, Bland JM: Effectiveness of acute postoperative pain management. I: Evidence from published data. Br J Anaesth 2002;89:409–423.
11. Svensson I, Sjostrom B, Haljamae H: Assessment of pain experiences after elective surgery. J Pain Symptom Manage 2000;20:193–201.
12. Apfelbaum JL, Chen C, Mehta SS, Gan TJ: Postoperative pain experience: Results from a national survey suggest postoperative pain continues to be undermanaged. Anesth Analg 2003;97:534–540.
13. Bruster S, Jarman B, Bosanquet N, et al: National survey of hospital patients. BMJ 1994;309:1542–1546.
14. Bostrom BM, Ramberg T, Davis BD, Fridlund B: Survey of post-operative patients' pain management. J Nurs Manag 1997;5:341–349.
15. McNeill JA, Sherwood GD, Starck PL, Thompson CJ: Assessing clinical outcomes: Patient satisfaction with pain management. J Pain Symptom Manage 1998;16:29–40.
16. Carroll KC, Atkins PJ, Herold GR, et al: Pain assessment and management in critically ill postoperative and trauma patients: A multisite study. Am J Crit Care 1999;8:105–117.
17. McNeill JA, Sherwood GD, Starck PL, Nieto B: Pain management outcomes for hospitalized Hispanic patients. Pain Manag Nurs 2001;2:25–36.
18. Blank FS, Mader TJ, Wolfe J, et al: Adequacy of pain assessment and pain relief and correlation of patient satisfaction in 68 ED fast-track patients. J Emerg Nurs 2001;27:327–334.
19. Corizzo CC, Baker MC, Henkelmann GC: Assessment of patient satisfaction with pain management in small community inpatient and outpatient settings. Oncol Nurs Forum 2000;27:1279–1286.
20. Jamison RN, Ross MJ, Hoopman P, et al: Assessment of postoperative pain management: Patient satisfaction and perceived helpfulness. Clin J Pain 1997;13:229–236.

21. Sherwood GD, McNeill JA, Starck PL, Disnard G: Changing acute pain management outcomes in surgical patients. AORN J 2003;77:374, 377–380, 384–390.
22. Yellen E, Davis GC: Patient satisfaction in ambulatory surgery. AORN J 2001;74:483–486, 489–494, 496–498.
23. Bauer KP, Dom PM, Ramirez AM, O'Flaherty JE: Preoperative intravenous midazolam: Benefits beyond anxiolysis. J Clin Anesth 2004;16:177–183.
24. Brander VA, Stulberg SD, Adams AD, et al: Predicting total knee replacement pain: A prospective, observational study. Clin Orthop 2003;(416):27–36.
25. Caumo W, Schmidt AP, Schneider CN, et al: Preoperative predictors of moderate to intense acute postoperative pain in patients undergoing abdominal surgery. Acta Anaesthesiol Scand 2002;46:1265–1271.
26. Daltroy LH, Morlino CI, Eaton HM, et al: Preoperative education for total hip and knee replacement patients. Arthritis Care Res 1998;11:469–478.
27. Doering S, Katzlberger F, Rumpold G, et al: Videotape preparation of patients before hip replacement surgery reduces stress. Psychosom Med 2000;62:365–373.
28. Juhl IU, Christensen BV, Bulow HH, et al: Postoperative pain relief, from the patients' and the nurses' point of view. Acta Anaesthesiol Scand 1993;37:404–409.
29. Kain ZN, Sevarino F, Alexander GM, et al: Preoperative anxiety and postoperative pain in women undergoing hysterectomy: A repeated-measures design. J Psychosom Res 2000;49:417–422.
30. Kain ZN, Sevarino F, Pincus S, et al: Attenuation of the preoperative stress response with midazolam: Effects on postoperative outcomes. Anesthesiology 2000;93:141–147.
31. Kalkman CJ, Visser K, Moen J, et al: Preoperative prediction of severe postoperative pain. Pain 2003;105:415–423.
32. Karling M, Renstrom M, Ljungman G: Acute and postoperative pain in children: A Swedish nationwide survey. Acta Paediatr 2002;91:660–666.
33. Lamontagne LL, Hepworth JT, Salisbury MH: Anxiety and postoperative pain in children who undergo major orthopedic surgery. Appl Nurs Res 2001;14:119–124.
34. McDonald S, Hetrick S, Green S: Pre-operative education for hip or knee replacement. Cochrane Database Syst Rev 2004;1:CD003526.
35. Messer B: Total joint replacement preadmission programs. Orthop Nurs 1998;17(Suppl):31–33.
36. Ozalp G, Sarioglu R, Tuncel G, et al: Preoperative emotional states in patients with breast cancer and postoperative pain. Acta Anaesthesiol Scand 2003;47:26–29.
37. Polomano RC, Heffner SM, Reck DL, et al: Evidence for opioid variability. Part 2: Psychosocial influences. Semin Perioper Nurs 2001;10:159–166.
38. Scott LE, Clum GA, Peoples JB: Preoperative predictors of postoperative pain. Pain 1983;15:283–293.
39. Sjoling M, Nordahl G, Olofsson N, Asplund K: The impact of preoperative information on state anxiety, postoperative pain and satisfaction with pain management. Patient Educ Couns 2003;51:169–176.
40. Winefield HR, Katsikitis M, Hart LM, Rounsefell BF: Postoperative pain experiences: Relevant patient and staff attitudes. J Psychosom Res 1990;34:543–552.
41. Bell ML, Reeves KA: Postoperative pain management in the non-Hispanic white and Mexican American older adult. Semin Perioper Nurs 1999;8:7–11.
42. Calvillo ER, Flaskerud JH: Evaluation of the pain response by Mexican American and Anglo American women and their nurses. J Adv Nurs 1993;18:451–459.
43. Dimmitt J: Rural Mexican-American and non-Hispanic white women: Effects of abuse on self-concept. J Cult Divers 1995;2:54–63.
44. Fenwick C, Stevens J: Post operative pain experiences of central Australian aboriginal women: What do we understand? Aust J Rural Health 2004;12:22–27.
45. Greer SM, Dalton JA, Carlson J, Youngblood R: Surgical patients' fear of addiction to pain medication: The effect of an educational program for clinicians. Clin J Pain 2001;17:157–164.
46. Bennett DS, Carr DB: Opiophobia as a barrier to the treatment of pain. J Pain Palliat Care Pharmacother 2002;16:105–109.
47. Beauregard L, Pomp A, Choiniere M: Severity and impact of pain after day-surgery. Can J Anaesth 1998;45:304–311.
48. Management approaches for improved patient outcomes. Orthop Nurs 2000;(19 Suppl):10–21.
49. Berge DJ, Dolin SJ, Williams AC, Harman R: Pre-operative and post-operative effect of a pain management programme prior to total hip replacement: A randomized controlled trial. Pain 2004;110:33–39.
50. Chung JW, Lui JC: Postoperative pain management: Study of patients' level of pain and satisfaction with health care providers' responsiveness to their reports of pain. Nurs Health Sci 2003;5:13–21.
51. Dalton JA, Blau W, Lindley C, et al: Changing acute pain management to improve patient outcomes: An educational approach. J Pain Symptom Manag 1999;17:277–287.
52. Dawkins S: Patient-controlled analgesia after coronary artery bypass grafting. Nurs Times 2003;99:30–31.
53. Devine EC, Bevsek SA, Brubakken K, et al: AHCPR clinical practice guideline on surgical pain management: Adoption and outcomes. Res Nurs Health 1999;22:119–130.
54. Gocen Z, Sen A, Unver B, et al: The effect of preoperative physiotherapy and education on the outcome of total hip replacement: A prospective randomized controlled trial. Clin Rehabil 2004;18:353–358.
55. Goldsmith DM, Safran C: Using the Web to reduce postoperative pain following ambulatory surgery. Proc AMIA Symp 1999:780–784.
56. Griffin MJ, Brennan L, McShane AJ: Preoperative education and outcome of patient controlled analgesia. Can J Anaesth 1998;45:943–948.
57. Harrington JT, Dopf CA, Chalgren CS: Implementing guidelines for interdisciplinary care of low back pain: A critical role for pre-appointment management of specialty referrals. Jt Comm J Qual Improv 2001;27:651–663.
58. LaMontagne LL, Hepworth JT, Cohen F, Salisbury MH: Cognitive-behavioral intervention effects on adolescents' anxiety and pain following spinal fusion surgery. Nurs Res 2003;52:183–190.
59. Ridge RA, Goodson AS: The relationship between multidisciplinary discharge outcomes and functional status after total hip replacement. Orthop Nurs 2000;19:71–82.
60. Shuldham CM, Fleming S, Goodman H: The impact of pre-operative education on recovery following coronary artery bypass surgery: A randomized controlled clinical trial. Eur Heart J 2002;23:666–674.
61. Teutsch C: Patient-doctor communication. Med Clin North Am 2003;87:1115–1145.
62. Watt-Watson J, Stevens B, Costello J, et al: Impact of preoperative education on pain management outcomes after coronary artery bypass graft surgery: A pilot. Can J Nurs Res 2000;31:41–56.
63. Watt-Watson J, Stevens B, Katz J, et al: Impact of preoperative education on pain outcomes after coronary artery bypass graft surgery. Pain 2004;109:73–85.
64. Nilsdotter AK, Petersson IF, Roos EM, Lohmander LS: Predictors of patient relevant outcome after total hip replacement for osteoarthritis: A prospective study. Ann Rheum Dis 2003;62:923–930.
65. Ostendorf M, Buskens E, van Stel H, et al: Waiting for total hip arthroplasty: Avoidable loss in quality time and preventable deterioration. J Arthroplasty 2004;19:302–309.
66. Bondy LR, Sims N, Schroeder DR, et al: The effect of anesthetic patient education on preoperative patient anxiety. Reg Anesth Pain Med 1999;24:158–164.
67. Camu F, Beecher T, Recker DP, Verburg KM: Valdecoxib, a COX-2-specific inhibitor, is an efficacious, opioid-sparing analgesic in patients undergoing hip arthroplasty. Am J Ther 2002;9:43–51.
68. Giraudet-Le Quintrec JS, Coste J, Vastel L, et al: Positive effect of patient education for hip surgery: A randomized trial. Clin Orthop 2003;414:112–120.
69. Holtzman J, Saleh K, Kane R: Effect of baseline functional status and pain on outcomes of total hip arthroplasty. J Bone Joint Surg Am 2002;84A:1942–1948.
70. Knutsson S, Engberg IB: An evaluation of patients' quality of life before, 6 weeks and 6 months after total hip replacement surgery. J Adv Nurs 1999;30:1349–1359.
71. Lilja Y, Ryden S, Fridlund B: Effects of extended preoperative information on perioperative stress: An anaesthetic nurse intervention for patients with breast cancer and total hip replacement. Intensive Crit Care Nurs 1998;14:276–282.
72. McGregor AH, Rylands H, Owen A, et al: Does preoperative hip rehabilitation advice improve recovery and patient satisfaction? J Arthroplasty 2004;19:464–468.
73. Meding JB, Anderson AR, Faris PM, et al: Is the preoperative radiograph useful in predicting the outcome of a total hip replacement? Clin Orthop 2000;376:156–160.
74. O'Connell T, Browne C, Corcoran R, Howell F: Quality of life following total hip replacement. Ir Med J 2000;93:108–110.

75. Scherak O, Kolarz G, Wottawa A, et al: [Effect of inpatient rehabilitation measures on patients with total hip endoprostheses—evaluation 15 months after operation. Acta Med Austriaca 1996;23:142–145.
76. Topol EJ: Failing the public health—rofecoxib, Merck, and the FDA. N Engl J Med 2004;351:1707–1709.
77. Lenzer J: US government agency to investigate FDA over rofecoxib. BMJ 2004;329:935.
78. Horton R: Vioxx, the implosion of Merck, and aftershocks at the FDA. Lancet 2004;364:1995–1996.
79. Couzin J: Drug safety: Withdrawal of Vioxx casts a shadow over COX-2 inhibitors. Science 2004;306:384–385.
80. Sibbald B: Rofecoxib (Vioxx) voluntarily withdrawn from market. CMAJ 2004;171:1027–1028.
81. Berenson A, Harris G, Meier B, Pollack AL: Despite warnings, drug giant took long path to Vioxx recall. NY Times, Nov 14, 2004:A1, A32.
82. Choi HK, Seeger JD, Kuntz KM: Effects of rofecoxib and naproxen on life expectancy among patients with rheumatoid arthritis: A decision analysis. Am J Med 2004;116:621–629.
83. Oakley G Jr: Lessons from the withdrawal of rofecoxib: Observational studies should not be forgotten. BMJ Dec 4 2004;329:1342.
84. Abenhaim L: Lessons from the withdrawal of rofecoxib: France has policy for overall assessment of public health impact of new drugs. BMJ 2004;329:1342.
85. Giaquinta D: Lessons learned after the withdrawal of rofecoxib. Manag Care Interface 2004;17:25–26, 46.
86. Dieppe PA, Ebrahim S, Martin RM, Juni P: Lessons from the withdrawal of rofecoxib. BMJ 2004;329:867–868.
87. Gallagher RM: Balancing risks and benefits in pain medicine: Wither Vioxx Pain Med 2004;5:329–330.
88. DeMaria AN: The fallout from Vioxx. J Am Coll Cardiol 2004; 44:2080–2081.
89. Kelly DJ, Ahmad M, Brull SJ: Preemptive analgesia. I: Physiological pathways and pharmacological modalities. Can J Anaesth 2001;48:1000–1010.
90. Suzuki H: Recent topics in the management of pain: Development of the concept of preemptive analgesia. Cell Transplant 1995;(Suppl 1):S3–S6.
91. Wilder-Smith CH, Hill L, Dyer RA, et al: Postoperative sensitization and pain after cesarean delivery and the effects of single IM doses of tramadol and diclofenac alone and in combination. Anesth Analg 2003;97:526–533.
92. Halbert J, Crotty M, Cameron ID: Evidence for the optimal management of acute and chronic phantom pain: A systematic review. Clin J Pain 2002;18:84–92.
93. Redmond M, Florence B, Glass PS: Effective analgesic modalities for ambulatory patients. Anesthesiol Clin North Am 2003;21:329–346.
94. Subramaniam B, Subramaniam K, Pawar DK, Sennaraj B: Preoperative epidural ketamine in combination with morphine does not have a clinically relevant intra- and postoperative opioid-sparing effect. Anesth Analg 2001;93:1321–1326.
95. Joshi GP: Postoperative pain management. Int Anesthesiol Clin 1994;32:113–126.
96. Wright BD: Clinical pain management techniques for cats. Clin Tech Small Anim Pract 2002;17:151–157.
97. Gottschalk A, Smith DS, Jobes DR, et al: Preemptive epidural analgesia and recovery from radical prostatectomy: A randomized controlled trial. JAMA 1998;279:1076–1082.
98. Katz J, Cohen L: Preventive analgesia is associated with reduced pain disability 3 weeks but not 6 months after major gynecologic surgery by laparotomy. Anesthesiology 2004;101:169–174.
99. Rosaeg OP, Krepski B, Cicutti N, et al: Effect of preemptive multimodal analgesia for arthroscopic knee ligament repair. Reg Anesth Pain Med 2001;26:125–130.
100. Sekar C, Rajasekaran S, Kannan R, et al: Preemptive analgesia for postoperative pain relief in lumbosacral spine surgeries: A randomized controlled trial. Spine J 2004;4:261–264.
101. Horattas MC, Evans S, Sloan-Stakleff KD, et al: Does preoperative rofecoxib (Vioxx) decrease postoperative pain with laparoscopic cholecystectomy? Am J Surg 2004;188:271–276.
102. Akarsu T, Karaman S, Akercan F, et al: Preemptive meloxicam for postoperative pain relief after abdominal hysterectomy. Clin Exp Obstet Gynecol 2004;31:133–136.
103. Trampitsch E, Pipam W, Moertl M, et al: [Preemptive randomized, double-blind study with lornoxicam in gynecological surgery.] Schmerz 2003;17:4–10.
104. Settecase C, Bagilet D, Bertoletti F, Laudanno C: [Preoperative diclofenac does not reduce pain of laparoscopic cholecystectomy.] Rev Esp Anestesiol Reanim 2002;49:455–460.
105. Oztekin S, Hepaguslar H, Kar AA, et al: Preemptive diclofenac reduces morphine use after remifentanil-based anaesthesia for tonsillectomy. Paediatr Anaesth 2002;12:694–699.
106. Gilabert Morell A, Sanchez Perez C: [Effect of low-dose intravenous ketamine in postoperative analgesia for hysterectomy and adnexectomy]. Rev Esp Anestesiol Reanim 2002;49:247–253.
107. Giannoni C, White S, Enneking FK: Does dexamethasone with preemptive analgesia improve pediatric tonsillectomy pain? Otolaryngol Head Neck Surg 2002;126:307–315.
108. Kokki H, Salonen A: Comparison of pre- and postoperative administration of ketoprofen for analgesia after tonsillectomy in children. Paediatr Anaesth 2002;12:162–167.
109. Reuben SS, Bhopatkar S, Maciolek H, et al: The preemptive analgesic effect of rofecoxib after ambulatory arthroscopic knee surgery. Anesth Analg 2002;94:55–59.
110. Nagatsuka C, Ichinohe T, Kaneko Y: Preemptive effects of a combination of preoperative diclofenac, butorphanol, and lidocaine on postoperative pain management following orthognathic surgery. Anesth Prog 2000;47:119–124.
111. Norman PH, Daley MD, Lindsey RW: Preemptive analgesic effects of ketorolac in ankle fracture surgery. Anesthesiology 2001;94:599–603.
112. Cabell CA: Does ketorolac produce preemptive analgesic effects in laparoscopic ambulatory surgery patients? AANA J 2000;68:343–349.
113. Ko JC, Miyabiyashi T, Mandsager RE, et al: Renal effects of carprofen administered to healthy dogs anesthetized with propofol and isoflurane. J Am Vet Med Assoc 2000;217:346–349.
114. Zacharias M, Hunter KM, Baker AB: Effectiveness of preoperative analgesics on postoperative dental pain: A study. Anesth Prog 1996; 43:92–96.
115. Likar R, Krumpholz R, Pipam W, et al: [Randomized, double-blind study with ketoprofen in gynecologic patients: Preemptive analgesia study following the Brevik-Stubhaug design.] Anaesthesist 1998; 47:303–310.
116. Likar R, Krumpholz R, Mathiaschitz K, et al: [The preemptive action of ketoprofen: Randomized, double-blind study with gynecologic operations.] Anaesthesist 1997;46:186–190.
117. Rockemann MG, Seeling W, Bischof C, et al: Prophylactic use of epidural mepivacaine/morphine, systemic diclofenac, and metamizole reduces postoperative morphine consumption after major abdominal surgery. Anesthesiology 1996;84:1027–1034.
118. Katz J, Jackson M, Kavanagh BP, Sandler AN: Acute pain after thoracic surgery predicts long-term post-thoracotomy pain. Clin J Pain 1996; 12:50–55.
119. Mezei M, Hahn O, Penzes I: [Preemptive analgesia—preoperative diclofenac sodium for postoperative analgesia in general surgery.] Magy Seb 2002;55:313–317.
120. Lakdja F, Dixmerias F, Bussieres E, et al: [Preventive analgesic effect of intraoperative administration of ibuprofen-arginine on postmastectomy pain syndrome.] Bull Cancer 1997;84:259–263.
121. Lambert A, Dashfield A, Cosgrove C, et al: Randomized prospective study comparing preoperative epidural and intraoperative perineural analgesia for the prevention of postoperative stump and phantom limb pain following major amputation. Reg Anesth Pain Med 2001;26:316–321.
122. Jin F, Chung F: Multimodal analgesia for postoperative pain control. J Clin Anesth 2001;13:524–539.
123. Paech MJ, Pavy TJ, Orlikowski CE, et al: Postcesarean analgesia with spinal morphine, clonidine, or their combination. Anesth Analg 2004; 98:1460–1466.
124. Stephens J, Laskin B, Pashos C, et al: The burden of acute postoperative pain and the potential role of the COX-2-specific inhibitors. Rheumatology (Oxford) 2003;42(Suppl 3):iii40–iii52.
125. Schumann R, Shikora S, Weiss JM, et al: A comparison of multimodal perioperative analgesia to epidural pain management after gastric bypass surgery. Anesth Analg 2003;96:469–474.
126. Ochroch EA, Mardini IA, Gottschalk A: What is the role of NSAIDs in pre-emptive analgesia? Drugs 2003;63:2709–2723.
127. Bardiau FM, Taviaux NF, Albert A, et al: An intervention study to enhance postoperative pain management. Anesth Analg 2003;96:179–185.
128. Anderson AD, McNaught CE, MacFie J, et al: Randomized clinical trial of multimodal optimization and standard perioperative surgical care. Br J Surg 2003;90:1497–1504.

129. Issioui T, Klein KW, White PF, et al: Cost-efficacy of rofecoxib versus acetaminophen for preventing pain after ambulatory surgery. Anesthesiology 2002;97:931–937.
130. Doyle E, Bowler GM: Pre-emptive effect of multimodal analgesia in thoracic surgery. Br J Anaesth 1998;80:147–151.
131. Skinner HB: Multimodal acute pain management. Am J Orthop 2004;33(Suppl):5–9.
132. Skinner HB, Shintani EY: Results of a multimodal analgesic trial involving patients with total hip or total knee arthroplasty. Am J Orthop 2004;33:85–92.
133. Kamming D, Chung F, Williams D, et al: Pain management in ambulatory surgery. J Perianesth Nurs 2004;19:174–182.
134. Rosenberg J, Kehlet H: Does effective postoperative pain management influence surgical morbidity? Eur Surg Res 1999;31:133–137.
135. Baker AB: Analgesia for day surgery. Med J Aust 1992;156:274–280.
136. McDonnell A, Nicholl J, Read SM: Acute pain teams and the management of postoperative pain: A systematic review and meta-analysis. J Adv Nurs 2003;41:261–273.
137. McDonnell A, Nicholl J, Read SM: Acute pain teams in England: Current provision and their role in postoperative pain management. J Clin Nurs 2003;12:387–393.
138. Loughrey JP, Fitzpatrick G, Connolly J, Donnelly M: High dependency care: Impact of lack of facilities for high-risk surgical patients. Ir J Med Sci 2002;171:211–215.
139. Schafheutle EI, Cantrill JA, Noyce PR: Why is pain management suboptimal on surgical wards? J Adv Nurs 2001;33:728–737.
140. Rawal N, Allvin R: [Postoperative pain an unnecessary suffering: A model of "emergency pain relief" implemented in Orebro.] Lakartidningen 2001;98:1648–1654.
141. Rawal N: 10 years of acute pain services—achievements and challenges. Reg Anesth Pain Med 1999;24:68–73.
142. Chen PP, Ma M, Chan S, Oh TE: Incident reporting in acute pain management. Anaesthesia Aug 1998;53:730–735.
143. Stomberg MW, Wickstrom K, Joelsson H, et al: Postoperative pain management on surgical wards—do quality assurance strategies result in long-term effects on staff member attitudes and clinical outcomes? Pain Manag Nurs 2003;4:11–22.
144. Goldstein DH, VanDenKerkhof EG, Blaine WC: Acute pain management services have progressed, albeit insufficiently in Canadian academic hospitals. Can J Anaesth 2004;51:231–235.
145. Stadler M, Schlander M, Braeckman M, et al: A cost-utility and cost-effectiveness analysis of an acute pain service. J Clin Anesth 2004;16:159–167.
146. Powell AE, Davies HT, Bannister J, Macrae WA: Rhetoric and reality on acute pain services in the UK: A national postal questionnaire survey. Br J Anaesth 2004;92:689–693.
147. Joranson DE: Are health-care reimbursement policies a barrier to acute and cancer pain management? J Pain Symptom Manage 1994;9:244–253.
148. Pain management: Theological and ethical principles governing the use of pain relief for dying patients. Task Force on Pain Management, Catholic Health Association. Health Prog 1993;74:30–39, 65.
149. Jordan-Marsh M, Hubbard J, Watson R, et al: The social ecology of changing pain management: Do I have to cry? J Pediatr Nurs 2004;19:193–203.
150. Middleton C: Barriers to the provision of effective pain management. Nurs Times 2004;100:42–45.
151. Watt-Watson J, Chung F, Chan VW, McGillion M: Pain management following discharge after ambulatory same-day surgery. J Nurs Manag 2004;12:153–161.
152. Manias E, Bucknall T, Botti M: Assessment of patient pain in the postoperative context. West J Nurs Res 2004;26:751–769.
153. MacLellan KL: Postoperative pain: Strategy for improving patient experiences. J Adv Nurs 2004;46:179–185.
154. Idvall E: Quality of care in postoperative pain management: What is realistic in clinical practice? J Nurs Manag 2004;12:162–166.
155. Chavis SW, Duncan LH: Pain management—continuum of care for surgical patients. AORN J 2003;78(3):382–386, 389–399; quiz 400–401, 403–404.
156. Rawal N: Treating postoperative pain improves outcome. Minerva Anestesiol 2001;67(Suppl 1):200–205.
157. Krenzischek DA, Windle P, Mamaril M: A survey of current perianesthesia nursing practice for pain and comfort management. J Perianesth Nurs 2004;19:138–149.

11 术后疼痛的临床评估

GABRIELA IOHOM

术后疼痛的临床评估除了进行疼痛测量，还应起到以下作用：
1. 协助术后疼痛的诊断和量化。
2. 选择适当的治疗方案。
3. 评估治疗效果。

在美国，疼痛得不到有效治疗的原因多为临床医师对疼痛及疼痛缓解的错误评估[1]。理想的疼痛评估需从多方面着手，然而受时间和人员因素限制，往往只能通过术后一段时间的记录来获取相关信息。应将疼痛作为第五项生命体征，至少每隔3~4 h，分别在休息和活动时进行一次疼痛评分。综合数据决定一个疼痛阈值，当分数超过此阈值时即应给予疼痛治疗。

全面的术后疼痛评估要求包括疼痛病史和体检。疼痛病史需包含疼痛的部位、强度、性质、当时疼痛状况、诱发和缓解因素、相关症状以及治疗措施。

患者自诉是最可靠的疼痛指标，因为它是患者自己的主观感受，而不是医师经过刻意处理的资料。同时，疼痛强度测量也不是将一名患者的疼痛与另一名患者进行比较，而是比较同一名患者在不同时间的疼痛强度[2]。

其次是必要的体检，尽管在紧急情况下受到时间的限制。患者往往通过语言和非语言方式来表达其疼痛强度及对镇痛的迫切要求。最恰当的方式是观察患者的动作及表情，有些体检可能会加重患者的疼痛[3]。

体检过程中应同时评估患者的一般身体情况，尤其是疼痛部位，并观察各种身体因素（即情绪、深呼吸、体位的改变）对疼痛的影响和（或）躯体功能的恢复情况（即情绪波动、日常生活自理能力）[4]。

对于不便于沟通的婴儿、儿童、老年人及心智障碍患者，可通过测量其生理指标（即心率、血压、呼吸）或观察其明显情绪反应（即哭闹、面部表情、退缩等行为）来评估其疼痛程度。患者痛苦行为越多，说明疼痛越严重。虽然这些措施只能对疼痛进行间接评估，但其作用在临床应用中已得到验证。

术后疼痛治疗是临床上的一个独立领域。术后急性疼痛的发生多是可预知的，其疼痛强度与手术部位有关。与其他类型的疼痛不同，它是短期的，并能在相对短的时间内逐渐好转。患者的情绪往往因为疼痛以及害怕迟迟得不到处理而处于焦虑状态。医师可以通过术前访视与患者或患者家属之间建立一种互利信关系，以便了解疼痛病史，并指导患者如何判断及处理疼痛。除了少数无法与之交流的患者可以用行为和（或）生命体征取代外，术后疼痛评估主要以患者自诉为依据。分别在静息和活动（如移动、深呼吸、咳嗽等）时按照以下方法实施：①根据手术类型和疼痛强度在固定的间隔时间有规律地进行评估；②对每例新报道的疼痛病例实行评估；③给予镇痛治疗后应间隔一段时间再进行评估（如给予地西泮后30 min或者口服镇痛药后1 h）[5]。在患者活动期间进行疼痛评估有利于提高临床调查的敏感性，例如两种药物对于患者在静息时的作用相同，但当患者做深呼吸或咳嗽等活动状态时却有可能大不相同[6]。

尽管手术创伤是引起术后疼痛最普遍和最明显的原因，但仍然存在许多潜在的可导致术后疼痛的诱因。

当患者出现突发的难以控制或复杂的疼痛时，我们应考虑可能出现了另一种疾病或并发症，如可能发生了室间隔综合征、腹膜炎或心绞痛等。此外，神经性疼痛可能表现为进行性疼痛加重，这种并发症由原发创伤所致，治疗难度较大，早期干预可能会有较好的效果[3]。

疼痛测量

疼痛是一种复杂多因素产生的症状，它不仅决定于组织的损伤和机体对伤害的感知，还与以往的疼痛经历、个人信念、情绪、环境等有关。目前还没有令人满意的客观测量疼痛的方法。患者的自诉是对疼痛最客观的描述。

理论上讲，术后疼痛的评估应该从多个角度进行，如强度、部位、对情绪的影响以及一系列相关症状。然而，这种多角度的评价方案对外科患者来说过于复杂，不便于广泛运用。临床上只适合采用简单的疼痛评估方法[7]。

根据所用维度数量的不同，自我描述测量方法又可分为单维和多维两种。

单维疼痛测量方法

直接分级法/口述分级评分法/口述描绘评分法

这是最古老的疼痛测量方法：给患者一张列有数个描述疼痛程度的词汇列表，让患者从中选出最能反映目前疼痛强度的一个词[8]。此表格通常包含2～7个词汇。

这种方法比较简单，患者只需用"是"或"否"回答，例如"你现在是否感觉疼痛？"。四级口述描绘评分法（verbal rating scale，VRS）是临床上常用的评价疼痛强度的方法，它选用了4个形容词：无、轻微、中等、重度。五级口述描绘评分法词汇包括轻微、不适、沮丧、恐惧和极其痛苦[9]。五级 VRS 同样也可用于疼痛缓解程度的评级，词汇有无、轻微、中度、良好、完全不疼[3]。

这种评分法的缺陷在于可选词汇有限、患者的主观偏倚和疼痛的非持续性，并且要求用统计学的非参数检验来进行分析。临床实践证实其与视觉模拟评分法（visual analogue scale，VAS）呈正相关[10]。

数字评分法

数字评分法（numerical rating scale，NRS）是最简单、最常用的方法[11]。数字刻度尺用"0～10"来描述，0表示不痛，10表示想像中最剧烈的疼痛。患者口头选出或书面画出（图11-1）最能描述其疼痛程度的数字。

NRS 的优点是简便、可重复、易领会，并且对疼痛的微小变化较敏感。小至5岁的儿童、只要会数数或对数字有一些认识的孩子（如知道8＞4）都能够采取此种方法[9]。NRS 与 VAS 相关性良好，尽管不是线性相关[12]。

视觉模拟评分法（VAS）

长期以来，一些精神病专家一直使用将主观感受（即抑郁、焦虑、恐惧、健康）通过视觉模拟评分法进行量化评分的方法[13,14]。Huskission[15,16]首先发现并确认了这种方法在疼痛评估中同样有效。它与口述 NRS 较相似。VAS 采用一条长 10 cm、两端分别标记"不痛"和"想像中最剧烈的疼痛"的直线，患者依据自己感受的疼痛程度在 VAS 线上某一点作一标记（图11-2）。通过测量标记点与直线起点的距离得出疼痛分值。不同方法结合使用可能会影响分值，例如"想像中最剧烈的疼痛"在 VAS 评分中可能仅被评为"严重疼痛"。VAS 可以设计成水平线，也可以是垂直线，均不影响评分结果[17]。尽管视觉模拟评分法是一种更有根据的评分方法，但与口述评分法相比所耗费的时间较多，因而在临床上并未得到广泛应用。

DeLoach 等[18]论述了麻醉可致患者术后认知能力

不痛 0 1 2 3 4 5 6 7 8 9 10 想像中最剧烈的疼痛

图 11-1 数字评分法(NRS)。

不痛 _____ 想像中最剧烈的疼痛

图 11-2 视觉模拟评分法（VAS）。

暂时减退，从而降低了 VAS 值与患者主观感受的相关性，导致临床测量值会有 ±20 mm 的误差。

VAS 值与疼痛呈线性相关，至少对轻至中度疼痛患者如此，因此 VAS 可以换算成一个比值。我们可以运用参数检验分析 VAS 值，证实该值的变化与痛觉强度变化的相关性[19]。

图像评分法

图像评分法与直接分级法相似，它由 4~6 个表情图组成，从高兴、微笑到伤心和泪流满面等不同的面容（图 11-3）。这种评分法是 VAS 的延伸，而且比 NRS 和 VAS 更简单实用。图像评分法更适合于那些不便于交流的人群（如 3 岁左右的儿童、老年人、智力低下、言语障碍或教育程度低的人）[9]。其缺点是患者会潜意识扰乱评估结果（即患者会倾向于选择中间的图像），并且需要特定的工具（即图表）。

多维疼痛调查工具

McGill 疼痛问卷 (McGill Pain Questionnaire, MPQ)

McGill 疼痛调查表（MPQ）是目前所使用的涉及内容最广泛的多维评分法之一[20]。方法是列出 20 组能描述疼痛特征的基础词汇供患者选择，从生理、情感和评价 3 个方面对疼痛进行较全面的评估。患者经讲解后从中选出最能表达他们疼痛的词（图 11-4）。从该调查表可以得到以下 3 个数值：

(1) 疼痛分级指数 (Pain Rating Index, PRI)：每组中的每一个词根据其表达的疼痛强度给予一个分值，所有分值之和即为 PRI 值。从 3 个方面进行评分分别得出 3 个分值。

(2) 选词数量 (number of words chosen, NWC)

(3) 现时疼痛强度指数 (Present Pain Intensity Index, PPII)：要求患者完成一个当前疼痛强度量表 (Present Pain Intensity Scale, PPIS)，该表由从"不疼"到"剧痛"等词汇构成。

MPQ 早期是为慢性疼痛一般评估而设计的，现已证实其在急性疼痛[21]尤其是术后疼痛的评估中同样有效[22]。

急性疼痛患者与慢性疼痛患者相比，从生理感觉角度评分所得分值偏高，而从情感角度评分所得分值偏低[21]。MPQ 调查表用于评价术后患者服用止痛药前后的疼痛变化时，至少其敏感性与 VRS 和 VAS 相近[22]。

简式 McGill 疼痛问卷 (short-form MPQ, SF-MPQ)

简式 MPQ（SF-MPQ；图 11-5）主要用于在短时间内获得患者信息，与 VAS 或 PPII 仅测量疼痛强度相比，它所获得的信息数量更多、范围更广[23]。MPQ 需 10 min 才能完成，而简式 MPQ 只需 2~5 min 即可。PPII 分为五级，用数字 1~5 表示，分别代表：1 轻微；2 不适；3 痛苦；4 恐惧；5 剧痛。VAS 和 PPII 只能提供疼痛强度的数据，不能提供疼痛的性质。构成简式 MPQ 的 15 个描述词多是根据生理和情感两方面选出的。最常用的生理描述词有：跳痛、放射痛、刺痛、锐痛、痉挛痛、捏痛、烧灼痛、隐痛、沉重痛、触痛、割裂痛；最常用的情感描述词有：筋疲力尽的、令人厌恶的、恐惧的、令人痛苦的。每个词根据其强度给予评分：0＝无、1＝轻微、2＝中度、3＝重度。因此，生理和情感可以从两方面分别评分，也可以算成总分。

简式 MPQ 与 MPQ 表中的疼痛等级指数密切相关[23]，而且对各种干扰因素、术后镇痛药物的作用和术中硬膜外药物的持续作用引起的临床变化都具敏感性[23,24]。成年人（包括老年患者）都能有效地完成此调查[25]。

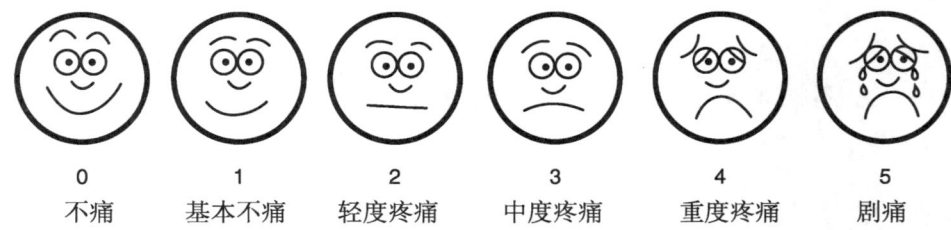

图 11-3 面部表情疼痛评分。(From Wong DL, Hockenberry-Eaton M, Wilson D, et al: Wong's Essentials of Pediatric Nursing, 6th ed. St. Louis, Mosby, 2001, p 1301.)

McGILL 疼痛问卷表

患者姓名 _____ 日期 _____ 时间 _____ am/pm

疼痛评估指数（PRI）：感觉（S）_____ 情感（A）_____ 评估（E）_____ 其他（M）_____
　　　　　　　　　　　　　　(1-10)　　　　　(11-15)　　　　　(16)　　　　　(17-20)

疼痛评估指数（总强度）PRI(T) _____ 现时疼痛强度（PPI）_____
　　　　　　　　　　　　　　　(1-20)

1	闪烁痛 ____ 颤动痛 ____ 脉动痛 ____ 搏动痛 ____ 跳动痛 ____ 重击痛 ____	11	疲劳 ____ 筋疲力尽 ____	
		12	厌烦 ____ 窒息 ____	
		13	可怕的 ____ 惊恐的 ____ 恐怖的 ____	
2	跳动痛 ____ 闪动痛 ____ 刺　痛 ____			
3	针刺痛 ____ 钻　痛 ____ 钻孔痛 ____ 刀割痛 ____ 枪刺痛 ____	14	惩罚感 ____ 严惩感 ____ 残忍的 ____ 邪恶的 ____ 致死的 ____	
		15	不幸的 ____ 盲目的 ____	
4	锐　痛 ____ 切割痛 ____ 撕裂痛 ____	16	讨厌的 ____ 麻烦的 ____ 悲惨的 ____ 剧烈的 ____ 不可忍受的 ____	
5	捏　痛 ____ 按压痛 ____ 咬　痛 ____ 痉挛痛 ____ 挤压痛 ____			
		17	扩散的 ____ 放射的 ____ 穿透的 ____ 刺穿的 ____	
6	牵拉痛 ____ 拉扯痛 ____ 扭曲痛 ____			
		18	绷紧的 ____ 麻木的 ____ 牵拉的 ____ 挤压的 ____ 撕裂的 ____	
7	热　痛 ____ 烧灼痛 ____ 烫伤痛 ____ 灸烤痛 ____			
		19	凉的 ____ 寒冷的 ____ 冰冻的 ____	
8	麻刺痛 ____ 痒　痛 ____ 刺　痛 ____ 蜇刺痛 ____			
		20	烦恼不已的 ____ 令人厌恶的 ____ 令人痛苦的 ____ 可怕的 ____ 非常剧烈的 ____	
9	钝　痛 ____ 酸　痛 ____ 伤　痛 ____ 隐　痛 ____ 胀　痛 ____			
		现时疼痛强度		
10	触痛 ____ 绷紧痛 ____ 擦痛 ____ 分裂痛 ____	0 1 2 3 4 5	无痛 ____ 轻微 ____ 不适 ____ 痛苦 ____ 恐惧 ____ 剧痛 ____	

短暂的 ____　节律的 ____　持续的 ____
瞬时的 ____　周期的 ____　稳定的 ____
暂时的 ____　间歇的 ____　不变的 ____

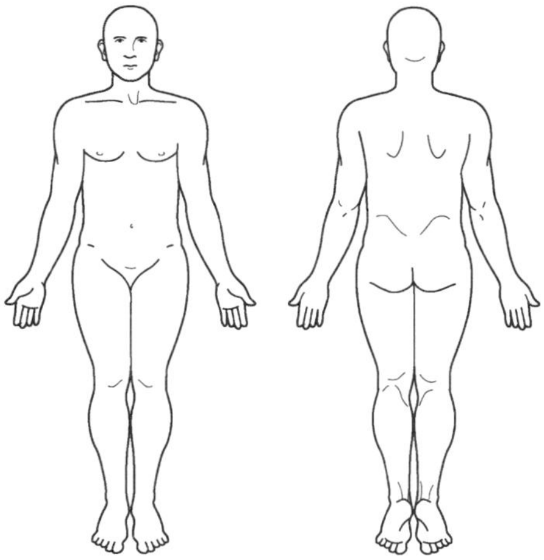

E = 外侧
I = 内侧

备注：

图 11-4　McGill 疼痛问卷表。(Reprinted from Turk DC, Melzack R [eds]: Handbook of Pain Assessment. Copyright 1992, The Guilford Press, New York.)

研究 #	
	日期:

简式McGill疼痛问卷

I 疼痛评定指数（PRI）：
　以下词语用来描绘平均疼痛。请选择最能表达你现在疼痛感觉的词汇，并在其对应栏中划（✓）。但请仅仅对于骨盆区域疼痛进行描述。

		无		轻微		中度		重度
a	跳痛	0		1		2		3	
	刺痛	0		1		2		3	
	刀割痛	0		1		2		3	
	锐痛	0		1		2		3	
	痉挛痛	0		1		2		3	
	绞痛	0		1		2		3	
	热灼痛	0		1		2		3	
	隐痛	0		1		2		3	
	胀痛	0		1		2		3	
	触痛	0		1		2		3	
	撕裂痛	0		1		2		3	
b	筋疲力尽的	0		1		2		3	
	厌烦的	0		1		2		3	
	恐惧的	0		1		2		3	
	受罪-惩罚感	0		1		2		3	

II 现时疼痛强度—视觉模拟评分法。在以下图表中标记出目前疼痛强度：

无痛 |—————————————————————————| 想像中最剧烈的疼痛

III 整体疼痛强度评估。请在你认为最能描述你疼痛强度的词汇栏中划（✓），但请仅仅描述您骨盆区域的疼痛。

评估		
0	无痛	
1	轻微	
2	不适	
3	痛苦	
4	恐惧	
5	剧痛	

IV 评分：

		评分
I-a	S-PRI（感觉疼痛评定指数）	
I-b	A-PRI（情感疼痛评定指数）	
I-a+b	T-PRI（总体疼痛评定指数）	
II	PPI-VAS（现时疼痛强度-视觉模拟评分）	
III	整体疼痛强度评估	

图 11-5　针对于骨盆区域疼痛的简式 McGill 疼痛问卷表（SF-MPQ）。(From www.med.umich.edu/obgyn/repro-endo/Lebovic-research/PainSurvey.pdf/)

定量感觉检测

定量感觉检测（quantitative sensory testing，QST，图11-6）是一种无创性躯体感觉检测方法。通过测试，我们可以了解疼痛从外周神经末梢（感受器）传至大脑(丘脑)的整个传导途径。各种疼痛的感受阈值和忍耐力大致平均地分布于人群中。在适当的实验条件下，给予标准化的有害刺激，将疼痛反应量化，从而获得客观的感觉和疼痛感知力的测量数据[26]。最常用的方法是机械刺激（即不同强度的Von Frey毛发静态感觉测试或振动感觉动态测试）或热刺激(使用Peltier探针使皮肤达到特定温度)。受试者汇报感觉阈值、痛觉阈值、疼痛的忍耐限度以及恰好区分不同刺激之间的界值。但该方法耗时过多，且需要患者完全配合，因此，目前仍然只限于研究使用。

目前已有一些研究术前实验性疼痛反应来预测术后疼痛的程度。例如，在截肢患者中，术前压迫痛阈与术后残肢痛和幻肢痛成反比[27]；术前热感觉定量测试可以预测剖宫产术后患者静止或活动时疼痛评分，以此可以解释54%以上的术后疼痛的变异性[28]；对于前交叉韧带修复术患者，术前对不同强度热刺激的反应，与其术后几周内关节疼痛等级强相关[29]；术前冷痛耐受力测试可预测腹腔镜胆囊切除术后疼痛[30]。总之，这些发现证明阈上实验性疼痛反应是患者术后急性疼痛强度的重要预测因子[26]。

临床上尚缺少模拟疼痛的设备。但是，可以预计QST将会成为一种越来越普遍的疼痛评估手段[26]。

镇痛需求

在临床研究中，也使用镇痛药的首次使用时间和使用剂量来对疼痛进行测量。目前已经应用的有患者自控镇痛装置（patient-controlled analgesia，PCA）。方法是在一段时间内通过PCA装置输入的镇痛药物剂量来评估疼痛强度[31]，所得到的数字性数据相对容易进行分析。结果提示，药物需求与给药比值能很好地反映患者对镇痛药的需求[32]。这种测量方法应用了计算机化的PCA装置，除了疼痛强度外还易受很多其他因素（即剂量变化、副作用、心理差异）影响。

疼痛测量小结

从全文来看，疼痛测量应贯穿于疼痛干预前和之后的多个时刻。理想情况下，可计算时间-镇痛效应曲线下面积。疼痛强度差异之和（summed pain intensity differences，SPID）或疼痛缓解措施[疼痛完全缓解（TOTPAR）]反映疼痛干预的累积效应。然而，它们并不能反映镇痛效应的起效和峰值，如果说这些数据是重要的，那么必须测量达到最大疼痛缓解（或疼痛减轻）时间以及疼痛恢复时间；SPID和TOTPAR可以通过以下公式来计算[33]：

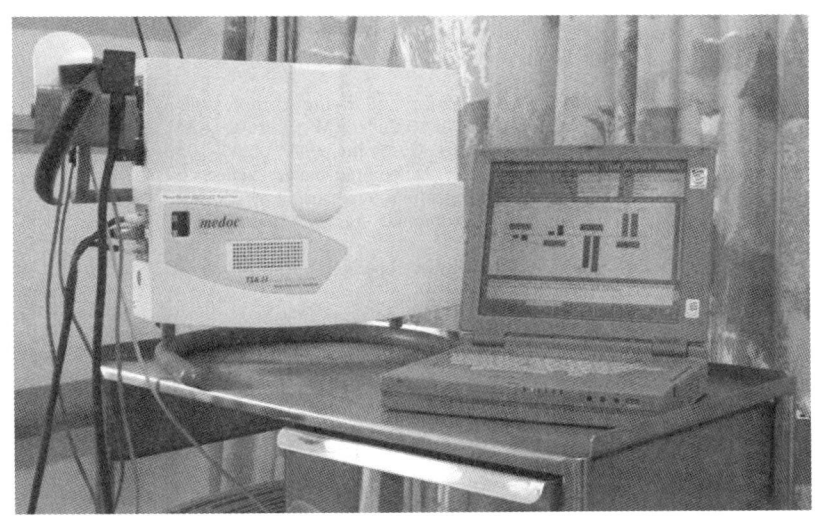

图11-6 定量感觉检测（QST）。图中所示为定量感觉测试仪，图片左上方是热电极和患者反应装置，它连接在一台可以显示测试结果的便携式计算机上。(From Heffernan A: Transcutaneous spinal electroanalgesia: Its effects in acute and chronic pain and healthy volunteers [Thesis]. Leicester, UK, Leicester University, 2002.)

$$\text{SPID} = \sum_{t=0-6}^{n} \text{PID}_t$$

$$\text{TOTPAR} = \sum_{t=0-6}^{n} \text{PR}_t$$

公式中,在不同的评估时间点 t ($t=0,1,2,n$),P_t 和 PR_t 分别代表对应时间点的疼痛强度和疼痛缓解程度;P_0 指 $t=0$ 时的疼痛强度;PIDt 指疼痛强度差值,用 (P_0-P_t) 来计算。

结论

对疼痛进行反复评估是提高急性疼痛治疗疗效的基础。重要的是疼痛评估的性能,而不是测量工具本身。测量应尽可能以患者主诉为主,因为护理人员往往容易低估患者的疼痛强度。由于术后机体功能的恢复与手术结果有关,因此,必须在静息和相关活动时分别进行疼痛评估。患者有得到恰当的疼痛治疗的权利,因而疼痛评估不再是可有可无的,而是必须进行的。

(陈 芳译 汤 媛 熊源长校)

参考文献

1. Max MB, Payne R, Edwards WT, et al: Principles of Analgesic Use in the Treatment of Acute Pain and Cancer Pain, 4th ed. Glenview, IL, American Pain Society, 1999.
2. Slezak J, Hacobian A: The history and clinical examination. In Ballantyne J, Fishman SM, Abdi S (eds): The Massachusetts General Hospital Handbook of Pain Management, 2nd ed. Philadelphia, Lippincott Williams & Wilkins, 2002, pp 37–46.
3. Hobbs GJ, Hodgkinson V: Assessment, measurement, history and examination. In Rowbotham DJ, Macintyre P (eds): Acute Pain. London, Arnold, 2003, pp 93–111.
4. Loeser JD: Medical evaluation of the patient with pain. In Loeser JD, Butler SH, Chapman CR, et al (eds): Bonica's Management of Pain, 3rd ed. Baltimore, Lippincott Williams & Wilkins, 2001, pp 267–279.
5. McCaffery M, Pasero C: Assessment: Underlying complexities, misconceptions, and practical tools. In McCaffery M, Pasero C (eds): Pain Clinical Manual, 2nd ed. St. Louis, Mosby Inc, 1999, pp 35–102.
6. Dahl JB, Rosenberg J, Hansen BL, et al: Differential analgesic effects of low-dose epidural morphine and morphine-bupivacaine at rest and during mobilization after major abdominal surgery. Anesth Analg 1992;74:362–365.
7. Benhamou D: Evaluation de la douleur postoperatoire. Ann Fr Anesth Reanim 1998;17:555–572.
8. Keele KD: The pain chart. Lancet 1948;3:6–8.
9. LeBel AA: Assessment of pain. In Ballantyne J, Fishman SM, Abdi S (eds): The Massachusetts General Hospital Handbook of Pain Management, 2nd ed. Philadelphia, Lippincott Williams & Wilkins, 2002, pp 58–75.
10. Stubhaug A, Breivik H: Post-operative analgesic trials: Some important issues. Baillieres Clin Anaesthesiol 1995;9:555–584.
11. Price DD, Bush FM, Long S, Harkins W: A comparison of pain measurement characteristics of mechanical visual analogue and simple numerical rating scales. Pain 2004;56:217–226.
12. Murphy DF, McDonald A, Power C, et al: Measurement of pain: A comparison of the visual analogue with a non visual analogue scale. Clin J Pain 1988;3:197–199.
13. Aitken RCB: A growing edge of measurement of feelings. Proc Roy Soc Med 1969;62:989–993.
14. Clarke PRF, Spear FG: Reliability and sensitivity in the self-assessment of well-being [abstract]. Br J Psychol Soc 1964;17:55.
15. Huskisson EC: Measurement of pain. Lancet 1974;2:1127–1131.
16. Scott J, Huskisson EC: Graphic representation of pain. Pain 1976;2:175–184.
17. Brievik EK, Skoglund LA: Comparison of present pain intensity assessments on horizontally and vertically orientated visual analogue scales. Methods Find Exp Clin Pharmacol 1998;20:719–724.
18. DeLoach LJ, Higgins MS, Caplan AB, Stiff JL: The visual analog scale in the immediate postoperative period: Intrasubject variability and correlation with a numeric scale. Anesth Analg 1998;86:102–106.
19. Myles PS, Troedel S, Boquest M, Reeves M: The pain visual analog scale: Is it linear or nonlinear? Anesth Analg 1999;89:1517–1520.
20. Melzack R: The McGill Pain Questionnaire: Major properties and scoring methods. Pain 1975;1:277–299.
21. Reading AE: A comparison of the McGill pain questionnaire in chronic and acute pain. Pain 1982;13:185–192.
22. Jenkinson C, Carroll D, Egerton M, et al: Comparison of the sensitivity to change of long and short form pain measures. Quality Life Res 1995;4:353–357.
23. Melzack R: The short-form McGill Pain Questionnaire. Pain 1987;30:191–197.
24. Lowe NK, Walker SN, McCallum RC: Confirming the theoretical structure of the McGill pain questionnaire in acute clinical pain. Pain 1990;46:53–60.
25. Gagliese L, Melzack R: Age differences in the quality of chronic pain: A preliminary study. Pain Res Manage 1997;2:157–162.
26. Edwards R, Sarlani E, Wesselmann U, Fillingim RB: Quantitative assessment of experimental pain perception: Multiple domains of clinical relevance. Pain 2005;114:315–319.
27. Nikolajsen L, Ilkjaer S, Jensen TS: Relationship between mechanical sensitivity and postamputation pain: A prospective study. Eur J Pain 2000;4:327–334.
28. Granot M, Lowenstein L, Yarnitzky D, et al: Postcesarean section pain prediction by preoperative experimental pain assessment. Anesthesiology 2003;98:1422–1426.
29. Werner MU, Duun P, Kehlet H: Prediction of postoperative pain by preoperative nociceptive responses to heat stimulation. Anesthesiology 2004;100:115–119.
30. Bisgaard T, Klarskov B, Rosenberg J, Kehlet H: Characteristics and prediction of early pain after laparoscopic cholecystectomy. Pain 2001;90:261–269.
31. Lehmann KA: Patient-controlled intravenous analgesia for postoperative pain relief. In Max MB, Portenoy RK, Laska E (eds): The Design of Analgesic Clinical Trials. Advances in Pain Research and Therapy, vol 18. New York, Raven Press, 1991, pp 481–506.
32. McCoy EP, Furness G: Forum: Patient-controlled analgesia with and without background infusion. Analgesia assessed using the demand: delivery ratio. Anaesthesia 1993;48:256–265.
33. McQuay H, Moore A: An Evidence-Based Resource for Pain Relief. Oxford, Oxford Medical Publications, 1998, pp 14–18.

12 术后急性疼痛的预测和预防：超前镇痛新进展

JOEL KATZ

目前，一种过时的疼痛理论仍然在指导术后急性疼痛的处理。该理论认为：当外周疼痛信号从受体传递到大脑中枢时，被动执行该传递过程的神经系统最终产生疼痛[1]。该观点从策略上导致了术后急性疼痛处理的不足，即总是在患者出现疼痛后才治疗。术后患者到达 PACU 时常常会感到极度疼痛，此时，患者往往需接受成倍剂量的阿片类药物才能将疼痛程度控制在可耐受水平。然而，基础研究和临床数据均显示：短暂的伤害性信号传入或直接损伤（例如切断组织、神经和骨骼）激活 C 纤维后会诱发长时程中枢神经功能的改变，该改变在有害刺激消除或损伤痊愈后仍可能持续存在[2,3]。这种认为神经系统外周与中枢之间存在动态相互作用机制的疼痛观点与以往有所不同，过去认为疼痛是因伤害性冲动从损伤部位直接传递到中枢后而产生的[1]。

所以，只有疼痛出现后才进行处理的习惯正逐渐被预防性治疗措施所取代，这些措施并不仅仅直接减少术中伤害性刺激并降低应激反应的程度，尽管这些作用也值得我们为之努力，其更重要的目的是在术前、术中和术后阻断伤害性刺激向上级中枢传导[4-6]。提出在疼痛出现之前进行预防性治疗的理论假设是：外周的伤害性信息（如术前疼痛、切皮、术中刺激、术后炎症反应、异位电活动等）传入脊髓会导致中枢神经系统的长时程敏化和高兴奋性，继而使传入的伤害性刺激冲动扩大化，使患者术后疼痛加剧，术后镇痛药需要量增加。如果在围手术期的不同时间及时采取预防措施，打断外周伤害性刺激冲动的释放及向脊髓不同位点的传导，则可阻断中枢敏感化的产生，从而降低术后疼痛的强度，并减少术后镇痛药的需要量。

术后急性疼痛预防措施针对的目标

围手术期可分为术前、术中和术后三期。不同时期均存在促进术后急性疼痛发展的因素。这些因素包括：①术前已经存在的有害刺激和疼痛；②术中皮肤、肌肉、神经及骨骼的切割、牵拉等有害刺激等；③术后伤口挛缩、炎症反应、损伤神经的异位神经活动等。这些因素均能促进外周和中枢敏感化的形成。所以，这些因素都是预防措施所针对的目标。这些因素在围手术期的作用及其相互影响取决于手术操作、组织损伤的范围及性质、手术时间长短、术后伤口处置、术前所用药物的药代动力学、术中追加镇痛药与否、术后镇痛方法和许多其他因素。将围手术期三个阶段的许多不良影响降到最低，则可降低术后外周和中枢敏感化的发生及持续存在的可能性，进而减少术后镇痛药的需要量。

图 12-1 描述了围手术期术前、术中和术后三期 8 个临床试验组应用镇痛药的情况。术前干预包括手术前数天和切皮前数分钟给药。术中干预包括切皮后立即给药和手术结束前（即皮肤缝合时）给药。术后干预包括手术结束后立即给药及术后数天连续给药。在每个时期镇痛药投放的时间安排上可能存在很大差异。这种潜在差异性在手术前和手术后阶段（例如时间范围从天到分钟）极为显著，但有证据显示：即使在手

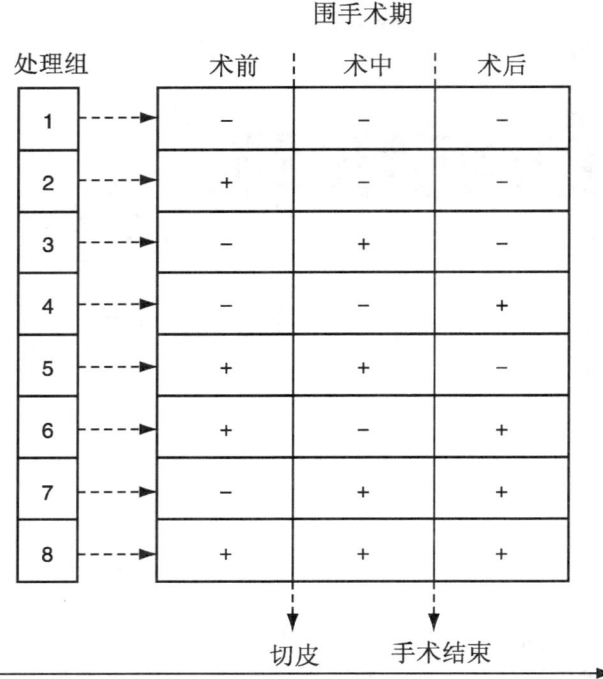

图 12-1 显示围手术期三个阶段（术前、术中和术后）镇痛药的随机给予情况（给予-+，不给予--）。根据不同阶段随机给予镇痛药（组）进行组合产生了 8 个不同的处理组和 28 种可能的两组研究设计。

术阶段，切皮后干预的时机（如从分钟到小时），组间差异相当大。

疼痛的预测

充分了解围手术期三个阶段和中枢敏感化形成的相关因素及其作用是预测患者是否会经历严重的急性术后疼痛及慢性术后疼痛的关键。回顾既往有关术后疼痛和麻醉的文献可以发现：从"现在痛"可以预测"将来痛"[7-9]。这一发现适用于所有的手术类型，无论手术时间长短。术前剧烈疼痛和持续长时间术前疼痛是发生严重的早期急性术后疼痛和慢性术后疼痛的高危因素[10-20]。冷压力试验或热痛阈刺激试验显示为高等级的术前痛、I 度烧伤疼痛等都预示在手术后会出现更严重的急性术后疼痛[21-23]。另外，剧烈的急性术后疼痛不仅预示出院后会出现疼痛[16,24]，也是促使慢性术后疼痛形成的危险因素之一[25-30]。

没有哪一个因素能像"现在痛"一样与将来疼痛的发生及发展有如此的相关性。一些研究认为：低龄[10,16]、女性[16]、焦虑[10,17]以及各种其他心理变量[7,31-34]对预测术后疼痛有一定意义，但是不具备从"现在痛"可以预测术后疼痛发生及疼痛强度的这种高度一致性。

在疼痛预测方面要确定些什么？是有关疼痛自身的强度、性质和持续时间，还是确定疼痛个体的敏感性、心理易损性及遗传倾向？减少手术诱发的中枢敏感化将会改变急性痛的过程，是否可降低术后慢性疼痛的发生率？什么因素在急性术后疼痛转变为慢性顽固性神经病理性疼痛中起重要作用？我们还不知道这些问题的答案，但与手术相伴的围手术期外周伤害性疼痛刺激与术后急性和慢性疼痛的强度和镇痛药的需要量相互关联。

超前镇痛的历史和发展

Crile 首先提出：手术刺激所引起的中枢神经系统的兴奋可能会增强术后急性疼痛[35]。Wall 随后表达了相同的观点[36]，并进一步指出："手术前的超前镇痛"可以阻断手术切口对中枢神经系统敏感化的诱导作用，从而降低急性术后疼痛的强度。自从疼痛与麻醉文献引入这个观点以后，基于已经证实及相矛盾的临床证据、基础研究的新进展和关键性的假设等，该观点不断被精炼和修正。这些研究提示：触发中枢敏感化形成的因素已不仅仅是外科切口创伤，还包括手术前有害刺激、术中刺激、手术后外周及中枢炎症介质及异位神经电活动等。

最新资料指出：全麻可以减弱伤害性刺激由外周向脊髓及大脑中枢的传导，但是不能阻断这个传导[37]。全身应用阿片类药物并不能充分高密度阻断脊髓伤害性神经元的兴奋，达不到防止中枢敏感化的目标[38]。这些发现还显示：即使手术中接受全身麻醉患者的意识已丧失，但全麻药或常规剂量的阿片类药物并不能显著影响脊髓背角神经元的兴奋过程。这些发现让我们更加重视术后疼痛及镇痛药需求量增加的问题。

超前镇痛的争议和迷惑

对超前镇痛定义的争论导致了许多新名词的产生[5,39-45]，包括创伤性休克防止法[46]、预先术前镇痛[36]、超前镇痛[47]、预防性镇痛[5,48]、平衡镇痛[49]、广义的超

图12-2 超前镇痛研究的试验设计与预期术后结果，即切皮前干预与切皮后而不是手术结束前同样干预的比较。这个设计曾经用于Katz等[52]的研究中，研究中两组经历侧位开胸手术的患者，一组在切皮前硬膜外注射芬太尼或盐水，另一组在切皮后给药。切皮前硬膜外注射芬太尼(G1)比切皮前注射盐水组(G2)手术后6h的疼痛程度明显减轻，在手术之后12～24h中吗啡的使用量明显下降。PACU，麻醉后监护病房。

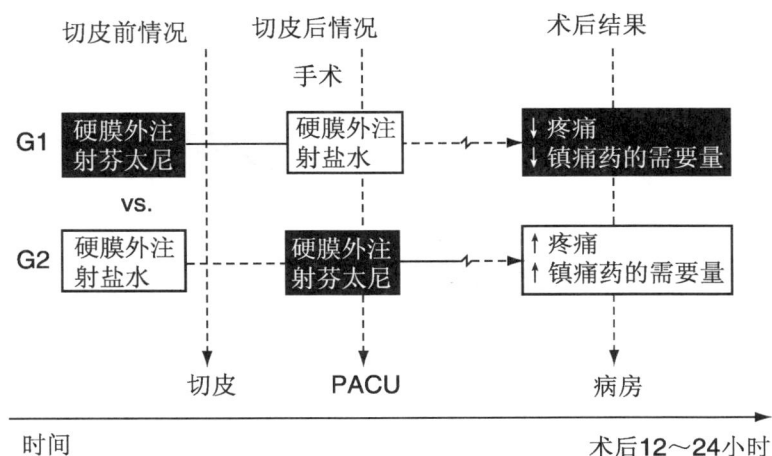

前镇痛[6]和保护性镇痛[50]等。实际上，正是这种争论才使超前镇痛的价值和意义得以发展和提高。

文献中有关超前镇痛的研究方法有两种比较通用[51]。经典超前镇痛研究要求两组患者接受同一镇痛处方治疗[47]，只是用药时间不同，一组在手术前，另一组在切皮后或手术后（治疗组合2：3和2：4，如图12-1示），两组间唯一不同是与切皮时间相关的药理学因素，即一组接受治疗是在手术前，另一组是在切皮后（图12-2，Katz及其同事的研究[52]）或手术后（图12-3，Dirking及其同事的研究[53]）。

仅限于切皮后或手术后分组处理的试验方法在方法学上具有一定吸引力，由于阳性结果的存在，该方法为我们观察处理效果及可能的作用机制提供了一个时间窗。另一方面，目前关于超前镇痛的认识极为有限而狭隘[3,5,41]，部分是因为我们对术前、术中、术后各阶段外周伤害性刺激传入与中枢敏感化形成及术后疼痛的相关程度并不清楚。超前镇痛狭隘的概念结合超前镇痛经典术前/术后设计研究假设：手术中对伤害性刺激信息的阻断比术后干预对手术后疼痛程度的影响更大，然而该设计方法并没有考虑其他一些可能合理的替代方法。对某些特定手术来说，切皮、术中创伤等操作所导致中枢敏感化（即在手术后处理组中）和手术后炎性伤害性信息传入和/或异位（即在手术前处理组中）程度相同，导致两组间术后疼痛程度和镇痛药的需要量无显著差异[4]。

两组研究在切皮前后或手术前后治疗组间术后疼痛程度或镇痛药需要量上未见明显差别，没有设计适当的对照组是该研究的内在缺陷（例如处理组合1，8，或如图12-1）。该研究的阴性结果提示：切皮后或手术后阻断伤害性刺激的传入对降低中枢敏感化有一定作用，而术前干预并非完全无效（例如图12-4和12-5，描述Katz等[54,55]和Gordon等[56]的研究）。随

图12-3 超前镇痛研究的试验设计与预期术后结果，即切皮前干预与(G1)与手术后完全同样干预(G2)的比较。预期结果是以经典的确定的超前镇痛假说为基础，即手术中有害传入促成术后疼痛和镇痛药应用的作用大于术后有害传入所致。Dirking等采用这一设计进行研究[53]，即将疝修补前15min腹股沟区域给予利多卡因阻滞患者与手术后立即给予相同处置给药的患者相比较。在手术前和手术后处理组中，疼痛和镇痛药的应用无明显差异，导致未产生预防效应的原因是无对照组（如图12-4和图12-5）。PACU，麻醉后监护病房。

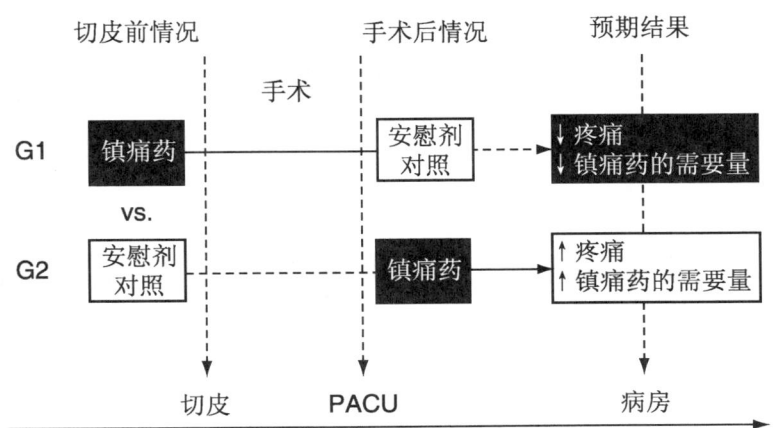

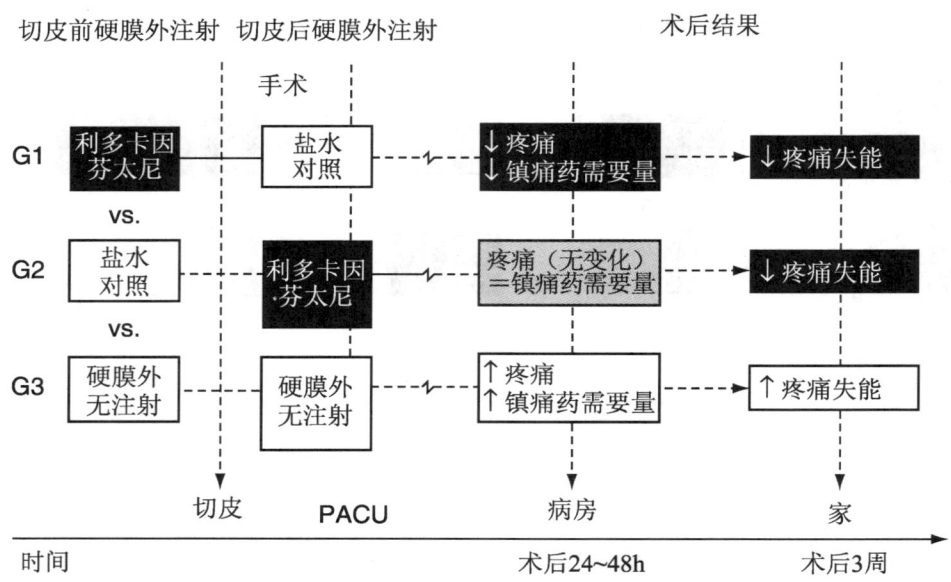

图 12-4 Katz 等[54,55]使用的试验设计指出了超前镇痛的两组研究设计上的内在缺陷（如图 12-2）。在女性妇科剖宫术切皮前（G1）而不是切皮后（G2）硬膜外注射利多卡因和芬太尼与硬膜外注射盐水的患者相比，吗啡用量和累积使用量下降，痛觉过敏减少[54]。3 周随访显示，两组中接受硬膜外镇痛组的疼痛失能率明显低于标准治疗组[55]。结果强调标准治疗对照组的重要性，以避免超前镇痛的两组研究（切皮前与切皮后）未能发现预期效应的问题。PACU，麻醉后监护病房。

后的研究重视了标准治疗对照组的重要性[54,55]。其他报道指出：对某些类型的手术，在术后数小时内阻断外周伤害性刺激的大量传入可以减少后续阶段的疼痛[54,55]，然而手术中阻断伤害性疼痛刺激却没有这样的效果（图 12-5）[56]。最近文献中针对超前镇痛的狭义概念提出了另一个重要观点：由于超前镇痛定义的不一致，导致人们的研究注意力偏离了某些重要的临床发现[4]。

为了最大限度地降低围手术期三个阶段伤害性刺激所诱发的中枢敏感化，已经研发了另一更具包容性的方法——预防性镇痛。与其他治疗和（或）安慰剂治疗或未治疗比较，采用预防性镇痛治疗的患者术后疼痛程度和（或）镇痛剂的消耗量明显减少，其持续效应超过预防用药物临床作用的持续时间（例如，图 12-1 中治疗组 1 与 2 和治疗组 1 和 5）。对预防用药物作用消失后的持续观察使我们确信：这种预防效应绝不是简单的药物镇痛作用。然而，由于治疗后情况的缺失，这样的试验设计不能提供与这些效应相关因

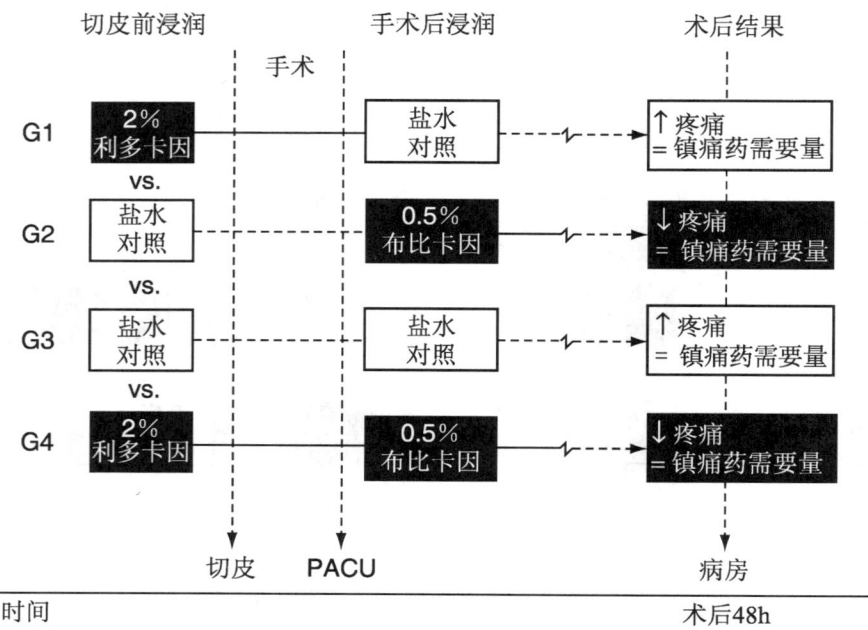

图 12-5 Gordon 等的设计方案评估了阻断或不阻断有害的术中和（或）术后传入对后期术后疼痛的相对作用[56]。在第三磨牙取出术后，随机双盲分别给予患者局部麻醉药（利多卡因或布比卡因）或盐水。研究结果证实采用预防性镇痛，注射布比卡因组（G2,G4）手术后 48h 的疼痛强度，比术前注射利多卡因组（G1）或盐水对照组（G3）明显降低。结果提示在第三磨牙取出术后数小时的外周伤害性疼痛刺激比手术中伤害性疼痛刺激促成更大范围的中枢敏感化和更强的后期术后疼痛，因为手术后局部麻醉药阻断比术中阻断更有效。PACU，麻醉后监护病房。

图 12-6 试验设计比较了两种不同的手术前干预与无处理的对照组的情况。这个设计曾用于 Tverskoy 等关于超预防性镇痛的首次前瞻性研究[57]。行腹股沟疝修补术患者随机分成 3 组：全身麻醉加局部麻醉药浸润麻醉组（G1），脊髓麻醉麻醉组（G2），或单纯全身麻醉组（G3）。虽然与对照组相比，浸润或脊髓麻醉可显著降低手术后 24h 活动性疼痛的强度，但是浸润组在所有组中疼痛最少。这种疼痛评分结果术后 10d 对手术切口机械压力反应的疼痛评分仍然显著。PACU，麻醉后监护病房。

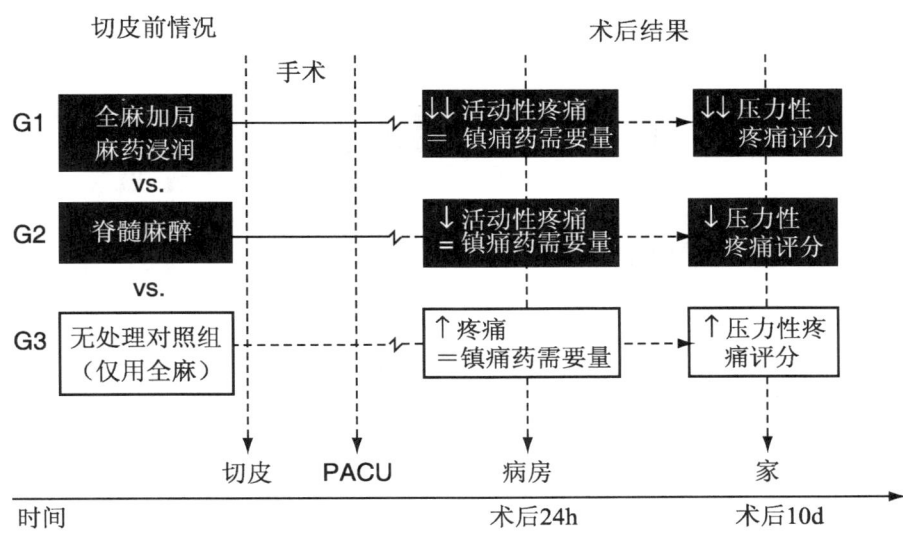

素及该效应大致持续时间范围的信息（如图 12-6 和 12-7 分别是 Tverskoy[57] 和 Reuben[58] 等采用该类设计的研究）。

证实预防效应并不要求在手术前就开始干预，治疗可以在手术过程中（例如图 12-1 中处理组 1 与 3）或手术后（例如图 12-1 中处理组 1 与 4）进行。例如，如果手术后给予拟研究的镇痛药而不是安慰剂，术后患者的疼痛程度/镇痛剂消耗量就会降低，而且该效应一直会持续至预防性镇痛药的作用消失之后（见图 12-8）[59]。预防性镇痛的焦点不在于麻醉干预的相关时机，而在于降低围术期伤害性刺激的强度，后者可导致外周及中枢敏感化，并增加术后疼痛的强度及镇痛药的需要量。

文献概要

以采用随机双盲研究的超前镇痛和预防性镇痛文献为基础的循证综述提示：超前镇痛[4,48,50,60,61] 和预防性镇痛[4,48,62] 对术后疼痛的预防意义与所采用的方法相关，尽管后者比前者的阳性证据更多。但更多关于超前镇痛的模糊结论可能提示这样一个事实：术中和术后伤害性信息的传入促发了中枢敏感化的形成，因此导致术前处理组与手术后处理组作用差异的缩小。

Katz[4] 和 McCartney[48] 采用以前超前镇痛的定义作为标准，评估了从 1987 年 12 月到 2002 年 4 月 175 项关于预防性镇痛和超前镇痛的随机双盲对照研究。研究者分析了所有应用过的药物，得出的结论认为：处

图 12-7 试验设计比较了手术前加手术后的干预与对照组的情况。如果手术前加手术后干预的情况表现比安慰剂对照组疼痛减轻和镇痛药需要量减少超过了目标镇痛药作用的持续时间，就证实有预防性镇痛。Reuben 等曾经用过这一设计[58]，随机将女性患者分成两组：根治性乳房切除术前晚服用文拉法辛（75 mg/d）或安慰剂（每天）两周。6 个月随访显示文拉法辛组的胸壁痛、臂痛和腋痛的发生率明显低于安慰剂组。PACU，麻醉后监护病房。

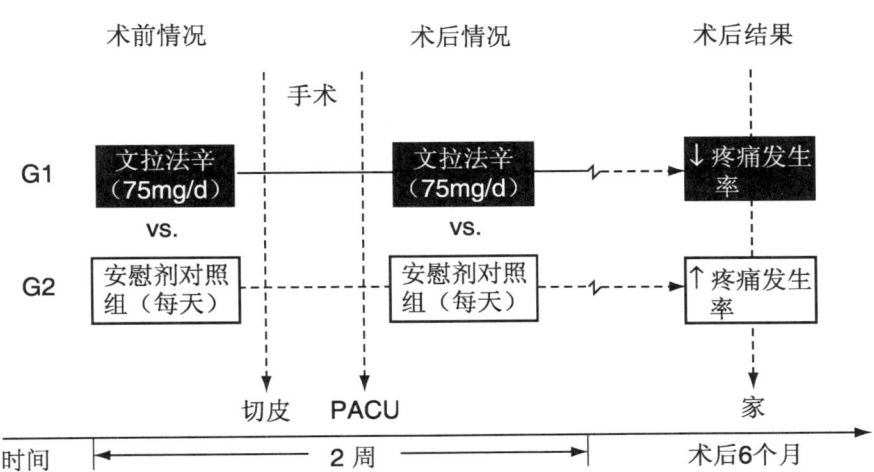

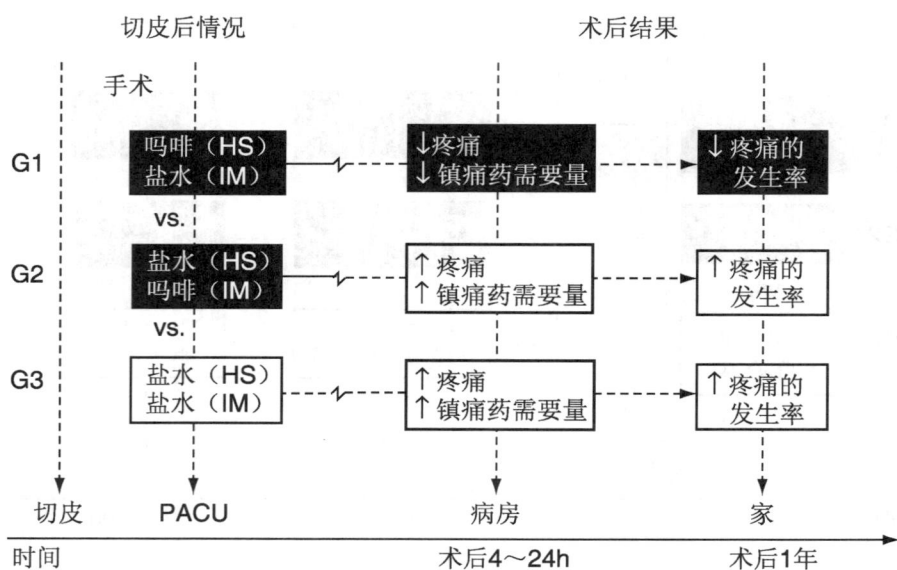

图 12-8 试验设计比较切皮后镇痛药干预与安慰剂或无处理对照。如果切皮后的情况比对照组疼痛减轻和（或）镇痛药需要量减少的时间超过了目标镇痛药作用的临床持续时间，就证实有预防性镇痛。Reuben 等曾经用这样的设计，他们在颈椎融合术时在髂骨移植骨片取出的位置(HS)注射吗啡而不是盐水，结果与接受肌注吗啡（G2）和接受盐水的安慰剂对照组(G3)比较，可减少短期疼痛和镇痛药需要量以及手术后 1 年供体部位的慢性疼痛发病率。研究表明，甚至在切皮后和骨移植物已经取出后给予止痛剂，仍能获得预防性镇痛（即文章中提到的外周伤害性疼痛损伤性刺激）。PACU，麻醉后监护病房。

理组预防性镇痛效果显著的比例明显高于非处理组（表 12-1）。扁桃体切除术[63-67]或腹股沟疝修补术[57,68-71]前应用局部麻醉药后，患者术后疼痛显著降低且持续时间超过了局部麻醉药作用时间。

关于定时给予阿片类药物及合用（或不用）局部麻醉药超前镇痛尚无定论，部分由于阿片类药物的急性耐受或阿片类药物所诱导的痛觉过敏可能会影响该结论[75-77]。一般而言，应用阿片类药物后所产生的与超前镇痛相关的术后疼痛减轻/镇痛药消耗量降低的作用很小。

几乎没有证据显示定时给予非甾体类抗炎药（NSAID）可产生超前镇痛或预防镇痛效果[4,48]。这个结论与 Moiniche 等[50]的荟萃分析结果相符，但是与随后 Ong 等[61]和 Dahl 及 Moiniche[60]的荟萃分析结论相矛盾。Ong 等[61]报道 NSAID 预防性镇痛效果指数为 0.39，而 Dahl 和 Moiniche[60]的分析显示：6/8 的研究证实在手术前给予 NSAID 比手术后给予更能降低术后疼痛。研究结果出现偏差的主要原因可能与采用不同时间段的文献有关。Ong 等[61]和 Dahl 与 Moiniche[60]报道的从 2001 年以来应用 NSAID 超前镇痛的重要研究数量增加了，而 katz[4,48]的综述只包括 2002 年 4 月以前的研究。

尽管 NSAID 对术后疼痛的预防有着潜在的重要意义，但是 Cox-2 抑制剂罗非昔布存在心血管栓塞事件的高风险[78-80]。因此，必须指出目前评估 NSAID 有效性的研究只有一项采用 Cox-2 抑制剂[81]。

Katz[4]、Katz 及 McCartney[48]的综述指出：预防性应用 NMDA 受体拮抗剂氯胺酮和右美沙芬具有重要意义。在 26 项预防性应用 NMDA 拮抗剂的临床试验中，73%（19 项）研究显示，疼痛强度显著下降和（或）镇痛药的需要量减少（表 12-1）。McCartney 等定性的系统性回顾研究也支持该结论[62]，在 McCartney 等的研究中，他们采用了更保守的试验方法评估了多种 NMDA 受体拮抗剂的预防性镇痛作用，结果显示术后患者的疼痛强度/镇痛药需要量均下降。研究结果还提示，在超过 NMDA 受体拮抗剂 5 个半衰期的时间点上仍然具有上述效果。共有 40 项研究报告（24 项使用氯胺酮、12 项使用右美沙芬，4 项应用镁剂）符合 McCartney 的入选标准。支持氯胺酮和右美沙芬具有预防性镇痛作用的证据非常有力，有 58% 和 67% 的研究证实了术后疼痛减轻和（或）镇痛药需要量减少，该效果的时间超过了药物作用的临床持续时间。4 项关于镁的研究报道不能提供该药具有预防性镇痛作用。荟萃分析指出：没有证据能显示 NMDA 受体拮抗剂具有超前镇痛效果[50,60,61]，这一发现与基础研究的结果具有一致性，即该类药物对中枢敏感化的预防和逆转效果相当[82]。

由于多模式镇痛的研究很少，各项临床研究所设计的给药途径、方式、剂量、频率和患者分布特点等差异较大，故对局部麻醉药、阿片类药物和 NSAID 联合应用时机的效能问题，目前尚无足够数据能得出可靠结论[4]。

表 12-1 根据所给药物进行超前和预防性镇痛的研究总结

药物	研究总数	超前镇痛效应(%)		预防性镇痛效应(%)		相反效应(%)	效应总数(%)
		阳性	阴性	阳性	阴性		
局部麻醉药*	65	8 (10.7)	16 (21.3)	27 (36.0)	18 (24.0)	6 (8.0)	75 (100)
阿片类药物	25	7 (25.0)	5 (17.9)	10 (35.7)	3 (10.7)	3 (10.7)	28 (100)
NSAID	25	3 (11.5)	12 (46.2)	1 (3.8)	8 (30.8)	2 (7.7)	26 (100)
NMDA 拮抗剂	31	5 (13.2)	6 (15.8)	19 (50.0)	7 (18.4)	1 (2.6)	38 (100)
可乐定	2	0 (0.0)	0 (0.0)	2 (100.0)	0 (0.0)	0 (0.0)	2 (100)
局部麻醉药和阿片类药物	21	4 (17.4)	5 (21.7)	7 (30.4)	6 (26.1)	1 (4.3)	23 (100)
多模式镇痛	6	2 (25.0)	0 (0.0)	2 (25.0)	3 (37.5)	1 (12.5)	8 (100)
总计†	175	29 (14.5)	44 (22.0)	68 (34.0)	45 (22.5)	14 (7.0)	200 (100)

* $P = 0.05$ 为 Fisher 精确检验预防性效应的阳性数据
† $P = 0.01$ 方差分析预防性效应的阳性数据。效应的总数超过了研究的数量是因为设计的试验是对超前性和预防性两种效应进行评估。见正文关于超前效应和预防效应的叙述。
NMDA，N- 甲基 -D- 天(门)冬氨酸；NSAID，非甾体类抗炎药物

Combined data from Katz J: Timing of treatment and pre-emptive analgesia. In Rice A, Warfield C, Justins D, et al: Clinical Pain Management: Acute Volume. London, Arnold, 2003, pp 113-162; and Katz J, McCartney CJL: Current status of pre-emptive analgesia. Curr Opin Anaesthesiol 2002;15:435-441.

结论

严重的术前疼痛是引发术后急性剧烈疼痛及促使术后慢性疼痛形成的高危因素。严重的急性术后疼痛预示出院后仍会疼痛，也是术后慢性疼痛形成的一个高危因素。这些发现已经促进临床预防并超前采用一些措施来阻断围手术期伤害性信息的传入，进而降低术后急性疼痛的强度，避免术后慢性疼痛的形成。

有证据显示：与超前镇痛的临床研究（如表 12-1 示）相比，预防性镇痛治疗对术后疼痛的预防作用显著。虽然被评估的 175 项临床试验的设计性质有相当大的差别[4,48]，但总的来说，这些措施可减少术后疼痛/镇痛药消耗量，而且这些措施的预防效果一直持续至镇痛药物作用消失后。根据切皮前或切皮后（或手术后）伤害性刺激的传入会导致术后痛觉致敏的观点，这些证明预防性镇痛具有一定优势的证据是可以理解和接受的[4]。根据部分研究结果可以推论：在切皮后或术后应用超前镇痛对降低术后中枢敏感化同样有益，但与预防性镇痛相比该益处则无法体现。超前镇痛研究的对照组不足/缺乏严重限制了对试验结果的正确解读，并导致了一些不成熟甚至错误的结论的产生，甚至有错误观点认为，手术前对伤害性刺激的阻断无临床益处。

切皮前/切皮后或手术后无标准治疗组或缺少对伤害性刺激完全阻断的治疗方案，均导致了目前试验设计的不完善，而继续应用这些不完善的试验设计来研究超前镇痛将会影响我们对超前镇痛的认识。许多领域已接受了超前镇痛的概念，但如果我们继续将超前镇痛的定义狭隘化，则一些难题将永远无法解决，我们也不能摆脱目前该领域研究比较混乱的状况，更不可能取得革命性的研究进展。如果要进一步认识术后疼痛的相关因素并正确评价一些临床措施的意义，还必须采用合理的对照研究。将来，我们的研究要集中在对围手术期三个阶段伤害性刺激的完全阻断，进而最大限度地预防手术诱发的痛觉敏感化。

社会心理因素在慢性疼痛的形成及维持中具有重要的作用[83-85]，所以在术前/术后应常规评估相关的心理、情感和生理变化，这些因素的评估对预测术后疼痛的严重性、康复质量及术后慢性疼痛的形成均具有重要意义。

（王 薇译 许 华 熊源长 邓小明校）

参考文献

1. Melzack R, Wall PD: The Challenge of Pain, 2nd ed. New York, Basic Books, 1988.
2. Woolf CJ, Salter MW: Neuronal plasticity: Increasing the gain in pain. Science 2000;288:1765–1769.

3. Coderre TJ, Katz J, Vaccarino AL, Melzack R: Contribution of central neuroplasticity to pathological pain: Review of clinical and experimental evidence. Pain 1993;52:259–285.
4. Katz J: Timing of treatment and pre-emptive analgesia. In Rice A, Warfield C, Justins D, et al (eds): Clinical Pain Management: Acute Volume. London, Arnold, 2003, pp 113–162.
5. Kissin I: Preemptive analgesia: Terminology and clinical relevance. Anesth Analg 1994;79:809.
6. Kissin I: Preemptive analgesia. Anesthesiology 2000;93:1138–1143.
7. Perkins FM, Kehlet H: Chronic pain as an outcome of surgery: A review of predictive factors. Anesthesiology 2000;93:1123–1133.
8. Katz J: Pain begets pain—predictors of long-term phantom limb pain and post-thoracotomy pain. Pain Forum 1997;6:140–144.
9. Dworkin RH: Which individuals with acute pain are most likely to develop a chronic pain syndrome? Pain Forum 1997;6:127–136.
10. Kalkman CJ, Visser K, Moen J, et al: Preoperative prediction of severe postoperative pain. Pain 2003;105:415–423.
11. Tasmuth T, Blomqvist C, Kalso E: Chronic post-treatment symptoms in patients with breast cancer operated in different surgical units. Eur J Surg Oncol 1999;25:38–43.
12. Jensen TS, Krebs B, Nielsen J, Rasmussen P: Immediate and long-term phantom limb pain in amputees: Incidence, clinical characteristics and relationship to pre-amputation limb pain. Pain 1985;21:267–278.
13. Nikolajsen L, Ilkjaer S, Kroner K, et al: The influence of preamputation pain on postamputation stump and phantom pain. Pain 1997;72:393–405.
14. Caumo W, Schmidt AP, Schneider CN, et al: Preoperative predictors of moderate to intense acute postoperative pain in patients undergoing abdominal surgery. Acta Anaesthesiol Scand 2002;46:1265–1271.
15. Scott LE, Clum GA, Peoples JB: Preoperative predictors of postoperative pain. Pain 1983;15:283–293.
16. Thomas T, Robinson C, Champion D, et al: Prediction and assessment of the severity of post-operative pain and of satisfaction with management. Pain 1998;75:177–185.
17. Harden RN, Bruehl S, Stanos S, et al: Prospective examination of pain-related and psychological predictors of CRPS-like phenomena following total knee arthroplasty: A preliminary study. Pain 2003;106:393–400.
18. Brander VA, Stulberg SD, Adams AD, et al: Predicting total knee replacement pain: A prospective, observational study. Clin Orthop 2003;416:27–36.
19. Liem MS, van Duyn EB, van der Graaf Y, van Vroonhoven TJ: Recurrences after conventional anterior and laparoscopic inguinal hernia repair: A randomized comparison. Ann Surg 2003;237:136–141.
20. Poobalan AS, Bruce J, King PM, et al: Chronic pain and quality of life following open inguinal hernia repair. Br J Surg 2001;88:1122–1126.
21. Bisgaard T, Klarskov B, Rosenberg J, Kehlet H: Characteristics and prediction of early pain after laparoscopic cholecystectomy. Pain 2001;90:261–269.
22. Granot M, Lowenstein L, Yarnitsky D, et al: Postcesarean section pain prediction by preoperative experimental pain assessment. Anesthesiology 2003;98:1422–1426.
23. Werner MU, Duun P, Kehlet H: Prediction of postoperative pain by preoperative nociceptive responses to heat stimulation. Anesthesiology 2004;100:115–119.
24. Beauregard L, Pomp A, Choiniere M: Severity and impact of pain after day-surgery. Can J Anaesth 1998;45:304–311.
25. Lau H, Patil NG, Yuen WK, Lee F: Prevalence and severity of chronic groin pain after endoscopic totally extraperitoneal inguinal hernioplasty. Surg Endosc 2003;17:1620–1623.
26. Callesen T, Bech K, Kehlet H: Prospective study of chronic pain after groin hernia repair. Br J Surg 1999;86:1528–1531.
27. Katz J, Jackson M, Kavanagh BP, Sandler AN: Acute pain after thoracic surgery predicts long-term post-thoracotomy pain. Clin J Pain 1996;12:50–55.
28. Hayes C, Browne S, Lantry G, Burstal R: Neuropathic pain in the acute pain service: A prospective survey. Acute Pain 2002;4:45–48.
29. Senturk M, Ozcan PE, Talu GK, et al: The effects of three different analgesia techniques on long-term postthoracotomy pain. Anesth Analg 2002;94:11–15.
30. Tasmuth T, Kataja M, Blomqvist C, et al: Treatment-related factors predisposing to chronic pain in patients with breast cancer—a multivariate approach. Acta Oncol 1997;36:625–630.
31. Jorgensen T, Teglbjerg JS, Wille-Jorgensen P, et al: Persisting pain after cholecystectomy: A prospective investigation. Scand J Gastroenterol 1991;26:124–128.
32. Borly L, Anderson IB, Bardram L, et al: Preoperative prediction model of outcome after cholecystectomy for symptomatic gallstones. Scand J Gastroenterol 1999;34:1144–1152.
33. Cohen L, Fouladi RT, Katz J: Preoperative coping strategies and distress predict postoperative pain and analgesic consumption in women undergoing abdominal gynecologic surgery. J Psychosom Res 2005;58:201–209.
34. Hanley MA, Jensen MP, Ehde DM, et al: Psychosocial predictors of long-term adjustment to lower-limb amputation and phantom limb pain. Disabil Rehabil 2004;26:882–893.
35. Katz J: George Washington Crile, anoci-association, and pre-emptive analgesia. Pain 1993;53:243–245.
36. Wall PD: The prevention of post-operative pain. Pain 1988;33:289–290.
37. Rundshagen I, Kochs E, Schulte am Esch J: Surgical stimulation increases median nerve somatosensory evoked responses during isoflurane-nitrous oxide anaesthesia. Br J Anaesth 1995;75:598–602.
38. Abram SE, Yaksh TL: Morphine, but not inhalation anesthesia, blocks post-injury facilitation: The role of preemptive suppression of afferent transmission. Anesthesiology 1993;78:713–721.
39. Taylor BK, Brennan TJ: Preemptive analgesia: Moving beyond conventional strategies and confusing terminology. J Pain 2000;1:77–84.
40. Futter M: Preventive not pre-emptive analgesia with piroxicam. Can J Anaesth 1997;44:101–102.
41. Katz J: Pre-emptive analgesia: Evidence, current status and future directions. Eur J Anaesthesiol Suppl 1995;10:8–13.
42. Kissin I: Preemptive analgesia: Why its effect is not always obvious. Anesthesiology 1996;84:1015–1019.
43. Yaksh TL, Abram SE: Preemptive analgesia: A popular misnomer, but a clinically relevant truth? APS J 1993;2:116–121.
44. Penning JP: Pre-emptive analgesia: What does it mean to the clinical anaesthetist? Can J Anaesth 1996;43:97–101.
45. Dionne R: Preemptive vs preventive analgesia: Which approach improves clinical outcomes? Compend Contin Educ Dent 2000;21:48,51–54,56.
46. Crile GW: The kinetic theory of shock and its prevention through anoci-association (shockless operation). Lancet 1913;185:7–16.
47. McQuay HJ: Pre-emptive analgesia. Br J Anaesth 1992;69:1–3.
48. Katz J, McCartney CJL: Current status of pre-emptive analgesia. Curr Opin Anaesth 2002;15:435–441.
49. Amantea B, Gemelli A, Migliorini F, Tocci R: Preemptive analgesia or balanced periemptive analgesia? Minerva Anestesiol 1999;65:19–37.
50. Moiniche S, Kehlet H, Dahl JB: A qualitative and quantitative systematic review of preemptive analgesia for postoperative pain relief: The role of timing of analgesia. Anesthesiology 2002;96:725–741.
51. Kissin I: Preemptive analgesia at the crossroad. Anesth Analg 2005;100:754–756.
52. Katz J, Kavanagh BP, Sandler AN, et al: Preemptive analgesia: Clinical evidence of neuroplasticity contributing to postoperative pain. Anesthesiology 1992;77:439–446.
53. Dierking GW, Dahl JB, Kanstrup J, et al: Effect of pre- vs postoperative inguinal field block on postoperative pain after herniorrhaphy. Br J Anaesth 1992;68:344–348.
54. Katz J, Cohen L, Schmid R, et al: Postoperative morphine use and hyperalgesia are reduced by preoperative but not intraoperative epidural analgesia: Implications for preemptive analgesia and the prevention of central sensitization. Anesthesiology 2003;98:1449–1460.
55. Katz J, Cohen L: Preventive analgesia is associated with reduced pain disability 3 weeks but not 6 months after major gynecologic surgery by laparotomy. Anesthesiology 2004;101:169–174.
56. Gordon SM, Brahim JS, Dubner R, et al: Attenuation of pain in a randomized trial by suppression of peripheral nociceptive activity in the immediate postoperative period. Anesth Analg 2002;95:1351–1357.
57. Tverskoy M, Cozacov C, Ayache M, et al: Postoperative pain after inguinal herniorrhaphy with different types of anesthesia. Anesth Analg 1990;70:29–35.
58. Reuben SS, Makari-Judson G, Lurie SD: Evaluation of efficacy of the perioperative administration of venlafaxine XR in the prevention of postmastectomy pain syndrome. J Pain Symptom Manage 2004;27:133–139.

59. Reuben SS, Vieira P, Faruqi S, et al: Local administration of morphine for analgesia after iliac bone graft harvest. Anesthesiology 2001;95: 390–394.
60. Dahl JB, Moiniche S: Pre-emptive analgesia. Br Med Bull 2004;71:13–25.
61. Ong KS, Lirk P, Seymour RA, Jenkins BJ: The efficacy of preemptive analgesia for acute postoperative pain management: A meta-analysis. Anesth Analg in press.
62. McCartney CJ, Sinha A, Katz J: A qualitative systematic review of the role of N-methyl-D-aspartate receptor antagonists in preventive analgesia. Anesth Analg 2004;98:1385–1400.
63. Agren K, Engquist S, Danneman A, Feychting B: Local versus general anaesthesia in tonsillectomy. Clin Otolaryngol 1989;14:97–100.
64. Jebeles JA, Reilly JS, Gutierrez JF, et al: The effect of pre-incisional infiltration of tonsils with bupivacaine on the pain following tonsillectomy under general anesthesia. Pain 1991;47:305–308.
65. Jebeles JA, Reilly JS, Gutierrez JF, et al: Tonsillectomy and adenoidectomy pain reduction by local bupivacaine infiltration in children. Int J Pediatr Otorhinolaryngol 1993;25:149–154.
66. Molliex S, Haond P, Baylot D, et al: Effect of pre- vs postoperative tonsillar infiltration with local anesthetics on postoperative pain after tonsillectomy. Acta Anaesthesiol Scand 1996;40:1210–1215.
67. Johansen M, Harbo G, Illum P: Preincisional infiltration with bupivacaine in tonsillectomy. Arch Otolaryngol Head Neck Surg 1996; 122:261–263.
68. Sinclair R, Cassuto J, Hogstrom S, et al: Topical anesthesia with lidocaine aerosol in the control of postoperative pain. Anesthesiology 1988;68: 895–901.
69. McLoughlin J, Kelley CJ: Study of the effectiveness of bupivacaine infiltration of the ilioinguinal nerve at the time of hernia repair for post-operative pain relief. Br J Clin Pract 1989;43:281–283.
70. Teasdale C, McCrum AM, Williams NB, Horton RE: A randomised controlled trial to compare local with general anaesthesia for short-stay inguinal hernia repair. Ann R Coll Surg Engl 1982;64:238–242.
71. Fischer S, Troidl H, MacLean AA, et al: Prospective double-blind randomised study of a new regimen of pre-emptive analgesia for inguinal hernia repair: Evaluation of postoperative pain course. Eur J Surg 2000;166:545–551.
72. Kissin I, Bright CA, Bradley EL Jr: The effect of ketamine on opioid-induced acute tolerance: Can it explain reduction of opioid consumption with ketamine-opioid analgesic combinations? Anesth Analg 2000;91: 1483–1488.
73. Li X, Angst MS, Clark JD: Opioid-induced hyperalgesia and incisional pain. Anesth Analg 2001;93:204–209.
74. Vinik HR, Kissin I: Rapid development of tolerance to analgesia during remifentanil infusion in humans. Anesth Analg 1998;86:1307–1311.
75. Celerier E, Laulin J, Larcher A, et al: Evidence for opiate-activated NMDA processes masking opiate analgesia in rats. Brain Res 1999;847: 18–25.
76. Celerier E, Rivat C, Jun Y, et al: Long-lasting hyperalgesia induced by fentanyl in rats: Preventive effect of ketamine. Anesthesiology 2000;92: 465–472.
77. Crain SM, Shen KF: Antagonists of excitatory opioid receptor functions enhance morphine's analgesic potency and attenuate opioid tolerance/dependence liability. Pain 2000;84:121–131.
78. Topol EJ: Rofecoxib, Merck, and the FDA. N Engl J Med 2004;351: 2877–2878.
79. Bombardier C, Laine L, Reicin A, et al: Comparison of upper gastrointestinal toxicity of rofecoxib and naproxen in patients with rheumatoid arthritis. VIGOR Study Group. N Engl J Med 2000;343:1520–1528.
80. Samad TA, Sapirstein A, Woolf CJ: Prostanoids and pain: Unraveling mechanisms and revealing therapeutic targets. Trends Mol Med 2002; 8:390–396.
81. Reuben SS, Bhopatkar S, Maciolek H, et al: The preemptive analgesic effect of rofecoxib after ambulatory arthroscopic knee surgery. Anesth Analg 2002;94:55–59.
82. Woolf CJ, Thompson SW: The induction and maintenance of central sensitization is dependent on N-methyl-D-aspartic acid receptor activation: Implications for the treatment of post-injury pain hypersensitivity states. Pain 1991;44:293–299.
83. Turk DC: Cognitive-behavioral approach to the treatment of chronic pain patients. Reg Anesth Pain Med 2003;28:573–579.
84. Dworkin RH, Turk DC, Farrar JT, et al: Core outcome measures for chronic pain clinical trials: IMMPACT recommendations. Pain 2005; 113:9–19.
85. Turk DC, Dworkin RH, Allen RR, et al: Core outcome domains for chronic pain clinical trials: IMMPACT recommendations. Pain 2003; 106:337–345.

13 急性疼痛服务

NARINDER RAWAL

手术后镇痛一直是一项重大的医疗挑战。围手术期镇痛的改善不仅是基于人道主义的原因，而且是减少术后病死率[1-4]和病残率[2]的基础。术后疼痛未缓解可能延缓患者出院和康复，而且可能影响患者实施康复治疗，从而导致预后不良。目前研究表明，尽管已采用有效的药物治疗，但是依然存在疼痛治疗不足。目前普遍认为，与其开发新型镇痛药物或技术解决镇痛不足这个问题，不如建立一个适当的组织机构应用现有的专业知识来解决[5]。

尽管20世纪70年代末就有一些评述主张成立一个镇痛组织来指导和管理镇痛的实施，并由其负责术后镇痛的教育与培训，但近10年后才出现专门处理住院患者术后疼痛的服务。许多医疗保健组织已经建议广泛应用急性疼痛服务（acute pain service，APS）[6-12]。此外，提供APS是当前皇家麻醉医师学会以及澳大利亚与新西兰麻醉医师学会培训的必需内容[13]。

急性疼痛服务的普及

在英国，外科与麻醉联合委员会工作报告组建议应该由一个包括专业护理成员在内的多学科联合小组来实施APS。他们还建议，这种服务应该全天候负责处理术后疼痛、在职培训护理和医疗人员以及研究调查与审核[7]。澳大利亚[6]、美国[8,10]、德国[9]、瑞典[11]的国家专业委员会先后提出了类似的建议，美国麻醉医师协会特别委员会更新了该建议[12]。英国开展了两项全国性调查，以明确工作报告组建议采纳程度[14,15]。调查结果显示，就应当如何构成APS存在很大的差异，而且一些医院仅拥有工作报告组所建议的部分内容[14,15]。表13-1显示欧洲、北美、澳大利亚和新西兰APS的普及状况[14-27]。

不同国家宣称其拥有相当数量的APS，但这并不意味不存在确定的相关标准。许多医院认为其服务足以满足患者的需求，尽管这些医院只拥有APS的部分内容。而且这些APS并没有明确其所提供服务的性质、服务的人员与设备、从事APS人员的培训与资格或APS的效果。例如，近期一项加拿大的调查显示医学院校附属医院拥有APS的百分比从1993年的53%上升至92%。但是单纯麻醉医师从事APS的比例从36%降至22%，这归咎于临床需求的不断增长和麻醉医师数量较少。只有44%的医疗中心拥有指定的APS医师，护理人员的比例仅为55%。而且，仅有29%的医疗中心宣称拥有正在应用的前瞻性数据收集系统。这项调查的研究者认为，并没有获得任何关于未接受APS的住院患者急性疼痛管理的信息，恰恰这些患者在术后患者总数中占了很大部分[26]。结合其他类似的调查[27,28]，这些加拿大研究者呼吁建立评价及比较APS作用的国家统一的明确标准。

急性疼痛服务的构成

"手术后疼痛"一文[7]划时代地发表后的20世纪90年代期间，术后疼痛管理的主要组织模式一直是APS，其主要在美国[21]得到不断发展，并逐渐引入英

表 13-1　APS* 普及率的全国性调查

研究	地区/国家	调查年份	普及率
Zimmerman 和 Stewart[16]	加拿大	1991	24/47 (53%)†
Goucke 和 Owe[17]	澳大利亚，新西兰	1992/1993	37/111 (33%)
Rawal 和 Allvin[18]	欧洲	1993	37/105 (34%)
Davies[19]	英国	1994	77/221 (35%)†
Windsor 等[15]	英国	1994‡	151/354 (43%)
Merry 等[20]	新西兰	1990	10/358 (3%)
Merry 等[20]	新西兰	1994	12/62 (19%)
Harmer 和 Davies[14]	英国	1996	17/22§
Ready[21]	美国	1995‖	97/221 (44%)†
Warfield 和 Kahn[22]	美国	1995	236/324 (73%)
Neugebauer 等[23]	德国	1995	126/300 (42%)
Stamer 等[24]	德国	1997	390/1000 (39%)
O'Higgins 和 Tucdey[25]	英国	1999	161/446 (36%)
Goldstein 等[26]	加拿大	2000‖	>49%**
Powell 等[27]	英国	2004	50/62 (93%)†
		2004	70/325 (83%)

*正式的"急性疼痛服务"负责准备的人员和资金。
†仅大学附属的。
‡1994 年完成的调查，其中包含 1990 年的资料。
§这部分调查仅包含 22 个床位≥150 个的公费 Crown Health Enterprises。
‖未声明的调查年代。
**240 名麻醉系导师中有 180 位确认一个急性疼痛小组，回顾病房中的硬膜外镇痛。

Adapted from Werner MU, S?holm L, Rotb?ll-Nielsen P, Kehlet H: Does an acute pain service improve postoperative outcome? Anesth Analg 2002;95: 1361-1372.

国。但是自从 1990 年以来，APS 的实施仍呈零碎无序状态，直到 20 世纪 90 年代末才有相继报道显示院内和院间 APS 的机构和功能在不断发生变化[27]。

尽管一致认为 APS 的主要功能之一是确保新型术后镇痛技术安全和有效地应用，如患者自控镇痛（PCA）和硬膜外镇痛，但是很多没有 APS 的医院可能也提供这些服务[29]。重要的是区分镇痛技术本身带来的益处与由 APS 专业人员提供更专业管理和教育所带来的益处。

虽然 APS 的数量在增长，但是仍有证据表明有些医院面临财政问题，可能仅提供"象征性"的服务。如今几乎没有学者研究 APS 的临床效能与效价。McDonnell 等[29]认为尽管他们的研究表明 APS 与许多动机有关，如保障术后疼痛管理良好，但是研究并没有探讨 APS 对患者预后的影响。

APS 的需求

Stamer 等[24]回顾了有关 APS 的文献，结论认为：虽然有指南，但是全世界大多数 APS 并不符合以下基本质量标准：

- 定期评估和记录疼痛评分，每天至少一次；
- 记录疼痛处理措施；
- 指定人员进行 APS；
- 对夜间和周末的术后疼痛处理制定相应的政策。

尽管每个机构对其 APS 要求都不一样，发表的标准修改后必须适应于当地情况，但是 APS 的主要内容应该包括以下几项[29]：

（1）指定人员 24h 负责 APS；在小型医院，一位

（2）规范静息和活动状态下疼痛评定，维持疼痛评分在预定的阈水平以下，记录评分（使疼痛水平可视化），为儿童和认知障碍患者采用适当的评分方法。

（3）主动与外科医师及病房护士合作，制订治疗方案和危急处理预案，以达到术后运动和功能恢复的预定目标。

（4）不断加强对病房护士的教育，以提供安全和效价良好的镇痛技术。

（5）给患者宣教疼痛监测和处理方法、目的、优点以及不良反应。

（6）定期核查外科病房镇痛技术的效价以及住院患者与门诊患者的满意度。

APS 可改善患者结局吗？

一般认为，APS 的引入使特殊镇痛技术的应用有所增加，如硬膜外、外周神经镇痛技术以及 PCA 在外科病房的应用。这些方法的运用对改善患者健康和减少术后发病率可能具有真正的推动作用。对安全性的评估是 APS 的一项重要任务，但是还不能确定 APS 在预防和减少这些事件中的作用[12,13]。这项空缺令人失望，因为实施和管理硬膜外镇痛及 PCA 是 APS 的重要内容。

一项研究报道显示，自从 APS 引入后，下呼吸道感染的发生率从 1.3%下降到 0.4%[30]。Tsui 等[31]调查了食管肿瘤进行食管切除术的患者。这些患者分成两组，APS 处理组（n = 299），传统处理的非 APS 组（n = 279）。APS 组患者接受以阿片类药物为主的术后硬膜外或静脉镇痛，非 APS 组患者接受间断吗啡肌内注射。结果 APS 组患者心肺并发症发生率明显低于非 APS 组，而且住院时间较短[31]。但是一些研究并未发现 APS 管理的患者住院时间有所缩短[13,32,33]。

2002 年的一篇文献综述中，Werner 等[13]研究了 44 个项目以及 4 项临床试验包含 84 097 例术后患者的 APS 和结局。研究结论认为 APS 的实施可使疼痛等级显著降低。术后严重呼吸抑制（需要纳洛酮逆转）发生率，静脉滴注吗啡为 0%～1.7%，PCA 为 0.1%～2.2%，脊髓使用阿片类药物为 0.1%～1.0%，硬膜外使用阿片类药物与局麻药混合液为 0%～0.5%；这证实了人们的一般观点，即任何途径给予阿片类药物的呼吸抑制发生率都极低，但是风险相近[13]。这项结果与 ASA 特别委员会的一份报告有共同之处，即支持麻醉医师在恰当和可行的情况下应用硬膜外麻醉、PCA 和区域阻滞技术。文献指出运用这三种镇痛方法的不良反应并不多于其他效果较差的方法[12]。Werner 等[13]也报道了 APS 的引入可能与术后恶心呕吐和尿潴留的发生率降低有关。但是，由于有关 APS 功能及其所提供服务的研究差异巨大，他们不能确定镇痛方法的不良反应、患者满意度或术后发病率[13]。如果能说服医院行政管理人员了解 APS 在可承担的费用内可显著改善结局，他们就更乐意投资了。

APS 的效价比高吗？

有必要对成本效益进行分析，包括并发症、不良反应以及后果衡量，以证明 APS 需求的正当性；但迄今为止并没有这类研究。术后疼痛管理的成本效益分析必须考虑镇痛药物、设备以及医护人员时间成本，在加强医疗病房（intensive care unit，ICU）、麻醉后加强监护病房（post-anesthesia care unit，PACU）和（或）外科病房的滞留时间以及术后发病率[13]。

Brodner 等[34]的研究显示多模式镇痛方案可改善镇痛、减少应激及早期拔管，从而减少大手术后即刻需进入 ICU 的患者数量。因为从高度依赖区域转出较早，结果每例患者净节省约 43 美元[34]。与代价高昂的多学科 APS 相比，数项其他研究提倡运用以护理人员为主、麻醉医师指导的低成本模式[5,35-37]。缺乏明确的对照及后果评估，妨碍了对急性疼痛处理的成本分析[38-41]。没有任何有效方法来评价不同镇痛水平的经济费用，而且也没有充分明确围手术期区域镇痛对经济学结果的影响[13]。目前没有任何证据表明以医师为基础的多学科 APS 比以专业护士为主、麻醉医师指导的 APS 更好或具有更高的效价比。虽然很难进行成本效益研究，但是非常需要这类研究。

如何进行 APS

开展一项疼痛管理程序的第一步是组织一个由有兴趣、有动力且代表患者医护不同专业技能和方法的个人组成的多学科团队。

教育

疼痛管理程序的一项最基础也是最必要的工作就是为患者和医疗保健提供者制定和实施教育计划。对于患者来说，应该在术前评估时就开展教育，其内容应该包括充分镇痛的重要性、医院工作人员提供有效疼痛控制的承诺、处理术后疼痛的不同方法、如何描绘疼痛强度的实用信息[如视觉模拟评分（visual analogue scale，VAS）或数字评分]以及当应用 PCA 和区域阻滞技术时如何参与疼痛管理计划[5,41,42]。

定义最大限度可接受的疼痛评分以及"使疼痛程度可视化"

因为缺乏正规的疼痛判定标准，许多医护人员始终认为无疼痛主诉的患者是没感到疼痛。因此，有必要来确定最大限度可接受的疼痛评分，并且在处理前后应大致记录疼痛强度。这些记录文件也为审核提供了资料，并有利于回顾和改善服务。传统上，患者一般认为术后疼痛是不可避免的；患者不可能了解到他们能期待接受到的镇痛服务标准以及有效镇痛的潜在益处。人们不应再忽略质量保证措施；应该告知患者其疼痛程度将被维持在预先设定的阈水平（通常为 10 分制 VAS 的 3 分）或该水平以下，如果疼痛评分超过该阈值将触发干预措施以减轻疼痛。从硬膜外镇痛或 PCA 转换为口服镇痛疗法过程中常见"镇痛间歇"。专业 APS 的质量改进可以缩短这种间歇，从而提高患者舒适度。

专职镇痛护士为主 APS 的发展

目前越来越明确的是，如果 APS 的目标在于改善所有外科手术（包括门诊手术）患者术后镇痛质量的话，则必须制定更简单、更廉价的 APS 模式。在俄勒冈州大学医院，以专职镇痛护士为基础、麻醉医师进行监督的模式是基于这样的概念而建立的：通过训练在职外科护理人员、经全身最佳方式使用阿片类药物以及在选择运用区域镇痛技术和 PCA 能显著改善术后镇痛效果[5]。这种模式的基础是每 3 小时规律性地评估 VAS 评分以记录每例患者疼痛强度，并且在生命体征表上记录处理效果。这项评估包括静息时和活动时以及在接受处理前后的疼痛程度。VAS 评分大于 3 分时要立即处理。

在这个组织中外科医师和病房护士的参与至关重要。专职镇痛护士或"急性疼痛护士"（acute pain nurse，APN）每天巡视所有外科病区；APN 的职责见表 13-2。在这个组织中，每个患者的处理都是根据麻醉医师、外科医师和病房护士联合制定的标准医嘱和方案。这样的安排便于病房护士必要时灵活地给予镇痛药物。麻

表 13-2 瑞典俄勒冈州大学附属医院的 APS 组织 *	
"负责疼痛处理"的医疗成员	责任
APS 主管	负责协调院内 APS 以及在职人员教学
麻醉领域	负责外科术前、术中及术后监护（包括术后疼痛）
"疼痛代表"的病房医师	为所在外科病房正式负责疼痛处理
	协助将镇痛整合到临床个体化手术操作中
"疼痛代表"的日班及夜班护士	负责执行疼痛管理的指导方针和病房常规监护 †
急性疼痛处理护士（专职疼痛处理护士）	每日巡视所有外科病房
	为年度核查收集数据（EDA、PCA、周围神经阻滞）
	为技术问题（EDA、PCA）"寻找故障"
	指引有问题的患者来麻醉科（和外科和麻醉科进行联系）
	对病房护士进行"床边"教学

* 每年这个组织令 16 000 名患者获益（VAS≤3 分），从 1991 年开始就已有满意效果。每名患者大概花费 3 美元（药物和设备费用除外）。
† 在标准医嘱基础上对患者进行处理，由麻醉科、外科和护理负责人联合作出进一步诊断。疼痛代表每 3 个月进行一次讨论来改进外科病房疼痛处理的常规操作。
EDA，硬膜外镇痛；PCA，患者自控镇痛。

醉医师全面负责患者的术前、围手术期和术后麻醉监护相关事宜，包括术后疼痛处理。麻醉科医师根据科室要求使用的"急性疼痛镇痛阶梯"，为患者选择具体疼痛治疗方法，如 PCA、硬膜外或外周神经阻滞。在规定的工作时间里，该麻醉医师负责会诊或急症处理；其他时间里，该麻醉医师随叫随到并负责相同的工作。这种模式能改善术后疼痛处理，见表 13-3。

基于每年的审核资料，各个外科病房的"疼痛代表"与麻醉医师和 APN 定期碰面，讨论改进工作。在上述组织中，唯一增加的就是 2 位 APN 的开支。在我们医院，每年实施约 16 000 台外科手术；我们这个组织低廉的花费（大约每例患者 3 美元，不包括药物和耗材费用）给所有这些患者都带来了好处。常规审核已经证实 90% 以上的患者已经达到了我们 APS 的目标。近年来麻醉医师被要求会诊或传呼的次数逐渐下降，现在每周会诊仅 1～2 次。但是，我们最近审核的资料显示夜间镇痛的需求比日间更大。

瑞典医学会已经接受这种组织模式的大体原则并推荐给国内医院[11]。对于药物种类、用药剂量、给药途径以及治疗持续时间的选择应该个体化[12]。

Bardiau 等[43]描述了根据我们的模式在一家比利时综合性医院实施 APS 的过程，这家医院拥有 1005 张床位，其中外科病房 240 张床位。这个过程在 3 年多的时间里分为 8 个步骤。这个计划期望能够改善所有外科住院患者的术后疼痛并一直维持这项服务。首先，成立一个疼痛处理委员会（pain management committee，PMC），包括麻醉医师、外科医师、药剂师和护士。第 2 个月，进行一项关于护士对术后护理的态度与知识的调查，包括 35 项的匿名问卷。第 3 个月，引进 10cmVAS 装置用于常规判定疼痛强度。随后的 6 个月时间里，设计一个基线调查（调查 I）来分析目前疼痛处置的实际情况。

在这 6 个月的调查后，根据 APN 和典型疼痛建立一个以专业护士为基础、麻醉医师监督的 APS 模式。标准化的治疗方案、每 4 小时定期按 VAS 评估疼痛强度、记录处理效果以及 APN 是这种模式的基础。PMC 制定一项临床制度，为术后疼痛处理创造一种最合适的方案。3 个月以后，对 671 例患者进行了第二项调查（调查 II），以评价 APS 实施的效果。最后，对 2383 例患者进行了第 3 次确定性调查（调查 III），以了解初始改进是否得以维持。

由于缺乏护理指南和疼痛处理方案，在对护士的调查中发现护士缺乏有效评估和处理疼痛的知识与技能。APS 实施后疼痛缓解程度大大改善。对乙酰氨基酚的消耗量明显增长。非甾体类抗炎药物的使用比例从调查 I 中的 20% 分别增长到调查 II 的 64% 和调查 III 的 99%。吗啡的使用量略有减少。这个项目的研究者的结论是，疼痛处理与护理实践的标准化以及有规律地反馈绩效是改善疼痛处理的基本要素。一个由外科医师、麻醉医师和护士组成的团队是改善疼痛治疗所必需的。现在需要进行成本效益分析来进一步证实这些结果[43]。

美国式 APS 的问题

美国大多数重要医疗机构的 APS 是以麻醉医师为基础的。综合性疼痛管理团队通常包括麻醉专家、麻醉住院医师、受过专业训练的护士、药剂师和理疗师。有时还包括生物医学者和输液泵配药人员。秘书和记帐人员也是美国式 APS 的一部分。由该团队成员定时访视和评估 APS 实施的患者。

以麻醉医师为基础的 APS 组织模式通常可提供"高科技"的疼痛管理服务，而且美国大多数 APS 基本上仅只有硬膜外镇痛和 PCA 服务。一个良好的 APS

表 13-3	如何改善术后疼痛管理？
在病房	"令疼痛程度可视化"（定期评估，记录）
	允许病房护士在标准方案基础上进行疼痛处理
外科医师	预定术后活动和功能恢复的目标
麻醉医师	根据不同个体来选择镇痛方式、进行教学、监督急性疼痛处理护士（APN）
APN	对病房护士进行床边教学；为硬膜外镇痛、PCA、周围神经阻滞等"排除故障"，定期巡视 APS
医院管理层	制定全院性的疼痛管理政策

组织应该为每例外科手术患者提供最佳的疼痛管理，包括儿童和门诊手术患者。美国式 APS 的费用极高而且日益受到医疗保健支付者的质疑。在许多医疗机构，PCA 的管理已被外科医师接管。美国许多 APS 规模正在缩小，预计将进一步缩减。

很显然，我们需要一种能为所有外科患者提供有效镇痛的新型 APS 模式。医疗保健组织认证联合委员会（Joint Commission on Accreditation of Healthcare Organizations，JCAHO）为美国一个制定医疗保健标准的独立非盈利组织，认识到了这种需求。在美国确定医疗保健机构的认证，部分要视其是否符合 JCAHO 的疼痛评估与护理标准。医疗保健机构必须认识到患者有权评估与处理其疼痛。JCAHO 的标准要求医院应该评估、处理和记录患者的疼痛，保证他们的工作人员能胜任疼痛评估与管理，对患者和家属进行有效疼痛管理的教育。医院还必须考虑到门诊手术患者需要了解出院后疼痛管理的信息和指导[41]。

病房护士作用的提升

外科病房护士负责评估每例患者的疼痛强度，给予规定的镇痛处理，并监测其镇痛效果和不良反应以及区域阻滞范围。研究证实护士在改善镇痛治疗效果中起到关键性作用[5,14,43,44]。临床专业护理人员或经过疼痛管理专业训练的 APN 越来越多地成为急性疼痛处理团队中的一部分。她们能够指导病房护士、提供必要的支持并帮助启动与监督镇痛工作。她们也促进外科医师、麻醉医师和病房护士间的合作。

如果要改善外科病房的术后疼痛管理，就必须提升护士的作用。在许多国家和医疗机构中，不允许病房护士经静脉内或硬膜外导管注射阿片类药物，于是每次 PCA 和硬膜外用药剂量需要调整时她们得求助于 APS 医师。这种要求浪费时间，不切实际，而且成本高，效益差，没有必要。随着患者自我处理能力的增加，这种对病房护士的限制看起来就很奇怪。在医院外，糖尿病儿童被允许自我注射可能是危险剂量的胰岛素，肿瘤患者被允许自己进行硬膜外和鞘内注射药物镇痛。家庭呼吸机、家庭透析、家庭 PCA 装置和非肿瘤患者阿片类药物的运用正日益被人们所接受。值得注意的是，许多医院允许助产士给分娩疼痛的产妇硬膜外导管"注满"药物，却不允许病房护士对术后疼痛进行相同处理。

许多国家和机构的充分证据表明，经过适当的教育与训练，病房护士能调整镇痛剂量、监测和管理镇痛方法，如外科病房的 PCA 和硬膜外镇痛。目前广泛地认识到疼痛管理中护士教育应是一项优先考虑的重要事情[5,14,41-43]。在我们的机构，已经允许病房护士静脉给予单次剂量的阿片类药物、设定 PCA 泵、经硬膜外导管内用药、减少或增加 PCA 或硬膜外药物用量（在医嘱范围内）。在 1991 年启动 APS 时还不允许护士实施以上工作。年度审核资料证实，通过 APN 定期指导和日常巡视，可使镇痛安全和有效。

外科医师的作用

尽管所有指南都强调以多学科联合的 APS 作为一种改善术后镇痛方法的重要性，但是尚无任何文献表明多学科小组中个体成员的确切作用。外科医师作用的重要性远大于药剂师；毫不夸张地说，没有外科医师参与的 APS 注定要失败。外科医师参与的重要性有以下几项理由：①制定所有镇痛技术的方案，这是由于大部分外科患者不需要硬膜外和 PCA 技术来获得有效镇痛；②制定达到术后活动和功能恢复预定目标的临床方案，以期减少住院时间；③制定门诊手术（占手术总量达 70%，且在不断升高）术后的疼痛管理方案；④为完成 APS 目标，改善病房护士的依从性，包括频繁的疼痛评估与文件记录[41]。

审核和持续性质量改善

评价疼痛管理质量和证实如硬膜外镇痛、PCA 和外周神经阻滞等技术的效价必须定期审核 APS。这种审核可发现必须重视的技术问题以及下次审核前必须改进的事宜。

2003 年，Taverner[44] 报道了英国北部和约克郡地区进行的审核，以评估术后疼痛管理的结局。这项研究包括了在该地区所有住院时间超过 2 周的外科手术患者，涉及 16 所医院，大至拥有 5500 张床位的教学医院，小至不超过 400 张床位的综合性区域医院。分别在恢复室 24h 及术后 7 天时静息与活动状态下测定疼痛评分，同时收集疼痛管理模式的资料。其结果显示尽管临床中有改进，并组成了急性疼痛管理团队，但是仍有很大比例的患者自述存在不能忍受的疼痛。疼痛管理团队并不能给术后患者提供更好的疼痛管理[44]。这一结果强调必须进行定期审核，以解决 APS 的问题，并明确其费用是否合理。

疼痛管理程序中最重要的活动之一就是对关于疼痛控制的机构制度和实践进行持续回顾并提供问题处理的机制。这个团队中的成员应该定期交流，提供正式的反馈意见，并探讨进一步改进的可能。这种交流是评估 APS 效率的重要场所，以重视临床实践问题，并寻找解决 APS 低效的方法[42]。总之，关于审核方面的文献十分有限。

展望

APS 的治疗目标不仅在于减轻疼痛程度，而且还包括促进患者舒适感和功能恢复。由于服务目标的扩展以及相关标准与期望的逐步提高，给麻醉医师在原本超负荷的工作基础上增加了新的负担[45]。在疼痛评估过程中人们发现相关标准正在不断改进。由于疼痛控制的改善，对其评估更加困难。尽管疼痛管理的目标仍是减轻疼痛强度，但仅在静息状态下评估疼痛程度是不够的；对腹部及胸部手术患者还必须评估活动时和咳嗽时的疼痛程度。

毋庸置疑，APS 具有主导性的教育作用。随着教育的成功开展，其他医疗保健提供者可能加入这一队伍中来。多学科联合的方法可能拓展 APS 在所有患者功能恢复方面的作用。这种作用的扩展可在改善患者所有医疗服务并使医院管理者认识到 APS 值得支持方面加倍获益[45]。

英国关于 APS 的未来方向尚有争议。有建议疼痛服务的发展应综合其他疼痛服务（慢性与姑息性治疗）、与危重护理团体合作[46]以及制定综合性术后康复程序[16]。关于工作时间以外护理的中心问题是争论 APS 的关键作用在于提供一种简易直接的患者保健服务，或是在于为教育和训练提供资源服务并促进实践活动。Powell 等[27]推测，如果 APS 成为一种良好的资源，并能广泛改善有关组织结构及有关人员的态度，以达到良好的疼痛管理，那么 APS 本身是否是一项日间服务就无所谓了，因为良好的服务应该是覆盖全天 24h[27]。然而，事实上，大多数患者在夜间感觉疼痛更为剧烈[47]，目前 APS 1 周 168h 中仅 50h 的"工作时间"模式注定会令许多患者处于疼痛折磨中[27]。

APS 的关键作用并不是提供一种简单、直接的患者护理服务，而是作为一种资源为教育和培训服务，并根据麻醉医师、外科医师和护士联合制定的规则和方案为促进临床实践服务。这些方案必须整合成为每种手术操作的临床预案。定期审核可显示能否达到 APS 的目标[41]。

已有一些人提出 APS 应该与其他疼痛服务（慢性疼痛、姑息性护理）相整合。除非团队中有一位麻醉医师仅负责 APS 才能实现这种建议，因为慢性疼痛与术后疼痛处理的临床实践完全不同。APS 麻醉医师应该参与术前、围手术期及术后期，包括麻醉实施和培训其他成员实施区域麻醉。并非所有慢性疼痛服务都由麻醉医师来实施；即使由麻醉医师实施，也很少涉及实施麻醉服务。因此，这些麻醉医师并不熟悉外科病房常规术后疼痛管理实践。所以，尚不明确建立一个更加综合性的服务机构是否能解决术后疼痛问题[27]。在我们医院，APS 组织与慢性疼痛管理组织是分开的。对于手术的慢性疼痛患者、药物滥用患者以及术后并发症可能必须长期镇痛的患者，这两个组织之间能保持良好的合作。作为规定，交接班时间是 7 天，即术后第 7 天后，慢性疼痛小组会接手术后疼痛的管理。

目前，通过网络很容易得到外科特殊操作的相关指南与建议，从各种信息中选出有用的信息[48,49]。APS 的作用就是将恰当的循证镇痛技术整合应用到每种外科手术操作中去。特殊手术操作的术后疼痛处理可望取得较以前常规"一种方法应付所有情况"的方法更好的结局。其临床实践模式的根本变化还需要根据临床证据提出明确建议。

PROSPECT[50]（出自特殊操作性术后疼痛处理）是一个基于网络的程序，可为每一种镇痛药、麻醉性治疗措施和用于特殊操作中的手术技术提供循证信息，允许临床医师根据信息作出治疗决定。这些证据来自于应用 Cochrane 方法的系统性文献综述，来自于可比性程序得出的可转换证据以及当前临床实践。特殊操作性镇痛方法不同于以前发表的急性疼痛指南中的处理方法，后者列举了各种术后疼痛的控制方法，但是并未建议何种特殊技术用于控制某种手术后的疼痛。PROSPECT 的一个重要特点是外科干预在术后疼痛与预后中的作用。腹腔镜下胆囊切除术和初次全髋置换术的处理建议可以在 PROSPECT 网上查到，而且麻醉医师和外科医师的 PROSPECT 工作组目前正在综述子宫切除术、结肠切除术、疝修补术和开胸手术的相关处理[51,52]。用于术后疼痛治疗的药物和方法日益增加，人们的主观努力（如 PROSPECT）以及人们越来越意识到特殊操作性镇痛的需求，都支持对这些药物和方法进行合理而有目标的使用。

Rosenquist 等[48]与美国退伍军人健康事务（Veterans Health Affair，VHA）质量和实施办公室协作，基于广泛电子检索得到的证据做成标准等级来论证关于术前和术后规范电子版和传统"书面"指南之间的内在关系。他们列出了一张表格，展示了根据具体手术的镇痛选择菜单。已确定了优先选择哪种特殊镇痛技术和药物种类。在 VHA 网站上可找到该指南[53]。与此相反的是，PROSPECT 网站提供镇痛和手术干预的最新文献和所有证据，允许每个用户自己决定来接收或修改 PROSPECT 小组提出的建议。这种修正是必要的，因为这涉及费用、可用的药物、传统疗法以及监管问题。

小结

外科手术患者关心的中心问题是免于术后疼痛，而且其减轻疼痛可能大大促进临床预后。然而，尽管很久以来已认识到这个问题，但在国际上术后疼痛处理不足一直是一个重大问题。从文献中我们清楚地认识到 APS 的介入已经提高了人们对术后镇痛技术能改善患者预后的认识。

日益明确的是，一个由专门医师和护士组成的团队是外科病房中术后急性疼痛管理程序良好运转的基本前提条件。尽管没有随机比较的文献，但是手术前后的研究支持 APS 减轻疼痛的效果，并提示不良反应也较少[12]。利用先进技术行区域麻醉（如导管）和 PCA 运转 APS 的医院数量不断增多。与此同时，尚无国家统一的 APS 应该采用的最佳组织结构意见。因此很明显，需要确切的规范来制定统一的国家标准，这样 APS 的绩效在每个医院都能通过国家审核来评估和比较。网络为基础的特殊手术操作的启动如 PROSPECT 可提供循证建议，允许临床医师来选择适当的药物与方法，这可能成为将来 APS 方案的一部分。

对于成功实施 APS，选择一种适当的组织结构可能与选择治疗方法一样重要。目前对于 APS 的标准包括人员配备、设备配备和组织模式，尚无统一意见。重要的是，要认识到质量改进工作的进行必须特别地适合于本地区情况，因为没有任何一种方法能保证成功适合于所有场合。应将有效的镇痛整合到一般外科护理中，以改善患者预后，这取决于外科医师与麻醉医师的紧密合作。APS 也必须证明其自身价值，并证实其所分配资源与专业技术的合理性。

（汪鼎鼎译　张伟时　邓小明校）

参考文献

1. Ballantyne JC, Carr DB, deFerranti S, et al: The comparative effects of postoperative analgesic therapies on pulmonary outcome: Cumulative meta-analyses of randomised, controlled trials. Anesth Analg 1998; 86:598–612.
2. Rodgers A, Walker N, Schug S, et al: Reduction of postoperative mortality and morbidity with epidural or spinal anaesthesia: Results from overview of randomised trials. BMJ 2000;321:1493.
3. Kehlet H, Holte K: Effect of postoperative analgesia reduces on surgical outcome. Br J Anaesth 2001;87:62–72.
4. Beattie WS, Badner NH, Choi P: Epidural analgesia reduces post-operative myocardial infarction: A meta-analysis. Anesth Analg 2001;93:853–858.
5. Rawal N, Berggren L: Organization of acute pain services—a low cost model. Pain 1994;57:117–123.
6. National Health & Medical Research Council of Australia: Acute Pain Management Scientific Evidence. Canberra, Australia, Ausinfo, 1999.
7. Royal College of Surgeons and College of Anaesthetists Working Party on Pain after Surgery: Pain after Surgery. London, Royal College of Surgeons, 1990.
8. US Department of Health and Human Services, Agency for Health Care Policy and Research: Acute Pain Management: Operative and Medical Procedures and Trauma. (Publication No. 92-0032.) Rockville, Md, AHCPR Publications, 1992.
9. Wulf H, Neugebauer E, Maier C: Die behandlung akuter perioperativer und posttraumatischer schmerzen: Empfehlungen einer interdisziplinaeren expertenkommission. New York, G Thieme, 1997.
10. Joint Commission on Accreditation of Healthcare Organizations: 1992 Hospital Accreditation Standards. Oakbrook Terrace, Ill, JCAHO, 2001.
11. Behandling av postoperativ smärta, riktlinjer och kvalitetsindikatorer [Treatment of postoperative pain, guidelines, and quality indicators]. Svenska Läkaresällskapet [Swedish Medical Association], Förlagshuset Gothia AB, Stockholm, 2001. Available at www.gothia.nu/
12. Practice guidelines for acute pain management in the perioperative setting: An updated report by American Society of Anesthesiologists Task Force on Acute Pain Management. Anesthesiology 2004;100: 1573–1581.
13. Werner MU, Søholm L, Rotbøll-Nielsen P, Kehlet H: Does an acute pain service improve postoperative outcome? Anesth Analg 2002;95: 1361–1372.
14. Harmer M, Davies KA: The effect of education, assessment and a standardised prescription on postoperative pain management: The value of clinical audit in the establishment of acute pain services. Anaesthesia 1998;53:424–430.
15. Windsor AM, Glynn CJ, Mason DG: National provision of acute pain services. Anaesthesia 1996;51:228–231.
16. Zimmerman DL, Stewart J: Postoperative pain management and acute pain service activity in Canada. Can J Anaesth 1993;40:568–575.
17. Goucke CR, Owe H: Acute pain management in Australia and New Zealand. Anaesth Intensive Care 1995;23:715–717.
18. Rawal N, Allvin R: Acute pain services in Europe: A 17-nation survey of 105 hospitals. The EuroPain Acute Pain Working Party. Eur J Anaesthesiol 1998;15:354–363.
19. Davies K: Findings of a national survey of acute pain services. Nurs Times 1996;92:31–33.
20. Merry A, Jugde MA, Ready B: Acute pain services in New Zealand hospitals: A survey. N Z Med J 1997;110:233–235.
21. Ready LB: How many acute pain services are there in the United States, and who is managing patient-controlled analgesia [letter]? Anesthesiology 1995;82:322.

22. Warfield CA, Kahn CH: Acute pain management: Programs in US hospitals and experiences and attitudes among US adults. Anesthesiology 1995;83:1090–1094.
23. Neugebauer E, Hempel K, Sauerland S, et al: [The status of perioperative pain therapy in Germany: Results of a representative, anonymous survey of 1,000 surgical clinics. Pain Study Group.] Chirurg 1998;69:461–466.
24. Stamer UM, Mpasios N, Stuber F, Maier C: A survey of acute pain services in Germany and a discussion of international survey data. Reg Anesth Pain Med 2002;27:125–131.
25. O'Higgins, Tuckey JP: Thoracic epidural anaesthesia and analgesia: United Kingdom practice. Acta Anaesthesiol Scand 2000;44:1087–1092.
26. Goldstein DH, Van Den Kerkhof EG, Blaine WC: Acute pain management services have progressed albeit insufficiently in Canadian academic hospitals. Can J Anesth 2004;51:231–235.
27. Powell AE, Davies HTO, Bannister J, Macrae WA: Rhetoric and reality on acute pain services in the UK: A national postal questionnaire survey. Br J Anaesth 2004;92:689–693.
28. Reference deleted.
29. McDonnell A, Nicholl J, Read S: Acute pain teams in England: Current provision and their role in postoperative pain management. J Clin Nurs 2003;12:387–393.
30. Wheatley RG, Madej TH, Jackson IJ, Hunter D: The first year's experience of an acute pain service. Br J Anaesth 1991;67:353–359.
31. Tsui SL, Law S, Fok M, et al: Postoperative analgesia reduces mortality and morbidity after esophagectomy. Am J Surg 1997;173:472–478.
32. Lempa M, Gerards P, Koch G, et al: Efficacy of an acute pain service: A controlled comparative study of hospitals. Langenbecks Arch Chir Suppl Kongressbd 1998;115:673–676.
33. Rose DK, Cohen MM, Yee DA: Changing the practice of pain management. Anesth Analg 1997;84:764–772.
34. Brodner G, Mertes N, Buerkle H, et al: Acute pain management: Analysis, implications and consequences after prospective experience with 6349 surgical patients. Eur J Anaesthesiol 2000;17:566–575.
35. Coleman SA, Booker-Milburn J: Audit of postoperative pain control: Influence of a dedicated acute pain nurse. Anaesthesia 1996;51:1093–1096.
36. Mackintosh C, Bowles S: Evaluation of a nurse-led acute pain service: Can clinical nurse specialists make a difference? J Adv Nurse 1997;25:30–37.
37. Bardiau FM, Braeckman MM, Seidel L, et al: Effectiveness of an acute pain service inception in a general hospital. J Clin Anesth 1999;11:583–589.
38. Stacey BR, Rudy TE, Nelhaus D: Management of patient-controlled analgesia: A comparison of primary surgeons and a dedicated pain service. Anesth Analg 1997;85:130–134.
39. Mackey DC, Ebener MK, Howe BL: Patient-controlled analgesia and the acute pain service in the United States: Health-Care Financing Administration policy is impeding optimal patient-controlled analgesia management [letter; comment]. Anesthesiology 1995;83:433–434.
40. Ready LB: Organization and operation of an acute pain service. In Ashburn MA, Fine PG, Stanley TH (eds): Pain Management and Anesthesiology. Dordrecht, The Netherlands, Kluwer Academic, 1998, pp 125–135.
41. Rawal N: Acute Pain Services revisited: Good from far, far from good [editorial]? Reg Anesth Pain Med 2002;27:117–121.
42. Blau WS, Dalton AB, Lindley C: Organization of hospital-based acute pain management programs. Southern Med J 1999;92:465–471.
43. Bardiau FM, Taviaux NF, Albert A, et al: An intervention study to enhance postoperative pain management. Anest Analg 2003;96:179–185.
44. Taverner T: A regional pain management audit. Nurs Times 2003;99:34–37.
45. Bonnet F: Postoperative pain management: A continuing struggle. ESA Newsletter 2004;17:8–9.
46. Counsell DJ: The acute pain service: A model for outreach critical care. Anaesthesia 2001;56:925–926.
47. Closs S, Briggs M, Everitt VE: Implementation of research findings to reduce postoperative pain at night. Int J Nurs Stud 1999;36:21–31.
48. Rosenquist RW, Rosenberg J: Postoperative pain guidelines. Reg Anesth Pain Med 2003;28:279–288. Available at www.oqp.med.va.gov/cpg/cpg.htm/
49. Rowlingson JC, Rawal N: Postoperative pain guidelines: Targeted to the site of surgery. Reg Anesth Pain Med 2003;28:265–267.
50. PROSPECT: Procedure-specific pain management. Available at www.postoppain.org/
51. Rawal N, McCloy RF, PROSPECT Working Group: Incisional and intraperitoneal local anaesthetics in laparoscopic cholecystectomy and abdominal hysterectomy: A systematic review. Reg Anesth Pain Med 2004;29:A307.
52. Fischer B, Camu F, PROSPECT Working Group: Comparative benefits of epidural analgesia following hysterectomy and colonic resection. Reg Anesth Pain Med 2004;29:A309.
53. U.S. Veterans Health Affairs, Office of Quality and Performance: Clinical Practice Guidelines: Postoperative Pain. Available at www.oqp.med.va.gov/cpg/PAIN/PAIN_base.htm/

14 阿片类药物的应用临床药理学

DAMIAN MURPHY

阿片类药物是临床最常用的一类镇痛药。很久以前古苏美尔人（Sumerian）就熟识了它们的药效，并已在很多文献中报道。阿片这个词就是起源于古希腊语"汁"，大概是由于这种药提炼自罂粟浆汁的缘故。阿片本身就包含了20种以上不同的生物碱。1803年，Serturner最早提纯出吗啡，随后其他阿片类衍生物相继问世，并很快应用于临床。阿片类物质是指一切含吗啡类成分的天然品及人工合成的衍生物。

阿片类镇痛药之所以在很多国家广泛使用，原因在于其生产容易，价格低廉，以及镇痛效果佳[1]。然而30年前的一份调查就已表明：由于医护人员对疼痛剧烈程度了解的欠缺，对药效持续时间评价过高以及对药物成瘾性的恐惧，导致大多数患者的镇痛药用量不足[2]。但从那时起，人们的认识并没有多大进步。即使在阿片类药物已广泛用于术后镇痛的今天，仍有60%以上的术后患者在忍受中到重度的疼痛[3]。

本章重点阐明阿片类药物的基本药理学以及详尽的围手术期临床应用。药物特点及围手术期应用将在其他章节详述。

阿片类镇痛药的作用机制

临床所用阿片类镇痛药是通过结合特定的膜受体即阿片受体（opioid receptor，OR）发挥作用。这些受体和公认的肽类递质[内源性阿片类肽（EOP）]组成内源性阿片系统（endogenous opioid system，EOS），在生理学其他功能上调控哺乳动物的伤害性痛觉传递[4]。

内源性阿片系统（EOS）

内源性阿片类肽是由蛋白原分子合成的，包括内啡肽类、强啡肽类和脑啡肽类。内源性阿片类肽存在于中枢和周围神经系统，以及心血管、胃肠道系统和免疫细胞中[5]。虽然内源性阿片肽发挥着作为神经递质或感觉传递的调质作用，但我们仍未了解它们确切的生理学作用。如对 μ 受体高选择性的其他内源性配基（内啡肽，endomorphin），就是在1997年发现的[6]。内啡肽-1和内啡肽-2都是只含4个氨基酸的多肽类，它们的具体作用不清，但可以肯定的是，它们在哺乳动物的伤害性疼痛调节中发挥着特殊的作用。

阿片类受体：中枢和外周定位

内源性阿片系统在30年前就确立了它在疼痛和疼痛治疗中的重要性。其中 μ 受体（MOR 或 OP_3）、κ 受体（KOR 或 OP_2）、δ 受体（DOR 或 OP_1）在中枢神经系统的分布是众所周知的[7]。第四个受体与传统的阿片类受体有较高的同源性，被命名为 ORL-1 或 OP_4。痛敏肽或孤啡肽-FQ定义为 ORL-1 的内源性配基，具有与强啡肽高度一致的序列同源性[8]。内源性阿片系统参与了生理学上的一些过程，其中包括疼痛的中枢调节，但并不涉及呼吸抑制[9]。实验表明 ORL-1 激动剂激活后导致脊髓镇痛和脊髓上的痛觉过敏。因此，以激活 ORL-1 受体而达到镇痛的方法并不可取，除非有更多的针对性的药理学实验支持。痛敏肽受体拮抗剂是候选的抗抑郁药和镇痛药。

MOR 广泛分布于大脑皮层、杏仁核、海马、丘脑、中脑、脑桥、骨髓和脊髓。KOR 分布大致相同，此外，还分布在下丘脑。DOR 分布不如它们广泛，仅出现在端脑和脊髓中。阿片类受体同样分布在周围神经系统，当局部给药时，也会产生镇痛作用[10]。外周给药的优点是可以避免中枢给药导致的不良反应，尤其是呼吸抑制。然而，通过不同途径和不同位点给予阿片的临床药效仍存在争议[11]。

阿片类受体最初是根据被激动剂激活或拮抗剂拮抗的药理学效应分类的。根据药理学基础研究，每一种阿片类受体的亚型已清楚分类。就 MOR 来说，两种主要亚型似乎间接镇痛（MOR-1）和导致呼吸抑制（MOR-2）。不幸的是，我们仍然缺乏针对 MOR-1 受体的特异性阿片剂。这种新药的研制将是疼痛研究的一大跨越。

三种主要的阿片类受体激活后产生的镇痛作用（见表 14-1）与其他药理学效应有关。有趣的是，KOR 受体激活后可出现烦躁和多尿，而不是呼吸抑制。

阿片类受体属于 G 蛋白偶联的受体家族，它们通过第二信使（环腺苷酸）和离子通道传输信号。阿片类受体激活减少了钙离子内流，因而减少了突触前兴奋性神经递质的释放（如 P 物质），促进钾离子外流，导致超极化和突触传递的减少。在脊髓回路中，阿片类受体可以调节 γ-氨基丁酸的传递抑制。这种阿片类的反抑制作用可能增强下行性抑制通道介导的伤害性反射传递的调节。

阿片类镇痛药通过激活一个或多个阿片类受体起效，其受体 MOR、DOR、KOR 已通过药理学（生物鉴定，立体特异性结合）和克隆方法定性。我们对阿片类受体的机制了解并不全面[12]，因为：（1）不同的药物可能既是激动剂，又是拮抗剂；（2）很难找到受体作用特异性强的阿片类药物（激动剂或拮抗剂）；（3）阿片类可能作用于一个以上的受体蛋白位点，介导构象改变。（4）受体经二聚作用构成复合体（如 MOR/MOR、DOR、KOR 和 MOR/DOR）。我们缺乏这些复合体的药理学方面的资料[13]。

阿片类镇痛药的分类

阿片类药物的临床分类是根据它们对不同受体的亲和力和药效而分。同样也可根据镇痛效果强弱而分（表 14-2）。

阿片类药物的药代动力学

药代动力学参数包括药物的吸收、分布、代谢和排泄的过程，对药物在临床上的正确使用极其重要。一般来讲，阿片类药物通过各种途径给药都能很好吸收。吸收图反映了各种可行的给药途径（皮下、椎管内、舌下、经鼻、吸入、肠外给药、口服和直肠给

表 14-1	不同阿片类受体激活的效应
受体类型	效应
μ（MOR）	脊髓上、脊髓、及外周镇痛
	呼吸抑制
	胃肠道：肠梗阻、便秘、恶心、呕吐
	瘙痒、尿潴留
	心血管抑制
	耐受性/依赖性
	镇静、欣快
	瞳孔缩小
κ（KOR）	脊髓水平镇痛
	烦躁
	镇静
	多尿
δ（DOR）	调节 MOR 受体
	脊髓和脊髓上镇痛

表 14-2	围手术期常用的阿片类镇痛药
激动剂	吗啡
	芬太尼
	阿芬太尼
	舒芬太尼
	哌替啶
	羟考酮
	海洛因
	瑞芬太尼
部分激动药	丁丙诺啡
激动-拮抗药	布托啡诺
	喷他佐辛
拮抗剂	纳洛酮
	纳曲酮

药）与口服吸收在释放模式上有很大相同。

药物从血到不同的组织和体腔，包括在骨骼肌和脂肪中的分布，取决于其脂溶性和pKa值。药物是否为脂溶性和在生理pH值下的解离度影响跨膜转运和与受体结合的能力。阿片类药物分子量相近，但脂溶性和pKa不同（pKa值越小，生理pH值下非游离酸的比例就越大）。非游离酸形式比离子更易透过细胞膜。因此，与其他pH在8~9之间的阿片类药物相比[13]，阿芬太尼（pKa 6.5）起效更快。脂溶性大多数由油/水分配系数决定（见表14-3）。阿片类药物的油/水分配系数值略有不同（吗啡1.4，舒芬太尼1.778）。数值越高，表明其亲脂性越好。高脂溶性的药物起效都很迅速，因为可以很快地由血浆到达活化位点[14]。

大多数阿片类药物有着相近的消除半衰期，同其表观分布容积（Vd）成正比，与清除率（Cl）成反比。表观分布容积大的药物如芬太尼，消除半衰期更长。相反清除迅速，表观分布容积小的瑞芬太尼半衰期很短。然而，由于阿片类药物广泛分布于体内，故单比较其半衰期并不能预测药物的持续时间[14]。

一个更有效的量度标准是时量相关半衰期，时量相关半衰期是指药物停止输注后中央室中的药物浓度下降50%需要的时间。当药物输注停止，外周室的药物重新分布到中央室去，从而延长了半衰期[16]，但阿片类药物的血浆水平和临床镇痛阈值之间的关系并不清楚[17]。临床上，阿片类药物的毒性主要与血浆浓度相关。

肝是阿片类药物代谢的主要场所。因为许多药物的肝清除率很高，所以肝血流量是代谢率的主要决定因素。与阿片类药物接触的机体器官（如肠、肺）发生生物转化较少，但这种情况并不是所有阿片类药物或给药途径都一样，如芬太尼经皮吸收并不发生代谢转化[18]。阿片类药物一般在肝内经历Ⅰ相和Ⅱ相反应，合成代谢产物才能产生药理学活性。

阿片类代谢产物的镇痛效果

吗啡代谢主要是与葡萄糖醛酸偶联，形成吗啡-3-葡萄糖醛酸（M3G）和吗啡-6-葡萄糖醛酸（M6G），一小部分脱甲基生成去甲吗啡。吗啡-6-葡萄糖醛酸是吗啡体内的主要代谢产物，给小鼠鞘内注射该药物时，显示出比吗啡强10~20倍的效能[19]。它在人体的镇痛效果尚未明确，因为不同的试验数据结果互相矛盾。在健康志愿者试验疼痛模型中，Lotsch

表14-3 阿片类药物的生化特点

阿片类药物	分子量 (kDa)	pKa	电离系数 (%)*	油/水分配系数†
吗啡	285	7.9	76	1.4
芬太尼	336	8.4	91	813
阿芬太尼	416	6.5	11	128
舒芬太尼	386	8.0	80	1.778
哌替啶	247	8.5	76	39

*电离系数指pH7.4时阿片类的电离百分比
†油/水分配系数指药物在pH7.4时在水相和油相分配之比。值越高，脂溶性越大；值越低，水溶性越大。

Modified from Gourlay G: Clinical Pharmacology of opioids in the treatment of pain. In Giamberardino MA (ed): Pain 2002-An Updated Review: Refresher Course Syllabus, 10th World Congress on Pain. Seattle, IASP Press, 2002, pp 381-394.

等[20]比较吗啡和安慰剂，发现吗啡-6-葡萄糖醛酸小剂量静脉输注效果并不明显[20]。在另一个手术后疼痛模型中，在皮肤缝合时，分别随机静脉给予吗啡（0.15 mg/kg）、安慰剂和吗啡-6-葡萄糖醛酸（0.1 mg/kg），在术后第一个24 h内，吗啡-6-葡萄糖醛酸和安慰剂组的镇痛需要量明显高于吗啡组[21]。相反，其他健康志愿者在不完全缺血疼痛[22]或电刺激[23]疼痛模型研究中表明，每70 kg 3.3~5 mg的吗啡-6-葡萄糖醛酸可以达到无痛的效果。总之，吗啡-6-葡萄糖醛酸是潜在的镇痛药，但临床应用价值尚待证实。

吗啡-3-葡萄糖醛酸对MOR受体并无亲和力，但过量吸食吗啡后产生的一些兴奋效应，如肌阵挛、惊厥和痛觉过敏可能与吗啡-3-葡萄糖醛酸有关。细胞色素P450 2D6有将可待因代谢产物转化为吗啡的作用。10%的白种人缺乏这种转化能力，我们称之为乏代谢者。这种人群即使注射镇痛剂量的可待因也不能有效镇痛[24]。

芬太尼的代谢产物认为是失活的，而哌替啶的代谢产物（如去甲哌替啶）不仅缺乏临床镇痛效果，而且重复给药或延长输注时间时可增加药物蓄积（尤其是老年人或肾功能损害患者），产生神经兴奋作用[25]。

影响阿片类药物药代动力学的因素

影响阿片类药物药代动力学并有临床意义的主要因素包括：年龄、性别、系统疾病、肥胖以及血浆蛋白浓度或结合力。

年龄

可以预言,由于年龄的差异,药物的作用可有较大变化和严重的临床后果。以下因素可以改变婴儿阿片类药物的持续时间及药效:(1)未成熟的细胞色素P450系统;(2)肾清除率减少(导致半衰期延长);(3)血脑屏障未成熟,导致大脑中药物浓度增高。有报道表明给予新生儿其他年龄组常规剂量的阿片类药物时,可导致癫痫发作[26]。因此,婴儿应用阿片类药物时更应谨慎控制剂量,并对药效进行跟踪评估。一些研究表明:吗啡静脉注射20 μg/(kg·h)可以有效控制3个月到14岁之间小儿的术后疼痛[27]。

一项前瞻性的随机双盲试验表明:van Dijk等[28]报道了持续或间断给1岁以下的开胸手术婴儿静注吗啡可以有效地镇痛。新生儿和1~6个月的婴儿对疼痛强度的差异性和吗啡的需要量迥然不同。新生儿疼痛评分较低,而1~6个月的婴儿对痛觉反应更大,需要更大的吗啡剂量。

与年轻人相比,老年人对阿片类药物很敏感,可能是由于老年人的清除率和表观容积分布降低,导致体内吗啡药物浓度增高,所以用药需要更加谨慎[29]。

性别

回顾动物和人类学研究的综述表明,阿片类对男性的镇痛效果比对女性更有效[30]。然而在1例疼痛模型中,对健康志愿者使用经皮电刺激疗法,Sarton等[31]证明了静注吗啡后(单次注射0.1 mg/kg后每小时0.03mg/kg静注)对女性的效果更佳,即使在起效和失效时间上都比男性慢。我们需要更多的对照研究来分析性别差异所带来的所需剂量的差别。

肝病和肾病

大多数阿片类代谢产物都是经肝代谢,经肾排泄。肾损害似乎并不会改变单次注射阿片类药物的药代动力学,但是持续输注会引起活性代谢产物的潜在积聚,导致药理学效应的增加。在这种情况下,M6G或去甲哌替啶更有可能蓄积,而非其母体化合物吗啡或哌替啶[32]。尽管丁丙诺啡、阿芬太尼、舒芬太尼、瑞芬太尼的药代动力学在肾功能衰竭患者体内几乎没有改变,但持续给予芬太尼会导致镇静时间延长。瑞芬太尼因为具有超短的半衰期,似乎是肾功能衰竭患者的合理选择。

患有肝损害的患者使用推荐剂量的阿片类药物镇痛时,似乎没有引起严重的临床问题[33]。但是动物研究表明,吗啡在没有肝功能的动物体内其半衰期延长,药效也增强了[34]。

在人体试验上则一直存在着矛盾的结论:一项研究表明,较正常对照组而言,肝硬化患者的吗啡血浆清除率降低,而半衰期延长[35]。另一项肝移植患儿的调查表明阿片类药物的药代动力学没有改变[36]。单次剂量芬太尼和舒芬太尼并不会影响肝肾衰竭患者的药代动力学,持续输注芬太尼会导致蓄积,延长药效[37]。阿芬太尼在肾功能衰竭患者身上的血浆清除率和清除减少,所以临床不建议使用[38]。瑞芬太尼是肝肾衰竭患者可选择的阿片类药物。

肥胖

肥胖的定义是指相对于瘦体质的身体脂肪或脂肪组织过量。常用体重指数(body mass index,BMI)评价肥胖程度。体重指数大于30认为是肥胖[39]。肥胖者较同龄、同性别、同身高的非肥胖者体质绝对量更大。我们对于肥胖对药代动力学影响的认识很有限,但是对肥胖患者谨慎应用窄治疗指数的药物似乎更加合理。瑞芬太尼,一种亲脂的阿片类,其药代动力学曾在24名接受择期手术的患者进行研究。其中12名瘦体质62(±14)kg,总体重可达113(±17)kg,另12名则为正常体重。结果表明,理想体重患者接受的瑞芬太尼剂量用于病态肥胖患者也是适用的[40]。一项详细的研究也表明,肥胖患者手术中芬太尼用量通常比实际体重估计的量要高[41],所以剂量应当参照理想体重患者。

血浆蛋白浓度或结合力

血浆蛋白浓度,尤其是α_1-酸性糖蛋白(α_1-acid glycoprotein,AAG),在创伤或手术后和慢性炎性紊乱和癌症时降低。因为大多数阿片类药物要与这类蛋白质结合,所以AAG减少的患者由于给药后游离型药物的血药浓度较高,故可能对阿片类药物很敏感。

给药途径

静脉

阿片类药物通过各种途径都能很好吸收。临床上一般静脉注射在起效时间上差别不大(2~5 min)。静脉途径比口服、肌内注射更易滴定。儿童大手术后采用静脉输注和间断注射，镇痛效果差别不大[28]。

肌内注射

药物的亲脂性是肌内注射后吸收起效快慢的决定因素。如果剂量和加药间隔时间完全个体化，肌内注射可提供良好的镇痛。然而，由于术后低温、低血容量、末梢血管收缩等因素，患者术后肌内注射吗啡的组织吸收率常变化很大[42]，再加上反复注射可产生肌肉痛，因此围手术期不主张肌内注射给药。

口服

大多数阿片类片剂的起效时间约 1 h。口服的生物利用度差异很大，芬太尼几乎是 0，而吗啡在 10%～50% 之间（见表 14-4）。食物尤其是高脂饮食，对吗啡的吸收率影响很大，饱食时吸收率慢于禁食状态，其他阿片类药物尚不明确[43]。

术后疼痛治疗时，口服是否有效取决于手术种类。Cochrane 数据库[44]一份综述表明，单次口服二氢可待因对不同手术后的急性疼痛无效。然而，根据多项研究数据合在一起的另一综述表明，单次服用羟考酮（5 mg 以上），伴或不伴对乙酰氨基酚，效应胜过安慰剂。基于以上结果，研究员建议联合用药效果等同于肌内注射吗啡加非甾体类抗炎药，但药物不良反应发生率更高[45]。围手术期口服阿片类药物适用于轻中度术后疼痛，但因其不良反应较多而被限用。

舌下给药

舌下给药可以经过黏膜进入体内循环，避免了肝的首过效应。影响吸收率的因素包括：pKa、脂溶性、分子量、弥散速度和口腔 pH 值[46]。芬太尼经口腔黏膜和唾液入肠道可以直接吸收，就像含棒棒糖一样[47]。由于此种途径药物不易大剂量释放，限制了它在术后急性疼痛的应用。

皮肤吸收

药物经皮肤给药后有两种转运形式：常规（被动）转运和电离子渗透（主动）转运。

常规被动转运

分子量小、亲脂性好、非游离性药物更易渗透细胞外膜，避免了首过代谢。影响敷用阿片类贴膜[透皮给药系统（transdermal delivery system，TDS）]因素包括：角质层的渗透性、皮温、贴膜位置、皮肤有无缺损、患者的年龄和种族。经皮芬太尼贴膜和丁丙诺啡是目前最常用于慢性疼痛的透皮给药系统的阿片类制剂。一旦使用，药物在皮内恒速释放蓄积达 12～16 h，这种蓄积像一种二次容器，保持血药浓度稳定大约 3 天左右[48]。芬太尼的表观终末半衰期为 15～24 h，所以当贴膜撕去后，体内仍保持相当可观的药物浓度。

TDS 并不主张用于术后，因为当再次给药时或疼痛消退后会导致呼吸抑制[49]。

表 14-4　阿片类药物药代动力学和代谢产物

阿片类	半衰期	等效静脉剂量 (mg/kg)	等效口服剂量 (mg/kg)	清除率 ml/(min·kg)	持续时间 (h)	口服吸收率 (%)	活化代谢产物
吗啡	2～4h	0.1	0.3～0.5	15	3～5	10～50	M6G
芬太尼	1.7(α)min	0.001	0.001～0.015，舌下	13	0.75～1	经皮，90	无
哌替啶	3～4h	1	1.5～2	12	2～3	30～60	去甲哌替啶
阿芬太尼	1.4(α)min	0.05	N/A	6	0.5	无	无
舒芬太尼	1.4(α)min	0.0001	N/A	12.7	1	无	无
可待因	3h	1.2	2		4～6	60～90	吗啡
羟考酮	2～6h	N/A	0.1	40	4～6	40～130	羟吗啡酮
瑞芬太尼	5min，与输注时间无关	(0.05～2) μg/(kg·h)	N/A	40	取决于输注时间	N/A	氧化亚氮

离子电渗疗法

离子电渗疗法的设计旨在克服角质层对药物吸收的屏障，电场的运用使带电的药物成分透过皮肤。在对600多名术后疼痛患者的研究表明：每10 min释放40 μg芬太尼效果等同于标准化的患者自控镇痛（patient-controlled analgesia，PCA）装置[50]。然而，其缺点在于恒定剂量释放，并不适用于年老和年幼的患者。

经鼻吸入

经鼻吸入的优点在于具有减轻给药痛苦、快速起效和患者自控等优点，目前已用于临床疼痛治疗。它避免了肝的代谢，达到与静脉注射类似的效果。然而，常规途径药物吸收率变化很大，最好的经鼻吸入药物就是分子量小的高脂溶性药物。芬太尼、舒芬太尼、哌替啶、海洛因和布托啡诺就有这种剂型。平均起效时间是12～22 min，达峰时间为24～60 min，表明在药代动力学和临床结果存在相当大的个体差异[51]。

尽管经鼻吸入阿片类药物可应用于门诊或住院患者以及慢性疼痛患者，但仍需要更好的临床剂型和设备问世。

直肠给药

直肠给药并不常用于术后镇痛，因为直肠给药吸收率变化极大，并且又取决于药品成分。药物在进入体循环和门脉循环前就已经吸收了，因此减少了首过代谢的浓度。一般直肠给药剂量同口服剂量。

皮下注射

皮下注射时，水溶性好的药物更易吸收。老年术后患者皮下注射效果类似肌内注射[52]，但水肿、低血压和外周循环不良时一般不宜使用。

椎管给药：硬膜外和鞘内给药

阿片类受体位点在脊髓背角，但不局限于浅层，同样也位于脊髓的黑质。这意味着椎管内给予阿片类药物必须要弥散至脊髓深层方发挥镇痛作用。药物的弥散取决于其分子量、浓度梯度、离子和非离子比率，特别是脂溶性。欧洲一些研究已证实吗啡和芬太尼硬膜外或鞘内给药可治疗术后疼痛[53]。

当阿片类药物直接注入脑脊液（cerebrospinal fluid，CSF）时，小剂量则可发挥镇痛作用，因为此处已无解剖屏障，而且血液再吸收很缓慢。然而，硬膜外腔给药时，药物必须透过硬脊膜才能到达脊髓结合阿片类受体[54]。硬膜外给药的全身吸收很迅速，亲脂药物的血药浓度与肌内注射效果等同。

在应用微量透析技术的猪模型中，可以持续测定硬膜外或鞘内间隙的阿片类药物浓度。Bernards等[55]证明了药物脂溶性与以下因素密切相关（1）硬膜外腔的滞留时间，（2）终末半衰期（即：脂溶性越好，半衰期越长）。

吗啡是最早也是最常见的椎管内应用的药物。它的长效作用会因为脑内再分配而导致严重的呼吸抑制等不良反应。临床上将大多数阿片类药物鞘内注射，能产生有效的镇痛作用，并且不良反应小。理想的鞘内阿片类药物应当能快速从CSF进入脊髓，并且清除率慢、中度或无脑内分布。

临床上不同阿片类药物的鞘内镇痛效应和持续时间与静脉给药相比差异很大，这主要归因于药物的作用持续时间和脑内扩散。这些因素受药物亲脂性（脂溶性药物较水溶性药物更易吸收入脊髓，见表14-3）、受体亲和力、内在活性及体循环内药物消除影响。

亲水性阿片类药物，如吗啡，CSF中清除缓慢，导致脑内药物浓度相对较高。在动物模型中，发现吗啡鞘内给药的作用较静脉更强。而芬太尼却相反，作用很弱[56]。亲脂类阿片类药物如芬太尼，由CSF迅速转运至脊髓中富含脂质的组织中，在多节段上快速发挥镇痛作用。在轴索上给予阿片类药物，在其作用终止时其新陈代谢如何尚不清楚。

因为硬膜外给药和静脉给药它们血浆水平，镇痛作用和不良反应都相似[55]，所以硬膜外给予亲脂性药物，其作用的确切位点尚不清楚，但一些研究提出了亲脂性药物的作用位点[57,58]。在一项10名志愿者的小型研究中，研究了硬膜外单次推药和输注芬太尼的镇痛效果。数据表明单次给药作用在脊髓机制，而输注则通过吸收入体循环和再分配起效[59]。虽然如此，尽管仍有部分药物在CSF中扩散并引起严重并发症，但亲脂化合物的镇痛调节作用还是主要通过体循环吸收而起效的[60]。

阿片类药物的不良作用

临床应用阿片类药物的最终目标就是仔细地滴定以有效控制疼痛,此外别无它用。传统的全身给药具有中枢和外周效应,这归因于阿片受体在体内的广泛分布。一般来说,虽然不良反应发生率和严重程度根据阿片种类、剂量、给药途径及患者不同而异,但其有效作用(镇痛)和不良反应是同时出现的。主要不良反应如下:

呼吸抑制

临床上真正的呼吸抑制发生率并不知道。据推测,治疗剂量的阿片类药物引起呼吸抑制的发生率,在不考虑给药途径时小于1%[61],然而并没有确切的证据表明各种阿片类药物、给药方案、给药途径以及同时在神经根和胃肠外使用阿片类药物(镇静与否)时呼吸抑制的发生情况。

一般来说,阿片类药物通过逐渐减少呼吸频率与潮气量来减少分钟通气量,主要效应在于降低了大脑髓质呼吸中枢对二氧化碳分压的反应性。给予阿片类药物后,出现二氧化碳曲线右移,斜坡下降。尽管静脉注射起效快的阿片类药物后,患者可能处于清醒状态却发生呼吸暂停,而呼吸频率减少发生较迟,这些并不是阿片类药物引起呼吸抑制的有效迹象[62]。

阿片类药还抑制对缺氧的呼吸反应。目前已在志愿者身上研究了鞘内与静脉注射相同镇痛剂量吗啡对缺氧后通气反应的相对影响[63],结果表明两者结果基本相同。鞘内给药反应持续较长(12 h以上),说明阿片类药物从中枢机制影响了通气。

阿片类药物引起的呼吸抑制是活化 MOR 介导的,动物实验证明 MOR 敲除小鼠,全身应用吗啡后,既没有呼吸抑制,也没有脊髓或脊髓上的抗伤害性感受[64]。因此,在疼痛缺失的情况下,阿片类介导的镇痛与呼吸抑制是不可分离的。然而,志愿者与疼痛患者的反应又不一致。呼吸中枢收到疼痛刺激信号后,可以减弱阿片类介导的呼吸抑制[65]。急性疼痛时,阿片类药物应当逐渐加量,不应害怕呼吸抑制而妨碍术后患者的镇痛。但药物滴定、剂量、给药间隔必须谨慎以降低风险[66]。

阿片类药物呼吸抑制的处理取决于严重程度,必要时静脉少量逐次给予纳洛酮(100~400 μg),或静脉输注,因为纳洛酮的半衰期明显比大多数阿片类药物短(参见第15章)。

瘙痒症

阿片类药物如吗啡和芬太尼静脉注射后可导致组胺释放,引起局部短暂瘙痒症。瘙痒症也是阿片类药物椎管内注射常见的不良反应之一,根据人群研究,发生率变异很大。其确切机制尚不清。存在几种假说,如与给予阿片类药相关的异常皮肤敏感性、瘙痒中枢的存在和脊髓背侧角异常神经元的活化[67]。瘙痒症的治疗尚有争论。很多药物治疗,如抗组胺剂、5-HT受体拮抗剂、阿片受体拮抗剂、丙泊酚、非甾体抗炎类药和氟哌啶醇都被评价过。不逆转镇痛或导致深度镇静的药物评价最好。对不同患者群[68](包括儿童[69]),昂丹司琼是治疗阿片类药物所导致瘙痒症的最有效药物之一,常规静脉注射 2~4 mg。

胃肠道效应

阿片类药物延迟胃排空,增加小肠和大肠蠕动时间,抑制肠液分泌和渗透。肠梗阻和便秘是阿片类药物治疗的常见不良反应。一些生理因素可以抑制或促进胃排空,交感兴奋和疼痛可延迟胃排空。阿片类药物减少胃酸分泌,增加胃窦张力。胃排空延迟有一些严重后遗症,包括口服药或营养素的吸收缓慢、恶心和增加误吸风险[70],全肠道平滑肌张力增加,胆汁胰液分泌减少。

虽然口服和肠外给药是阿片类药物引起胃肠蠕动延迟的主要原因,但一些研究表明硬膜外和鞘内给药也可延迟胃排空[71]。研究表明局麻下辅以神经安定术进行剖腹手术的患者,较全身或硬膜外给予阿片类药物的患者,胃肠功能恢复更快[72]。

硬膜外给药延迟胃排空的机制不清,因为药物对全身和局部的影响还不完全明确。术后肠梗阻是多因素的,而阿片类药物发挥重要作用[73]。阿片类受体分布于肠腔,而阿片类药物引起的胃肠道抑制作用,是阿片类药物与胃肠道与中枢神经系统 MOR 结合的结果。中枢与外周神经系统 MOR 受累的比例与剂量相关。阿片类药物导致的胃排空和胃肠蠕动延迟可以被阿片类受体拮抗剂逆转,如甲基纳曲酮,这表明其作用机制主要在外周[74,75]。与安慰剂组行肠道手术或根治性子宫全切的患者比较,使用作用在外周的新型 MOR

拮抗剂 alvimopan，不能透过血脑屏障，但可以促进胃肠恢复，缩短住院时间[76]。

治疗剂量的阿片类增加胆道张力，缘于 Oddi 括约肌的痉挛或收缩，影响可以长达 12 h 以上。阿片类对括约肌作用很复杂，小剂量纳洛酮、硝酸甘油可以缓解临床症状[77]。没有迹象表明等效镇痛剂量的哌替啶在治疗胆绞痛或肾绞痛方面优于其他阿片类药物。

泌尿系统不良反应

阿片类增加输尿管和膀胱收缩的张力和幅度，但因人而异。尽管机制不明，但内源性阿片系统似乎通过骶段脊髓水平副交感输出来调控膀胱的生理功能[78]。

椎管内给药后的尿潴留比肌内注射或静脉给予等效剂量发生率更高，说明椎管内给药的机制与药物的全身吸收并不等同[79]。人体研究显示，硬膜外注射吗啡导致膀胱逼尿肌 15 min 内松弛，且持续数小时，纳洛酮可逆转。其他阿片药物试验提示：鞘内注射亲脂类药物可能对术后膀胱排空的影响更小[80]。术后延迟膀胱排空的其他因素包括：患者的血容量、术式和手术部位以及促抗利尿激素活化的因子[81]。

恶心呕吐

术后恶心呕吐（postoperative nausea and vomiting，PONV）是术后常见的棘手问题，尽管是多因素所致，但术中和术后使用阿片类药物对 PONV 的发生意义重大。然而，目前尚不清楚[82,83]位于化学感受器触发区（chemoreceptor trigger zone，CRTZ）和相关髓质中心的阿片类受体是如何影响 PONV 发生的。PONV 与给药途径关系不大，因为硬膜外和鞘内给药发生率与静脉给药相同[84]。椎管内给药后，阿片类药物向头侧扩散很可能是其机制。与 PONV 发生相关的因素还包括：疼痛、高血压、术式、活动、胃胀气、胃排空延迟和性别（女性多见）。

心血管系统不良反应

仰卧位时，阿片类药物对人体血压、心率和心律影响最小。立位后可能产生直立性低血压。其他不良反应见于冠心病患者，治疗剂量可降低氧耗、心排出量、左室压力和舒张压[85]。吗啡注射后可引起组胺释放，导致低血压[86]。阿片类药物通常引起外周动静脉血管的舒张，所以血容量过低的患者注射阿片类药物要注意。芬太尼和其他短效阿片类药物单用或在其他可刺激迷走神经的手术（如喉镜检查）应用时，可引起心动过缓。部分激动剂和激动-拮抗剂复合物很少用于术后急性疼痛，此章不详述。

小结

阿片类药物的临床应用药理学比较复杂，要考虑到个体差异性以及影响药代动力学和药效学的种种因素。吗啡始终是评价其他药物的标准，尽管与其他强效药物镇痛效果相当。疼痛的出现改变了阿片类药物的临床应用药理学特点，必须根据疼痛强度及患者实际情况加药。最常见的镇痛不足的原因就在于对阿片类药物不良反应的恐惧。然而，我们不能因为害怕呼吸抑制就限制阿片类药物的合理使用。我们应采用滴定法，使给药剂量、间隔时间和追加剂量最优化，为围手术期患者提供良好的个体化镇痛。

（吴　倩译　熊源长校）

参考文献

1. Arner S, Bolund C, Rane A, et al: Narcotic analgesics in the treatment of cancer and postoperative pain. Acta Anaesthesiol Scand 1982; 26(Suppl 74):1–78.
2. Marks RM, Sacher EJ: Under treatment of medical inpatients with narcotic analgesics. Ann Intern Med 1973;78:173–181.
3. Apfelbaum JL, Chen C, Matha SS, et al: Postoperative pain experience results from a national pain survey suggest postoperative pain continues to be undermanaged. Anesth Analg 2003;97:534–550.
4. Vaccarino AL, Kastin AJ: Endogenous opiates. Peptides 2000;21: 1975–2034.
5. Zadina JE, Hackler L, Ge LJ, Kastin AJ: A potent and selective endogenous agonist for the mu-opiate receptor. Nature 1997;386:499–502.
6. Horvath G: Endomorphin-1 and endomorphin-2: Pharmacology of the selective endogenous mu-opioid receptor agonists. Pharmacol Ther 2000;88:437–463.
7. Mansour A, Khachaturian H, Lewis ME, et al: Anatomy of CNS opioid receptors. Trends Neurosci 1988;11:308–314.
8. Darland T, Heinricher MM, Grandy DK: Orphanin FQ/nociceptin: A role in pain and analgesia, but so much more. Trends Neurosci 1998; 21:215–221.
9. Calo G, Guerrini R, Rizzi A, et al: Pharmacology of nociceptin and its receptor: A novel therapeutic target. Br J Pharmacol 2000;129: 1261–1283.
10. Stein C, Yassouridis A: Peripheral morphine analgesia. Pain 1997;71: 119–121.
11. Picard PR, Tramer MR, McQuay HJ, Moore RA: Analgesic efficacy of peripheral opioids (all except intra-articular): A qualitative systematic review of randomised controlled trials. Pain 1997;72:309–318.
12. Kosterlitz HW, Paterson SJ: Opioid receptors and mechanism of opioid analgesia. In Benedetti C, Chapman CR, Giron G (eds): Advances in Pain Research and Therapy, vol 14. New York, Raven Press, 1989, pp 37–43.

13. Levac, BAR, O'Dowd BF, George SR: Oligomerization of opioid receptors: Generation of novel signalling units. Curr Opin Pharmacol 2002; 2:76–81.
14. Bovill JG: Pharmacokinetics of opioids. In Bowdle TA, Hortia A, Kharasch ED (eds): The Pharmacological Basis of Anaesthesiology. New York, Churchill Livingstone, 1994, pp 37–81.
15. Thompson JP, Rowbotham DJ: Remifentanil: An opioid for the 21st century. Br J Anaesth 1996;76;341–343.
16. Hughes MA, Glass PSA, Jacobs JR: Context sensitive half time in a multicompartment model for intravenous anaesthetic drugs. Anesthesiology 1992;76:334–341.
17. Dalhstrom B, Tamsen A, Paalzow L, et al: Patient controlled analgesic therapy. Part IV: Pharmacokinetic and analgesic plasma concentrations of morphine. Clin Pharmacokinet 1982;7:266–279.
18. Gourlay GK: Treatment of cancer pain with transdermal fentanyl. Lancet Oncol 2001;2:165–172.
19. Sullivan AF, McQuay HJ, Baily D, et al: The spinal antinociceptive actions of morphine metabolites morphine 6 glucuronide and normorphine in the rat. Brain Res 1989;482:219–224.
20. Lotsch J, Kobal G, Stockmann, et al: Lack of analgesic activity of morphine-6-glucuronide intravenous administration in healthy volunteers. Anesthesiology 1997;87:1348–1358.
21. Motamed C, Mazoit X, Ghanouchi K, et al: Pre-emptive intravenous morphine-6-glucuronide is ineffective for postoperative pain relief. Anesthesiology 2000;92:355–360.
22. Buetler TM, Wilder-Smith OGH, Aebi S, et al: Analgesic actions of i.v. morphine-6-glucuronide in healthy volunteers. Br J Anaesth 2000;84:97–99.
23. Penson RT, Joel SP, Bakhshi K, et al: Randomised placebo controlled trial of the activity of the morphine glucuronides. Clin Pharmacol Ther 2000;68:667–676.
24. Desmeules J, Gascon MP, Dayer P, Magistris M: Impact of environmental and genetic factors on codeine analgesia. Eur J Clin Pharmacol 1991; 41:23–26.
25. Danziger LH, Martin SJ, Blum RA: Central nervous system toxicity associated with meperidine use in hepatic disease. Pharmacotherapy 1994;14:235–238.
26. Koren G, Butt W, Pape K, et al: Morphine induced seizures in newborn infants. Vet Hum Toxicol 1985;27:519–520.
27. Lynn Am, Opheim KE, Tyler DC: Morphine infusions after paediatric cardiac surgery. Crit Care Med 1984;12:863–866.
28. van Dijk M, Bouwmeester NJ, Duivenvoorden HJ, et al: Efficacy of continuous versus intermittent morphine administration after major surgery in 0–3 year old infants: A double-blind randomised controlled trial. Pain 2002;98:305–313.
29. Kaiko RF, Walssenstein SL, Rogers AG, et al: Narcotics in the elderly. Medi Clin North Am 1982;66:1079–1089.
30. Keat B, Sarton E, Dahan A: Gender differences in opioid mediated analgesia: Animal and human studies. Anesthesiology 2000;93:539–547.
31. Sarton E, Olofsen E, Den Hartigh J, et al: Sex differences in morphine analgesia: An experimental study in healthy volunteers Anesthesiology 2000;93:670–675.
32. Angst MS, Buhrer M, Lotsch J: Insidious intoxication after morphine treatment in renal failure: Delayed onset of morphine-6-glucuronide action. Anesthesiology 2000;92;1473–1476.
33. Patwardhan RV, Johnson RF, Hoyumpa A, et al: Normal metabolism of morphine in cirrhosis. 1981;81:1006–1011.
34. Greene NM, Hug CC: Pharmacokinetics. In Kitaha LM, Collins JG (eds): Narcotic Analgesics in Anesthesiology. Baltimore, Williams & Wilkins, 1982, pp 1–41.
35. Hasselstrom J, Eriksson LS, Person A, et al: The metabolism and bioavailability of morphine in patients with liver cirrhosis. Eur J Pharmacol 1990;29:289–297.
36. Davis JP, Stiller RL, Cook DR, et al: Effects of cholestatic hepatic disease and chronic renal failure on alfentanil pharmacokinetics in children. Anesth Analg 1989;68:579–583.
37. Davies G, Kingswood C, Street M: Pharmacokinetics of opioids in renal dysfunction. Clin Pharmacokinet 1996;31:410–422.
38. Hohne C, Donaubauer B, Kaisers U: Opioids during anaesthesia in liver and renal failure. Anaesthesist 2004;53:291–303.
39. National Institutes of Health: Clinical guidelines on the identification, evaluation, and treatment of overweight and obesity in adults. Bethesda, Md, Department of Health and Human Services, National Institutes of Health, National Heart, Lung, and Blood Institute, 1998.
40. Egan TD, Huizinga B, Gupta SK, et al: Remifentanil pharmacokinetics in obese versus lean patients. Anesthesiology 1998;89:562–573.
41. Shibutani K, Inchiosa MA, Sawada K, et al: Accuracy of pharmacokinetic models for predicting fentanyl concentrations in lean and obese surgical patients: Deviation of dosing weight. Anesthesiology 2004; 101:603–613.
42. Forrest J: Pharmacology of opioids. In Acute Pain Pathophysiology and Treatment. Ontario, Canada, Manticore, 1998, pp 77–98.
43. Kaiko RF: The effect of food intake on the pharmacokinetics of sustained-release morphine sulphate capsules. Clin Ther 1997;19:296–303.
44. Edwards JE, Moore RA, McQuay HJ: Single dose dihydrocodeine for acute postoperative pain. Cochrane Database Syst Rev 2000;(4):CD002760.
45. Edwards JE, Moore RA, McQuay HJ: Single dose oxycodone and oxycodone plus paracetamol (acetaminophen) for acute postoperative pain. Cochrane Database Syst Rev 2000;(4):CD002763.
46. Ripamonti C, Bruera E: Rectal, buccal and sublingual narcotics for the management of cancer pain. J Palliative Care 1991;7:30–35.
47. Schechter NL, Weisman SJ, Rosenblum M, et al: The use of oral transmucosal fentanyl citrate for painful procedures in children. Paediatrics 1995;95:335–339.
48. Varel JR, Shafter SL, Hwang SS, et al: Absorption characteristics of transdermally applied fentanyl. Anesthesiology 1989;70:928–934.
49. Sandler AN, Baxter AD, Katz J: A double blind patient controlled trial of transdermal fentanyl after abdominal hysterectomy. Anesthesiology 1994;81:1169–1180.
50. Viscusi E, Reyonlds L, Chung F, et al: Patient controlled transdermal fentanyl HCl vs intravenous morphine pump for postoperative pain. JAMA 2004;291:1293.
51. Dale O, Hjortkjaer R, Kharasch ED: Nasal administration of opioids for pain management in adults. Acta Anesthesiol Scand 2002;46:759–770.
52. Semple TJ, Upton RN, Macintyre PE, et al: Morphine blood concentrations in elderly postoperative patients following administration via an indwelling subcutaneous cannula. Anaesthesia 1997;52:318–323.
53. Rawal N, Alllvin RL: Epidural and intrathecal opioids for postoperative pain in Europe—a 17 nation questionnaire study of selective hospitals. Euro Pain Study Group on Acute Pain. Acta Anesthesiol Scand 1996; 40:1119–1126.
54. Nordberg G: Pharmacokinetic aspects of spinal morphine analgesia. Acta Anesthesiol Scand Suppl 1984;79:1–38.
55. Bernards CM, Shen DD, Sterling ES, et al: Epidural cerebrospinal fluid and plasma pharmacokinetics of epidural opioids. Part 1: Difference among opioids. Anesthesiology 2003;99:455–465.
56. Abram SE, Mampilly GA, Milsavljevic D: Assessment of the potency and intrinsic activity of systemic versus intrathecal opioids in the rat. Anesthesiology 1997;87:127–134.
57. D'Angelo R, Gerachner JC, Eisenach J, et al: Epidural fentanyl produces labor analgesia by a spinal mechanism. Anesthesiology 1998;88:1519–1523.
58. Salomaki TE, Latinen JO, Nuutinen LS: A randomised double blind comparison of epidural versus intravenous infusion for analgesia after thoracotomy by rostral spread. Anesthesiology 1991;75:790–795.
59. Ginosar Y, Riley ET, Angst MS: The site of action of epidural fentanyl in humans: The difference between infusion and bolus administration. Anesth Analg 2003;97:1428–1438.
60. Eisenach JC: Lipid soluble opioids do move in cerebrospinal fluid. Reg Anesth Pain Med 2001;26:296–297.
61. Rygnestad T, Borchgrevink PC, Eide E: Postoperative epidural infusion of morphine and bupivacaine is safe on surgical wards: Organisation of the treatment, effects and side effects of 2000 consecutive patients. Acta Anesthesiol Scand 1997;41:868–876.
62. Babenco HD, Conard PF, Gross JB: The pharmacodynamic effect of a remifentanil bolus on ventilatory control. Anesthesiology 2000;92:393–398.
63. Bailey PL, Lu JK, Pace NL, et al: Effects of intrathecal morphine on the ventilatory response to hypoxia. N Engl J Med 2000;343:1228–1234.
64. Dahan M, Sarto E, Teppema L, et al: Anaesthetic potency and influence of morphine and sevoflurane on respiration in mu opioid receptor knockout mice. Anesthesiology 2001;94:824–832.
65. Borgbjerg FM, Nielsen K, Franks J: Experimental pain stimulates respiration and attenuates morphine-induced respiratory depression:

A controlled study in human volunteers. Pain 1996;64:123–128.
66. Hopf HW, Weitz S: Postoperative pain management. Arch Surg 1994;129:128–132.
67. Szarvas S, Harmon D, Murphy D: Neuraxial opioid-induced pruritus: A review. J Clin Anesth 2003;15:234–239.
68. Borgeat A, Stirnemann HR: Ondansetron is effective to treat spinal or epidural morphine-induced pruritus. Anesthesiology 1999;90:432–436.
69. Arai L, Stayer S, Schwartz R, Dorsey A: The use of ondansetron to treat pruritus associated with intrathecal morphine in two paediatric patients. Paediatr Anesth 1996;6:337–339.
70. Nimmo WS: The effects of anaesthesia on gastric motility and emptying. Br J Anaesth 1984;56:29–36.
71. Thoren T, Wattwil M: The effects on gastric emptying on thoracic epidural analgesia with morphine or bupivacaine. Anesth Analg 1988;67:687–694.
72. Jorgensen H, Wetterslev J, Moiniche S, Dahl JB: Epidural local anaesthetics versus opioid-based analgesic regimens on postoperative gastrointestinal paralysis, PONV and pain after abdominal surgery. Cochrane Database Syst Rev 2000;(4):CD001893.
73. Luckey A, Livingston E, Tache Y: Mechanism and treatment of postoperative ileus. Arch Surg 2003;128:206–214.
74. Murphy D, Sutton JA, Prescott LF, Murphy MB: Opioid induced changes in gastric emptying: A peripheral mechanism in man. Anesthesiology 1997;87:765–770.
75. Yuan CS, Foss JF: Oral methylnaltrexone for opioid-induced constipation. JAMA 2000;284:1383–1384.
76. Wolff BG, Michelassi F, Tood M, et al: Alvimopan, a novel peripheral acting μ opioid antagonist. Ann Surg 2004;240:728–735.
77. Isenhower HL, Muller BA: Selection of narcotic analgesic for pain associated with pancreatitis. Am J Health Syst Pharm 1998;55:480–486.
78. Malinovsky LM, Le Normand L, LePage JY, et al: The urodynamic effects of intravenous opioids and ketoprofen in humans. Anesth Analg 1998;87:456–461.
79. Peterson TK, Husted SE, Rybo L, et al: Urinary retention during i.m. and extradural morphine analgesia. Br J Anaesth 1982;54:1175–1178.
80. Lui S, Chiu AA, Carpenter RL, et al: Fentanyl prolongs lidocaine spinal anaesthesia without prolonging recovery. Anesth Analg 1995;80:730–734.
81. Rawal N, Mollefors KM, Axelsson K, et al: An experimental study of urodynamic effects of epidural morphine and naloxone reversal. Anesth Analg 1983;62:641–647.
82. Andrews PLR: Physiology of nausea and vomiting. Br J Anaesth 1992;69:2S–19S.
83. Hornby PJ: Central neurocircuitry associated with emesis. Am J Med 2001;111(Suppl 8A):106S–112S.
84. Correll DJ, Viscusi ER, Grunwald Z, Moore JH Jr: Epidural analgesia compared with intravenous morphine patient-controlled analgesia: Postoperative outcome measures after mastectomy with immediate TRAM flap breast reconstruction. Reg Anesth Pain Med 2001;26:444–449.
85. Estafanous F (ed): Opioids in Anaesthesia II. London, Butterworth-Heinemann, 1990, pp 93–109.
86. Rosow CE, Moss J, Philbin DM, et al: Histamine release during morphine and fentanyl anaesthesia. Anesthesiology 1982;56:93–96.

15 阿片类镇痛药在围手术期的应用

COLIN J. L. McCARTNEY · AHTSHAM NIAZI

麻醉医师的主要职责是处理疼痛；自从麻醉学专业开始为此目标而努力以来，人们就一直在应用阿片类镇痛药。阿片类镇痛药仍然是处理术后中度至重度疼痛的主要药物；尽管开发了一些新型阿片类药物，但吗啡仍是衡量比较所有其他阿片类药物的"金标准"。然而，每种阿片类药物在一定临床条件下以及特殊给药途径下，可能都有其特定优点。急性疼痛处理中，阿片类药物通常都用于包括非甾体类抗炎药（nonsteroidal anti-inflammatory drug，NSAID）、对乙酰氨基酚、局部麻醉技术以及其他镇痛辅助药物在内的多模式镇痛方案中[1]。这种方案既可改善疼痛控制水平，也可减少阿片类药物的用量，从而降低阿片类药物相关的不良作用。

国际疼痛研究协会（International Association for the Study of Pain，IASP）对疼痛的定义为：一种与急性或潜在组织损害相关的不愉快的感觉与情感体验，或对这种损害的描述[2]。术后疼痛是典型伤害性感受，是由组织损伤及创伤后炎症反应所致。这种类型的疼痛常常对阿片类药物治疗反应良好。术后疼痛偶尔是神经性疼痛，特别是发生周围神经或中枢神经直接损伤时。神经性疼痛通常被描述为放射样（电击样）或烧灼样疼痛；与伤害性感受疼痛不同，既往一般认为阿片类镇痛药对神经性疼痛治疗效果差。但是，目前这种观念已经受到挑战，许多研究已经证实阿片类药物有利于神经性疼痛患者[3,4]。

本章将对阿片类药物用于围手术期镇痛有利作用的证据加以综述，并分析特殊阿片类药物通过各种途径给药的优缺点，讨论新型镇痛技术，如口服阿片类药物控释剂及外周给予阿片类药物的应用。

方法

通过 Medline 资料库检索出 1966—2004 年 12 月的文献，进行系统性综述。检索词包括：阿片类药物、吗啡、芬太尼、氢吗啡酮、羟考酮、二醋吗啡、口服、静脉内、硬膜外、鞘内、经皮、外周、关节内、控释。同时也检索 Cochrane 数据库和牛津疼痛网站的相关资料。主要包括有关疼痛评价的随机双盲研究。当无较高质量证据时，应用其他相关研究来解答特殊问题；在需要使用这类文献之处，在文中特别注明。

经静脉、肌肉以及口服给予阿片类药物处理急性疼痛的数据以需要治疗的人数（number needed to treat，NNT）和需要伤害的人数（number needed to harm，NNH）来表示。阿片类药物经其他给药途径的资料以百分比和发生频率来表示。NNT 用于测量两种干预治疗结果的比较，它是治疗组与对照组相比，绝对风险下降值的倒数[5]。假设一项曲马多研究中，其使用曲马多后剧烈疼痛风险从不应用曲马多时的 0.3 下降至 0.05，则其绝对风险下降值为 0.25（0.3-0.05），这样 NNT 则为 1÷0.25，或者为 4。

临床上，NNT 为 4 意味着用曲马多治疗 4 例患者可预防 1 例疼痛。然而，几乎没有研究能证明单用一种治疗方法能 100% 缓解疼痛，因此计算疼痛缓解 50% 的 NNT 更容易。采用 NNT 概念也能计算和表达不良事件的发生情况，这就是所谓的 NNH。NNT 的应用有限，因为其一般指在某个时间点进行单次用药干预的作用，可能并不能精确反映治疗作用当时的质量。但是，它是证实不同治疗相对效率的有用工具。

静脉内阿片类药物的治疗

旁注 15-1 总结了以下部分。

吗啡

吗啡仍是衡量阿片类镇痛药效果的金标准，肌内注射 10 mg 疼痛缓解 50% 疼痛的 NNT 是 2.9[6]。但是，未见计算静脉使用吗啡 NNT 的研究。人们在现代急性疼痛治疗中一般认为吗啡重复肌内给药可带来注射痛，因而并不理想；任何可能情况下，都应采用静脉内给药途径[7]。下面详细论述对吗啡与其他阿片类药物镇痛作用和副作用进行比较的许多研究。

哌替啶

目前不推荐全身应用哌替啶来处理术后疼痛，因为其不良作用（心动过速、高血压、神经毒性代谢产物蓄积）的发生率较高，且与其他强效阿片类药物如吗啡和氢吗啡酮相比并无优势[8]。

对其他阿片类药物不耐受或过敏的患者，至少 100 mg 的哌替啶确实能产生镇痛作用（体重 70 kg，NNT 为 2.9）[9]，且作用持续时间（2～3 h）比吗啡短，因此间隔 4 h 给药就会出现镇痛不全窗口[8]。哌替啶治疗胆源性绞痛或肾性绞痛的效果在临床上并不优于其他阿片类药物。术后长时间用药可带来一些缺点，包括其代谢产物去甲哌替啶有蓄积的可能，其神经毒性（引起癫痫）是哌替啶的 2～3 倍，血浆半衰期 14～48h。哌替啶是最易引起老年人谵妄的阿片类药物，特别是使用 PCA 时[8]。已有哌替啶与单胺氧化酶抑制剂之间存在致命性相互作用的报道[8]。总之，胃肠外给予阿片类药物不适合选择哌替啶，因为其作用持续时间短、存在抗胆碱能作用以及神经毒性的可能。已证实，哌替啶的 NNH 为 2.9，而吗啡 NNH 为 9.1[9]，也说明哌替啶副作用更大。对吗啡不耐受或过敏的术后疼痛患者，应用不良反应发生率较低的药物，如氢吗啡酮，可能对患者更有利。

氢吗啡酮

该药是一种半合成的吗啡衍生物。对体重 70 kg 的患者，胃肠外约 2 mg 氢吗啡酮与 10 mg 吗啡等效；也就是说，氢吗啡酮的效能大约是吗啡的 5 倍[10]。静脉内给药时，氢吗啡酮起效迅速（5 min 内），短时间达到峰效应（10～20 min），半衰期较短（3～4 h）[11]。氢吗啡酮的主要代谢产物 3-葡萄糖苷酸氢吗啡酮不具有镇痛作用，对大鼠有神经兴奋作用[12]，在肾损害患者体内可能蓄积[13]。一般认为，尽管缺乏随机研究的支持，但静脉内氢吗啡酮对老年患者及肾损害患者的不良作用较少。Rapp 等[14]将 18～65 岁下腹部或骨盆手术的 61 例患者随机分为两组，使用等效剂量的氢吗啡酮或吗啡静脉 PCA。结果显示两组镇痛作用相当，但是吗啡组患者认知障碍较少。目前尚无关于氢吗啡酮与其他阿片类药物用于肾功能损害患者术后镇痛的随机双盲研究。

芬太尼

Janssen 制药公司于 20 世纪 50～60 年代致力于研发合成比吗啡和哌替啶的镇痛活性与效能更强而不良作用更少的阿片类镇痛药，芬太尼是该公司合成的一系列阿片类药物中的一种。芬太尼在结构上与哌替啶类似[15]。胃肠外给药时，芬太尼的镇痛效能是吗啡的 80～100 倍，因此 100 μg 芬太尼相当于 10 mg 吗啡。静脉给药时，芬太尼起效快于吗啡[15]，麻醉后恢复室（post-anesthesia care unit，PACU）中，常常单次静脉注射芬太尼 0.25～0.5 μg/kg，用于患者麻醉恢复后立即镇痛。芬太尼达峰时间（5 min）允许其每 5 min 重复注射 1 次，这样有助于达到充分镇痛的血药浓度。

旁注 15-1　静脉内阿片类药物
中、重度疼痛时，吗啡依然是静脉阿片类药物镇痛金标准；等效镇痛剂量的氢吗啡酮为良好的替代药物
短效阿片类药物可能有利于门诊手术患者，因为其能有效缓解疼痛，且恶心与呕吐发生率较低
曲马多可有效地缓解术后轻、中度疼痛，严重不良反应发生率低，因此受到临床医师青睐
哌替啶并不优于吗啡和其他阿片类药物，且存在诸多缺点

芬太尼能用于 PCA 装置或持续滴注，提供术后镇痛作用[15]。

曲马多

曲马多是一种作用于中枢神经系统的不典型阿片类药物，为人工合成的可待因 4-苯基-乙哌双酮的类似物。曲马多对 μ、κ 及 δ 阿片受体的亲和力较弱[16]，体重 70 kg 患者静注 50～150 mg 曲马多的镇痛效能相当于静注吗啡 5～15 mg[17]。曲马多对轻中度疼痛具有镇痛作用。

短期使用曲马多耐受性良好，主要不良反应有头晕、恶心、镇静、口干以及出汗，呼吸抑制不常见[16]。曲马多可能引起癫痫发作，尤其用于癫痫患者以及合用促惊厥药物时（如单胺氧化酶抑制剂、三环类抗抑郁药和选择性 5-羟色胺摄取抑制剂），应慎用于头部损伤的患者[17]。

门诊手术中胃肠外阿片类药物的应用

门诊手术后患者不能达到出院标准的主要原因是存在疼痛和恶心[18]。Claxton 等[19]观察了 58 例门诊手术后静脉使用吗啡或芬太尼控制疼痛的患者，结果吗啡组疼痛缓解的质量与时间更佳，但是该组患者回家后恶心和呕吐发生率较高（59% vs 24%，$P = 0.01$）。另一项多中心大样本研究包括 2438 例 18 岁或 18 岁以上的患者（1496 例门诊患者，942 例住院患者），比较了静脉瑞芬太尼与芬太尼，并探讨了手术对血流动力学的影响以及术后恢复情况。结果显示瑞芬太尼组患者血流动力学变化较小，出院较早[20]。

有研究对其他短效阿片类药物（如阿芬太尼和舒芬太尼）与芬太尼进行了比较，以确定经历麻醉的门诊患者术后恶心与呕吐的发生率。在 274 例患者中对等效剂量芬太尼、阿芬太尼与舒芬太尼进行的研究显示，阿芬太尼麻醉手术后恶心与呕吐的发生率最低[21]。因此，较短效阿片类镇痛药因不良反应较少，尤其用于多模式镇痛时，可能更适用于门诊手术患者。

口服阿片类药物疗法

旁注 15-2 总结了以下内容。

> **旁注 15-2　口服阿片类药物**
>
> 所有口服阿片类药物应该尽可能采用多模式镇痛疗法，包括对乙酰氨基酚、NSAID，必要时采用其他辅助药
>
> 阿片类药物治疗从静脉向口服用药过渡时，可应用 CR 制剂，必要时每 2h 间断应用按需剂量的 IR 制剂
>
> 变换给药途径时应加强注意，以防止用量过大或用量不足
>
> 复合镇痛药，如对乙酰氨基酚复合羟考酮或可待因，可用于轻至中度疼痛

即释剂

阿片类镇痛药吗啡、氢吗啡酮、羟考酮、右丙氧芬、二氢可待因、可待因以及曲马多都常口服给药，并有即释（immediate-release，IR）制剂（表 15-1）。

可待因与右丙氧芬（60～65 mg）的镇痛作用均较弱，NNT 分别是 16.7 和 7.7[22,23]。二氢可待因单独使用时镇痛作用也较弱，其镇痛效果弱于布洛芬，后者 NNT 为 2.4[24]。然而，曲马多是一种有效镇痛剂，100 mg 剂量时 NNT 为 4.6，出现眩晕的 NNH 为 11，出现恶心的 NNH 是 7～8[22]。羟考酮 5mg 与安慰剂无差异，15mg 可为腹部和妇科手术提供有效的术后镇痛作用（NNT 2.4）[25]，但是嗜睡显著（NNH 3.3）。口服阿片药的 NNT 比较见于表 15-2。

可待因是一种药物前体，其必须通过肝细胞色素 P450 2D6（CYP 2D6）代谢为吗啡，才具有镇痛作用[26]。人群中 7%～10% 的个体不表达功能性 CYP 2D6，故这些患者应用可待因不能发挥镇痛作用。可待因的大多数不良反应（镇静、头晕、烦躁不安、恶心、瘙痒）是由该药物前体（可待因）及其活性代谢产物（吗啡）所介导的，因此，这些患者应用可待因后无镇痛作用，但是可出现不良反应[26]。

以体重 70 kg 患者为例，即释剂常用剂量为：吗啡 5～10 mg，羟考酮 5～10 mg，氢吗啡酮 1～2 mg。

控释剂

数种阿片类药物（吗啡、氢吗啡酮、羟考酮、可待因、曲马多）有口服控释（controlled-release，CR）制剂，该制剂能明显延长药物血浆半衰期，维持更长的无痛时间[25,27]。这些药常常每 8～12 h 给予一次固定剂量。芬太尼也有皮肤贴，需要每 72 h 更换 1 次。对

表 15-1 围手术期常用阿片药物的等效镇痛剂量（体重 70 kg 的个体）

药物	口服	静脉内/肌内	患者自控镇痛（单次注射）	硬膜外（单次注射）	鞘内	备注
吗啡	10~30mg/2~3h	10~15mg/3~4h	1~2mg	1~4 mg	100~300μg	中重度疼痛的金标准；肾功能损害者活性代谢产物蓄积
可待因	30~60mg/4h	15~60mg/4h	只用于肌内注射，不用于PCA	不使用	不使用	用于轻、中度疼痛；常用固定剂量的口服制剂；人群中10%个体不能将其转变为吗啡
氢吗啡酮	2~3mg	2~3mg/4h	0.2~0.4mg	0.5~1mg	100~200μg	口服生物利用度较高；硬膜外或鞘内给药的不良反应少于其他阿片类药物
二醋吗啡	N/A	5~10mg	0.5~1mg	2~3mg[98]	200~300μg[99]	
芬太尼	N/A	20~50μg单次注射，麻醉后恢复室术后疼痛时可每5min一次，总量可达150μg	20~50μg	50~100μg 单次注射	12.5~25μg 单次注射	不推荐经皮给药；硬膜外或鞘内给药时存在早期呼吸抑制的风险
羟考酮	10~20mg	—	—	不使用	不使用	可使用控释剂
曲马多	50~150mg/4~6h	50~100mg/4~6h	20mg	不推荐	不推荐	可使用缓释剂
哌替啶	100~300mg/3h	100mg*	10mg	不推荐	不推荐	口服生物利用度低；毒性代谢产物：去甲哌替啶

* 首个 24h 总剂量不超过 1000mg，之后每天 600mg。老年人和肾功能损害患者应减量。

需要或可能需要多次应用阿片类药物 IR 制剂（每日超过 4 次）的患者可应用 CR 制剂。

对于耐受口服用药的患者，CR 制剂能够与静脉内或口服 IR 阿片类药物联合使用。这些患者 CR 阿片类药物的初始剂量应根据其静脉内或 IR 制剂的最近 24 h 使用量进行计算。静脉内阿片药物用量需要先换算成口服等效剂量（吗啡、羟考酮或氢吗啡酮）。阿片类药物每日需要总量的 50%～75% 以 CR 制剂，分 2~3 次给予患者[28]，再调整静脉内或口服 IR 阿片类药物用量，以达到良好的疼痛控制。如果患者正在口服阿片类药物 IR 制剂，则同样计算出每日阿片类药物剂量，将其每日总量的 50%～75% 分 2~3 次以 CR 制剂给予，再按需给予 IR 制剂，以取得良好效果。应用 CR 制剂后，根据镇痛效果、阿片类药物相关不良反应以及 IR 制剂进一步需求量来增加或减少 CR 制剂剂量。

许多研究证实，常规疼痛处理方案中加用 CR 制剂具有显著的优势，包括镇痛效果改善、阿片类药物总需求量（CR+IR）减少以及阿片类药物相关不良反应较少[25,29-33]。然而，对于首次使用阿片类药物的患者，必须注意不加限制 CR 制剂用量的情况，因为有报道患者使用透皮芬太尼贴剂后出现严重呼吸系统的不良反应[34,35]。本章不讨论阿片类药物耐受患者围手术期镇痛问题。

联合使用阿片类镇痛药

只要患者能进饮液体，曲马多、可待因以及羟考酮都可与对乙酰氨基酚和（或）阿司匹林联合用于住院和门诊手术患者。

联合应用镇痛药对于轻中度疼痛有效，其对应 NNT 分别为：阿司匹林 650 mg + 可待因 60 mg 的 NNT 是 5.3[22]，对乙酰氨基酚 + 可待因 60 mg NNT 是 2.2[36]，对乙酰氨基酚 + 右丙氧芬 NNT 是 4.4[37]，对乙酰氨基酚 + 曲马多 NNT 是 2.7[38]。羟考酮 5 mg 与对乙酰氨基酚 325 mg 联合应用（NNT 2.5）的效果等同于

表 15-2 常用口服阿片类药物和复合镇痛药缓解至少 50% 疼痛所需治疗人数（NNT）

药物和用量	NNT（50%缓解疼痛）
可待因 60 mg	16.7
右丙氧芬 65 mg	7.7
曲马多 100 mg	4.6
对乙酰氨基酚 1000 mg/650mg + 可待因 60 mg	2.2/4.2
羟考酮 5 mg + 对乙酰氨基酚 325 mg	2.5
对乙酰氨基酚 1000 mg + 右丙氧芬 65 mg	4.4
阿司匹林 650 mg + 可待因 60 mg	5.3
对乙酰氨基酚 1000 mg/650 mg	3.8/4.6

15 mg 羟考酮，而不良反应并不多于对照组。增加羟考酮（10 mg）或对乙酰氨基酚剂量（500 mg 或 1000 mg）并不增强镇痛效果，反而增加不良反应的发生率，如嗜睡（NNH 2.1）、眩晕、恶心和呕吐（NNH 8.4）（表 15-2）[39]。

阿司匹林或对乙酰氨基酚每日最大剂量可能限制其联合镇痛药的使用。因此，在治疗急性轻至中度疼痛时，宜根据个体需要给予对乙酰氨基酚固定剂量（每 6 小时 650～1000 mg），在此基础上，联合口服阿片类药物来控制疼痛。

椎管内阿片类药物的治疗

1979 年，报道了首例鞘内和硬膜外使用阿片类药物[40,41]。此后，人们通过椎管内途径几乎应用了所有阿片类药物。总的来说，与静脉给药相比，椎管内给予较少量阿片类药物即可获得有效的镇痛作用，这是因为注射部位靠近作用位点（脊髓）。与常规给药途径相比，椎管内应用阿片类药物有可能引起更高的不良反应发病率[42]。尽管如此，椎管内给予阿片类药物还是具有明显优势，支持围手术期椎管内应用阿片类药物。

硬膜外给予阿片类药物

旁注 15.3 总结了以下部分。

旁注 15-3 硬膜外阿片类药物

- 硬膜外给予亲脂性阿片类药物（芬太尼、舒芬太尼）主要通过全身再分布起作用
- 硬膜外给予亲水性阿片类药物（吗啡、二醋吗啡、氢吗啡酮）在脊髓作用位点产生镇痛作用
- 手术部位以下水平通过硬膜外给予吗啡可提供有效持久的镇痛作用

硬膜外使用阿片药物优点

硬膜外使用阿片类药物的优点在于产生镇痛作用的同时，无运动或交感阻滞作用[43]。与常规肌内注射相比，硬膜外应用阿片类药物可使胸部和上腹部手术患者呼吸峰流速恢复时间明显缩短，肺部并发症（肺不张及肺实质浸润）减少以及住院时间缩短[44]。与全身麻醉及术后胃肠外应用阿片类药物相比，腹部、胸部或血管大手术的高危患者接受硬膜外麻醉及术后硬膜外应用局麻药和（或）阿片类药物，术后并发症发生率和死亡率降低，结果改善（住院时间较短，费用较低）[44]。外周血管疾病患者接受主动脉旁路手术后，应用患者自控硬膜外镇痛（patient-controlled epidural analgesia，PCEA）可显著减少术后血栓形成、感染及心血管并发症[44]。对于接受大手术的高危患者，应用局麻药和（或）阿片类药物的硬膜外镇痛是首选方法，其效价比也理想[44]。

哪种阿片类药物产生的椎管内镇痛效果最好？

当经硬膜外途径单给予一种镇痛药时，亲脂性阿片类药物如芬太尼、舒芬太尼和阿芬太尼会重新分布到血液和硬膜外脂肪组织[44,45]，主要产生全身性镇痛作用。硬膜外单次注射芬太尼似乎具有（有限的）脊髓作用，因此与静脉内给予同等剂量药物相比，其缓解短期疼痛（小于 1 h）可能更有效[46]。亲水性药物与硬膜外脂肪结合较少，较少吸收入血；阿片类药物，如吗啡[47]和氢吗啡酮[48]，经硬膜外腔给予较小剂量所产生的镇痛效果优于或等同于静脉给予同等剂量。表 15-3 列出具体阿片类药物产生椎管内脊髓介导镇痛作用的可能。

文献资料显示，最适用于硬膜外持续滴注的阿片类药物是氢吗啡酮，与吗啡相比，该药可取得良好镇痛效果，且不良反应较少[49-51]。但是，硬膜外吗啡具有作用时间长的优点[52]，单次剂量 2～4 mg 产生镇痛效

表 15-3 术后疼痛处理中各种阿片类药物产生椎管介导镇痛作用的可能性

阿片类药物	给药途径	
	硬膜外给药	鞘内给药
吗啡	高	高
氢吗啡酮	高	高
二醋吗啡	高	高
阿芬他尼	可忽略	未知
芬太尼	低	中等
舒芬太尼	可忽略	中等
哌替啶*	未知	未知

*因为局部麻醉药的作用,很难确定该药椎管内选择性。

Modified from Bernards CM: Understanding the physiology and pharmacology of epidural and intrathecal opioids. Best Pract Res Clin Anaesthesiol 2002;16:489-505.

果能达到至少 12 h。吗啡与氢吗啡酮的镇痛效果相近,但是氢吗啡酮似乎起效较快,持续时间更短[53]。一项关于硬膜外持续应用吗啡和氢吗啡酮的比较性研究显示,吗啡引起的瘙痒发生率是氢吗啡酮的 4 倍[49]。吗啡引起的恶心和呕吐发生率为 17%～34%[54],通常发生在用药 4～6 h 后吗啡向头侧扩散时[55]。

给药平面是否有意义?

许多研究者对给药平面(如腰段或胸段)是否会影响阿片类药物向头侧扩散以及药物镇痛效能与毒性提出疑问。数项研究证实,亲脂性阿片类药物(芬太尼和丁丙诺啡)经两种平面持续给药所产生的镇痛效果无差异,提示可能与这些药物吸收入血以及发挥脊髓以上镇痛作用有关。然而,Grant 等[56]将 20 例开胸手术患者随机分为腰段或胸段硬膜外给予吗啡,结果证实两组疼痛评分或不良作用无差异,但是腰段组吗啡需要量较大。该研究提供的有限证据表明,远离手术切口平面经硬膜外给予亲水性阿片类药物(如吗啡)具有镇痛作用。

硬膜外阿片类药物和局麻药

评价术后疼痛的研究表明,椎管内联合使用局麻药与亲水性阿片类药物可显著改善术后镇痛效果[57,58]。这种方法可提供有效的镇痛作用,同时减少每种药物所需用量,减少不良反应。但是,术后疼痛时硬膜外局麻药滴注时,加用亲脂性阿片类药物如芬太尼或舒芬太尼的镇痛效果并不优于单纯使用局麻药,而阿片类药物相关不良反应的风险增加[59-61]。表 15-4 为推荐的阿片类药物单次注射和持续输注方案。

鞘内给予阿片类药物

尽管鞘内应用阿片类药物由于全身吸收而需要较大剂量亲脂性阿片类药物才能产生有效的镇痛作用,但所有鞘内给予的阿片类药物都存在脊髓介导的机制(旁注 15-4)。静脉内或鞘内途径给予等效价吗啡与芬太尼可证实这种特性。尽管静脉内芬太尼与吗啡的效价比是 100:1,但是鞘内应用的效价比约为 8:1(即需要 25 μg 芬太尼才能产生与 200 μg 吗啡相同的镇痛效果)。作用持续时间也相差甚大,吗啡作用持续时间长达 24 h,而芬太尼只有 2～3 h。亲水阿片类药物在脑脊液(CSF)中向头侧扩散,与脊髓以上受体结合而产生镇痛作用,此时脊髓介导的镇痛作用正在下降[45]。鞘内给予阿片类药物可减少局麻药用量,从而减弱运动

表 15-4 70kg 患者硬膜外阿片类药物的建议用药方案*

药物	溶液	单次注射	基础输注	PCEA 单次注射量
氢吗啡酮	0.015～0.03mg/ml	0.2～1mg	0.15～0.3mg/h	0.15～0.3mg/10～20min
氢吗啡酮 0.015～0.03 mg/ml + 布比卡因 0.0625%～0.125%	—	—	5～10ml/h	2～4ml/15～20min
芬太尼	5～10μg/ml	25～50μg	50～100μg/ml	10～15μg/10～15 min
芬太尼 2～4μg/ml + 布比卡因 0.0625%～0.125%	—	—	5～10ml/h	2～4ml/15～20min
吗啡	0.1mg/ml	2～4mg	0.5～0.8mg/h	0.2～0.3mg/10～15min
舒芬太尼	1μg/ml	2.5～5μg	5～10μg/h	2～4μg/5～10min

*通过胸段或腰段硬膜外导管给药剂量。

Modified from de Leon-Casasola OA, Lema MJ: Potoperative epidural opioid analgesia: What are the choices? Anesth Analg 1996;83:867-875.

> **旁注 15-4　鞘内阿片类药物**
>
> 鞘内应用亲脂性阿片类药物（芬太尼，舒芬太尼）可通过脊髓与全身机制产生镇痛作用。鞘内应用小剂量阿片类药物可减少局麻药剂量，从而减轻运动神经的阻滞
>
> 鞘内应用亲水性阿片类药物（吗啡，二醋吗啡，氢吗啡酮）主要作用于脊髓位点，镇痛作用与不良作用起效缓慢
>
> 骨盆及下肢手术后鞘内注射吗啡（100～200 μg）可提供有效的镇痛作用，但是其不良反应多于二醋吗啡（200 μg）

神经的阻滞，这对门诊手术患者尤为重要[62]。

鞘内使用亲水性阿片类药物如吗啡（0.1～0.4 mg）可提供有效而持久的镇痛作用。Rathmell 等[63]比较了 120 例全髋和全膝关节成形术后患者鞘内分别给予 0.1mg、0.2mg、0.3 mg 的吗啡或安慰剂的效果。结果显示，鞘内吗啡的镇痛作用长达 24 h，且 0.2 mg 和 0.3 mg 的剂量最有效。0.3 mg 组恶心发生率显著增高，所有使用吗啡的患者都出现了明显的瘙痒，并需要治疗。由于全髋关节成形术比全膝置换术术后疼痛持续时间短，且强度较弱，因此鞘内注射较小剂量阿片类药物即可充分镇痛，尤其是老年患者[64]。

鞘内注射二醋吗啡（0.2 mg）也可产生持久镇痛作用，而瘙痒和嗜睡少于吗啡[65]。氢吗啡酮的特性与二醋吗啡相似。Drakeford 等[66]比较了鞘内丁卡因复合 0.14 mg 氢吗啡酮、0.5 mg 吗啡或安慰剂在全髋和全膝关节成形术中的作用，结果显示加入两种阿片类药物可明显改善镇痛时间与镇痛质量，但两种阿片类药物的镇痛效果或不良事件无差异。

椎管内阿片类药物与呼吸抑制

椎管内（硬膜外或鞘内）应用阿片类药物可产生一些不良反应（表 15-5），其中最具临床意义的是呼吸抑制[67]。椎管内阿片类药物引起的呼吸抑制程度呈剂量依赖性；但其他危险因素是联合胃肠外应用阿片类药物或镇静剂；老年患者似乎特别易于发生（旁注 15-5）。鞘内或硬膜外给予常规剂量阿片类药物后引起需要治疗的呼吸抑制发生率与肌内或静脉内应用阿片类药物治疗相近（0.1%～1%）[68,69]。

呼吸抑制可分为早期呼吸抑制和迟发型呼吸抑制两种类型。早期呼吸抑制通常发生在椎管内应用阿片类药物 2 h 以内，因此其诊断和治疗通常都是在手术室或恢复室内进行。这种呼吸抑制通常与使用亲脂性阿片类药物有关，主要是由于药物全身吸收所致，因为血药浓度与呼吸抑制程度呈正比[70,71]。许多呼吸抑制的报道都与硬膜外大剂量应用芬太尼和舒芬太尼有关；鞘内给药，特别是应用较小剂量阿片类药物，该并发症并不常见[69]。

迟发型呼吸抑制的特征是给予亲水性阿片类药物后 6～12 h 发生，发生缓慢但进行性加重（而不是突然迅速发生）[72]。呼吸抑制的发生时间大约与 CSF 从胸腰段脊髓水平流到脑干的时间相一致[45]。大多数报道与硬膜外或鞘内使用吗啡有关[73-76]，但给予大剂量亲脂性阿片类药物也可诱发迟发性呼吸抑制。尚未见有硬膜外或鞘内最后一次使用吗啡超过 24 h 后发生呼吸抑制的报道，大量研究提示，硬膜外或鞘内最后一次使用吗啡超过 12 h 后发生呼吸抑制极为罕见[74]。

硬膜外或鞘内注射阿片类药物后呼吸抑制的监测与诊断需要护理人员具备适当的监护水平并具有一定的风险意识。需监测的项目及监测时间还存在争议。有关监测恰当类型和持续时间尚有争议。人们已试用呼吸监测方法如脉搏氧饱和度和二氧化碳波形，但是因假报警过于频繁而并不可靠[77]。大量经验提示，第一个 24 h 内每小时监测一次呼吸频率和镇静水平就足以检测出呼吸抑制的发生[77]。持续给予阿片类药物的患者应每 4 h 监测 1 次，直至治疗结束；第一个 24 h 辅助给氧并密切观察可能对高风险患者有利。过度镇静状态可能是提示呼吸抑制的一项良好临床指征，特别是呼吸频率减少至 10 次/分钟以下时[77-79]。

静脉纳洛酮可迅速逆转阿片类药物引起的呼吸抑制。但是必须小心避免完全拮抗其镇痛作用，纳洛酮剂量应以 0.1 mg 递增。通常需反复注射或滴注，因为纳洛酮作用时间为 35～45 min[80]，显著短于大多数椎管内阿片类药物的作用时间。研究表明，纳洛酮输注速率在 2～5 μg/（kg·h）时可逆转呼吸抑制，而并不拮抗镇痛作用[81]。当发生呼吸抑制时，麻醉医师在现场至关重要。

阿片类药物介导外周镇痛作用

炎症期间，外周感觉纤维和免疫细胞表达阿片样受体和内源性阿片类物质[82,83]。许多研究评估了阿片类药物用于外周神经和关节腔的镇痛作用。尽管许多研究认为外周应用阿片类药物具有镇痛优势，但是与全

表 15–5	鞘内与硬膜外应用阿片类药物的常见不良反应
不良反应	发生率（%）
瘙痒	11～44[48]
恶心和呕吐	17～34[53]
尿潴留	33～50[105]
呼吸抑制	0.1～1*
精神状态改变：镇静、嗜睡	—

* 等同于静脉或肌内注射阿片类药物后的呼吸抑制风险。

旁注 15–5　椎管内应用阿片类药物后呼吸抑制风险增加的因素

- 年龄大
- 同时胃肠外使用阿片类药物或镇静药
- 大剂量阿片类药物
- 重复单次注射
- 合并呼吸疾病或 ASA 大于 3 级
- 胸部手术或长时间手术

旁注 15–6　椎管内阿片类药物与呼吸抑制

椎管内应用阿片类药物的呼吸抑制发生率在 0.1%～1%，其与其他胃肠外给药相似

亲脂性阿片类药物主要通过全身吸收，因此呼吸抑制可能出现早且快（<2 h），通常与硬膜外应用大剂量亲脂性阿片类药物有关

亲水性阿片类药物由于其在 CSF 中向头侧扩散，因此可能产生延迟性或缓慢发生的呼吸抑制（>2 h），且通常发生在 6~12 h 之间，但是给药后长达 24 h 也能发生

围手术期椎管内应用阿片类药物的所有患者都应在适当环境给予适当监测，且麻醉医师能随时赶到

身应用阿片类药物进行对照的研究很少。没有这种对照，就不可能推断外周阿片类药物是否具有真正的外周作用，或实际上是药物吸收入血进入 CNS 所产生的镇痛作用。如果不良反应较少，真正外周介导的阿片类药物镇痛作用可能具有优势；如果这种镇痛作用由中枢所介导，则无任何明显优势。

外周神经部位阿片类药物的作用

初级传入纤维上的阿片样受体是由脊髓背根神经节转运到炎症部位神经纤维末梢上的；然而，尽管沿

表 15–6	15 项外周神经应用阿片类药物的研究结果（不包括曲马多和丁丙诺啡）
总结果	8 项肯定
	7 项否定
全身对照研究结果*	6 项全身对照研究：
	4 项肯定
	2 项否定
	9 项无全身对照的研究：
	4 项肯定
	5 项否定

轴突转运，这些受体仍然不易与激动剂相互作用。1997 年和 2000 年两项系统性回顾可能解释其中原因，结果显示局麻药中加入阿片类药物用于外周神经阻滞并无任何改善镇痛的效果[84,85]。最近总结有关外周神经应用阿片类药物（不包括丁丙诺啡和曲马多）的研究显示其镇痛作用仍有争议（表 15–6）[86-90]。另外，Choyce 和 Peng 等[91]综述了阿片类药物在静脉区域麻醉中的应用，结果同样令人失望。外周神经给药具有镇痛作用的两种阿片类药物是丁丙诺啡和曲马多。Candido 等[92]在腋路阻滞时将 0.3mg 丁丙诺啡加入甲哌卡因与丁卡因混合液中，结果表明其镇痛持续时间较腋路阻滞加肌注同样剂量丁丙诺啡几乎延长 100%。该研究支持较早两项无全身对照的有关丁丙诺啡研究结果[93,94]。

Kapral 等[95]将 100 mg 曲马多作为辅助用药加入甲哌卡因用于腋路阻滞。将 60 例患者随机分为 3 组：第一组应用 1%甲哌卡因＋2 ml 生理盐水；第二组应用 1%甲哌卡因＋100 mg 曲马多；第三组应用 1%甲哌卡因＋2 ml 生理盐水＋静脉 100mg 曲马多。该研究结果显示腋路曲马多组的运动与感觉阻滞持续时间均显著长于静脉内曲马多组和对照组（$P<0.01$）。随后，Robaux 等[96]应用安慰剂以及 40mg、100mg 和 200mg 曲马多加入固定剂量的 1.5%甲哌卡因中进行了腋路阻滞时曲马多的剂量–反应研究；结果发现 200 mg 曲马多的镇痛效果最好，而不良作用不增加。然而，该研究并没有比较静脉内使用曲马多的作用。

阿片类药物关节腔内注射及其他外周给药途径

阿片类激动剂到达炎症组织内，与感觉末梢上的阿片样受体结合，产生镇痛作用[97]。在人体，阿片类

药物注入已有炎症的关节腔内（intra-articular，IA）可产生镇痛作用。1997年，Kalso等[98]系统检验了IA阿片类药物的作用，结果显示IA注射1~5 mg吗啡可产生长时间镇痛，且无明显不良作用。然而，该研究没有确定剂量-反应关系。随后的研究支持上述结果，表明IA注射吗啡[99,100]、曲马多[101]、丁丙诺啡[102]和舒芬太尼[103]均具有镇痛作用。

Reuben等[104]的一项研究显示颈椎融合手术时，在取髂骨部位骨内注射吗啡（5mg）者急性疼痛发生率和慢性疼痛发生率（术后1年时进行评价）均显著低于肌注吗啡和安慰剂（5%分别比37%、33%）。

旁注15.7总结了以上讨论。

小结

除微创手术外，阿片类镇痛药仍然是术后疼痛治疗方案中不可或缺的一部分。

吗啡仍然是最好的静脉阿片类药物，然而羟考酮等药物在口服给药时具有药代动力学优势。

权衡利弊，椎管内给予阿片类药物可产生显著的镇痛作用。椎管内给予二醋吗啡和氢吗啡酮似可取得最佳镇痛效果，且不良作用最少。

总的来讲，尚未观察到外周神经应用阿片类药物的优势，但是曲马多和丁丙诺啡复合局部麻醉药用于外周神经阻滞时可产生外周介导的镇痛作用。已证实关节腔内注射吗啡可产生镇痛作用。

采用多模式镇痛方法包括应用对乙酰氨基酚、NSAID，必要时给予其他辅助药物如NMDA受体拮抗剂、$α_2$激动剂和抗惊厥药物，都能进一步加强阿片类药物的镇痛优势，并显著减少其不良反应。

旁注 15-7　外周给予阿片类药物

外周已有炎症时，关节腔内注射吗啡剂量高达5 mg可产生明显镇痛作用

骨移植供体取骨部位骨内注射吗啡5 mg可能减轻急性与慢性骨移植性疼痛

外周神经阻滞时，局麻药中加入曲马多200 mg或丁丙诺啡0.3 mg可加强局麻药的作用

（圣　奎译　刘　毅　邓小明校）

参考文献

1. Kehlet H, Dahl JB: The value of "multimodal" or "balanced analgesia" in postoperative pain treatment. Anesth Analg 1993;77:1048–1056.
2. Pain terms: A list with definitions and notes on usage. Recommended by the IASP Subcommmittee on Taxonomy. Pain 1979;6:249–252.
3. Kalso E, Edwards JE, Moore RA, et al: Opioids in chronic non-cancer pain: Systematic review of efficacy and safety. Pain 2004;112:372–380.
4. Watson CP, Watt-Watson JH, Chipman ML: Chronic noncancer pain and the long term utility of opioids. Pain Res Manag 2004;9:19–24.
5. Cook RJ, Sackett DL: The number needed to treat: A clinically useful measure of treatment effect. BMJ 1995;310:452–454.
6. McQuay HJ, Carroll D, Moore RA: Injected morphine in postoperative pain: A quantitative systematic review. J Pain Symptom Manage 1999;17:164–174.
7. Bollish SJ, Collins CL, Kirking DM, et al: Efficacy of patient-controlled versus conventional analgesia for postoperative pain. Clin Pharm 1985;4:48–52.
8. Latta KS, Ginsberg B, Barkin RL: Meperidine: A critical review. Am J Ther 2002;9:53–68.
9. Smith LA, Carroll D, Edwards JE, et al: Single-dose ketorolac and pethidine in acute postoperative pain: Systematic review with meta-analysis. Br J Anaesth 2000;84:48–58.
10. Lawlor P, Turner K, Hanson J, et al: Dose ratio between morphine and hydromorphone in patients with cancer pain: A retrospective study. Pain 1997;72:79–85.
11. Coda BA, O'Sullivan B, Donaldson G, et al: Comparative efficacy of patient-controlled administration of morphine, hydromorphone, or sufentanil for the treatment of oral mucositis pain following bone marrow transplantation. Pain 1997;72:333–346.
12. Wright AW, Mather LE, Smith MT: Hydromorphone-3-glucuronide: A more potent neuro-excitant than its structural analogue, morphine-3-glucuronide. Life Sci 2001;69:409–420.
13. Dean M: Opioids in renal failure and dialysis patients. J Pain Symptom Manage 2004;28:497–504.
14. Rapp SE, Egan KJ, Ross BK, et al: A multidimensional comparison of morphine and hydromorphone patient-controlled analgesia. Anesth Analg 1996;82:1043–1048.
15. Peng, PW, Sandler H, Alan NA: Review of the use of fentanyl analgesia in the management of acute pain in adults. Anesthesiology 1999;90:576–599.
16. Shipton EA: Tramadol—present and future. Anaesth Intensive Care 2000;28:363–374.
17. Lee CR, McTavish D, Sorkin EM: Tramadol: A preliminary review of its pharmacodynamic and pharmacokinetic properties, and therapeutical potential in acute and chronic pain states. Drugs 1993;46:313–340.
18. Chung F, Mezei G: Factors contributing to a prolonged stay after ambulatory surgery. Anesth Analg 1999;89:1352–1359.
19. Claxton AR, McGuire G, Chung F, et al: Evaluation of morphine versus fentanyl for postoperative analgesia after ambulatory surgical procedures. Anesth Analg 1997;84:509–514.
20. Twersky RS, Jamerson B, Warner DS, et al: Hemodynamics and emergence profile of remifentanil versus fentanyl prospectively compared in a large population of surgical patients J Clin Anesth 2001;13:407–416.
21. Langevin S, Lessard MR, Trepanier CA, et al: Alfentanil causes less postoperative nausea and vomiting than equipotent doses of fentanyl or sufentanil in outpatients. Anesthesiology 1999;6:1666–1673.
22. Moore RA, McQuay HJ: Single-patient data meta-analysis of 3453 postoperative patients: Oral tramadol versus placebo, codeine and combination analgesics. Pain 1997;69:287–294.
23. Collins SL, Edwards JE, Moore RA, et al: Single-dose dextropropoxyphene in post-operative pain: A quantitative systematic review. Eur J Clin Pharmacol 1998;54:107–111.
24. Collins SL, Moore RA, McQuay HJ, et al: Oral ibuprofen and diclofenac in post-operative pain: A quantitative systematic review. Eur J Pain 1998;2:285–291.
25. Sunshine A, Olson NZ, Colon A, et al: Analgesic efficacy of controlled-release oxycodone in postoperative pain. J Clin Pharmacol 1996;36:595–603.

26. Cleary J, Mikus G, Somogyi A, et al: The influence of pharmacogenetics on opioid analgesia: Studies with codeine and oxycodone in the Sprague-Dawley/Dark Agouti rat model. J Pharmacol Exp Ther 1994;271:1528–1534.
27. Hale ME, Fleischmann R, Salzman R, et al: Efficacy and safety of controlled-release versus immediate-release oxycodone: Randomized, double-blind evaluation in patients with chronic back pain. Clin J Pain 1999;15:179–183.
28. Ginsberg B, Sinatra RS, Adler LJ, et al: Conversion to oral controlled-release oxycodone from intravenous opioid analgesic in the postoperative setting. Pain Med 2003;4:31–38.
29. Bourke M, Hayes A, Doyle M, et al: A comparison of regularly administered sustained release oral morphine with intramuscular morphine for control of postoperative pain. Anesth Analg 2000;90:427–430.
30. Cheville A, Chen A, Oster G, et al: A randomized trial of controlled-release oxycodone during inpatient rehabilitation following unilateral total knee arthroplasty. J Bone Joint Surg Am 2001;83A:572–576.
31. Kampe S, Warm M, Kaufmann J, et al: Clinical efficacy of controlled-release oxycodone 20 mg administered on a 12-h dosing schedule on the management of postoperative pain after breast surgery for cancer. Curr Med Res Opin 2004;20:199–202.
32. Kaufmann J, Yesiloglu S, Patermann B, et al: Controlled-release oxycodone is better tolerated than intravenous tramadol/metamizol for postoperative analgesia after retinal surgery. Curr Eye Res 2004;28:271–275.
33. Reuben SS, Connelly NR, Maciolek H: Postoperative analgesia with controlled-release oxycodone for outpatient anterior cruciate ligament surgery. Anesth Analg 1999;88:1286–1291.
34. Sandler A: Transdermal fentanyl: Acute analgesic clinical studies. J Pain Symptom Manage 1992;7:S27–S35.
35. Sandler AN, Baxter AD, Katz J, et al: A double-blind, placebo-controlled trial of transdermal fentanyl after abdominal hysterectomy: Analgesic, respiratory, and pharmacokinetic effects. Anesthesiology 1994;81:1169–1180.
36. Smith LA, Moore RA, McQuay HJ, et al: Using evidence from different sources: An example using paracetamol 1000 mg plus codeine 60 mg. BMC Med Res Methodol 2001;1:1.
37. Collins SL, Edwards JE, Moore RA, et al: Single-dose dextropropoxyphene in post-operative pain: A quantitative systematic review. Eur J Clin Pharmacol 1998;54:107–112.
38. Edwards JE, McQuay HJ, Moore RA: Combination analgesic efficacy: Individual patient data meta-analysis of single-dose oral tramadol plus acetaminophen in acute postoperative pain. J Pain Symptom Manage 2002;23:121–130.
39. Edwards JE, Moore RA, McQuay HJ: Single dose oxycodone and oxycodone plus paracetamol (acetaminophen) for acute postoperative pain. Cochrane Database Syst Rev 2000;4:CD002763.
40. Behar M, Magora F, Olshwang D, et al: Epidural morphine in treatment of pain. Lancet 1979;1(8115):527–529.
41. Wang JK, Nauss LA, Thomas JE: Pain relief by intrathecally applied morphine in man. Anesthesiology 1979;50:149–151.
42. Morgan M: The rational use of intrathecal and extradural opioids. Br J Anaesth 1989;63:165–188.
43. de Leon-Casasola OA, Lema MJ: Postoperative epidural opioid analgesia: What are the choices? Anesth Analg 1996;83:867–875.
44. Rawal N: Opioids and non opioids' efficacy, safety and cost benefit. Pain Reviews 1996;3:31–62.
45. Bernards CM: Understanding the physiology and pharmacology of epidural and intrathecal opioids. Best Pract Res Clin Anaesthesiol 2002;16:489–505.
46. Ginosar Y, Riley ET, Angst MS: The site of action of epidural fentanyl in humans: The difference between infusion and bolus administration. Anesth Analg 2003;97:1428–1438.
47. Kilbride MJ, Senagore AJ, Mazier WP, et al: Epidural analgesia. Surg Gynecol Obstet 1992;174:137–140.
48. Liu S, Carpenter RL, Mulroy MF, et al: Intravenous versus epidural administration of hydromorphone: Effects on analgesia and recovery after radical retropubic prostatectomy. Anesthesiology 1995;82:682–688.
49. Chaplan SR, Duncan SR, Brodsky JB, et al: Morphine and hydromorphone epidural analgesia: A prospective, randomized comparison. Anesthesiology 1992;77:1090–1094.
50. Goodarzi M: Comparison of epidural morphine, hydromorphone and fentanyl for postoperative pain control in children undergoing orthopaedic surgery. Paediatr Anaesth 1999;9:419–422.
51. Halpern SH, Arellano R, Preston R, et al: Epidural morphine vs hydromorphone in post-caesarean section patients. Can J Anaesth 1996;43:595–598.
52. Celleno D, Capogna G, Sebastiani M, et al: Epidural analgesia during and after cesarean delivery: Comparison of five opioids. Reg Anesth 1991;16:79–83.
53. Brose WG, Tanelian DL, Brodsky JB, et al: CSF and blood pharmacokinetics of hydromorphone and morphine following lumbar epidural administration. Pain 1991;45:11–15.
54. Rauck RL: Epidural and spinal narcotics. American Society of Anesthesiologists' Annual Refresher Course Lectures 1991;274:1–7.
55. Tawfik MO: Mode of action of intraspinal opioids. Pain Rev 1994;1:275–294.
56. Grant GJ, Zakowski M, Ramanathan S, et al: Thoracic versus lumbar administration of epidural morphine for postoperative analgesia after thoracotomy. Reg Anesth 1993;18:351–355.
57. Crews JC, Hord AH, Denson DD, et al: Comparison of the analgesic efficacy of 0.25% levobupivacaine combined with 0.005% morphine, 0.25% levobupivacaine alone, or 0.005% morphine alone for the management of postoperative pain in patients undergoing major abdominal surgery. Anesth Analg 1999;89:1504–1509.
58. Dahl JB, Rosenberg J, Hansen BL, et al: Differential analgesic effects of low-dose epidural morphine and morphine-bupivacaine at rest and during mobilization after major abdominal surgery. Anesth Analg 1992;74:362–365.
59. Berti M, Casati A, Fanelli G, et al: 0.2% ropivacaine with or without fentanyl for patient-controlled epidural analgesia after major abdominal surgery: A double-blind study. J Clin Anesth 2000;12:292–297.
60. Finucane BT, Ganapathy S, Carli F, et al: Prolonged epidural infusions of ropivacaine (2 mg/mL) after colonic surgery: The impact of adding fentanyl. Anesth Analg 2001;92:1276–1285.
61. Scott DA, Blake D, Buckland M, et al: A comparison of epidural ropivacaine infusion alone and in combination with 1, 2, and 4 microg/mL fentanyl for seventy-two hours of postoperative analgesia after major abdominal surgery. Anesth Analg 1999;88:857–864.
62. Ben David B, Solomon E, Levin H, et al: Intrathecal fentanyl with small-dose dilute bupivacaine: Better anesthesia without prolonging recovery. Anesth Analg 1997;85:560–565.
63. Rathmell JP, Pino CA, Taylor R, et al: Intrathecal morphine for postoperative analgesia: A randomized, controlled, dose-ranging study after hip and knee arthroplasty. Anesth Analg 2003;97:1452–1457.
64. Murphy PM, Stack D, Kinirons B, et al: Optimizing the dose of intrathecal morphine in older patients undergoing hip arthroplasty. Anesth Analg 2003;97:1709–1715.
65. Husaini SW, Russell IF: Intrathecal diamorphine compared with morphine for postoperative analgesia after caesarean section under spinal anaesthesia. Br J Anaesth 1998;81:135–139.
66. Drakeford MK, Pettine KA, Brookshire L, et al: Spinal narcotics for postoperative analgesia in total joint arthroplasty: A prospective study. J Bone Joint Surg Am 1991;73:424–428.
67. Chaney MA: Side effects of intrathecal and epidural opioids. Can J Anaesth 1995;42:891–903.
68. Leon-Casasola OA, Parker B, Lema MJ, et al: Postoperative epidural bupivacaine-morphine therapy: Experience with 4,227 surgical cancer patients. Anesthesiology 1994;81:368–375.
69. Rygnestad T, Borchgrevink PC, Eide E: Postoperative epidural infusion of morphine and bupivacaine is safe on surgical wards: Organisation of the treatment, effects and side-effects in 2000 consecutive patients. Acta Anaesthesiol Scand 1997;41:868–876.
70. Koren G, Sandler AN, Klein J, et al: Relationship between the pharmacokinetics and the analgesic and respiratory pharmacodynamics of epidural sufentanil. Clin Pharmacol Ther 1989;46:458–462.
71. Whiting WC, Sandler AN, Lau LC, et al: Analgesic and respiratory effects of epidural sufentanil in patients following thoracotomy. Anesthesiology 1988;69:36–43.
72. Stenseth R, Sellevold O, Breivik H: Epidural morphine for postoperative pain: Experience with 1085 patients. Acta Anaesthesiol Scand 1985;29:148–156.

73. Gustafsson LL, Schildt B, Jacobsen K: Adverse effects of extradural and intrathecal opiates: Report of a nationwide survey in Sweden. Br J Anaesth 1982;54:479–486.
74. Rawal N, Arner S, Gustafsson LL, et al: Present state of extradural and intrathecal opioid analgesia in Sweden: A nationwide follow-up survey. Br J Anaesth 1987;59:791–799.
75. Krenn H, Jellinek H, Haumer H, et al: Naloxone-resistant respiratory depression and neurological eye symptoms after intrathecal morphine. Anesth Analg 2000;91:432–433.
76. Neustein SM, Cottone TM: Prolonged respiratory depression after intrathecal morphine. J Cardiothorac Vasc Anesth 2003;17:230–231.
77. Mulroy MF: Monitoring opioids. Reg Anesth 1996;21(Suppl):89–93.
78. Etches RC, Sandler AN, Daley MD: Respiratory depression and spinal opioids. Can J Anaesth 1989;36:165–185.
79. Ready LB, Loper KA, Nessly M, et al: Postoperative epidural morphine is safe on surgical wards. Anesthesiology 1991;75:452–456.
80. Stoelting RK: Opioid antagonists. In Pharmacology and Physiology in Anesthetic Practice, 3rd ed. Philadelphia, Lippincott Williams & Wilkins, 1999, pp 106–107.
81. Rawal N, Schott U, Dahlstrom B, et al: Influence of naloxone infusion on analgesia and respiratory depression following epidural morphine. Anesthesiology 1986;64:194–201.
82. Brack A, Rittner HL, Machelska H, et al: Control of inflammatory pain by chemokine-mediated recruitment of opioid-containing polymorphonuclear cells. Pain 2004;112:229–238.
83. Likar R, Mousa SA, Philippitsch G, et al: Increased numbers of opioid expressing inflammatory cells do not affect intra-articular morphine analgesia. Br J Anaesth 2004;93:375–380.
84. Murphy DB, McCartney CJ, Chan VW: Novel analgesic adjuncts for brachial plexus block: A systematic review. Anesth Analg 2000;90:1122–1128.
85. Picard PR, Tramer MR, McQuay HJ, et al: Analgesic efficacy of peripheral opioids (all except intra-articular): A qualitative systematic review of randomised controlled trials. Pain 1997;72:309–318.
86. Reuben SS, Connelly NR, Maciolek H: Postoperative analgesia with controlled-release oxycodone for outpatient anterior cruciate ligament surgery. Anesth Analg 1999;88:1286–1291.
87. Fanelli G, Casati A, Magistris L, et al: Fentanyl does not improve the nerve block characteristics of axillary brachial plexus anaesthesia performed with ropivacaine. Acta Anaesthesiol Scand 2001;45:590–594.
88. Karakaya D, Buyukgoz F, Baris S, et al: Addition of fentanyl to bupivacaine prolongs anesthesia and analgesia in axillary brachial plexus block. Reg Anesth Pain Med 2001;26:434–438.
89. Likar R, Koppert W, Blatnig H, et al: Efficacy of peripheral morphine analgesia in inflamed, non-inflamed and perineural tissue of dental surgery patients. J Pain Symptom Manage 2001;21:330–337.
90. Nishikawa K, Kanaya N, Nakayama M, et al: Fentanyl improves analgesia but prolongs the onset of axillary brachial plexus block by peripheral mechanism. Anesth Analg 2000;91:384–387.
91. Choyce A, Peng P: A systematic review of adjuncts for intravenous regional anesthesia for surgical procedures. Can J Anaesth 2002;49:32–45.
92. Candido KD, Winnie AP, Ghaleb AH, et al: Buprenorphine added to the local anesthetic for axillary brachial plexus block prolongs postoperative analgesia. Reg Anesth Pain Med 2002;27:162–167.
93. Candido KD, Franco CD, Khan MA, et al: Buprenorphine added to the local anesthetic for brachial plexus block to provide postoperative analgesia in outpatients. Reg Anesth Pain Med 2001;26:352–356.
94. Viel EJ, Eledjam JJ, De La Coussaye JE, et al: Brachial plexus block with opioids for postoperative pain relief: Comparison between buprenorphine and morphine. Reg Anesth 1989;14:274–278.
95. Kapral S, Gollmann G, Waltl B, et al: Tramadol added to mepivacaine prolongs the duration of an axillary brachial plexus blockade. Anesth Analg 1999;88:853–856.
96. Robaux S, Blunt C, Viel E, et al: Tramadol added to 1.5% mepivacaine for axillary brachial plexus block improves postoperative analgesia dose-dependently. Anesth Analg 2004;98:1172–1177.
97. Mousa SA, Zhang Q, Sitte N, et al: β-endorphin-containing memory-cells and mu-opioid receptors undergo transport to peripheral inflamed tissue. J Neuroimmunol 2001;115:71–78.
98. Kalso E, Tramer MR, Carroll D, et al: Pain relief from intra-articular morphine after knee surgery: A qualitative systematic review. Pain 1997;71:127–134.
99. Brandsson S, Karlsson J, Morberg P, et al: Intraarticular morphine after arthroscopic ACL reconstruction: A double-blind placebo-controlled study of 40 patients. Acta Orthop Scand 2000;71:280–285.
100. Rasmussen S, Larsen AS, Thomsen ST, et al: Intra-articular glucocorticoid, bupivacaine and morphine reduces pain, inflammatory response and convalescence after arthroscopic meniscectomy. Pain 1998;78:131–134.
101. Alagol A, Calpur OU, Kaya G, et al: The use of intraarticular tramadol for postoperative analgesia after arthroscopic knee surgery: A comparison of different intraarticular and intravenous doses. Knee Surg Sports Traumatol Arthrosc 2004;12:184–188.
102. Varrassi G, Marinangeli F, Ciccozzi A, et al: Intra-articular buprenorphine after knee arthroscopy: A randomised, prospective, double-blind study. Acta Anaesthesiol Scand 1999;43:51–55.
103. Vranken JH, Vissers KC, de Jongh R, et al: Intraarticular sufentanil administration facilitates recovery after day-case knee arthroscopy. Anesth Analg 2001;92:625–628.
104. Reuben SS, Vieira P, Faruqi S, et al: Local administration of morphine for analgesia after iliac bone graft harvest. Anesthesiology 2001;95:390–394.
105. Petersen TK, Husted SE, Rybro L, et al: Urinary retention during i.m. and extradural morphine analgesia. Br J Anaesth 1982;54:1175–1178.
106. Leon-Casasola OA, Parker B, Lema MJ, et al: Postoperative epidural bupivacaine-morphine therapy. Experience with 4,227 surgical cancer patients. Anesthesiology 1994;81:368–375.
107. Rygnestad T, Borchgrevink PC, Eide E: Postoperative epidural infusion of morphine and bupivacaine is safe on surgical wards: Organisation of the treatment, effects and side-effects in 2000 consecutive patients. Acta Anaesthesiol Scand 1997;41:868–876.

16 患者自控镇痛

JEREMY N. CASHMAN

患者自控镇痛（patient-controlled analgesia，PCA）最初是用来更准确地测量患者镇痛需求的一种研究工具[1]。几乎与此同时，人们关注到术后疼痛不能有效缓解，促使人们探寻更为有效的阿片类镇痛药的给药途径和方法，包括PCA[2]。最早PCA装置之一是在静脉输液管上安上机械性弹簧夹子，患者捏紧该夹子可使盐酸哌替啶从药袋中流出[3]。当患者镇静后，患者就会自己松开夹子，药物停止流动。然而，在PCA成为认可的技术之前，输液泵经历了按时和按需的发展过程。1976年，PCA技术在英国用于临床，Cardiff Palliator成为第一个市售的PCA装置[4]。自此，PCA装置变得越来越精细，具有复杂的计算机控制泵，安全水平明显提高，具有数据输出能力。然而，也研制出来了"科技含量低"的一次性弹性定量PCA装置[5]。

目前，PCA在缓解术后疼痛方面得到广泛认可，常在急性疼痛服务小组的监督下应用。1995年，有2/3的欧洲医院使用PCA来缓解术后疼痛[6]，现在这个数据可能大大提高了。1999年发表的由美国23家医院实施的一项前瞻性多中心研究的报道中，Miaskowski等[7]指出，在接受急性疼痛服务治疗的2824例患者中，有3/4患者使用PCA。研究者观察到这种以麻醉为基础的急性疼痛服务可改善术后疼痛处理的质量，降低不良反应发生率，提高患者满意评分，使患者更早出院（Ⅲ类证据）；见旁注16-1[7]。

旁注 16-1　证据分级

Ⅰ类——从系统性回顾±荟萃分析中获得的证据
Ⅱ类——从一项或多项随机对照试验中获得的证据
Ⅲ类——从非随机对照试验、队列研究或病例对照研究中获得的证据
Ⅳ类——专家意见、描述性研究或专家委员会的报告

基本原理

PCA包括患者根据自己需要，自己间断地给予预定剂量的镇痛药（通常为一种阿片类药物）。护士控制、父母控制以及配偶控制的镇痛方式也有报道。最常用的给药途径是静脉内给药，但是也能经皮下、硬膜外以及鼻内给药。PCA得以应用的理论基础之一是阿片类药物在其低于镇静剂量下具有镇痛作用的特别现象。PCA是根据一个简单反馈环的概念，即患者感受到疼痛时就可触发给予一次按需剂量的镇痛药。如果疼痛没有充分缓解，则再次触发给予按需剂量；但是如果疼痛缓解满意，就不再需要按需剂量，直到出现下次疼痛。然而，患者镇痛的下次按需剂量的给予受到患者所经历药物不良反应的影响，如恶心、呕吐、幻觉和瘙痒。如果这些不良反应极其严重，可能引起患者不再要求应用任何按需剂量的镇痛药。

药代动力学和药效动力学

阿片类药物的药代动力学与药效动力学差异巨大，

表 16-1	用于患者自控镇痛的阿片类药物的药代动力学变量		
	分布容积 (L/kg)	清除率 [ml/(min·kg)]	消除半衰期 (h)
阿芬太尼	0.8	6.0	1.6
芬太尼	4.0	13.0	3.5
氢吗啡酮	4.1	22.0	3.1
哌替啶	4.0	12.0	4.0
吗啡	3.5	15.0	3.0
羟考酮	2.6	9.7	3.7
曲马多	2.9	6.0	7.0

加上治疗指数狭小,所以这种差异要求用药量因人而异。一项研究显示,术后患者哌替啶的最低有效镇痛浓度(minimum effective analgesic concentration, MEAC)相差3倍(III类证据)[8]。PCA的理论基础是患者逐步增加阿片类药物的剂量,以使血浆药物浓度达到镇痛效果良好而不良反应最小[1]。所有常用阿片类药物药代动力学与药效动力学特性都适合于PCA[9]。表16-1总结了用于PCA的阿片类药物药代动力学变量。

用于PCA的不同阿片类药物的效能没有显著差异(II类证据)[10]。吗啡最常用于PCA,而芬太尼因其缺乏活性代谢产物而可能更适合用于肾功能受损的患者。相反,如有可能,最好避免应用哌替啶,因其存在去甲哌替啶毒性的可能。

给药途径

PCA通常经静脉给药,但是也能经皮下、硬膜外和鼻内给药。与静脉给药相比,通过PCA皮下给药需要更高的阿片类药物浓度(见后)。除了皮下给药需要较高的药物浓度外,这两种给药途径的镇痛效果相当,恶心与呕吐的发生率无任何差异(II类证据)[11,12]。虽然一些学者认为患者硬膜外自控镇痛(patient-controlled epidural analgesia, PCEA)费用较昂贵且技术更复杂,其应用并不合理[14],但是PCEA还是越来越普及[13]。通常PCEA背景输注速率低(仅为每小时最大单次给药总剂量的30%),锁定时间较长(长达30 min)。经鼻定量喷雾的给药方式成功地用于脂溶性阿片类药物,如芬太尼、二醋吗啡和布托啡诺(III类证据)[15]。该系统简单,但是可选的不同镇痛药剂量有限或监测选择有限。

剂量参数

单次给药剂量

单次给药剂量是指患者每次按压时PCA泵所给的药物总量。单次给药剂量的多少影响PCA的成功:太少,镇痛不全;太大,并发症过多。单次给药的最佳剂量是能够提供满意的镇痛效果,但无过多并发症的药物剂量;对于吗啡来说,最佳剂量是1mg,但是如果该剂量被证实太小,那么患者能通过增加按压次数来部分地补偿(II类证据)[16]。单次给药剂量的多少可能需要根据患者治疗后的疼痛评分进行调整。研究提示,PCA单次输注引起吗啡血药浓度的迅速变化可能导致恶心呕吐等不良反应。但是,延长单次剂量给药的持续时间并不会减少不良反应(II类证据)[17]。

锁定间隔时间

锁定间隔时间是指PCA装置在单次给药后不再输注药物的时间。锁定间隔时间应该足够长,以让患者判断疼痛是否得到充分缓解。锁定间隔时间的长短受所用药物、单次给药剂量大小以及给药途径的影响。研究显示,锁定间隔时间通常在5~10 min之间,但是几乎所有探讨锁定间隔时间影响的研究均显示有明显差异(II类证据)[18,19]。表16-2和16-3显示不同阿片类药物的推荐单次给药剂量和锁定间隔时间。

负荷剂量

负荷剂量是指达到镇痛效果所需镇痛药的首次剂量。不同患者的负荷剂量相差很大,但似乎确实与随后的镇痛药用量有关。因此,负荷剂量多少和第一个30 min内的镇痛评分对于预测个体疼痛管理可能很有价值(II类证据)[20]。

背景输注

连续背景输注是指以恒速输注镇痛药,其中能通过单次给药进行补充。人们期望连续背景输注给药可改善成人的镇痛质量,但是实际上连续背景输注给药并不明显改善镇痛效果或睡眠质量,反而增加阿片类药物的用药总量,并增加不良反应风险

表 16-2　静脉自控镇痛中阿片类药物单次给药剂量、锁定间隔时间及背景输注速率指南

	药物浓度 (mg/ml)	单次给药剂量 (mg)	锁定间隔时间 (min)	背景输注速率 (mg/h) *
芬太尼	0.01	0.01~0.02	5~10	0.02~0.1
氢吗啡酮	0.2	0.1~0.5	5~10	0.2~0.5
哌替啶	10	5~15	5~12	5~40
吗啡	1	0.5~3.0	5~12	1~10
羟吗啡酮	0.25	0.2~0.4	8~10	0.1~1.0

* 不建议 PCA 常规应用背景输注给药（见正文）。

表 16-3　皮下患者自控镇痛中阿片类镇痛药的单次给药剂量、锁定间隔时间指南

	药物浓度 (mg/ml)	单次给药剂量 (mg)	锁定间隔时间 (min)
氢吗啡酮	1.0	0.2	15
吗啡	5.0	1.0	10
羟吗啡酮	1.5	0.3	10

（Ⅱ类证据）[21-24]。连续背景输注给药也增加呼吸抑制的风险，因此不建议常规用于成人。然而，连续背景输注给药可能适用于某些患者。例如，对正在使用阿片类药物以及可能对阿片类药物产生一定耐药的患者，可使用连续背景输注替代阿片类药物维持给药（Ⅳ类证据）[25]。如果患者接受背景输注给药，而不再需要单次给药，说明背景输注速率太高。

相反，连续背景输注给药有益于小儿（Ⅱ类证据），尽管其理想输注速度尚有一些争议[26]。与没有背景输注给药或以 10μg/(kg·min) 的背景输液相比，吗啡以极低剂量背景输注速率[4μg/(kg·min)]结合PCA的患者睡眠更好，低氧较少，恶心与呕吐较少（Ⅱ类证据）[27]。其他研究也发现吗啡背景输注速率稍加快，高达 16μg/(kg·min) 下，镇痛效果更好，而不良反应不增加（Ⅱ类证据）[26-28]。再增高背景输注速率至 20μg/(kg·min) 时镇痛效果不再有改善，但是低氧血症、过度镇静、恶心与呕吐发生率大于单用 PCA 方案（Ⅱ类证据）[29]。

剂量限值

剂量限值是指在一定时间内不管患者需求次数多少，患者所能接受的最大药物剂量。尚无真正的证据表明限定剂量可改善 PCA 安全。

注射次数／按压次数

注射次数／按压次数更常记录为按压次数／注射次数或需求次数／给药次数，指患者已经接受的成功注射镇痛药的次数与患者需求单次注射镇痛总次数之比。它能用于表达镇痛是否充分[30]；需求次数／给药次数之比超过 3∶1，则提示输注泵程序设置不当（通常是锁定间隔时间太长）或者患者理解差。

管理

患者的选择和教育

PCA 能用于治疗成人和 5 岁以上儿童的急性术后疼痛以及创伤、产科和一些内科急症诸如镰刀细胞危象以及恶性疼痛。旁注 16-2 概括了应用PCA 的一些适应证和禁忌证。某些患者担心药物过量、成瘾、与护士缺乏沟通以及机械故障。手术前对PCA 的使用进行指导不仅有助于减少患者这些顾虑，而且有助于减少 PCA 阿片类药物的用量，从而降低不良反应的严重性（Ⅱ类证据）[31-33]。

工作人员的 PCA 教育和指导

PCA 的有效应用需要仪器的充分维护、合理的使用方案和标准化的监测记录。为了安全使用 PCA，参与评估和治疗过程中的所有人员都应该接受有关 PCA 使用和危险性知识的良好培训。患者和病房医护人员缺乏 PCA 相关知识确实显示不出 PCA 的好处（Ⅳ类证据）[34]。

> **旁注 16-2　患者自控镇痛（PCA）的适应证和禁忌证**
>
> **适合使用 PCA 的患者**
> - 接受了重大手术，并正在禁食（NPO）的患者
> - 已明确"易发生"疼痛的患者
> - 禁忌肌内注射和（或）硬膜外镇痛的患者（如凝血功能障碍）
> - 强烈要求并接受过 PCA 使用教育的患者
>
> **可能不适合使用 PCA 的患者**
> - 拒绝接受该技术的患者
> - 即使适当解释后也不能理解 PCA 概念的患者
> - 曾对阿片类药物引起严重不良反应或过敏的患者
> - 有完全控制 PCA 想法的患者
> - 小于 5 岁的儿童
> - 发育迟缓的儿童
> - 意识不清的儿童

显然对 PCA 有效性、安全性和不良反应的监测很重要。应该经常评估患者，包括疼痛评分（休息和运动时）、镇静评分、呼吸频率、阿片类药物消耗量（按压次数/注射次数）、任何不良反应及其严重性、PCA 泵程序的任何改变。PCA 应该持续用到患者已经规律性口服镇痛药后。另外，在考虑停用 PCA 前，设定一个阈值，低于该阈值时就必须减少阿片类药物用量，可有所帮助。

效能

镇痛

通过 PCA 给予阿片类镇痛药的镇痛效果显著优于传统给药方法（Ⅰ类证据）[35-37]。然而，总的用药量并无显著差异（Ⅰ类证据）[35,36]。虽然 PCA 比肌内注射镇痛的疼痛评分低，镇痛效果好，但不如硬膜外镇痛效果好（Ⅰ类证据）[37]。

患者满意度

患者似乎知道手术后会有一定的疼痛，应用 PCA 的患者即使 PCA 不能完善镇痛（Ⅱ类证据）[38-40]，其满意度仍高于常规给药技术（Ⅰ类证据）[35,36]。而且，接受过传统肌内注射镇痛的患者压倒性地首选 PCA（Ⅳ类证据）[41]。患者满意度与疼痛本身的剧烈程度无关，而与控制疼痛缓解的感觉显著相关[32,42]。根据术后疼痛评分可以看出，即便镇痛结果并不总是成功的，但是患者仍对医护人员为缓解其疼痛所做的努力感到满意。另一个患者表现出较高满意的可能原因是由于害怕冒犯为他们术后护理的医护人员。

安全性

呼吸抑制

人们应用许多标准来定义呼吸抑制，包括呼吸频率、经皮氧饱和度、动脉血气分析和应用呼吸兴奋剂的必要性。其中，呼吸频率是最常用的指标。一项全欧洲急性疼痛服务调查显示，81% 的医院常规测定呼吸频率，而只有 41% 的医院测定氧饱和度（Ⅳ类证据）[43]。最常用呼吸频率低于 10 次/分钟，氧饱和度低于 90% 来定义呼吸抑制。与传统的阿片类药物给药途径相比，应用 PCA 的患者通气更好（Ⅰ类证据）[35]。PCA 的呼吸抑制发生率是 1.2%，表现为呼吸频率降低。动脉血氧饱和度下降的发生率虽然较高，但仍低于阿片类药物肌内注射的镇痛方法（Ⅰ类证据）[44]。

血流动力学抑制

吗啡经 PCA 和肌内注射以及经硬膜外给药均能导致血压下降（低血压）。但是，低血压可能是诸多因素的结果，而不仅因为镇痛。定义低血压的方法有多种：收缩压低于术前稳定值的 20%～30% 以上，收缩压绝对值低于 80～100 mmHg，收缩压/舒张压低于 90/60 mmHg。PCA 的低血压发生率低于 1%，要低于肌内注射和硬膜外给药镇痛（Ⅰ类证据）[44]。

耐受性

恶心和呕吐

大量调查报告认为恶心呕吐的发生与 PCA 有关。总体发生率似乎在 20% 以内（Ⅰ类证据）[45,46]。人们已经采取多种方法来减少术后恶心呕吐（postoperative nausea and vomiting, PONV）的发生，包括在 PCA 输注液中加入止吐药。人们试用过异丙嗪、赛克力嗪、氟哌利多、昂丹司琼以及格拉司琼。然而，

PCA 唯一有效的止吐药是氟哌利多（Ⅰ类证据）[47]。最佳剂量是每 1 mg 吗啡中加入 0.05 mg 氟哌利多（Ⅰ类证据）[48]。然而，临床上在 PCA 输注液中加入止吐药的方法并不普及，100 例患者中仅有 30 例从中受益（Ⅰ类证据）[47]，相反，每 100 例患者有 70 例可能发生氟哌利多的不良反应。

镇静

术后患者经常出现镇静，并不只与 PCA 有关。然而，与 PCA 相关的过度镇静可能提示即将发生呼吸抑制[41]。在遍及欧洲的调查中，82%的急性疼痛服务机构常规评估镇静情况（Ⅳ类证据）[43]。另一项大型回顾性研究显示，与PCA相关的过度镇静发生率为 5%，但是作者并未试图找出镇静与呼吸抑制之间的相关性（Ⅰ类证据）[46]。与 PCA 有关的其他心理影响有梦魇、幻觉以及恐慌发作。

瘙痒症

瘙痒症是一种较常见的不良反应，发生于 14%的 PCA 患者（Ⅰ类证据）[46]。其严重程度不一，难以处理，可能对常规治疗如抗组胺药无效。阿片类药物拮抗剂如纳洛酮和纳曲酮以及纳布啡和氟哌利多可有效预防瘙痒（Ⅰ类证据）[49]。

尿潴留

PCA 对尿潴留的影响尚有争议。一项大型回顾性研究表明，PCA 引起的尿潴留发生率是肌内注射镇痛的 6 倍（Ⅲ类证据）[45]。但是另一项回顾性研究显示，PCA 与肌内注射镇痛的尿潴留发生率极相近（Ⅰ类证据）[46]。

肠道功能

PCA 对肠道功能的影响也存有争议。所报道的半数研究认为，PCA 可增加延迟性术后肠梗阻的风险，另半数研究认为无任何差异。然而，腹部手术后患者使用 PCA 缓解胀气痛可能延长肠道动力的恢复时间。

危险性

现代 PCA 泵技术高超，且高度可靠，罕见给药失误。一项研究显示，使用 PCA 事故发生率为 1.2%，其中 52%是由于操作者失误，36%与机器有关，12%为药物不良反应[50]。操作者错误包括编程错误、PCA 机器设置问题以及患者选择不当或患者相关性错误。PCA 技术方面的机械故障可分类为输注过快、输注过慢或虹吸作用。旁注 16-3 总结了 PCA 相关的危险性。

早期的 PCA 机器中，静态电子放电可导致用于控制注射驱动的软件受损。现在这不再是个问题。另外，在静脉输液管上常规应用防逆流瓣以避免阿片类药物逆流，而把药物正确注入 PCA 泵并且检查注射器或贮液室有无裂隙可避免虹吸作用。

最后，有一项研究显示 PCA 的使用显著增加了腹部手术后伤口院内感染。其机制尚不明了，可能涉及许多复杂因素（Ⅳ类证据）[51]。

泵的更换

为防止发生机械故障，应该常规维护 PCA 泵。应该评估每个泵的可能寿命（通常为 8 年）；超过预计时间，应该仔细检查 PCA 泵[52]。英国健康药物和医疗产品管理部门（Medicines and Healthcare Products Regulatory Agency，MHRA）发布了一个指南，规定了更换输液泵的时间标准（这也适用于 PCA 泵）（旁注 16-4）。

旁注 16-3	与 PCA 有关的危险性

用药错误
泵的编程失误
错误触发
药物蓄积
泵失灵
输注过慢、输注过快、虹吸作用
输注系统缺陷
逆流
临床判断错误
患者选择不当
变态反应
对阿片类药物特别敏感
恶意地重新设置泵程序

| 旁注 16-4 | 决定患者自控镇痛泵更换时间的标准 |

外形及损伤程度超出可修理的范围
长期不可靠
淘汰
没有零件可换
出现效价比更高或临床更有效的泵

与患者自控镇痛相关的死亡

幸运的是，PCA 相关性死亡极为罕见。PCA 相关性死亡主要是由于药物过量，可能是因为编程失误或者泵失灵，但常有其他促发因素如低血容量[53-55]。根据一项报道，使用某种特殊 PCA 装置长达 12 年的 2200 万例患者中，有 5 例患者因该 PCA 而死亡，原因都是编程失误[54]。该报道的作者估计编程失误导致死亡的可能性与一种全身麻醉药引起死亡的可能性极为相近（1：300 000）。还要特别指出的是，这些数据与某种特殊 PCA 泵有关，该泵软件设计中设置了默认药物浓度，这可导致给药过量；目前该软件设计已升级。

小结

I 类证据支持以下有关 PCA 的声明：

- 阿片类药物经 PCA 给药的镇痛效果优于传统给药方法。
- 患者对 PCA 的满意度高于传统镇痛技术。
- PCA 应用阿片类药物时呼吸抑制发生率低于肌内注射阿片类药物镇痛。
- PCA 应用阿片类药物时低血压发生率低于肌内注射阿片类药物镇痛。
- 氟哌利多可有效防治 PCA 应用阿片类药物诱发的呕吐。

II 类证据支持以下声明：

- 静脉 PCA 与皮下 PCA 的镇痛效果相同。
- 低剂量连续背景输注对儿童有益。
- 在 PCA 输注液中加入止吐药对 30% 的患者有益。

（韩　烨译　翟　蓉　邓小明校）

参考文献

1. Sechzer PH: Objective measurement of pain. Anesthesiology 1968; 29:209–210.
2. Harmer M, Rosen M, Vickers MD: Patient-controlled analgesia: Proceedings of the First International Workshop on Patient-Controlled Analgesia. Oxford, Blackwell Scientific Publications, 1985.
3. Scott JS: Obstetric analgesia: A consideration of labor pain on a patient-controlled technique for its relief with meperidine. Am J Obstet Gynecol 1970;106:959–978.
4. Evans JM, McCarthy JP, Rosen M, Hogg MIJ: Apparatus for patient-controlled administration of intravenous narcotics during labour. Lancet 1976;1(7949):17–18.
5. Sawaki Y, Parker RK, White PF: Patient and nurse evaluation of patient-controlled analgesia delivery systems for postoperative pain management. J Pain Symptom Manag 1992;7:443–453.
6. Rawal N: Post-operative Pain Management: Into the 21st Century. EuroPain Opinion Leader Meeting Report. Paris, European Society of Anaesthesiology, 1995.
7. Miaskowski C, Crews J, Ready LB, et al: Anesthesia based pain services improve the quality of postoperative pain management. Pain 1999; 80:23–29.
8. Austin KL, Stapleton JV, Mather LE: Relationship between blood meperidine concentration and analgesic responses: A preliminary report. Anesthesiology 1980;53:460–466.
9. Upton RN, Semple TJ, Macintyre PE: Pharmacokinetic optimisation of opioid treatment in acute pain therapy. Clin Pharmacokinet 1997; 33:225–244.
10. Woodhouse A, Ward M, Mather L: Inter-subject variability in post-operative patient-controlled analgesia (PCA): Is the patient equally satisfied with morphine, pethidine and fentanyl? Pain 1999;80: 545–553.
11. Dawson L, Brockbank K, Carr EC, Barrett RF: Improving patients' post-operative sleep: A randomised control study comparing subcutaneous with intravenous patient-controlled analgesia. J Adv Nurs 1999;30: 875–881.
12. Urquhart ML, Klapp K, White PF: Patient-controlled analgesia: A comparison of intravenous versus subcutaneous hydromorphone. Anesthesiology 1989;69:428–432.
13. Wigfull J, Welchew E: Survey of 1057 patients receiving postoperative patient-controlled epidural analgesia. Anaesthesia 2001;56:471–476.
14. Ammar AD: Postoperative epidural analgesia following abdominal aortic surgery: Do the benefits justify the costs? Ann Vasc Surg 1988; 12:359–363.
15. Toussaint S, Maidl J, Schwagmeier R, Striebel HW: Patient-controlled intranasal analgesia: Effective alternative to intravenous PCA for postoperative pain relief. Can J Anaesth 2000;47:299–302.
16. Owen H, Plummer JL, Armstrong I, et al: Variables of patient-controlled analgesia. 1: Bolus size. Anaesthesia 1989;44:7–10.
17. Woodhouse A, Mather LE: The effect of duration of dose delivery with patient-controlled analgesia on the incidence of nausea and vomiting after hysterectomy. Br J Clin Pharmacol 1998;45:57–62.
18. Ginsberg B, Gil KM, Muir M, et al: The influence of lockout intervals and drug selection on patient-controlled analgesia following gynecological surgery. Pain 1995;62:95–100.
19. Badner NH, Doyle JA, Smith MH, Herrick IA: Effect of varying intravenous patient-controlled analgesia dose and lockout interval while maintaining a constant hourly maximum dose. J Clin Anesth 1996;8:382–385.
20. Stamer UM, Grond S, Maier C: Responders and non-responders to post-operative pain treatment: The loading dose predicts analgesic needs. Eur J Anaesthesiol 1999;16:103–110.
21. Owen H, Szekely SM, Plummer JL, et al: Variables of patient-controlled analgesia. 2: Concurrent infusion. Anaesthesia 1989;44:11–13.
22. Parker RK, Holtmann B, White PF: Effect of nighttime opioid infusion with PCA therapy on patient comfort and analgesic requirements after abdominal hysterectomy. Anesthesiology 1992;76:362–367.
23. Owen H, Plummer J: Patient-controlled analgesia: Current concepts in acute pain management. CNS Drugs 1997;8:203–218.
24. Sidebotham D, Dijkhuizen MR, Schug SA: The safety and utilization of patient-controlled analgesia. J Pain Symptom Manag 1997;14:202–209.

25. Macintyre P, Ready LB: Acute pain management: A practical guide. London, WB Saunders, 1996.
26. Berde CB, Lehn BM, Yee JD, et al: Patient controlled analgesia in children and adolescents: A randomized, prospective comparison with intramuscular administration of morphine for post-operative analgesia. J Pediatr 1991;118:460–466.
27. Doyle E, Harper I, Morton NS: PCA with low dose background infusions after lower abdominal surgery in children. Br J Anaesth 1993;71:818–822.
28. Gaukroger PB, Tomkins DP, van der Walt JH: Patient controlled analgesia in children. Anaesth Intensive Care 1989;17:264–268.
29. Doyle E, Robinson D, Morton NS: Comparison of PCA with and without a background infusion after lower abdominal surgery in children. Br J Anaesth 1993;71:670–673.
30. McCoy EP, Furness G, Wright PM: Patient-controlled analgesia with and without background infusion: Analgesia assessed using the demand:delivery ratio. Anaesthesia 1993;48:256–260.
31. Kluger MT, Owen H: Patients' expectations of patient-controlled analgesia. Anaesthesia 1990;45:1072–1074.
32. Chumbley GM, Hall G, Salmon P: Patient-controlled analgesia: An assessment by 200 patients. Anaesthesia 1998;53:216–221.
33. Lam KK, Chan MT, Chen PP, Kee WD: Structured preoperative patient education for patient-controlled analgesia. J Clin Anesth 2001;13:465–469.
34. Coleman SA, Booker-Milburn J: Audit of postoperative pain control: Influence of a dedicated pain nurse. Anaesthesia 1997;51:1093–1096.
35. Ballantyne JC, Carr DB, Chalmers TC, et al: Postoperative patient-controlled analgesia: Meta-analysis of initial randomised control trials. J Clin Anesth 1993;5:182–193.
36. Walder B, Schafer M, Heinzi I, Tramer MR: Efficacy and safety of patient-controlled opioid analgesia for postoperative pain. Acta Anaesthesiol Scand 2001;45:795–804.
37. Dolin SJ, Cashman JN, Bland JM: Effectiveness of acute postoperative pain management. I: Evidence from published data. Br J Anaesth 2002;89:409–424.
38. McArdle CS: Continuous and patient controlled infusions. In Doyle E (ed): International Symposium on Pain Control. (Royal Society of Medicine International Congress and Symposium Series No. 123.) London, Royal Society of Medicine, 1986, pp 17–22.
39. Wheatley RG, Madej TH, Jackson IJ, Hunter D: The first year's experience of an Acute Pain service. Br J Anaesth 1991;67:353–359.
40. Donovan B: Patient attitudes to postoperative pain relief. Anaesth Intensive Care 1983;11:125–128.
41. Ready LB: Patient-controlled analgesia—does it provide more than comfort? Can J Anaesth 1990;37:719–721.
42. Pellino TA, Ward SE: Perceived control mediates the relationship between pain severity and patient satisfaction. J Pain Symptom Manag 1998;15:110–116.
43. Rawal N, Allvin R: Epidural and intrathecal opioids for postoperative pain management in Europe—a 17-nation questionnaire study of selected hospitals. Euro Pain Study Group on Acute Pain. Acta Anaesthesiol Scand 1996;40:1119–1126.
44. Cashman JN, Dolin SJ: Respiratory and haemodynamic effects of acute postoperative pain management: Evidence from published data. Br J Anaesth 2004;93:212–223.
45. Werner MU, Soholm L, Rotboll-Nielsen P, Kehlet H: Does an acute pain service improve postoperative outcome? Anesth Analg 2002;95:1361–1372.
46. Dolin SJ, Cashman JN: Tolerability of acute postoperative pain management: Nausea, vomiting, sedation, pruritus and urinary retention. Evidence from published data. Br J Anaesth 2005;95:584–591.
47. Tramer MR, Walder B: Efficacy and adverse effects of prophylactic antiemetics during patient-controlled analgesia therapy: A quantitative systematic review. Anesth Analg 1999;88:1354–1361.
48. Culebres X, Corpatuaux JB, Gaggero G, Tramer M: The antiemetic efficacy of droperidol added to morphine patient-controlled analgesia: A randomised, controlled, multicenter dose-finding study. Anesth Analg 2003;97:816–821.
49. Kjelberg F, Tramer MR: Pharmacological control of opioid-induced pruritus: A quantitative systematic review of randomised trials. Eur J Anaesthesiol 2001;18:346–357.
50. Oswalt KE, Shrewsbury P, Stanton-Hicks M: The incidence of medication mishaps in 3,299 PCA patients. Pain 1990;5(Suppl):S152.
51. Horn SD, Wright HL, Couperus JJ, et al: Association between patient-controlled analgesia pump use and postoperative surgical site infection in intestinal surgery patients. Surg Infect 2002;3:109–118.
52. Medicines and Healthcare Products Regulatory Agency: Bulletin DB2003(02)—Infusion Systems. Available at www.mhra.gov.uk/home/idcplg?IdcService=SS_GET_PAGE&nodeId=233
53. Grey TC, Sweeney ES: Patient-controlled analgesia [letter]. JAMA 1988;259:2240.
54. Doyle DJ, Vicente KJ: Electrical short circuit as a possible cause of death in patients on PCA machines: Report on an opiate overdose and a possible preventive remedy. Anesthesiology 2001;94:940.
55. Vicente KJ, Kada-Bekhaled K, Hillel G, et al: Programming errors contribute to death from patient-controlled analgesia: Case report and estimate of probability. Can J Anaesth 2003;50:328–332.

17 区域麻醉和外周神经阻滞技术

BRIAN KINIRONS · DOMINIC HARMON

区域麻醉已经引起人们的再次关注，临床应用也日益增多。区域麻醉能在患者清醒的情况下提供完善的镇痛。近年来新药的出现、设备设计的改进以及成像技术的应用都改善了区域麻醉的质量与安全。持续输注技术允许一边调整输注速率一边观察效果，有利于所输注药物浓度与联合用药的调整。区域麻醉领域的一项主要进展是患者可以在家中实施自控区域麻醉。

人们长期以来一直认为区域麻醉在高危手术患者中具有重要作用[1]。尽可能缩小麻醉范围对于心肺储备功能下降的患者可能具有优势。应用区域麻醉可以避免全身麻醉相关并发症。本章讨论区域麻醉和术后疼痛管理的4个特殊问题，并且验证这些问题答案的现有证据。

是否有证据表明：与全麻相比，椎管内麻醉可以降低高危患者并发症发病率和死亡率？

为了验证这个问题，让我们选择一个明确定义的手术组：因髋部骨折行手术而接受麻醉的患者。髋部骨折是一种常见病，估计到2050年全世界可能有高达630万例患者。该估计对任何医疗体系都具有重要意义[2]。

髋部骨折患者通常合并重要心肺疾病，这些患者重要并发症发病率和死亡率可能与手术有关。其中20%患者术后1年内死亡[3]，而幸存者中有1/4需要长期的较高级别的护理，大部分患者日常生活活动受限[4]。死亡原因包括感染、静脉血栓形成、肺炎、肺栓塞、心肌缺血或梗死、脑血管意外以及褥疮。

证据

关于区域麻醉在降低发病率和死亡率方面是否优于全麻的争论由来已久。早在1933年，Nygaard[1]就证实腰麻并发症少于开放乙醚麻醉。

方法设计缺陷以及统计功效不足使现有研究结果的说服力有限。据估计用30天死亡率作为观察结果指标，假设死亡率在4.8%，并预测发现25%的差异，那么需要研究的对象为13 000～14 000例患者。这可解释为什么一些荟萃分析不可能证实区域麻醉后死亡率有所下降。

1992年，Sorenson和Pace第一个报道了比较全麻与区域麻醉下髋部骨折手术的荟萃分析[5]。这项荟萃分析对13项随机对照的股骨颈骨折手术修复患者的区域麻醉与全麻进行了比较（样本量为2000例）。观察结果指标是1个月时的死亡率、静脉血栓形成的发生率以及失血情况。虽然这项荟萃分析显示在1个月时两组死亡率无显著差别，但是全麻患者发生深静脉血栓形成（deep vein thrombosis，DVT）的可能性比区域麻醉组高4倍。这项荟萃分析的局限包括数项研究中的患者资料有重复，并且大多数患者没有接受任何DVT的预防措施。

Urwin等[6]随后作了一项类似的荟萃分析，回顾了15项随机对照试验，包括2126例患者。观察结果包括1个月死亡率、DVT发生率、失血情况、低血压发生率、心肌梗死、充血性心力衰竭、尿潴留、呕吐、肺炎、术后低氧血症、谵妄和肾功能衰竭。与Sorenson和Pace[5]的研究结果不同，Urwin等发现区域麻醉组患者在1个月时的死亡率低于全麻组[分别是49/766和76/812；比数比（OR）为0.68，95%可信区间（CI）为0.49～0.97]。这些回顾性资料显示区域麻醉组DVT发生率有所下降（30%比47%）。区域麻醉组致命性肺栓塞发生率也明显下降。除了全麻手术时间短于区域麻醉外，全麻无任何优势。

O'Hara等[7]回顾性分析了1983—1993年间美国20所医院所有髋关节骨折手术修复患者（9425例）的结局。主要观察指标是术后7日和1个月的死亡率，次要观察指标包括充血性心力衰竭、心肌梗死、院内肺炎和认知功能改变。研究者结论认为麻醉技术的选择与死亡率或发病率之间无任何关联[7]。他们还提示术前并存疾病以及ASA（American Society of Anesthesiologists Physical Status，ASA-PS）分级在决定结局方面可能更为重要。这项研究的局限性在于该研究为非随机性，是观察性资料，依靠医疗病史记录进行回顾，所以结果取决于围手术期记录的准确性。

Rodgers等[8]回顾性分析了全部被随机分配或未分配接受椎管内阻滞的患者结局。观察指标为死亡率、DVT、肺炎、呼吸抑制、心肌梗死、肾功能衰竭和肺栓塞。尽管研究人群不全为矫形外科手术，但是接受椎管内麻醉组患者是否总体死亡率下降1/3（OR为0.68，95%CI为0.49～0.96）。手术类型以及患者是否接受硬膜外麻醉或脊蛛网膜下腔麻醉与该死亡率下降无关。术后死亡率下降与是否继续应用区域阻滞技术也无关。但是Rodgets等[8]证实椎管内麻醉组DVT、术后肺炎、肾功能衰竭、心肌梗死、失血并发症以及呼吸抑制的发病率均有所下降。

尽管Cochrane数据库较早统计显示髋部骨折手术患者区域麻醉组死亡率有所下降[9]，但是随后的回顾性分析对该结果的统计学意义表示质疑[8]。然而，区域麻醉组患者术后谵妄发生率确实较低。

结论

目前尚无充分的资料确切认为此类手术人群区域麻醉更具优势，尚需大型多中心研究去解答这一问题。现有证据已经明确的是，髋部骨折采用手术修复的患者采用椎管内神经阻滞可降低静脉血栓形成的发生率。尽管Urwin等[6]和Rodgers等[8]的研究结果提示区域麻醉可降低术后1个月时的死亡率，但是Cochrane数据库系统回顾显示，区域麻醉降低死亡率的影响并不显著。没有任何确凿证据提示两种麻醉方法术后1年死亡率有差异。根据现有证据，最佳实践指南仍然主张该手术人群患者选用区域麻醉[11-13]。因为已经证明椎管内阻滞可降低该高危人群静脉血栓形成的发生率，所以主张髋部骨折手术修复患者应用这种麻醉方法似乎合理。

在外周神经阻滞中，是否有证据建议应用辅助药？

人们一直在局部麻醉溶液中联合应用辅助药物，认为这样可产生协同作用。这些辅助药物本身可能就具有局部麻醉作用，或在外周神经上可能有其靶点。其理想的临床作用不仅延长阻滞时间，而且能改善外周神经阻滞效果。这里不讨论碱化局麻药的效果以及肾上腺素的添加作用。必须阐明近期应用的一些其他辅助药的作用。这些药物为阿片类药物、可乐定、新斯的明和曲马多。

证据

阿片类药物

Picard等[14]荟萃分析了外周神经阻滞时辅助使用阿片类药物的效果。所分析的26项研究中有10项显示术中或术后阻滞效果改善，但是无一项研究认为这种明显改善作用与临床有关。研究者进一步认为设计较差的研究更可能得出加用阿片类药物效果较好的结果。结论是尚无证据支持外周神经阻滞时加用阿片类药物。

Murphy等[15]系统地回顾了臂丛阻滞时添加不同辅助药的结果。这些辅助药包括阿片类药物、可乐定、曲马多和新斯的明。结果显示，当前可用文献因研究设计不完善(缺乏系统的阿片类药物对照组)或缺乏足够说服力，而价值有限。关于阿片类药物辅助应用，他们认为与没有全身阿片类药物对照的研究相比，设定一个全身阿片对照组的研究更不可能证实其协同镇痛作用。他们得出结论，尚无充分证据能支持阿片类药物可以作为臂丛阻滞的辅助用药。该结论与先前

Picard[14]所报道的一致。根据这些分析结果，我们认为尚无充分证据支持阿片类药物作为神经丛阻滞的辅助用药。

可乐定

在脑干神经核、脊髓和初级传入神经元中都发现存在α_2受体，这提示可乐定同时具有外周与中枢作用[16]。虽然可乐定的确切机制尚不明了，但是已经提出多种假设。可乐定可能修饰局部麻醉药的构成、改变局麻药的药代动力学特征，或可能对神经具有直接药理作用[17]。目前已知可乐定可减少交感神经发出的冲动[18]。多项研究证实，中枢或外周给予可乐定可延长麻醉与镇痛的时间，并强化局麻药的阻滞作用（并不延长运动阻滞的时间）[17,19]。Murphy等[15]在一项系统性综述中报道的6项研究中有5项认为，加用可乐定可延长臂丛神经阻滞的镇痛时间。他们得出结论，加用可乐定达150 μg可延长镇痛时间，但不增加其不良反应。因此，证据支持可乐定辅助用于神经丛阻滞（表17-1）[20-27]。

新斯的明

鞘内注射新斯的明可产生镇痛作用[28]，一般认为这是由于脊髓背角γ-氨基丁酸释放增加所致[29]。关于新斯的明辅助用于外周神经丛阻滞的资料有限。Bone等[26]在臂丛阻滞中将新斯的明加入甲哌卡因中，发现术后第一个24h内对镇痛药的需求较少。相反，Bouaziz等[27]报道新斯的明并不延长腋路阻滞的感觉阻滞时间。而且，新斯的明组患者恶心和（或）呕吐发生率明显高于对照组。研究者进一步推测，在新斯的明具有治疗作用的研究中，该治疗作用可能是由于手术部位局部所给予的新斯的明所致[27]。目前尚无充分证据建议新斯的明辅助用于外周神经阻滞中（见表17-1）。

曲马多

曲马多同时具有中枢和外周作用[30]。它既是一种μ受体弱激动剂[31]，又可抑制突触对去甲肾上腺素的再摄取，并促进5-羟色胺的释放[32]。这些神经递质在调节疼痛下行通路中有重要作用[33]。人们还一直推测曲马多可能具有局部麻醉作用[34]，α_2受体拮抗剂[35]可逆转曲马多的镇痛作用，这提示曲马多可间接地激活突触后α_2受体。Kapral等[36]报道了评价曲马多作为臂丛阻滞辅助药效果的第一个研究。他们证实100 mg曲马多加入1%甲哌卡因40 ml中可明显延长臂丛阻滞的作用时间[30]。Kapral等[36]的研究中有一组全身给予曲马多，结果证实全身给药组与对照组之间的阻滞时间无显著差异，从而推测曲马多的作用是通过外周神经局部介导的。一项精妙的动物研究结果支持曲马多的这种局部麻醉作用[37]。Robaux等[38]分别将40mg、100mg或200mg曲马多分别加入1%甲哌卡因40 ml用于臂丛阻滞，以研究其剂量-效应关系。结果显示，当加入曲马多时术后镇痛需求呈剂量依赖性下降[38]。但Mannion等[39]在腰大肌阻滞中辅助应用0.5mg/kg曲马多却并未证实其镇痛效果更好。目前有关曲马多用作神经丛阻滞辅助药的资料有限（表17-2），需要进一步研究才能作出明确的建议。

表 17-1 应用可乐定和新斯的明作为臂丛神经阻滞辅助药物的研究

研究	技术	辅助药物	系统对照	结果
Eledjam 等[20]	锁骨上	可乐定，150μg	否	延长镇痛
Singelyn 等[21]	腋路	可乐定，150μg	是	延长镇痛
Gaumann 等[22]	腋路	可乐定，150μg	否	无差异
Buttner 等[23]	腋路	可乐定，120μg 和 240μg	否	延长镇痛
Singelyn 等[24]	腋路	可乐定，0.1~0.5μg/kg	否	延长镇痛
Bernard 和 Macaire[25]	腋路	可乐定，30μg、90μg 和 300μg	否	延长镇痛
Iskandar 等[17]	肱骨中路	可乐定，50μg	否	延长镇痛
Erlacher 等[19]	腋路	可乐定，150μg	否	延长镇痛
Bone 等[26]	腋路	新斯的明，500μg	否	镇痛改善
Bouaziz 等[27]	腋路	新斯的明，500μg	是	无差异

表 17-2　应用曲马多作为神经丛阻滞的辅助药物的研究

研究	操作	曲马多剂量	全身对照	结果
Kapral 等[36]	腋路	100 mg	是	延长镇痛时间
Robaux 等[38]	腋路	40、100 或 200 mg	否	延长镇痛时间
Mannion 等[39]	腰大肌	1.5 mg/kg	是	无差异

是否有证据建议应用区域麻醉减少术后认知功能障碍？

一项包括约 1200 例 60 岁以上患者的大型国际多中心试验表明，术后 1 周约 25.8%的患者出现术后认知功能障碍（postoperative cognitive dysfunction，POCD），术后 3 个月有 9.9%的患者出现POCD（同期对比，非手术对照组发生率在 1 周、3 个月时分别为 3.4%、2.8%）[40]。POCD 是远期结局的一项独立预测因子[41]。术后谵妄与死亡率和重要并发症发生率较高、住院时间较长和出院需要康复设备的比例较高独立相关[41]。

POCD 的一般病因学尚不明了，然而，现有研究支持多因素所致。老年患者[44]和术前认知或一般情况较差的患者[41]通常为高危 POCD 患者[44-46]。特定手术操作与 POCD 发病率较高有关[47]。体外循环下[48]心脏手术、胸部或主动脉瘤手术患者是 POCD 的较高危人群。一些特殊亚群患者为 POCD 较高危人群。老年矫形手术患者 POCD 总体发病率可能高达 7.5%～17.5%[49]，然而髋部骨折患者 POCD 发生率大大增高（28%～50%）[47-50]。术中促发 POCD 的因素尚不明了[51]。麻醉持续时间较长与 POCD 发病率较高有关[52]。现在可以确定某些药物与 POCD 的发生，特别是术后谵妄独立相关。精神活性药物如抗胆碱能药[44]、哌替啶[43]以及苯二氮卓类[43]的应羃与 POCD[43-45]的发生显著相关。另一项研究显示除外哌替啶的阿片类药物以及抗胆碱能药物与谵妄无关[54]。术后感染和呼吸合并症的存在也与 POCD 的发生有关[40]。

虽然许多 POCD 高危因素可能是不能改变的因素（即年龄增大、已有认知损害以及共存疾病严重），但是其他一些因素如疼痛控制差以及出现呼吸并发症确实可能与 POCD 发生率较高有关。一种可能的治疗方法是在多模式治疗中应用围手术期硬膜外镇痛（以局麻药为主的方案）。这种治疗方法可能减少 POCD 的一些已知危险因素，如降低呼吸并发症发生率[55]，提供更好的术后疼痛控制[56]，改善患者结局（如睡眠）[57]。这些因素可能促发 POCD 或术后谵妄[58]。

证据

Wu[59]所系统回顾的 19 项试验中，有 18 项未能证实术中全麻与区域麻醉之间对患者术后认知功能方面有差别。相对简单的单一干预措施，如术中椎管内麻醉，可能对复杂的围手术期并发症如 POCD 影响小，而 POCD 为多因素引起。不同于对其他器官系统的有益作用，术中椎管内麻醉对认知功能并无明显的直接生理益处，而且由于其作用时间有限，不可能提供充分的术后疼痛控制，而研究显示术后疼痛是发生 POCD 的一项因素[60]。

研究设计方面的问题

研究-设计方面的问题可能是目前研究结果不明确的原因。几乎所有比较术中椎管内麻醉与全身麻醉影响的试验在围手术期都常规应用苯二氮卓类药物，而苯二氮卓类与 POCD 发生显著相关[43]。

另一个可能的问题是当前试验中普遍缺乏术后镇痛。尚未严格地研究术后镇痛对精神功能的影响，但是人们已经认识到术后疼痛水平越高，POCD（特别是谵妄）的发生率越高[60]。因此，从理论上说，术后疼痛控制可能影响 POCD 发生率，而 POCD 的发生在术后 3 日内达到高峰[39]。而且，不同镇痛方案对术后认知功能的影响可能有所不同；某些类型的镇痛方案（如以局部麻醉药为主的硬膜外镇痛）不仅镇痛效果优于全身应用阿片类药物[56]，而且可避免阿片类药物的全身不良反应，而后者与 POCD 的发生有关[43]。最后，如同几乎所有的"区域对全身"麻醉的试验一样，没有一项随机对照试验是盲法研究，从而可能导致结果偏倚[57]。

该领域将来的研究将探讨认知功能损害水平（用适当的神经心理学试验来评估）与临床认知功能下降的相关性[61]。外周神经阻滞是区域麻醉实践的一部分。将来的研究还必须证明外周神经阻滞在减轻高危患者术后认知功能障碍中的作用。

是否有证据建议应用区域麻醉技术来减少术后肺部并发症？

当评价区域麻醉技术对术后肺部并发症的影响时，必须考虑以下两个问题：
1. 所选用的术后镇痛措施是否影响肺的结局？
2. 是否有降低术后肺部并发症发病率的更有效的术后镇痛措施？

肺功能障碍的病因

术后常见肺部并发症，可能与显著的病死率和病残率有关（图17-1），特别是上腹部和胸部手术后。术后肺功能障碍的病理生理学是多因素的，不仅由于手术创伤所致，而且与麻醉本身有关。全麻可引起呼吸抑制，功能残气量与肺容积减少。肌肉分离切口的手术创伤可能加剧这种肺功能下降，因为这种手术可引起呼吸肌群功能下降。术后镇痛不充分可限制患者深呼吸或咳嗽的能力，从而使患者易发生肺不张、肺炎以及继发性呼吸衰竭。内脏手术可能导致膈神经损害，从而引起膈肌功能障碍。各种原因引起的通气/灌注比例失调可导致低氧血症，后者可能损害认知功能，并影响伤口愈合。

证据

诸多因素限制了证据的解释。这些因素包括研究群体的多样性、不同的硬膜外技术与输注方案、阻滞平面不一致以及呼吸并发症的定义不一。而且，偏倚和小样本很难得出确切的结论。

Jayr等[63]所报道的是评价硬膜外镇痛影响的最大规模的研究之一。研究包括153例上腹部手术患者。在实施标准化全身麻醉后，术后随机接受皮下吗啡注射或硬膜外布比卡因与吗啡。肺功能测定包括动脉血氧分压（arterial partial pressure of oxygen，PaO_2）、肺功能检查和胸片。虽然硬膜外组患者疼痛明显减轻，但是两组肺部并发症发生率相近[63]。

Ballantyne等[64]荟萃分析了7种不同镇痛治疗对肺结局的影响。他们比较了硬膜外阿片类药物、硬膜外局部麻醉药、硬膜外阿片类药物联合局部麻醉药、肋间神经阻滞、胸膜内滴注局部麻醉药、胸部与腰部硬膜外的比较、切口浸润对切口无浸润，有创伤渗出对无创伤渗出。结局评估指标包括第一秒用力呼气量（forced expiratory volume in 1 second，FEV_1）、用力肺活量（forced vital capacity，FVC）、潮气量（vital capacity，VC）、呼气流速峰值（peak expiratory flow rate，PEFR）、PaO_2、肺不张和肺炎。与全身应用阿片类药物相比，硬膜外阿片类药物、硬膜外局部麻醉药以及硬膜外阿片类药物联合局部麻醉药物均可降低肺不张、肺部感染以及肺部并发症的发生率。硬膜外局部麻醉药组PaO_2较高。硬膜外腔加用阿片类药物可改善镇痛效果，但并不能证实其能改善肺功能（FEV_1和FVC）。肋间神经阻滞、切口浸润和胸膜内局部麻醉药滴注不能改善肺部结局。胸部硬膜外导管放置无任何益处。尽管这项荟萃分析支持硬膜外镇痛的应用，但提示更好的疼痛控制并不总是与肺功能常规指标的改善有关。

在随后的一项系统性回顾分析中，Rodgers等[65]对与椎管内阻滞有关的术后发病率和死亡率的减低进行了荟萃分析。他们证实接受椎管内麻醉的所有手术患者并发症发病率和死亡率都明显下降，而且椎管内阻滞患者术后肺炎较少[65]。这些研究人员还发现有一些证据支持肺炎成比例地减少与胸部硬膜外麻醉有关。随机接受椎管内神经阻滞的患者呼吸抑制发生率减少了59%。这种减少与患者是否同时接受全身麻醉无关。Rodgers等[65]的研究结果支持Ballantyne荟萃分析所建议的应用硬膜外镇痛[64]。

Kehlet和Holte[66]研究了术后镇痛对手术后果的影响。结果支持腹部大手术后应用局部麻醉药或者局部麻醉药与阿片类药物混合液行硬膜外镇痛，以减少术后肺部并发症发生率。

总之，有充分的证据支持应用硬膜外镇痛，以尽量减少术后肺部并发症。

（程 琛译 马 宇 邓小明校）

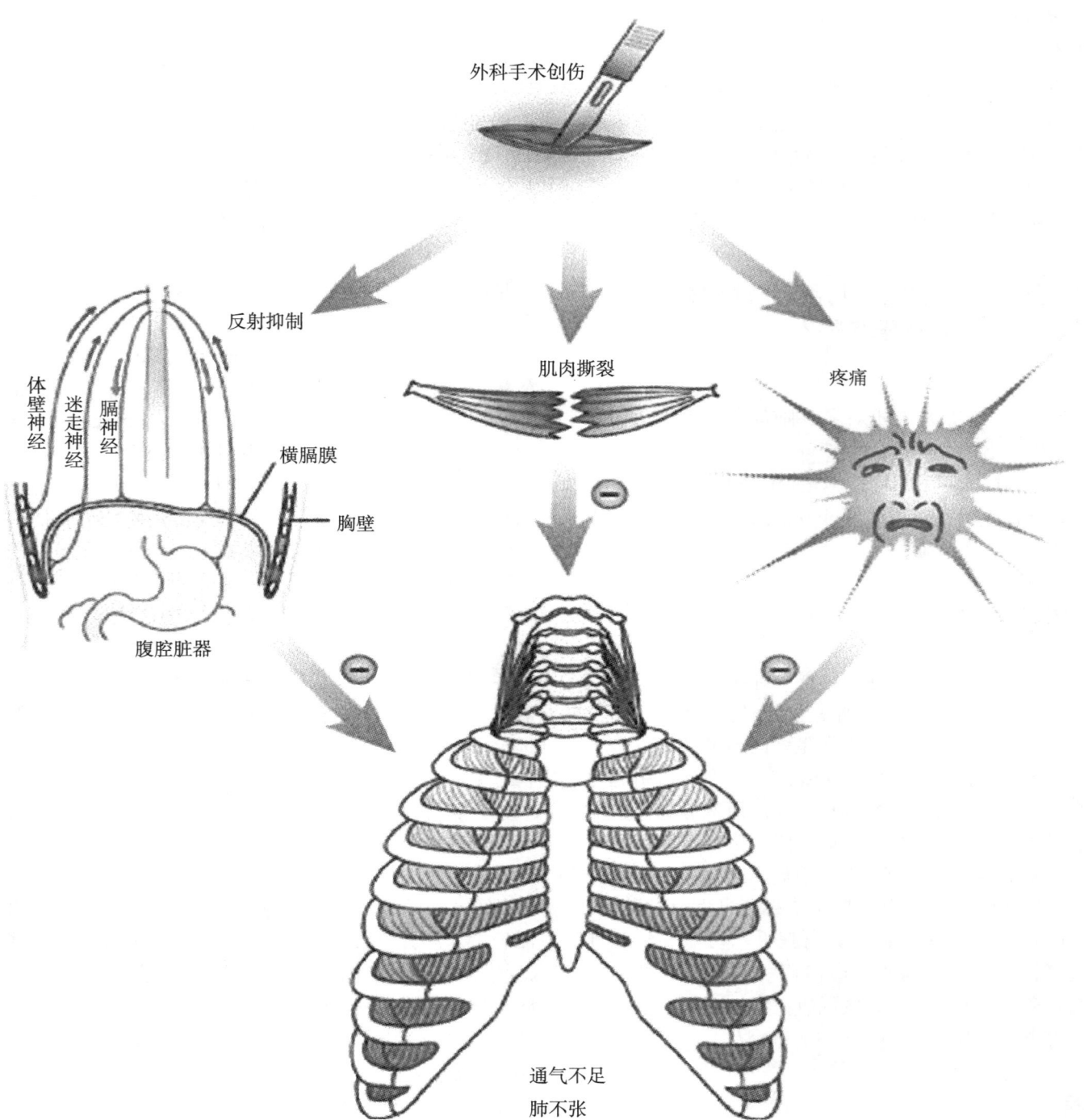

图 17-1 手术创伤后造成呼吸肌功能障碍的因素。手术创伤通过内脏和躯体神经介导刺激了中枢神经系统（CNS）反射；这些反射可引起膈神经和支配呼吸肌的其他神经反射抑制。呼吸肌的机械紊乱可损害其工作效率，而疼痛造成了呼吸肌运动的自限。这些因素都能引起肺容量降低，造成通气不足和肺不张。(From Warner DO: Preventing postoperative pulmonary complications: The role of the anaesthesiologist. Anesthesiology 2000;92:1467-1472.)

参考文献

1. Nygaard KK: Routine spinal anaesthesia in provincial hospital: With comparative study of postoperative complications following spinal and general ether anesthesia. Acta Chir Scand 1936;78:379–446.
2. Melton LJ. Hip fractures: A world-wide problem of today and tomorrow. Bone 1993;14(Suppl 1):S1–S8.
3. Schurch M-A, Rizzoli R, Mermillod B, et al: A prospective study on the socio-economic aspects of fracture of the proximal femur. J Bone Miner Res 1996;11:1935–1942.
4. Hochberg MC, Williamson J, Skinner EA, et al: The prevalence and impact of self-reported hip fracture in elderly community-dwelling women: The women's Health and Aging Study. Osteoporos Int 1998;8:385–389.
5. Sorenson RM, Pace NL: Anaesthetic techniques during surgical repair of femoral neck fractures: A meta-analysis. Anesthesiology 1992;77:1095–1104.
6. Urwin SC, Parker MJ, Griffiths R: General versus regional anaesthesia for hip fracture surgery: A meta-analysis of randomized trials [erratum in Br J Anaesth 2002;88:619]. Br J Anaesth 2000;84:450–455.
7. O'Hara DA, Duff A, Berlin JA, et al: The effect of anesthetic technique on postoperative operative outcomes in hip fracture repair. Anesthesiology 2000;92:947–957.
8. Rodgers A, Walker N, Schug S, et al: Reduction in postoperative mortality and morbidity with epidural or spinal anaesthesia: Results from overview of randomised trials. BMJ 2000;231:1493–1497.
9. Parker MJ, Urwin SC, Handoll HH, Griffiths R: General versus spinal/epidural anaesthesia for hip fracture in adults. Cochrane Database Syst Rev 2000;2:CD000521.
10. Parker MJ, Handoll HH, Griffiths R: Anaesthesia for hip fracture surgery in adults. Cochrane Database Syst Rev 2004;4:CD000521.
11. Gillespie WJ: Extracts from "clinical evidence": Hip fracture. BMJ 2001;322:968–975.
12. March LM, Chamberlain AC, Cameron ID, et al: How best to fix a broken hip. Fractured Neck of Femur Health Outcomes Project Team. Med J Aust 1999;170:489–494.
13. Chilov MN, Cameron ID, March LM: Evidence-based guidelines for fixing broken hip: An update. Med J Aust 2003:179:489–493.
14. Picard PR, Tramer MR, McQuay HJ, Moore RA: Analgesic efficacy of peripheral opioids (all except intra-articular): A qualitative systematic review of randomised controlled trials. Pain 1997;72:309–318.
15. Murphy DB, McCarthy CJ, Chan VW: Novel analgesic adjuncts for brachial plexus block: A systemic review. Anesth Analg 2000;90:1122–1128.
16. Elliott JA, Smith HS. α$_2$-Agonists. In Smith HS (ed): Drugs for Pain. Philadelphia, Hanley & Belfus, 2003, pp 191–200.
17. Iskandar H, Guillaume E, Dixmerias F, et al: The enhancement of sensory blockade by clonidine selectively added to mepivacaine after midhumeral block. Anesth Analg 2001;93:771–775.
18. Eisenach JC, Tong C: Site of hemodynamic effects of intrathecal α$_2$-adenergic agonists. Anesthesiology 1991;74:766–771.
19. Erlacher W, Schusching C, Koinig H, et al: Clonidine as adjunct for mepivacaine, ropivacaine and bupivacaine in axillary, perivascular brachial plexus block. Can J Anaesth 2001;48:522–525.
20. Eledjam JJ, Viel E, Charavel P, du Caliar J: Brachial plexus block with bupivacaine: Effects of added alpha-adrenergic agonists. Comparison between clonidine and epinephrine. Can J Anaesth 1991;38:870–875.
21. Singelyn FJ, Dangoisse M, Bartholomee S, Gouverneur JM: Adding clonidine to mepivacaine prolongs the duration of anesthesia and analgesia after axillary brachial plexus block. Reg Anesth 1992;17:148–150.
22. Gaumann D, Forster A, Griessen M, et al: Comparison between clonidine and epinephrine admixture to lidocaine in brachial plexus block. Anesth Analg 1992;75:69–74.
23. Buttner J, Ott B, Klose R: Der einflub von clonidinzusatz zu mepivacain. Anaesthesist 1992;41:548–554.
24. Singelyn FJ, Gouverneur JM, Robert A: A minimum dose of clonidine added to mepivacaine prolongs the duration of anesthesia and analgesia after axillary brachial plexus block. Anesth Analg 1996;83:1046–1050.
25. Bernard JM, Macaire P: Dose-range effects of clonidine added to lidocai for brachial plexus block. Anesthesiology 1997;87:277–284.
26. Bone HG, Van Aken H, Booke M, et al: Enhancement of axilla brachial block anaesthesia by coadministration of neostigmine. Anes
28. Hood DD, Eisenach JC, Tuttle R: Phase 1 safety assessment of intrathecal neostigmine methylsulphate in humans. Anesthesiology 1995;82:331–343.
29. Cohen SP, Abdi S: Clinical applications of spinal analgesia. In Smith HS (ed): Drugs for Pain. Philadelphia, Hanley & Belfus, 2003, pp 339–351.
30. Smith HS: Miscellaneous analgesic agents. In Smith HS (ed): Drugs for Pain. Philadelphia, Hanley & Belfus, 2003, pp 271–287.
31. Collart L, Luthy C, Dayer P: Partial inhibition of tramadol antinociceptive effect by naloxone in man. Br J Clin Pharmacol 1993;35:73P.
32. Raffa RB, Friderichs E, Reimann E, et al: Opioid and nonopioid components independently contribute to the mechanism of action of tramadol, an "atypical" opioid analgesic. J Pharmacol Exp Ther 1992;260:275–285.
33. Iosifescu DV, Alpert JE, Fava M: Antidepressants: Basic mechanisms and pharmacology. In Smith HS (ed): Drugs for Pain. Philadelphia, Hanley & Belfus, 2003, pp 215–222.
34. Mert T, Gunes Y, Guven M, et al: Comparison of nerve conduction blocks by an opioid and a local anesthetic. Eur J Pharmacol 2002;439:77–81.
35. Desmeules JA, Piguet V, Collart L, Dayer P: Contribution of monoaminergic modulation to the analgesic effect of tramadol. Br J Clin Pharmacol 1996;41:7–12.
36. Kapral S, Gollman G, Waltl B, et al: Tramadol added to mepivacaine prolongs the duration of axillary brachial plexus blockade. Anesth Analg 1999;88:853–856.
37. Tsai YC, Chang PJ, Jou IM: Direct tramadol application on sciatic nerve inhibits spinal somatosensory evoked potentials in rats. Anesth Analg 2001;92:1547–1551.
38. Robaux S, Blunt C, Viel E, et al: Tramadol added to 1.5% mepivacaine for axillary brachial plexus block improves postoperative analgesia dose dependently. Anesth Analg 2004;98:1172–1177.
39. Mannion S, O'Callaghan S, Murphy DB, Shorten GD: Tramadol as adjunct to psoas compartment block with levobupivacaine 0.5%: A randomized double-blinded study. Br J Anaesth 2005;94:352–356.
40. Moller JT, Cluitmans P, Rasmussen LS, et al: Long-term postoperative cognitive dysfunction in the elderly ISPOCD1 study: ISPOCD investigators. International Study of Post-Operative Cognitive Dysfunction. Lancet 1998;351:857–861.
41. Inuoye SK, Schlesinger MJ, Lydon TJ: Delirium: A symptom of how hospital care is failing older persons and a window to improve quality of hospital care. Am J Med 1999;106:565–573.
42. Inouye SK, Charpentier PA: Precipitating factors for delirium in hospitalized elderly persons: Predictive model and interrelationship with baseline vulnerability. JAMA 1996;275:852–857.
43. Marcantonio ER, Juarez G, Goldman L, et al: The relationship of postoperative delirium with psychoactive medications. JAMA 1994;272:1518–1522.
44. Dyer CB, Ashton CM, Teasdale TA: Postoperative delirium: A review of 80 primary data-collection studies. Arch Intern Med 1995;155:461–465.
45. Litaker D, Locala J, Franco K, et al: Preoperative risk factors for postoperative delirium. Gen Hosp Psychiatry 2001;23:84–89.
46. Ancelin ML, de Roquefeuil G, Ledesert B, et al: Exposure to anaesthetic agents, cognitive functioning and depressive symptomatology in the elderly. Br J Psychiatry 2001;178:360–366.
47. Zakriya KJ, Christmas C, Wenz JF Sr, et al: Preoperative factors associated with postoperative change in confusion assessment method score in hip fracture patients. Anesth Analg 2002;94:1628–1632.
48. Arrowsmith JE, Grocott HP, Reves JG, Newman MF: Central nervous system complications of cardiac surgery. Br J Anaesth 2000;84:378–393.
49. Fisher BW, Flowerdew G: A simple model for predicting postoperative delirium in older patients undergoing elective orthopedic surgery. J Am Geriatr Soc 1995;43:175–178.
50. Marcantonio ER, Flacker JM, Wright RJ, Resnick NM: Reducing delirium after hip fracture: A randomized trial. J Am Geriatr Soc 2001;49:516–522.
51. Marcantonio ER, Lee G, Orav JE, et al: The association of intraoperative factors with the development of postoperative delirium. Am J Med 1998;105:380–384.

52. Goldstein MZ, Young BL, Fogel BS, Benedict RH: Occurrence and predictors of short-term mental and functional changes in older adults undergoing elective surgery under general anaesthesia. Am J Geriatr Psychiatry 1998;6:42–52.
53. Berggren D, Gustafson Y, Eriksson B, et al: Postoperative confusion after anesthesia in elderly patients with femoral neck fractures. Anesth Analg 1987;66:497–504.
54. Schor JD, Levkoff SE, Lipsitz LA, et al: Risk factors for delirium in hospitalized elderly. JAMA 1992;267:827–831.
55. Ballantyne JC, Carr DB, deFerranti S, et al: The comparative effects of postoperative analgesic therapies on pulmonary outcome: Cumulative meta-analyses of randomized, controlled trials. Anesth Analg 1998; 86:598–612.
56. Dolin SJ, Cashman JN, Bland JM: Effectiveness of acute postoperative pain management. I: Evidence from published data. Br J Anaesth 2002;89:409–423.
57. Wu CL, Fleisher LA: Outcomes research in regional anesthesia and analgesia. Anesth Analg 2000;91:1232–1242.
58. Hanania M, Kitain E: Melatonin for treatment and prevention of postoperative delirium. Anesth Analg 2002;94:338–339.
59. Wu CL, Hsu W, Richman JM, Raja SN: Postoperative cognitive function as an outcome of regional anesthesia and analgesia. Reg Anesth Pain Med 2004;29:257–268.
60. Lynch EP, Lazor MA, Gellis JE, et al: The impact of postoperative pain on the development of postoperative delirium. Anesth Analg 1998; 86:781–785.
61. Flacker JM, Marcantonio ER: Delirium in the elderly: Optimal management. Drugs Aging 1998;13:119–130.
62. Warner DO: Preventing postoperative pulmonary complications: The role of the anaesthesiologist. Anesthesiology 2000;92:1467–1472.
63. Jayr C, Thomas H, Rey A, et al: Postoperative pulmonary complications: Epidural analgesia using bupivacaine and opioids versus parenteral opioids. Anesthesiology 1993;78:666–676.
64. Ballantyne JC, Carr DB, deFerranti S, et al: The comparative effect of postoperative analgesic therapies on pulmonary outcome: Cumulated meta-analyses of randomized controlled trials. Anesth Analg 1998; 86:598–612.
65. Rodgers A, Natalie W, Schug S, et al: Reduction of postoperative mortality and morbidity with epidural or spinal anaesthesia: Results from overview of randomised trials. BMJ 2000;321:1493–1497.
66. Kehlet H, Holte K: Effect of postoperative analgesia on surgical outcome. Br J Anaesth 2001;87:62–72.

18 非甾体类抗炎药在术后镇痛中的应用

JAMES HELSTROM · CARL E. ROSOW

非甾体类抗炎药（nonsteroidal anti-inflammatory durg，NSAID）是全球最常用的处方镇痛药。NSAID除了能很好地缓解急慢性疼痛外，还能起到有效的抗炎作用。NSAID的镇痛作用呈剂量相关性，但其镇痛作用有限，因此在围术期经常被用作阿片类镇痛药或区域麻醉的辅助用药。尽管这类药物偶尔可能引起如出血、肾功能不全等不良反应，但与其他镇痛药物相比，它的显著优势在于不会引起呼吸抑制或肠梗阻。

有关NSAID的临床文献很多，本文主要围绕NSAID作为围术期镇痛药物进行相关药理学阐述。第一部分简要回顾NSAID药理学、环氧合酶异构体以及可选用的药品。第二部分阐述NSAID在各种术后镇痛中镇痛效果的证据。最后一部分概述NSAID的毒性，这往往是临床中是否使用这些药物的决定因素。遗憾的是，大多数NSAID毒性研究都是针对长期应用，而这些数据于围手术期短期使用的相关性常不明确。选择性环氧合酶-2（Cox-2）抑制剂的心血管风险导致罗非昔布和伐地考昔从美国市场退出，这种情形仍在继续。一般来说，我们所说的NSAID指非选择性环氧合酶抑制剂（或所有抑制剂，而不管其选择性）。所谓"考昔类"特指对Cox-2异构体具有高选择性的药物。

NSAID的药理学

环氧合酶-1和环氧合酶-2

NSAID可逆地抑制环氧合酶（前列腺素内过氧化物合酶），该酶介导前列腺素（PG）和血栓烷A_2（TXA_2）的产生。环氧合酶的底物是花生四烯酸，是磷脂酶A_2分解细胞膜磷脂产生的一种脂肪酸。花生四烯酸也可以作为5-脂氧合酶的初始原料，是炎性介质白三烯家族合成的第一步。前列腺素是自分泌激素，在多种组织中具有介导生理功能的作用，例如维持胃黏膜屏障、调节肾血流、调节内皮细胞张力。TXA_2可促进血小板聚集。另外，前列腺素还起着整合炎症和伤害反应的作用，可导致组织局部水肿，并使局部伤害性感受器敏化[1]。环氧合酶有三种同工酶，但第三种尚未完全认识且未得到广泛认同。Cox-1和Cox-2是由位于不同染色体的基因所表达的，具有不同的组织细胞分布及各自特异的底物和功能。Cox-1的作用是促使构成型PG的合成，以维持内环境的稳态。正常情况下，许多组织[中枢神经（CNS）和肾除外]不出现Cox-2，但是炎症、发热、疼痛和各种细胞因子可诱导该酶的产生。Cox-3可能介导乙酰氨基酚的中枢镇痛作用，似是Cox-1基因表达的变异蛋白产物。Cox-1和Cox-2可分为结构型和诱导型，但这显然过于简单化，因为有证据表明在炎症反应中，Cox-2表达稳定，而Cox-1表达上调。

165

作用机制

对环氧合酶的抑制作用为 NSAID 的镇痛、抗炎及毒性作用提供了一个简单但并不完善的解释。前列腺素 E_2（PGE_2）产生于组织创伤的部位，并且使外周传入伤害性感受器对缓激肽、P 物质以及其他疼痛因子的作用敏化[2]。这形成了疼痛过敏状态，此时对后来的疼痛刺激反应强度增大和（或）疼痛阈值下降[3]。NSAID 并没有提高正常的疼痛阈值，但是可以使组织创伤后的疼痛过敏反应恢复正常，这主要是通过降低外周 PG 而实现的[4]。NSAID 也抑制了一系列与 PG 无关的炎症反应过程，例如抑制中性粒细胞超氧化物的产生和单核细胞磷脂酶 C 的活性[5]。值得注意的是，NSAID 的抗炎、镇痛作用与环氧合酶抑制效应之间的关系并不密切，描述如下：

- 镇痛剂量的阿司匹林（650mg，3～4h 一次，口服）抑制肾和血小板中 PG 合成，但不抑制炎症[6]。
- 双氯芬酸和吲哚乙酸是比阿司匹林更强的外周 PG 合成抑制剂，然而两者在第三磨牙拔除术患者的镇痛效能并不优于阿司匹林[7]。相反，萘普生和阿扎丙宗抑制 PG 合成的作用较弱，但是镇痛效能较强。
- 第三磨牙拔除后微量渗析导管植入表明酮咯酸减轻疼痛的剂量并不降低组织 PGE_2 的浓度[8]。

参与疼痛过敏反应的脑和脊髓 PG 为结构型和诱导型[9]。在脊髓标本中已经提取到前列腺素[10,11]，而鞘内注射 PGE2 可诱发痛觉过敏[12]。重复刺激或应用细胞因子可诱发痛觉过敏，同时伴随脊髓 Cox-2 信使 RNA（mRNA）的上调[13,14]。鞘内注射 NSAID 或考昔类可阻抑这种痛觉过敏，但是 Cox-1 特异性抑制剂却没有效果。提示 Cox-2 可能在中枢敏化作用中处于主导地位[16]。

NSAID 的一般特性

这里讨论的并不是个别药物的特性，因为这些在标准药理学教科书中就有论述。NSAID 是一类有许多共同特征的化学异构体。一般说来，药物的选择取决于药代动力学（包括可应用的剂型）和对 Cox-1 或 Cox-2 的选择性。围术期疼痛最常用 NSAID 的效能差异很大，但是一般半衰期较短，因此重复给药后起效较快，并迅速达到稳定的药物浓度（表 18-1）。长效 NSAID（如吡罗昔康，半衰期 57h）治疗慢性疼痛更有利，服药间隔较长，可提高患者的依从性。肠道外剂型 NSAID（如酮咯酸）对急性外科疼痛很有利。大多数 NSAID 口服生物利用度极好，并经肝代谢清除。多数 NSAID 与蛋白质具有高度亲和力，其中一些药物（如阿司匹林）临床剂量范围可使蛋白结合饱和——这意味着增加剂量可能导致游离药物浓度增高[17,18]。多数 NSAID 呈弱酸性，在生理 pH 值下大部分离子化。因为细胞内 pH 与细胞外炎症环境相比呈相对弱碱性，细胞内外离子梯度的产生促进了 NSAID 进入细胞[17]。非选择性 NSAID 对 Cox-1 和 Cox-2 抑制相对比率差异巨大，而且在体内不同区域影响 PG 合成的程度不同[19]。

术后镇痛的临床效能

概述

对大多数手术，口服和肠道外 NSAID 都是有效的术后镇痛药物。事实上，这些药物都已经在经典的第三磨牙拔除术后镇痛治疗中与安慰剂进行过对照研究。对这种轻中度疼痛，在局麻药药效消退后单独给予 NSAID，通常直接通过疼痛评分改变即可评价镇痛效能。对更严重的疼痛，NSAID 与阿片类药物联合应用，评估对"阿片类药物用量节省作用"（opioid-sparing）的程度。

表 18-1　常规治疗剂量下 NSAID 半衰期及血浆浓度

药品	半衰期（h）	血浆浓度（μM）*
萘普生	14	1.3
布洛芬	2	38～111
非诺洛芬	3	89.5
酮洛芬	2	9.4
吲哚美辛	4	1.4
舒林酸	7†	14.6‡
双氯芬酸	1	6.1
酮咯酸	5	8.0

*Data from Cryer B, Feldman M: Cyclooxygenase-1 and cyclooxygenase-2 selectivity of widely used nonsteroidal anti-inflammatory drugs. Am J Med 1998;104:413-421.

† 母体药物的半衰期。

‡ 有活性的硫化代谢产物的浓度。

对"阿片类药物用量节省作用"的研究设计与解释必须小心谨慎。在这些研究中，阿片类药物一般是通过滴定方式给予，在达到患者舒适后，停止给药，直至患者再次需要镇痛。在给予 NSAID 或者对照药物后，阿片类药物通过患者自控镇痛（PCA）装置的按需静脉阿片类药物用量给药，以维持满意的镇痛。这些研究的问题见图 18-1。阿片类药物有陡坡状的浓度–反应曲线，这意味着镇痛充分和镇痛不足的阿片类药物浓度差别很小（图 18-1 中的 A）。因而，阿片类药物作用的轻微改变（通过 NSAID 的增强作用）即可使镇痛变得完善（图 18-1 中的 B）。实验结果很显然表明 NSAID 发挥了大部分镇痛效果，但是很多镇痛效果实际上是阿片类药物的作用。"阿片类药物用量节省作用"的研究已用于支持一个错误理论，即各种 NSAID 在中重度术后疼痛的镇痛效能与吗啡相似（见附页）。

以下内容描述了有关 NSAID 在多种临床急性疼痛中应用的文献。镇痛效能的讨论限制在某些研究设计合理、实施良好的手术——即有足够的随机对照研究（RCT）数量，研究结果可以用做临床实践的参考。证据的强度按下列标准进行分类[20]：

A 级——基于良好和一致科学证据的建议。
B 级——基于有限或不一致科学证据的建议。
C 级——基于共识观点或专家意见的建议。

胸科手术

后外侧胸廓切开术是创伤最大的手术之一，典型切口是从第二或第三胸段皮节开始，并向前扩展，跨越更多皮节。术后不适是由于手术切口和肋骨疼痛，伴有潮式呼吸、肺部体征和分泌物。手术结束时通常放置两个大口径引流管，其中之一从胸前进入，放入后胸底部，可能引起胸膜痛，甚至硬膜外阻滞下也可产生疼痛[21]。除此之外，胸廓切开术常由于心包或横膈胸膜反射引起严重同侧肩痛，这是膈神经介导的牵涉痛[22]。在 1200 例后外侧胸廓切口的患者中，大部分患者在术后即时需要额外的镇痛治疗[23]。

因为胸廓切开术后疼痛相当严重，所以不考虑单独使用 NSAID 进行术后镇痛（旁注 18-1）。作为包括阿片类药物和（或）区域麻醉等多模式镇痛治疗的一部分，双氯芬酸、吲哚美辛、酮咯酸、吡罗昔康和替诺昔康已经在一些小型 RCT 进行了研究（表 18-2）。最终评价指标通常为切口疼痛视觉模拟评分（visual analogue scale，VAS）、阿片类药物用量及肺功能指数。尚无应用 NSAID 药物对胸廓切开术后同侧肩部疼痛进行镇痛治疗的研究。这些试验结果总结如下：

- 双氯芬酸[24,25]和吲哚美辛[26,27]可减少胸廓切开术后阿片类药物的用量和 VAS 疼痛评分。持续静脉注射双氯芬酸与肋间神经（T_3～T_7）阻滞合用可以在术后第一天减少吗啡用量 60%，第二天减少 76%，并在术后 20h、24h 时显著缓解肩部疼痛。

- 酮咯酸肌内注射与肋间神经阻滞和肌内注射阿片全碱合用可以减少紧急镇痛药的需求（即治疗急性疼痛所需的额外镇痛药）；但是阿片类药物的使用量或

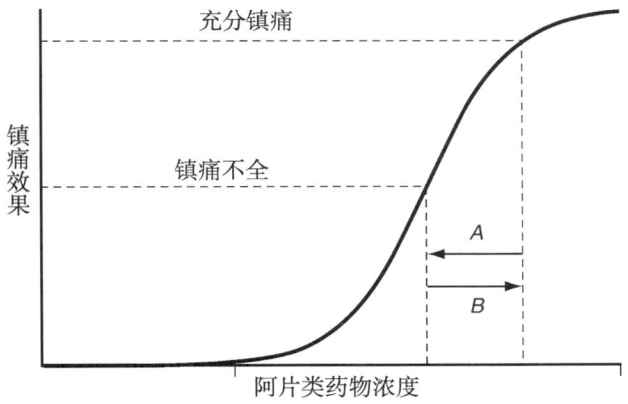

图 18-1　NSAID 的效果可能通过"阿片类药物节省作用"而被夸大（详见正文）。A.代表阿片类药物血浆浓度的轻微下降即可以从充分镇痛变为镇痛不全。B.代表药物血浆浓度相应的轻微升高即可从镇痛不全重新达到充分镇痛。

旁注 18-1　NSAID 在胸科手术中的应用

NSAID 与阿片类药物节省作用有关，并可轻度改善胸廓切开术后疼痛（B 级证据）；但这种镇痛效能绝不会强于单用阿片类药物（A 级证据）。将 NSAID 加入胸段硬膜外镇痛中没有益处。有关 NSAID（和减少阿片类药物）治疗对肺功能影响的研究病例数太少，以致不能得出相应结论。一项研究表明，一种 Cox-2 优先抑制剂尼美舒利能降低胸廓切开术后吗啡的需要量。在视频辅助胸腔镜手术中，NSAID 能够降低阿片类药物的需要量，但不能增强镇痛效果或改善肺功能（B 级证据）。关于 NSAID 治疗同侧肩部疼痛的资料不充分。

表 18-2　NSAID 对胸廓切开术后的镇痛效

研究	病例数	NSAID	区域阻滞	↓疼痛	↓阿片类药物	RCT
Perttume 等[24]	30	双氯芬酸	肋间	是	是	是
Rhodes 等[25]	44	双氯芬酸	肋间	是	是	是
Murphy&Medley[50]	50	吲哚美辛		是*	是*	否
Pavy 等[27]	60	吲哚美辛		是	是	是
Power 等[28]	75	酮咯酸	肋间	否	否	是
Merry 等[31]	20	替诺昔康		否	是	是
Merry 等[32]	45	替诺昔康	硬膜外、肋间	是	是	是
Bigler 等[33]	28	吡罗昔康	硬膜外	否	否	是
Singh 等[29]	62	酮咯酸	硬膜外	是	是	是
Carretta 等[240]	30	酮咯酸		否	是	是

* 历史对照。
RCT，随机对照试验。

疼痛评分并无差异[28]。静脉注射酮咯酸和在硬膜外用药中加入布比卡因可以同等程度降低患者自控硬膜外镇痛中氢吗啡酮的需要量[29]。在此项研究中，酮咯酸组术后呼气峰流速明显较高，但仍低于基线值。有一项研究表明，操作前给予酮咯酸和吗啡，在拔除胸导管时可以产生相同的镇痛效果[30]。

• 在胸段硬膜外麻醉的情况下加用静脉注射或口服替诺昔康[31,32]或吡罗昔康[33]可以减轻静息痛，但是并不能改善咳嗽引发的疼痛或肺功能。

视频辅助胸腔镜手术（video-assisted thoracoscopic surgery，VATS）是一种肺活检和小范围肺组织切除术的常见操作。它较胸廓切开术的创伤小，组织损伤也较小。尽管有关胸腔镜术后镇痛是否有益未达成共识，但据肋间神经阻滞或硬膜外阻滞和阿片类药物紧急使用的情况来看，VATS 确实较胸廓切开术后疼痛轻[34]。有一项研究评估了 30 例 VATS 术后 48h 静脉注射双氯芬酸或酮咯酸的镇痛效能[35]。NSAID 两组与安慰剂组相比，吗啡消耗量均有降低；VAS 评分或肺功能改变无差异。

研究也提示，中枢 Cox-2 在介导胸廓切开术后疼痛中起作用。有一项研究测定了 30 例胸廓切开术后患者脑脊液 PGE_2 主要代谢产物 6-酮基 $PGF_{1\alpha}$ 的水平。该代谢产物在术后升高 4 倍，这种改变可被一种 Cox-2 优先抑制剂尼美舒利所抑制。疼痛评分和吗啡需求量在尼美舒利组中都降低[36]。

妇科腹腔镜

腹腔镜手术可能比实施剖腹手术的疼痛程度轻[37,38]，出院早[39]，并发症少[40]。然而文献综述提示，它的优点并不一致，或并不像预期得那么多[41]。腹腔镜术后疼痛可能与切口或腹部膨胀相关，或可以产生肩部放射痛；这由多种原因所致。重要因素是残气量、气腹产生的压力和气体注入的速度。腹部膨胀能造成血管撕裂、神经牵拉以及炎性介质的释放，从而导致疼痛。同时，碳酸聚集或组织缺血导致的腹膜内酸中毒也可导致疼痛[42]。腹腔镜术后肩部疼痛与胸廓切开术后肩部疼痛相似，是膈肌激惹后膈神经传入所致的牵涉痛。腹腔镜术后有 35%～63% 的患者出现肩部疼痛，多数发生在术后第二天，而内脏痛主要是在术后第一天[43]。

妇科腹腔镜用于输卵管或卵巢诊断及操作。输卵管结扎术为最常见手术，可以通过几种办法完成，采用无菌夹闭术术后不适较少[44]。局部 PG 释放可能影响输卵管或卵巢手术后内脏痛的程度。输卵管中 $PGF_{2\alpha}$ 浓度约比血浆高 10 倍，卵巢卵泡中的 PGE_2 和 $PGF_{2\alpha}$ 含量也很高[45]。因此，输卵管和卵巢腹腔镜操作可能导致 PG 的释放，所以可以推测 NSAID 对这种类型的疼痛特别有效。

奇怪的是，NSAID 在这些情况下并不一定有效

旁注 18-2	NSAID 在妇科腹腔镜手术中的应用

在妇科腹腔镜手术中，围手术期给予 NSAID 与安慰剂相比，能够轻度改善术后疼痛评分并少量减少对镇痛后的紧急需求（B 级证据）。单独应用 NSAID 比长效阿片类药物的效果差（A 级证据）。在诊断性腹腔镜手术中，NSAID 的效能可能较高（B 级证据）。酮咯酸是研究最多的 NSAID，多数研究提示，其效果优于安慰剂（B 级证据）；在酮咯酸给药时间与术后疼痛或阿片类药物紧急需求的关系方面的证据不足（B 级证据）。除了吡罗昔康贴片外（B 级证据），NSAID 对术后肩部疼痛无效。

（旁注 18-2）。相关试验众多，但手术类型、给予 NSAID 时机和疼痛评估方法有所不同，具体总结如下：

- 有关酮咯酸的研究最多，包括 7 项前瞻性研究，350 多例患者（表 18-3）。Green 等[46]对 126 例诊断性腹腔镜检查或输卵管结扎术患者，在手术结束前 30min 分别注射安慰剂或酮咯酸，进行比较性研究。在诊断性腹腔镜手术酮咯酸组患者入苏醒室时，疼痛评分、剧烈疼痛芬太尼需要量、下床活动时间和转出苏醒室时间均明显缩短，但在输卵管结扎术组并无差异。Shapiro 和 Duffy[47]在 40 例输卵管结扎术妇女中也没有发现酮咯酸可以产生阿片类药物节省作用或疼痛状态减轻。DeLucia 和 White[48]报道，非特异性腹腔镜手术术前肌内注射酮咯酸可减轻术后疼痛，减少芬太尼的应用。随后，Pandit 等[49]在几乎同样的人群却得出相反的结论。最后，Compbell 等[50]在 72 例腹腔镜术患者术后皮下滴注酮咯酸或安慰剂 24~36h，研究其镇痛效能。结果安慰剂组芬太尼和可待因的使用显著大于酮咯酸组，酮咯酸组疼痛评分有优于安慰剂组的倾向；有趣的是，诊断性腹腔镜术和输卵管结扎术组的疼痛评分一样。

- 对于术后疼痛程度或需要紧急应用阿片类药物方面，萘普生[51,52,53]、双氯芬酸[54,55]和替诺昔康[56,57]并不一定优于安慰剂。

- 塞来昔布和帕瑞考昔各有一项前瞻性研究报道。与安慰剂相比，塞来昔布并不能减轻伤口疼痛或减少镇痛药需求量[58]。帕瑞考昔对输卵管结扎术患者镇痛效果弱于酮咯酸，但在这项研究中没有安慰剂组[59]。

- 有关 NSAID 与阿片类药物的前瞻性对照研究的结果不明确或效果不理想。例如输卵管结扎术后的即时痛，NSAID 效果差于吗啡[60]、羟考酮[61]和曲马多[62]。但是，有一项研究发现酮咯酸和哌替啶疗效一样[63]。术前给予布洛芬患者在苏醒期感到舒服的程度优于术中给予芬太尼[64]，这可能是由于苏醒期芬太尼时效已过。在腹腔镜的小操作中，替诺昔康比腹腔注射布比卡因或静脉注射芬太尼效果差[65]。

一些研究探讨了 NSAID 治疗腹腔镜术后肩部疼痛的效果。Edwards 等[55]发现，诊断性腹腔镜或输卵管结扎术术后肩部疼痛中，双氯芬酸和安慰剂的治疗效果无差异。尽管总体疼痛评分降低，但吲哚美辛[66]和萘普生[53]在肩部疼痛治疗中前者无明显疼痛减轻，而后者疼痛较明显。塞来昔布可显著减轻腹腔镜术后肩部疼痛，但总体疼痛评分和镇痛药需求与安慰剂患者并无显著差异[58]。吡罗昔康贴片较肩胛上神经阻滞更能有效缓解门诊腹腔镜手术后 6h、12h 时的疼痛，且镇痛药需求量减少[67]。

表 18-3	妇产科腹腔镜术后酮咯酸镇痛效能				
研究	病例数	对照物	↓疼痛	↓阿片类药物	RCT
Ng 等[59]	36	帕瑞考昔	是	否	是
Campbell 等[50]	72	安慰剂	否	是	是
DeLucia & White[48]	76	安慰剂	是	是	是*
Green 等[46]	80	安慰剂	是	是	是
Shapiro & Duffy[47]	40	安慰剂	否	否	是
Pandit 等[49]	54	安慰剂	否	否	是*
Prados&Blaylock[241]	57	安慰剂	否	否	是*

*摘要。
RCT，随机对照试验。

> **旁注 18-3** NSAID 在腹腔镜胆囊术中的应用
>
> NSAID 在腹腔镜下胆囊切除术后减轻疼痛和减少镇痛药物需求方面的效果确切（A 级证据），但是并不能改善术后肺功能。考昔类仍需要进一步研究，但帕瑞考昔/伐地考昔可减轻术后疼痛和减少阿片类药物用量（B 级证据）。

> **旁注 18-4** NSAID 在非腹腔镜妇科手术中的应用
>
> 在诊断性宫腔镜检查术中应用 NSAID 无效，但是术后应用有效（B 级证据）。在开腹的妇科手术中，NSAID 与阿片类药物和（或）硬膜外镇痛联合应用有效（B 级证据）。

腹腔镜胆囊切除术

如上所述，尽管有些研究表明，腹腔镜比开放手术疼痛较轻且肺功能恢复较好，但是腹腔镜术后镇痛的益处并没有被广泛认同[68]。非选择性 NSAID 和考昔类用于腹腔镜胆囊切除术术后疼痛治疗的研究众多，较妇科术后镇痛更为确实（旁注 18-3）。围术期应用酮咯酸[69,70]、双氯芬酸[71]、吲哚美辛[72]、罗非昔布[73]和帕瑞考昔/伐地考昔合剂[74]较安慰剂均能有效缓解术后疼痛和（或）降低镇痛药需求（见表 18-4）。Lane 等[70]研究了 125 例患者（术前或术后）肌内注射酮咯酸的效果，发现该药物的效果优于哌替啶。Liu 等[75]研究了术前给予酮咯酸对术后镇痛和通气的影响。酮咯酸组疼痛和肺功能数项指标明显改善。从疼痛和镇痛药物用量方面来看，利多卡因/替诺昔康混合剂腹腔内注射的效果优于利多卡因腹腔注射和替诺昔康静脉注射[76]。一项研究表明，193 例患者术前静脉注射帕瑞考昔，术后口服 4d 伐地考昔，既可减少吗啡用量，又可减轻阿片类药物的相关症状[74]。罗非昔布术前用药可以减少转出麻醉后恢复室（post anesthesia care unit，PACU）后需要阿片类药物的患者数量，但在住院时间上无明显差异[73]。

非腹腔镜妇科手术

人们评价了 NSAID 治疗非腹腔镜妇科操作引起的不适感，包括子宫镜检查术、子宫内膜活检术、子宫切除术以及宫颈扩张与刮宫术（旁注 18-4）。宫腔镜内膜活检术最常见的失败原因就是疼痛[77]。操作疼痛包括子宫颈扩张和进入、子宫膨胀以及内膜活检。研究提示，宫腔镜检查的不适可能与 PG 介导的子宫收缩有部分关系[78]，表示 NSAID 可能在对该操作性疼痛有效。

尽管 NSAID 在子宫镜检查时并不能有效地减轻疼痛，但术后镇痛治疗中也许有效。术前应用甲灭酸[78]或双氯芬酸[79]不能减轻子宫颈或子宫操作引发的疼痛，但甲灭酸可减少苏醒患者的不适感。在减轻术中或术后疼痛方面，术前口服右酮洛芬的效果不如子宫颈内注射甲哌卡因[80]。在 60 例不孕妇女检查手术中，术前使用萘普生可减轻子宫镜/腹腔镜检查术后的疼痛[53]。

从其他妇科操作获得的数据已经基本证实了子宫镜检查的结果。在宫颈扩张与子宫内膜刮除术、圆锥

表 18-4　腹腔镜胆囊切除术 NSAID 镇痛效能

研究	病例数	NSAID	对照物	疼痛↓	阿片类药物↓	RCT
Forse 等[72]	52	吲哚美辛（I）	酮咯酸（K）	是（I=K）	是（I=K）	是
Fredman 等[69]	60	双氯芬酸（D）	酮咯酸	是（D=K）	是（D=K）	是
Wilson 等[71]	55	双氯芬酸	安慰剂	是	否	是
Yeh 等[242]	88	替诺昔康	安慰剂	否	否	是
Elhakim 等[69]	90	替诺昔康（腹腔内）	安慰剂	是	是	是
Munro 等[243]	37	替诺昔康	安慰剂	否	是	是
Lane 等[70]	125	酮咯酸	安慰剂	是	是	是
Liu 等[75]	60	酮咯酸	安慰剂	是	是	是
Horattas 等[73]	116	罗非昔布	安慰剂	是	是	是
Gan 等[74]	193	帕瑞考昔+伐地考昔	安慰剂	是	是	是

RCT，随机对照试验。

活检术和外阴激光手术进行丙泊酚-氧化亚氮全身麻醉时，酮咯酸并不足以替代芬太尼，并且酮咯酸与芬太尼联合应用也不能缩短苏醒时间或减少术后不良反应[81]。子宫切除术、腹腔镜术和剖宫产后中重度疼痛，单独口服氟比洛芬的镇痛效果不如肌内注射吗啡[82]。妇科重大手术前给予替诺昔康的患者，自控给予布比卡因/芬太尼混合液硬膜外注射次数显著减少[83]。术后给予帕瑞考昔可显著减少术后第一个24h内吗啡PCA用量[84]。

产科手术

产科使用NSAID的指征包括外阴切开术、产后阴道撕裂、剖宫产和子宫痉挛的疼痛治疗（旁注18-5）。外阴切开术和子宫痉挛已被作为镇痛药效能模型进行了大量研究，而且对区分中枢和外周作用的镇痛药具有很好的敏感性[85]。外阴切开术和子宫痉挛可能在本质上代表不同性质的疼痛状态，因为阿司匹林对两者都有效，而可待因对子宫痉挛性疼痛无效[86]。对两种疼痛都有效的药物是处理产后疼痛的理想药物。其他研究结果总结如下：

- 已证明萘普生对产后子宫疼痛（包括痉挛痛）优于可待因和安慰剂[87]。
- Sunshine等[88,89]在两项研究中以阿司匹林和安慰剂为对照探讨了酮洛芬和吲哚洛芬对临产者中重度外阴切开术后、子宫痉挛或剖宫产切口疼痛的治疗效果。

> **旁注 18-5　NSAID 在产科手术中的应用**
>
> NSAID能够降低阴式分娩、外阴切开术和剖宫产术后的疼痛（B级证据）；NSAID也能缓解剖宫产术后子宫痉挛性疼痛（B级证据）。NSAID不应该在剖宫产前常规注入，因为它会导致胎儿动脉导管过早闭合（C级证据）。在正常围手术期应用情况下，NSAID不会在乳汁中集聚（B级证据）。

两者的镇痛效果显著优于安慰剂，而且酮洛芬比阿司匹林具有更快更持久的镇痛效果。

- 一项各种妇产科手术疼痛的研究表明，布洛芬单用和与可待因合用有效，包括用于外阴切开术后疼痛[90]。

NSAID对减轻剖宫产术后疼痛和子宫痉挛以及减少阿片药物用量方面的效果确切。表18-5列出了剖宫产全身麻醉或区域麻醉中NSAID合用或未用椎管内阿片类药物的相关镇痛研究。

在产前或产后使用NSAID可能产生一系列不良反应。其抑制子宫收缩作用和血小板功能抑制作用可能导致大出血，而且NSAID由母体向胎儿转移可能影响胎儿的动脉导管。其抑制子宫收缩作用的剂量似低于引起未成熟动脉导管闭合的剂量[91]。研究证实，吲哚美辛具有防止早产的作用，但未证实有引起未成熟动脉导管闭塞的作用[92]。NSAID在母乳中未检测到，所以一般认为其对母乳喂养的婴儿没有危害。

表 18-5　剖宫产 NSAID 镇痛效能

研究	病例数	NSAID	对照物	麻醉方式	↓疼痛	↓阿片类药物	RCT
Rorarius 等[244]	90	双氯芬酸	酮洛芬和安慰剂	任意	是	是	是
Elhakim 等[245]	50	替诺昔康	安慰剂	全麻	是	是	是
Bush 等[246]	50	双氯芬酸	安慰剂	全麻	是	是	是
Pavy 等[247]	50	酮咯酸	安慰剂	任意	否	是	是
Lowder 等[248]	44	酮咯酸	安慰剂	任意	是	是	是
Wilder 等[249]	120	双氯芬酸	曲马多和安慰剂	脊髓麻醉	是	是	是
Olofsson 等[250]	50	双氯芬酸	安慰剂	脊髓麻醉	是	是	是
Lim 等[251]	48	双氯芬酸	安慰剂	任意	否	是	是
Dennis 等[252]	50	双氯芬酸	安慰剂	脊髓麻醉	否	是	是
Cardoso 等[253]	120	双氯芬酸 q8h	双氯芬酸 PRN	脊髓麻醉	q8h>PRN*	是	是
Sun 等[254]	120	双氯芬酸	安慰剂	硬膜外	否	否	是

* 双氯芬酸每8h给予（q8h）的镇痛效果优于必要时给药的效果（PRN）。
RCT，随机对照试验。

矫形外科手术

人们对 NSAID 用于各种矫形外科手术的治疗进行了广泛的研究，包括关节置换术、关节镜检查和脊柱手术（旁注 18-6）。除了相当大的组织创伤外，许多手术涉及已有严重炎症的组织。不像其他的临床情况，矫形外科手术患者术前常应用 NSAID，因此这些残留的镇痛作用或毒性可能误认为是围手术期治疗。已经证实，NSAID 通过口服、直肠、静脉注射以及关节注射可发挥良好的药物效果。它们已经联合用于全身麻醉、脊麻和硬膜外麻醉中，但是几乎尚无文献表明可辅助用于局部阻滞。

关节镜手术

大量数据表明，NSAID 对关节镜术后疼痛有效（表 18-6）。这些结果归纳如下：

> **旁注 18-6** NSAID 在矫形外科手术中的
>
> NSAID 对于关节镜后疼痛具有确切效果（A 级证据），给药时间对于短时效 NSAID 双氯芬酸的镇痛效果没有影响。很多直接的比较研究表明各种 NSAID 具有相似的效能，并且等效于或优于口服阿片类药物（A 级证据）。在脊柱手术和全关节置换术中，NSAID 能够有效地降低疼痛评分，并减少阿片类药物的需要量（A 级证据）。尚无充分资料证实考昔类在脊柱手术中效果，但是这类药物在全关节置换术中有效（B 级证据）。

- Code 等[94]随机分配 66 例患者术前使用萘普生或安慰剂。NSAID 组在住院期间以及出院后 24h 的术后疼痛较轻，而且出院后镇痛药用量减少。
- Ogilvie-Harris 等[95]研究了关节镜下半月板切除术后随机分组接受萘普生或安慰剂的患者。与安慰剂相比，萘普生明显减轻静息痛和运动痛，并能减少镇痛药的使用量，且滑膜炎和渗出物也较少。

表 18-6 关节镜术中 NSAID 的镇痛效能

研究	病例数	NSAID	对照药物	↓疼痛	↓阿片类药物	RCT
Dahl 等[105]	61	布洛芬	对乙酰氨基酚	是	是	是
Reuben 等[199]	60	罗非昔布	安慰剂	是	是	是
Rautoma 等[255]	200	双氯芬酸	安慰剂	是	否	是
Hoe-Hansen 等[256]	41	酮洛芬	安慰剂	是	是	是
Code 等[94]	66	萘普生	安慰剂	是	是	是
Sandin 等[97]	64	双氯芬酸	安慰剂	是	否	是
Nelson 等[96]	67	双氯芬酸	安慰剂	是	是	是
Rasmussen 等[257]	120	萘普生	安慰剂	是	否	是
Smith 等[258]	60	酮咯酸	安慰剂	否	否	是
Arviddson 等[259]	40	吡罗昔康	安慰剂	是	N/A	是
Ogilvie-Harris 等[95]	139	萘普生	安慰剂	是	N/A	是
Norris 等[98]	127	双氯芬酸	安慰剂	否	否	是
Pedersen 等[260]	87	萘普生	安慰剂	否	是	是
Morrow 等[261]	71	双氯芬酸（D）	酮咯酸（K）	D=K	D=K	是
Berti 等[101]	45	右酮洛芬	酮洛芬	是	否	是
Dennis 等[100]	40	酮咯酸（K）	双氯芬酸（D）	(K=D)	(K=D)	是
Van Lancker 等[106]	100	替诺昔康	安慰剂	否	否	是
Barber 等[103]	125	酮咯酸（K）	氢可酮（H）	K>H	K>H	是
White 等[104]	252*	酮咯酸（K）	氢可酮（H）& 安慰剂	K=H	K=H	是
Twersdy 等[262]	69	酮咯酸（K）	芬太尼（F）	早期 F>K；后期 K>F	N/A	是
Laitennen 等[102]	75	吲哚美辛（I）	双氯芬酸 & 羟考酮（O）	D>I = O	D>I = O	是
Mcloughlin 等[263]	60	双氯芬酸	芬太尼 & 安慰剂	D = F	D = F	是
Drez 等[264]	52	萘普生（N）	右丙氧芬（P）	N > P	N = P	是
Morrow 等[265]	60	吡罗昔康（P）	布比卡因（B）	P+B > P	P+B > P	是
Gurkan 等[266]	40	双氯芬酸	布比卡因 & 安慰剂	是	是	是

*包括腹腔镜患者。
RCT，随机对照试验。

- 数项研究比较了术前与术后使用 NSAID 的疗效，但结论相悖。3 项双氯芬酸的研究认为，给药时间对于出院前的镇痛效果没有影响[96-98]。一项关于罗非昔布的 60 例患者的研究发现，在首次使用阿片类药物的时间、24h 止痛剂的用量和运动时的疼痛方面，术前给药的效果优于术后给药[99]。这种差异可能与药代动力学有关，因为双氯芬酸（半衰期 1h）达到峰稳态浓度的时间远远快于罗非昔布（半衰期 17h）。

- 双氯芬酸与酮咯酸比较以及酮洛芬与右酮洛芬比较研究证实，这些非选择性 NSAID 之间药效相等；双氯芬酸在缓解疼痛和镇痛药需求方面优于吲哚美辛[102]。

- 各类镇痛药交叉研究表明，NSAID 的疗效与氢可酮/对乙酰氨基酚联合应用相同[103,104]，优于羟考酮[102]和对乙酰氨基酚[101,105,106]。Barber 和 Gladu 发现对于前交叉韧带重建术后的即刻疼痛，酮咯酸的镇痛效果优于氢可酮[103]。White 等[104]研究了 68 例关节镜手术后中度或重度疼痛的患者，随机使用酮咯酸或氢可酮/对乙酰氨基酚，在任意时间点上这两种治疗方法的镇痛效果均无差异。

对关节内注射 NSAID 与关节内注射安慰剂和局麻药物合用或不合用阿片类药物，以及静脉注射 NSAID 进行了比较，结果如下：

- 2 项近 150 例患者的研究证明，关节腔内注射替诺昔康疗效优于静脉注射[107,108]。关节腔内注射布比卡因或吗啡分别添加替诺昔康[108]或酮咯酸[109]在降低术后疼痛评分方面优于非 NSAID 个体化治疗。

- Izdes 等[100]在经滑膜活检证实的关节炎患者中证实，在布比卡因中添加吡罗昔康进行关节内注射是有益的；对于活检结果炎症为阴性的患者无益。

脊椎手术

NSAID 在各种脊柱外科手术中都有效，包括椎间盘切除术、椎板切除术和固定术（表 18-7），总结如下：

（1）与安慰剂相比，吡罗昔康[111]、替诺昔康[112]和吲哚美辛[113,114]在脊柱手术中的镇痛效果更好，并降低阿片类药物的需求。

（2）在脊柱固定术[115,116]和椎间盘切除术[117]中，酮咯酸合用静脉注射阿片类药物（使用 PCA）的镇痛效果优于单独应用 PCA。

（3）考昔类的疗效不确定。罗非昔布或塞来昔布在缓解椎间盘切除术后的疼痛和降低阿片类需求方面与安慰剂无差异[118,119]；但是在脊柱固定术后，考昔类和阿片类药物 PCA 联合应用的镇痛效果优于单独使用阿片类药物 PCA[120]。

关节成形术

在关节置换手术中，对非选择性 NSAID 和考昔类与安慰剂、鞘内和静脉内注射阿片类药物以及其他药物的镇痛效果进行了比较研究，结果如下（表 18-8）：

- 布洛芬[121]、罗非昔布[122]、伐地考昔[123]和帕瑞考

表 18-7	脊柱手术中 NSAID 的镇痛效能						
研究	病例数	NSAID	对照药物	↓疼痛	↓阿片类药物	RCT
Pookarnjanamorako 等[111]	50	吡罗昔康	安慰剂	是	是	是
De Decker 等[112]	60	吡罗昔康（P）	替诺昔康（T）& 安慰剂	P 是，T 是	P 是，T 是	是
Mack 等[267]	30	酮咯酸（K）	布比卡因（B）	K = B	K = B	是
Le Roux & Samudrala[117]	55	酮咯酸	安慰剂	是	是	是
Reuben 等[115]	70	酮咯酸	安慰剂	是	是	是
Rosenow 等[268]	96	氟诺昔康（L）	吗啡（M）	L = M	N/A	是
Reuben 等[116]	80	酮咯酸	安慰剂	是	是	是
Fletcher 等[269]	60	酮洛芬	安慰剂	是	否	是
Nissen 等[114]	56	吲哚美辛	安慰剂	是	是	是
McGlew 等[113]	100	吲哚美辛	安慰剂	是	是	是
Thienthong 等[270]	56	氟诺昔康	安慰剂	否	否	是

RCT，随机对照试验。

表 18-8 关节置换术中 NSAID 的镇痛效能

研究	病例数	NSAID	对照药物	↓疼痛	↓阿片类药物	RCT
Bugter 等[127]	50	布洛芬	安慰剂	否	否	是
Iohom 等[129]	30	右酮洛芬	安慰剂	是	是	是
Silvanto 等[271]	64	双氯芬酸（D）	酮洛芬（Ke）& 安慰剂	D 是，Ke 是	D 是，Ke 是	是
Zhou 等[272]	164	酮咯酸	安慰剂	否	否	是
Kostamovaara 等[273]	85	酮咯酸（K）	双氯芬酸 & 酮洛芬（Ke）	K=D=Ke	K=D=Ke	是
Eggers 等[274]	101	替诺昔康	安慰剂	否	是	是
Beattie 等[275]	130	酮咯酸	安慰剂	是	是	是
Etches 等[126]	174	酮咯酸	安慰剂	是	是	是
Fragen 等[276]	59	酮咯酸	安慰剂	否	是	是
Dahl 等[121]	123	布洛芬	安慰剂	是	是	是
Hommeril 等[128]	32	酮洛芬（Ke）	硬膜外吗啡（M）	Ke=M	Ke=M	是
Boeckstyns 等[130]	81	吡罗昔康	安慰剂	是	是	是
Anderson 等[131]	60	双氯芬酸	安慰剂	是	是	是
Segstro 等[132]	50	吲哚美辛	安慰剂	是	是	是
Buvanendran 等[122]	70	罗非昔布	安慰剂	是	是	是
Malan 等[124]	201	帕瑞考昔	安慰剂	是	是	是
Rasmussen 等[125]	208	帕瑞考昔（P）	酮咯酸（K）& 安慰剂	P 是，K 是	P 是，K 是	是
Reuben 等[277]	100	罗非昔布	安慰剂	是	否	是

RCT，随机对照试验。

昔[124,125]与安慰剂相比，镇痛效果更好，并能减少阿片类药物的使用。

• Etehes 等[126]对 174 例患者持续滴注酮咯酸，发现酮咯酸比安慰剂镇痛效果更好，镇静作用更少，并能减少吗啡和止吐药的需求。

• 在 208 例实施全膝关节置换手术的患者中，静脉注射酮咯酸（30 毫克）和帕瑞考昔（20mg 或 40mg）与安慰剂和吗啡（4mg）进行比较，发现较高剂量帕瑞考昔与酮咯酸的效果一样，并优于吗啡和安慰剂。

NSAID 在关节手术中与鞘内和静脉内注射阿片类药物合用的研究结果总结如下：

• 鞘内注射吗啡加口服布洛芬[127]并不能改善镇痛效果或减少阿片类药物需求。

• 静脉注射酮洛芬在全膝关节或全髋关节成形术的镇痛效果与硬膜外注射吗啡（4mg）效果相当，但是前者不良反应较少[128]。

• Iohom 等[129]在应用布比卡因和吗啡脊髓麻醉下行全髋关节成形术的患者中研究了手术前后口服右酮洛芬的效果。与安慰剂组相比，NSAID 组疼痛较轻，阿片类药物的需求较少，恶心和镇静较轻，血浆内白细胞介素-6 的浓度较低。

• 在丁丙诺啡[130]、阿片全碱[131]和吗啡 PCA[132]中添加 NSAID 的镇痛效果优于单纯吗啡 PCA，且阿片类药物的需求量较少。

毒性

正如前面所讨论的，前列腺素（PG）的合成包括诱导型和结构型，后者在维持各种组织内稳态功能方面发挥关键作用。NSAID 是环氧合酶抑制剂，可以通过影响 PG 的重要生理作用而产生不良效应。因为 PG 在肾、血管和胃肠中起着重要作用，所以 NSAID 对这些组织产生明显不良反应就不足为奇了。NSAID 对骨质生长的影响并未引起注意，但这类药物对矫形外科手术可能有特殊的影响。不良反应如支气管痉挛、CNS 毒性（头痛、眩晕、无菌性脑膜炎）、肝炎、皮肤反应以及变态反应不在本节讨论，因为这些反应与围术期使用 NSAID 无特别关系。

肾毒性

PG 产生于肾皮质和髓质[133]。皮质 PG 产生于肾小球及入球和出球小动脉，其功能是调节去甲肾上腺素、血管紧缩素Ⅱ和血管加压素对肾血流量和肾小球的滤过作用[134]。髓质 PG 主要在集合管产生，调节水和电解质转运。尽管 Cox-2 对内稳态的确切影响尚不明了，但是两种环氧合酶异构体均在肾实质表达（旁注 18-7）[135]。

肾小球小动脉是肾小球血浆流量的主要阻力部位，也是肾小球滤过率（GFR）的主要决定因素。在清醒血容量正常状态下，心血管、肝、内分泌及肾功能正常的患者内源性 PG 合成在调控 GFR 方面并不起重要作用。然而，在出现急性或慢性血容量减少时，肾 PG 在维持 GFR 方面起到关键作用[136]。在这种情况下，肾血流和 GFR 的维持就需要依赖于 PG 合成（"前列腺素依赖性"）[134]。已经研究了大多数 NSAID 对尿液 PG 排出的影响。除了舒林酸，抗炎剂量 NSAID 对尿液 PG 排出的抑制程度大于 50%。肾 PG 合成的最大抑制时间发生在给药后 24～48h 内，停药后 72h 内可以完全逆转[136]，但是剂量-反应关系的相关研究尚未见报道。

一些特殊手术群体围手术期急性肾衰竭（acute renal failure，ARF）的危险增加，因此可能易发生 NSAID 诱发的肾损害。在一项 10 865 例心血管、普通外科或胆管外科患者的系统回顾性研究表明，术前存在肾损害、老年及左心功能障碍者是最容易出现围术期 ARF[137]。一些小型研究报道，在肝硬化/腹水或充血性心力衰竭（CHF）的患者，使用 NSAID 会导致肾功能明显恶化[138-139]。这些发现似乎确定 PG 依赖患者特别易发生 NSAID 相关肾毒性。迄今为止，尚未大范围围手术期人群证实类似的毒性，相关研究总结如下：

- 一项大型研究回顾性评价了 10 219 例肠道外应用酮咯酸的患者，并与 10 145 例应用阿片类药物的患者进行比较[140]。重要的是，两组基础肾功能状态没有进行匹配。酮咯酸和阿片类药物组术后 ARF 病例分别是 109 例和 113 例（1.07%比 1.11%，无统计学差异）。

旁注 18-7　NSAID 和肾毒性

肾功能正常患者围手术期应用 NSAID 能够产生短暂性肌酐清除率降低，但是通常不会导致血浆肌酐水平显著上升（A 级证据）。大量回顾性研究提示酮咯酸与阿片类药物相比，并没有增加急性衰竭（ARF）的危险（B 级证据），但有些小样本研究表明有一些关联。考昔类的试验表明其对肾功能的影响与非选择性 NSAID 相似（B 级证据）。

两组 ARF 总体危险升高与很多因素相关（原有肾脏疾病、肝硬化、癌症、氨基糖苷类药物治疗和转入内科监护室及重症监护室），但是酮咯酸治疗与相关诱发因素均无关。长时间酮咯酸治疗（>5d）可能与危险性增加相关[优势比（OR）2.08，95%可信区间（CI）1.08～4.00；P=0.03]。

- 一项荟萃分析对 19 项 NSAID 研究中 1204 例肾功能正常的患者进行了研究。术后第一天肌酐清除率总体下降 18%（下降 16ml/min；95%CI：5～28ml/min），但血清肌酐浓度没有增加。这种现象在多次使用 NSAID 后明显，而单次剂量后并不明显。

考昔类对肾影响的研究提示，这些药物对肾功能的影响与非选择性同类药物相似。对罗非昔布和吲哚美辛在老年（65～85 岁）患者中的应用进行了研究。与安慰剂相比，两者都能短暂性显著减少肾小球滤过率和肌酐清除率，但肾功能标准指数无任何差异[142]。另一项研究显示，塞来昔布或萘普生对肾电解质代谢的影响相近[143]。

胃肠道毒性

胃 PG 通过多种机制在维持胃肠道（GI）黏膜屏障中起到核心作用。PGE_2 和 PGI_2 刺激碳酸氢盐的分泌；增加黏液分泌和厚度，特别是在创伤后；增加黏膜层血流；减少氢离子产生[144]。前列腺素通过氢离子-钾离子-三磷酸腺苷酶（$H^+K^+ATPase$）泵负反馈抑制作用抑制胃壁细胞氢离子的产生[145]。它们还增加黏膜血流，从而快速地清除穿过黏膜下屏障的氢离子。当这种代偿性血管扩张失去时，胃会受到侵蚀[146]。胃十二指肠 PG 合成主要是 Cox-1 的功能[147,148]。然而，Cox-2 mRNA 在溃疡愈合边缘和胃黏膜受有害物质刺激后，其表达上调，提示这种异构体可能具有一定作用[149]。

NSAID 通过直接与间接作用对胃十二指肠黏膜造成伤害（"双重损伤"假说）（旁注 18-8）[150]。直接损害是因为 NSAID 可以直接透过黏膜层造成上皮黏膜的"漏洞"。质子通过直接通道造成胃十二指肠实质损伤。间接作用是由于 PG 抑制和上述细胞保护作用减弱所致。几种非选择性 NSAID 的体外试验表明 PG 抑制与胃黏膜损伤程度相关[151]。长期使用非选择性 NSAID 造成的胃十二指肠损伤能导致出血、溃疡和穿孔，这是美国报道此类药物最常见的不良反应之一[152]。除了

> **旁注 18-8　NSAID 和胃肠道毒性**
>
> NSAID 的胃肠道（GI）不良事件的可能性甚至限制了它的治疗过程（B 级证据）。具有危险因素的患者是可预先评估的，这些患者应用 NSAID 需要小心或避免应用（C 级证据）。米索前列醇、H_2 拮抗剂和质子泵抑制剂可降低所有患者 GI 不良反应风险（A 级证据）。考昔类可降低长期应用有关 GI 出血的风险（A 级证据）；围手术期应用的潜在益处还不清楚，应用这些药物时需要权衡可能出现的心血管安全性问题。

既往有 GI 出血或消化性溃疡病史之外，最重要的危险因素似有老年、心血管疾病和同时使用糖皮质激素。

有理由认为，围手术期短期使用 NSAID 治疗也可能发生某些 GI 毒性。内镜检查已经证明单次口服镇痛剂量的阿司匹林（650mg）可很快造成胃十二指肠损伤。12 例健康者服药后 2h 内均出现明确的胃黏膜下出血，24h 内均出现侵蚀损害[153]。第二次服用阿司匹林只会造成出血范围轻度扩大。一项 5 例志愿者的试验表明在 1h 内出现胃窦和胃底部多发性瘀斑，24h 时 80% 的病变仍然存在。

在一项以肠道外阿片类药物治疗为配对对照的 10 272 例患者的大型队列研究中，评估了肠道外给予酮咯酸后，术后 GI 和手术部位出血的发生率[155]。酮咯酸治疗发生 GI 毒性的相对危险为 1.30（95% CI 1.11～1.52）。剂量增加、治疗时间延长和患者年龄也是重要因素。15 项安慰剂对照研究表明，围术期 NSAID 治疗（2～7d）未发现危险性增加，但 48h 以内的并发症未做统计[156]。

长期服用 NSAID 药物时，预防 NSAID 诱发 GI 损伤的保护方案有效，但是对于短期治疗的预防效果尚不明确。米索前列醇（PGE1）作为前列腺素替代治疗可以降低溃疡穿孔和胃梗阻的发病率 90%；但是患者经常因为腹泻和胃肠胀气而中断治疗[157]。雷尼替丁——H_2 拮抗剂的治疗可以减少十二指肠溃疡发生率，但不降低胃溃疡发生率[158,159]。质子泵抑制剂奥美拉唑在防治长期服用 NSAID 相关的消化性溃疡方面优于米索前列醇和雷尼替丁[160,161]。但没有证据表明围手术期的这种相互作用。

万络（普伐他汀）胃肠结果调查研究（VIGOR）和塞来昔布关节炎长期治疗安全性研究（CLASS）已经证明，考昔类可保持胃 PG 合成，毫无疑问其慢性 GI 毒性少于非选择性 NSAID[162,163]。这些资料引发了关于这类药物应用利弊的激烈争论。因为围手术期短期应用 NSAID 无显著 GI 毒性，所以难以推测考昔类的优势。

心血管毒性

血栓栓塞事件

Cox-1 和 Cox-2 既存在于健康内皮细胞中，也存在于动脉硬化斑块中[164,165]。循环中的 TXA_2（包括来源于血小板）只由 Cox-1[166]，而 Cox-2 是 PGI_2 的主要来源[167]。细胞因子、剪切力和氧化以及低密度脂蛋白（LDL）[168]可上调 Cox-2 mRNA，反映动脉硬化的慢性炎症特征[169]。

全面得出非选择性 NSAID 心血管毒性的结论非常困难（旁注 18-9）。萘普生在动物模型中发现对缺血心肌具有保护作用，但是其他 NSAID，例如甲氯灭酸盐和吲哚美辛却没有类似作用[170]。多项病例对照回顾性观察研究调查了萘普生和其他 NSAID 的心血管风险[171-176]。除了 Solomon 等[172]的一项研究外，没有研究报告萘普生较安慰剂更具有心脏保护作用，尽管有 2 项研究报道萘普生较其他 NSAID 心血管风险小[174,175]。在 Solomon 的研究中，萘普生在两种性别的所有年龄人群中均具有心脏保护作用，但是其他 NSAID 无相应益处。有趣的是，非选择性 NSAID 在其 Cox-2 抑制作用最大剂量 1/5 时即可导致心血管危险性增加（OR 1.25, 95% CI 1.08～1.45）。

考昔类诱发的心血管毒性事件仍在发生。如上所述，罗非昔布和伐地考昔都已退出美国市场，但它们仍可能在严格的管制下重新引入。这些药物与心血管发病率和死亡率过高明确相关（后面讨论），但是该问题的严重程度以及发生机制尚不明确。在最简单的模型中，选择性 Cox-2 抑制剂导致血栓形成和其他心血

> **旁注 18-9　NSAID 和血栓栓塞事件**
>
> NSAID 似不增加心血管危险，但仅有阿司匹林具有心脏保护作用（A 级证据）。萘普生可能具有一定益处（B 级证据）。考昔类，包括罗非昔布、塞来昔布和伐地考昔都能增加心肌梗死、脑卒中和心血管死亡的风险（A 级证据）。在冠状动脉重建术患者中，帕瑞考昔和伐地考昔治疗在术后 10 天即可出现这种危险。证据提示这是考昔类药物的作用，但机制尚不清楚。考昔类并不比其他 NSAID 更有效，因此在特殊患者群体应用时必须要特别注重证据来判断它的益处。

管发病率是由于该药使 TXA₂ 引发的血管收缩和血小板聚集作用增强，并消除了 PGI₂ 的保护作用。结果总结如下：

- 考昔类确实可减少肾功能健康人群尿液中前列腺环素代谢产物的分泌[177]，但 PGI₂ 并不是维护健康人群内皮细胞功能的重要因素[178]。在严重动脉硬化和血小板激活患者 PGI₂ 生物合成增加[179]。这些发现提示 Cox-2 的部分防御机制可能是通过增加 PGI2 的产生，从而限制血小板激活。

- 从理论上讲，考昔类具有一定的保护作用，因为 Cox-2 参与炎性前列腺素类物质的产生，如 PGE₂ 和 PGH₂[167,168]。这些 PG 可促进基质金属蛋白酶的释放，易造成早期斑块形成、破裂和血小板活化[180,181]。

长期应用考昔类的毒性研究使人们认识到其心血管毒性作用，而 2005 年的一项大型研究提示围术期短期使用此类药物同样会产生相似毒性[182]。首个有关考昔类与心血管安全性问题的报道源自 VIGOR 研究，这是一项大型罗非昔布和萘普生长期应用研究[162]。罗非昔布 GI 毒性较小，但是在包括心肌梗死在内的所有血栓事件的危险性都显著升高。因为研究本身没有设置安慰组，所以有很多权威人士认为试验数据也可以通过萘普生的保护效果来解释。VIGOR 研究中的心血管事件没有得到另一项大型试验 CLASS[163] 的证实，后者对照研究了塞来昔布与布洛芬以及双氯芬酸在 8059 例类风湿性关节炎或骨关节炎患者中的治疗作用。值得特别强调的是，上述两项研究均未将心血管毒性作为主要终点。

自 2000—2004 年试图阐述考昔类药物心血管安全性的试验结果未获得确定性结果，结果如下：

- 观察性研究通常提示危险性增加[183,184]。
- 塞来昔布和美洛昔康在严重的冠状动脉疾病患者提示有益[185,186]。
- 两项大型关于罗非昔布的荟萃分析研究得出完全不同的结论。Konstam 等研究 28 000 余例患者（>14 000 患者具有年龄风险）服用罗非昔布对照安慰剂和非萘普生的 NSAID，未发现有过多心血管事件的证据[187]。Jüni 等对包括 20 000 余例患者的 18 项随机对照试验分析研究的结果提示罗非昔布可引起心血管事件增加[188]。

2004 年 9 月，万洛对腺瘤性息肉的预防试验（APPROVe）提前终止。在与安慰剂对照的 2586 例患者中，意外地发现罗非昔布使心血管事件的危险性增加了一倍（危险率 1.92，95%CI 1.19~3.11），特别是心肌梗死和缺血性脑卒中[189]。重要的是，明显增高的风险性只在使用 18 个月后发生。在这个结果公布后，生产万洛的 Merck 制药厂将该药撤出市场，并且对塞来昔布对腺瘤性息肉的预防研究（APC）进行了相似的试验观察[190]。在 APC 研究中，2035 例患者每天两次服用塞来昔布 200mg 或 400mg，或服用安慰剂。塞来昔布导致剂量相关的各种心血管死亡率、心肌梗死、脑卒中和充血性心力衰竭增加（相对整体危险性 2.8，95%CI 1.3~6.3）。这项试验同样提前终止了。

Nussmeier 等[182] 报道了一项多中心研究结果，1671 例患者在冠状动脉搭桥术后给予安慰剂或伐地考昔及其静脉用前体药物帕瑞考昔 10d[182]。在 30d 以上的评估期内，伐地考昔和帕瑞考昔的心脏事件发生率将近是安慰剂的 4 倍，包括心肌梗死、心搏骤停、脑卒中和肺栓塞（表 18-9）。这是首次明确证明即使在围术期短期使用考昔类也会增加不良结局的风险性。

高血压

NSAID 对血压（BP）的影响已得到很好地证实（旁注 18-10）。在志愿者，静脉滴注吲哚美辛可以升高平均动脉压大约 10 mmHg，并导致全身血管阻力升高 30%[191,192]。这种升高几乎完全可用肾和内脏血管张力增加来解释，通常在输注后 2~3min 内出现。心排出量显著下降可能是后负荷增加和心率降低共同作用所致[193]。

研究发现，许多 NSAID 都会减弱抗高血压药物的作用，包括 β 受体阻断剂、血管紧张素转化酶（ACE）抑制剂、噻嗪类利尿剂、哌唑嗪和肼苯哒嗪[194,195]。考昔类似乎具有相似的作用[196]。VIGOR 试验中罗非昔布治疗组患者比萘普生治疗组血压明显升高[162]。CLASS 试验中高血压的发生率和高血压的恶化情况在塞来昔布组与布洛芬组或双氯芬酸组相似[163,197]。在 1092 例接受抗高血压治疗的老年患者中进行了 6 周罗非昔布和塞来昔布的头对头对照研究。罗非昔布组 BP 增高 >20mmHg（并且收缩压 ≥140mmHg）的患者

旁注 18-10　NSAID 和高血压

在经治和未经治的高血压患者中，非选择性 NSAID 和考昔类能够导致血压轻微上升（B 级证据）。这种作用与长期或短期病死率和病残率的相关性尚不明了。

表 18-9 冠状动脉搭桥术后 30 日期间的心血管事件

治疗*	病例数	事件数量（%）	危险率（95%CI）	P
安慰剂	548	3(0.5)	—	—
安慰剂+伐地考昔	544	6(1.1)	2.0(0.5~8.1)	0.31
帕瑞考昔+伐地考昔	544	11(2.0)	3.7(1.0~13.5)	0.03
考昔类联合	1088	17(1.6)	2.9(0.8~9.9)	0.08

* 患者接受阿片类药物治疗后，在术后晨起接受下列 3 项治疗中的 1 项：（1）静脉给予安慰剂 3d，然后口服安慰剂至术后第 10d；（2）静脉给予安慰剂 3d，然后口服伐地考昔 10d；（3）静脉给予帕瑞考昔 3d，然后口服法地考昔 10d。
CI, 可信区间。
Modified from Nussmeier NA, Whelton AA, Brown MT, et al: Complications of the COX-2 inhibitors parecoxib and valdecoxib after cardiac surgery.N Engl J Med 2005;352:1081-1091.

数显著多于塞来昔布组；这种作用在血管紧张素转换酶抑制剂和 β 受体阻断剂治疗组更为显著[198]。

这种血压升高对围术期心血管（和脑血管）危险性的影响尚未有相关报道。舒张压下降 5~6mmHg 可以在 5 年时间内分别减少脑卒中 35%~45% 和冠心病 20%~25% 的发病率。但是围术期使用 NSAID 药物引发的此种程度的血压急性升高是否会导致危险性增加尚不明确。

充血性心力衰竭

NSAID 可导致左心室功能障碍患者失代偿。心排出量的下降可减少有效循环血量[200]，从而导致肾交感神经张力增高并激活肾素-血管紧张素系统。在这种情况下，肾血流和 GFR 依赖于 PG 合成[134]。Cox-1 和/或 Cox-2 抑制作用能通过血管显著收缩或促发肾性肾功能障碍来增加前负荷。

关于 NSAID 与失代偿性心力衰竭之间的相互关系尚无前瞻性研究（旁注 18-11）。但是，有很多观察性研究提示 NSAID 可增加易感患者 CHF 的危险性。已经诊断 CHF 患者前一周使用 NSAID，其病情恶化需要住院的优势比是 2.1（95% CI 1.2~3.3）[201]。CHF 发作后的患者给予 NSAID 可增加失代偿危险性（3.8，95% CI 1.1~12.7）[202]。考昔类尽管可能有相似的肾水钠潴留效应，但无类似的研究报道。

出血

环氧合酶可催化产生 PGH2，其是生成 TXA$_2$ 的底物。Cox-1 存在于血小板结构内，NSAID 可抑制 Cox-1，导致血小板聚集受限，并导致不同程度的出血时间延长（旁注 18-12）。因为血小板没有细胞核，所以不能上调 Cox-2[203]，因此选择性 Cox-2 抑制剂不会影响血小板活性。一般来说，NSAID 可引起中度、剂量依赖性的出血时间延长，并可能不超过正常上限[204]。环氧合酶抑制剂与围术期出血之间的研究多数来自阿司匹林。尽管 NSAID 和阿司匹林都抑制 PG 合成，但是阿司匹林不可逆地抑制乙酰化环氧合酶丝氨酸上的羟基，导致整个血小板生存期的活性和 TX-A2 生成受到持续抑制。相比之下，NSAID 可逆地抑制环氧合酶，因此在药物清除后，血小板功能可恢复至基础水平[203]。较长效 NSAID，如吡罗昔康，在停药数日内还能抑制血小板聚集功能[205]。

患者围术期使用 NSAID 增加出血的情况包括潜在的凝血疾病、嗜酒史、同时使用抗凝药物；研究结果描述如下[303]：

- 阿司匹林能促发临界凝血疾病的患者出现临床出血，并且实际上一直用于血小板-血管壁异常（如 Willebrand 病[206]和骨髓增生疾病）的辅助诊断[207]。

- 在阿司匹林和 NSAID 的作用下，酒精可显著延长出血时间[208]。这种现象的机制尚不清楚，但可能与增强前列腺素对血小板聚集抑制作用有关[209,210]。

- 许多 NSAID 与蛋白高度结合，并可将华法林从白蛋白结合部置换出来，因此使血浆游离华法林浓度升高。目前尚无研究确定这种作用与临床出血的相关性。

欧洲 49 个中心共 11 245 例患者参与了有关酮咯酸与术后止血功能之间关系的前瞻性研究[211]。研究对比了酮咯酸、双氯芬酸或酮洛芬在大手术中手术部位

旁注 18-11 NSAID 和充血性心力衰竭

观察性研究支持非选择性 NSAID 与充血性心力衰竭症状恶化有关（B 级证据）。无考昔类的相关资料。

旁注 18-12 NSAID 和出血

NSAID 影响血小板的聚集并延长凝血时间。考昔类不影响凝血。大样本研究表明应用酮咯酸、双氯芬酸和酮洛芬不会增加围手术期出血的风险（A 级证据），但在泌尿外科和耳鼻喉科手术中三种药物均会增加出血风险（B 级证据）。接受 NSAID 治疗的患者并无出血倾向，但进行耳鼻喉科手术时需要再次手术来控制出血的可能性会增加（B 级证据）。一项大型监测研究表明在应用酮咯酸的患者和应用阿片类药物的患者出血情况无区别（B 级证据）。短期应用阿司匹林（A 级证据）和长期应用 NSAID（B 级证据）的患者，采用椎管内镇痛和麻醉是安全的。

出血的危险性，包括了腹部、矫形外科、妇科、泌尿外科和整形 / 眼、鼻、咽喉科（ENT）手术。NSAID 类药物在危险性方面无差异，11 245 例患者中有 117 例（总体 1.04%）出现了术后出血的证据。同时接受低分子量肝素或肝素治疗增加危险性，整形 /ENT、妇科和泌尿外科手术出现手术部位出血的风险性较大。在酮咯酸上市后，对其围术期出血危险性进行了一项 10 272 例患者的治疗调查[155]。与阿片类药物治疗组相比，手术部位出血的校正后多变量优势比无差异。老年患者用药或注射较大剂量时，危险性可能轻度增加（统计学无差异）。

另外一些试验研究了 NSAID 导致出血的风险是否受特殊手术部位的影响。口腔和生殖泌尿道是溶解纤维蛋白活性的集中部位，因此在这些部位手术时，使用抗血小板制剂会导致出血危险性增高[203]。此外，有些手术（如眼科手术），即使是少量出血也会造成严重并发症。结果总结如下：

- 一项回顾性研究发现经尿道前列腺切除术中，如果患者术前使用阿司匹林和 NSAID，则需要较多的输血量[212]。
- 阿司匹林可以增加体外震波碎石、前列腺活检和经尿道膀胱肿瘤切除术后的出血[213]。
- 一项荟萃分析研究了 7 项有关成人和儿童扁桃体切除术（505 例患者）的出血风险。术后出血发生率无差异。但是 NSAID 治疗的患者需要再次手术止血的发生率较高（OR 2.3，3.9%CI 1.3～11.5；P=0.02）。需要止血的患者数量为 29（95% CI 17～44）[214]。
- 一项对 25 项扁桃体切除术研究进行的系统性定量分析得出了相似的结论。NSAID 并不增加出血量、术后出血发生率和延长住院日，但是需要再次手术止血率显著增高（OR 2.3，95%CI 1.12～4.83）。需要止血的患者数量为 60（95% CI 34～227）[215]。
- 对各种类型儿科手术 NSAID 使用情况的一项综述中有 4 项研究中术后出血的发生率显著增高[216]。有趣的是，其中 3 项研究与应用酮咯酸治疗扁桃体切除术后疼痛有关。
- 持续应用阿司匹林治疗与白内障手术术中出血增加无关[217]。

矫形外科手术通常会短期和长期使用 NSAID，特别需要手术修复的慢性关节炎患者，更需长期使用 NSAID。关于出血危险性的结论不一致，如下：

- 一项关于全髋成形术的回顾性研究对照比较了 76 例服用 11 种不同 NSAID 药物至术前 24h 的患者和 89 例术前至少 48h 停用 NSAID 药物的患者[218]。两组患者在术中输液量、输血量、术后伤口引流量、血细胞比容最大下降或住院日方面均无差异。但术前 24h 停用 NSAID 组术后低血压和 GI 出血的发生率较高，特别是使用半衰期长于 6h 的此类药物时。
- 另一项全髋手术研究将 25 例患者随机分成两组，术前给予 2 周布洛芬治疗的患者围术期平均失血量较安慰剂对照组高 45%（1161±472ml 比 796±337ml）[219]。
- 最后一项髋关节手术研究发现，接受阿司匹林治疗的患者尽管出血时间显著延长，但围术期失血量无明显增加[220]。
- 在膝关节镜手术中，术前萘丁美酮治疗对止血功能影响很小。

最后，美国区域麻醉学会（ASRA）总结如下：接受 NSAID 和阿司匹林治疗的患者区域麻醉下脊髓或硬膜外血肿的危险性并不增加[222]。在孕妇低剂量阿司匹林协作研究（Collaborative Low-dose Aspirin Study in Pregnancy, CLASP）中，1422 例高危产科患者每天给予 60mg 阿司匹林，所有患者都应用硬膜外麻醉，均未发生神经系统后遗症[223]。在一项硬膜外糖皮质激素注射的研究中，1214 例患者均无出血报道，其中 32% 的患者正在服用 NSAID[224]。

骨生长抑制作用

前列腺素在骨折后骨修复过程中起到重要的作用。骨修复包含了下列3个主要步骤：①类骨基质的产生；②基质矿化形成编织骨；③编织骨痂的吸收和再塑形并产生皮质骨以达到必要的骨形状和完整性[225]。损伤后，局部缺氧和炎症导致成骨细胞增生并移行到骨折部位。成骨细胞形成的胶原基质为骨再生提供了一个支架，以及自分泌物质，如前列腺素在骨形成和吸收的平衡中起到了决定性作用[226]。在兔创伤性骨折模型中，PGE_2 升高；这种升高被认为是促进骨形成[227]。大鼠在给予非选择性 NSAID 后骨折实验模型的愈合时间延长并且骨不连的发生率增高[228,229]，而且此效应仅在治疗后3天即可观察到[230]。Coxib 对这些模型显示有巨大的影响，提示 Cox-2 在这个进程中具有重要的作用[231]。实际上在 Cox-2 敲除小鼠中（同源 Cox-2 基因敲除）胫骨稳定性骨折的愈合相对 Cox-1 敲除小鼠和野生型小鼠显著延迟。

骨愈合和环氧合酶抑制剂（旁注 18-13）的临床数据主要是回顾性研究。Giannoudis 等[233]发现 NSAID 服用者在股骨干骨折髓内钉术后骨不连的发生率增高十倍。使用 NSAID 平均 21 周者，应用的时间越长，骨折患者最终愈合时间越长[234]。Glassman 等[235]回顾性地评价了在脊柱矫形融合术后给予酮咯酸的效果，结果发现在酮咯酸组无论是吸烟者还是不吸烟者骨不连的发生率均显著增高。

在98例移位型和非移位型 Colles'，骨折的患者中进行了氟比洛芬前瞻性双盲安慰剂对照的实验研究[236]。在一年的随访中，两组之间在骨折愈合时间和骨愈合率上没有显著差异。但在非移位型骨折中安慰剂组骨折完美愈合率较 NSAID 使用组显著增高。

到目前为止临床有关 NSAID 治疗对骨生长的影响的最多经验在于防治异位骨化，这在髋关节成形术中

旁注 18-13　NSAID 和骨愈合

动物模型表明 NSAID 和考昔类均会对骨折后骨愈合产生负面作用。Cox-1 和 Cox-2 都起到很重要的作用。临床研究表明可能会增加骨的不愈合率，但大多为回顾性研究资料（B 级证据）。一项回顾性研究表明 NSAID 对 Colles 骨折愈合无影响。在髋部手术或创伤后应用 NSAID 可以预防异位骨形成（A 级证据）。

约三分之一的患者出现[237]。异位骨化是一种骨组织外异常的骨质形成。通常是手术切除激活了静止的成骨干细胞，导致类骨样组织和异位骨形成。一项对13个随机实验的研究发现每100例患者围手术期使用 NSAID 使用可以防治1到2例严重的异位骨化和10～20例轻中度异位骨化。在一些动物模型中，平均治疗时间为5周，显著长于骨愈合不良者[230]。

问题是 NSAID 对骨形成的抑制效应是否有益。这种影响可能导致无菌性假体松动，特别是没有应用骨水泥的髋关节成形术患者。少量的前瞻性研究对此进行了关注。Wurnig 等[238]对80例接受了预防性吲哚美辛的治疗的患者和82例作为对照组而未给予药物治疗的患者进行了前瞻性研究以评估异位骨化。作者在6年后的随访中并未发现在无骨水泥干周围有射线透射性的增强或其他放射学改变。相似的结果在另外一项研究中得到证实，提示 NSAID 可能不会造成假体周围骨组织成骨不良[239]。

总结与结论

已经证明 NSAID 是具有多种作用的围术期有效镇痛剂，而严重副作用发生率相对较低。它们的治疗效果在于机体接受疼痛刺激后抑制其炎症和痛觉过敏的发展。同时，对外周组织和 CNS 环氧合酶异构体的抑制是保证治疗效果的前提。目前市场上许多种 NSAID 半衰期短和经胃肠外给药的剂型适用于围术期大多数患者的治疗。对于许多种轻中度疼痛，这类药物单独使用即可发挥良好的镇痛效果。对于较严重的疼痛，NSAID 经常与阿片类药物或区域/局部麻醉联合应用。

业已证明，在腹腔镜检查、分娩、剖宫产和矫形外科手术如关节镜和全关节成形术后，NSAID 的镇痛效果非常好。对于胸廓切开术和剖腹手术等其他更严重疼痛的手术，效果不确切。NSAID 对术中疼痛的缓解似乎无效。

因为前列腺素在肾、血小板、脉管系统和 GI 中发挥着重要的作用，所以 NSAID 也会导致这类组织的一些不良反应。尽管相关文献指出，在短期治疗中很少见到严重的毒性作用，但在临床决定是否使用 NSAID 时，还是要考虑其相关毒性作用。虽然肾衰竭的风险可能并不因为使用 NSAID 而增加，但是在治疗低血容量和伴有肾损伤的患者时，必须十分谨慎。

同样，在已有溃疡或 GI 出血或接受糖皮质激素治疗的患者避免使用 NSAID，则 GI 毒性风险也很低。NSAID 降低血小板的聚集功能，延长出血时间，但是在大部分外科手术的实施过程中并不会造成显著出血。出血风险在泌尿道手术、ENT 手术，包括扁桃体切除术中似乎更大。虽然 NSAID 可升高血压和加剧充血性心力衰竭的症状，但是围术期使用非选择性的此类药物与心血管危险性无关。只有阿司匹林确定具有心脏保护效应。

毫无疑问，考昔类对血小板和 GI 的影响更小，但是它们可增加心肌梗死、脑卒中和心血管死亡的危险。在一些高危患者，甚至是 10d 的短期治疗即会发生这类不良反应。这类药物已面临禁用的处境——塞来昔布剂量和适应证已受到严格限制，罗非昔布和伐地考昔是否会被重新使用还不清楚。目前几种考昔类的毒性已得到证明，因此得出这一结论——即应观察这类药物的类效应，是合理。因为与其他 NSAID 相比，考昔类并无更佳镇痛效果，使用它们的唯一指征是对出血高危或 GI 毒性患者进行长期治疗。目前，尚无任何证据显示在外科手术中应用考昔类治疗利大于弊。

附录

目前，直接比较一种 NSAID 与一种阿片类药物镇痛效果的研究几乎没有。因为不同人群疼痛强度可能不可比，所以参考多个安慰剂对照研究，容易导出错误的结论。本章完成后，有一项随机双盲研究发表了，该研究直接比较了 1003 例术后中重度疼痛患者静脉注射吗啡（0.1mg/kg）和酮咯酸（30mg）的镇痛效果[278]。虽然吗啡的不良反应更多，但其镇痛效果优于酮咯酸。在吗啡中加用酮咯酸氨可显著降低吗啡剂量及不良反应发生率。

（项明琼 陈界石译 许 涛 邓小明校）

参考文献

1. Vane JR, Bakhle YS, Botting RM: Cyclooxygenases 1 and 2. Annu Rev Pharmacol Toxicol 1998;38:97–120.
2. Lim RK: Pain. Annu Rev Physiol 1970;32:269–288.
3. Chapman V, Dickenson AH: The spinal and peripheral roles of bradykinin and prostaglandins in nociceptive processing in the rat. Eur J Pharmacol 1992;219:427–433.
4. Biemond P, Swaak AG, Penders JA, et al: Superoxide production by polymorphonuclear leucocytes in rheumatoid arthritis and osteoarthritis: In vivo inhibition by the antirheumatic drug piroxicam due to interference with the activation of the NADPH-oxidase. Ann Rheum Dis 1986; 45:249–255.
5. Bomalaski JS, Hirata F, Clark M: Aspirin inhibits phospholipase C. Biochem Biophys Res Commun 1986;139:115–121.
6. Abramson SB, Weissman G: The mechanisms of action of nonsteroidal anti-inflammatory drugs. Arthritis Rheum 1989;32:1–9.
7. McCormack K, Brune K: Dissociation between the antinociceptive and anti-inflammatory effects of the nonsteroidal anti-inflammatory drugs: A survey of their analgesic efficacy. Drugs 1991;41:533–547.
8. Gordon SM, Brahim JS, Rowan J, et al: Peripheral prostanoid levels and nonsteroidal anti-inflammatory drug analgesia: Replicate clinical trials in a tissue injury model. Clin Pharm Ther 2002;72:175–183.
9. Svensson CI, Yaksh TL: The spinal phospholipase-cyclooxygenase - prostanoid cascade in nociceptive processing. Annu Rev Pharmacol Toxicol 2002;42:553–583.
10. Dirig DM, Yaksh TL: In vitro prostanoid release from spinal cord following peripheral inflammation: Effects of substance P, NMDA and capsaicin. Br J Pharmacol 1999;126:1333–1340.
11. Malmberg AB, Yaksh TL: Cyclooxygenase inhibition and the spinal release of prostaglandin E2 and amino acids evoked by paw formalin injection: A microdialysis study in unanesthetized rats. J Neurosci 1995;15:2768–2776.
12. Minami T, Uda R, Horiguchi S, et al: Allodynia evoked by intrathecal administration of prostaglandin E2 to conscious mice. Pain 1994;57: 217–223.
13. Ichitani Y, Shi T, Haeggstrom JZ, et al: Increased levels of cyclooxygenase-2 mRNA in the rat spinal cord after peripheral inflammation: An in situ hybridization study. Neuroreport 1997;8:2949–2952.
14. Samad TA, Moore KA, Sapirstein A, et al: Interleukin-1 beta-mediated induction of COX-2 in the CNS contributes to inflammatory pain hypersensitivity. Nature 2001;410:471–475.
15. Yaksh TL, Dirig DM, Conway CM, et al: The acute antihyperalgesic action of NSAIDs and release of spinal PGE2 is mediated by the inhibition of constitutive spinal COX-2 but not COX-1. J Neurosci 2001;21: 5847–5853.
16. Malmberg AB, Yaksh TL: Hyperalgesia mediated by spinal glutamate or substance P receptor blocked by spinal cyclooxygenase inhibition. Science 1992;257:1276–1279.
17. Brooks PM, Day RO: Nonsteroidal anti-inflammatory drugs—differences and similarities. N Engl J Med 1991;324:1716–1725.
18. Moote C: Efficacy of nonsteroidal anti-inflammatory drugs in the management of postoperative pain. Drugs 1992;44(Suppl 5):14–30.
19. Cryer B, Feldman M: Cyclooxygenase-1 and cyclooxygenase-2 selectivity of widely used nonsteroidal anti-inflammatory drugs. Am J Med 1998; 104:413–421.
20. Ebell MH, Siwek J, Weiss BD: Strength of recommendation taxonomy (SORT): A patient-centered approach to grading evidence in the medical literature. Am Fam Physician 2004;69:548–556.

21. Sandler AN: Post-thoracotomy analgesia and perioperative outcome. Minerva Anesthesiol 1999;65:267–274.
22. Scawn NDA, Pennefather SH, Soorae A, et al: Ipsilateral shoulder pain after thoracotomy with epidural analgesia: The influence of phrenic nerve infiltration. Anesth Analg 2001;93:260–264.
23. Loan WB, Morrison JD: The incidence and severity of postoperative pain. Br J Anesth 1967;39:695–698.
24. Perttunen K, Kalso E, Heinonen J, Salo J: IV diclofenac in post-thoracotomy pain. Br J Anesth 1992;68:474–480.
25. Rhodes M, Conacher I, Morritt G, Hilton C: Nonsteroidal antiinflammatory drugs for postthoracotomy pain: A prospective controlled trial after lateral thoracotomy. J Thorac Cardiovasc Surg 1992;103:17–20.
26. Murphy DF, Medley C: Preoperative indomethacin for pain relief after thoracotomy: Comparison with postoperative indomethacin. Br J Anaesth 1993;70:298–300.
27. Pavy T, Medley C, Murphy DF: Effect of indomethacin on pain relief after thoracotomy. Br J Anaesth 1990;65:624–627.
28. Power I, Bowler GMR, Pugh GC, Chambers WA: Ketorolac as a component of balanced analgesia after thoracotomy. Br J Anaesth 1994;72:224–226.
29. Singh H, Bossard RF, White PF, Yeatts RW: Effects of ketorolac versus bupivacaine coadministration during patient-controlled hydromorphone epidural analgesia after thoracotomy procedures. Anesth Analg 1997;84:564–569.
30. Puntillo K, Ley SJ: Appropriately timed analgesics control pain due to chest tube removal. Am J Crit Care 2004;13:292–301.
31. Merry AF, Wardall GJ, Cameron RJ, et al: Prospective, controlled, double-blind study of IV tenoxicam for analgesia after thoracotomy. Br J Anaesth 1992;69:92–94.
32. Merry AF, Sidebotham DA, Middleton NG, et al: Tenoxicam 20 mg or 40 mg after thoracotomy: A prospective, randomized, double-blind, placebo-controlled study. Anaesth Intensive Care 2002;30:160–166.
33. Bigler D, Moller J, Kamp-Jensen M, et al: Effect of piroxicam in addition to continuous thoracic epidural bupivacaine and morphine on postoperative pain and lung function after thoracotomy. Acta Anaesthesiol Scand 1992;36:647–650.
34. Landreneau RJ, Hazelrigg SR, Mack MJ, et al: Postoperative pain-related morbidity: Video-assisted thoracic surgery versus thoracotomy. Ann Thorac Surg 1993;56:1285–1289.
35. Perttunen K, Nilsson E, Kalso E: IV diclofenac and ketorolac for pain after thorascopic surgery. Br J Anaesth 1999;82:221–227.
36. McCrory C, Fitzgerald D: Spinal prostaglandin formation and pain perception following thoracotomy: A role for cyclooxygenase-2. Chest 2004;125:1321–1327.
37. Barkun JS, Barkun AN, Sampalis JS, et al: Randomized controlled trial of laparoscopic versus mini cholecystectomy: A national survey of 4292 hospitals and an analysis of 77604 cases. Lancet 1992;340:1116–1119.
38. Tate JJ, Chung SCS, Dawson J, et al: Conventional versus laparoscopic surgery for acute appendicitis. Br J Surg 1993;80:761–764.
39. McMahon AJ, Russell IT, Baxter JN, et al: Laparoscopic versus minilaparotomy cholecystectomy: A randomized trial. Lancet 1994;343:135–138.
40. Stiff G, Rhodes M, Kelly A, et al: Long-term pain: Less common after laparoscopic than open cholecystectomy. Br J Surg 1994;81:1368–1370.
41. Laparoscopic cholecystectomy in PROSPECT: Procedure-specific pain management. Available at www.postoppain.org/frameset.htm
42. Willis VL, Hunt DR: Pain after laparoscopic cholecystectomy. Br J Surg 2000;87:273–284.
43. Joris J, Thiry E, Paris P, et al: Pain after laparoscopic cholecystectomy: Characteristics and effect of intraperitoneal bupivacaine. Anesth Analg 1995;81:379–384.
44. Chi IC, Cole LP: Incidence of pain among women undergoing laparoscopic sterilization by electrocoagulation, the spring-loaded clip, and the tubal ring. Obst Gynecol 1979;137:397–401.
45. Alexander JI. Pain after laparoscopy. Br J Anesth 1997;79:369–378.
46. Green CR, Pandit SK, Levy L, et al: Intraoperative ketorolac has an opioid-sparing effect in women after diagnostic laparoscopy but not after laparoscopic tubal ligation. Anesth Analg 1996;82:732–737.
47. Shapiro MH, Duffy BL: Intramuscular ketorolac for postoperative analgesia following laparoscopic sterilisation. Anaesth Intensive Care 1994;22:22–24.
48. DeLucia JA, White PF: Effect of intraoperative ketorolac on recovery after outpatient laparoscopy. Anesthesiology 1991;75:A13.
49. Pandit SK, Kothary SP, Lebenbom-Mansour DO, et al: Failure of ketorolac to prevent severe post-operative pain following outpatient laparoscopy. Anesthesiology 1991;75:A33.
50. Campbell L, Plummer J, Owen H, et al: Effect of short-term ketorolac infusion on recovery following laparoscopic day surgery. Anaesth Intensive Care 2000;28:654–659.
51. Dunn TJ, Clark VA, Jones G: Preoperative oral naproxen for pain relief after day-case laparoscopic sterilization. Br J Anaesth. 1995;75:12–14.
52. Comfort VK, Code WE, Rooney ME, Yip RW: Naproxen premedication reduces postoperative tubal ligation pain. Can J Anaesth 1992;39:349–352.
53. Van EE R, Hemrika DJ, van der Linden CT: Pain relief following day-case diagnostic hysteroscopy-laparoscopy for infertility: A double-blind randomized trial with preoperative naproxen versus placebo. Obstet Gynecol 1993;82:951–954.
54. Hovorka J, Kallela H, Kortilla K: Effect of intravenous diclofenac on pain and recovery profile after day-case laparoscopy. Eur J Anaesthesiol 1993;10:105–108.
55. Edwards ND, Barclay K, Catling SJ, et al: Day case laparoscopy: A survey of postoperative pain and an assessment of the value of diclofenac. Anaesthesia 1991;46:1077–1080.
56. Windsor A, McDonald P, Mumtaz T, Millar JM: The analgesic efficacy of tenoxicam versus placebo in day case laparoscopy: A randomised parallel double-blind trial. Anaesthesia 1996;51:1066–1069.
57. Colbert SA, McCrory C, O'Hanlon DM, et al: A prospective study comparing intravenous tenoxicam with rectal diclofenac for pain relief in day case surgery. Eur J Anaesthesiol 1998;15:544–548.
58. Phinchantra P, Bunyavehchevin S, Suwajanakorn S, Wisawasukmongchol W: The preemptive analgesic effect of celecoxib for day-case diagnostic laparoscopy. J Med Assoc Thai 2004;87:283–288.
59. Ng A, Temple A, Smith G, Emembolu J: Early analgesic effects of parecoxib versus ketorolac following laparoscopic sterilization: A randomized controlled trial. Br J Anaesth 2004;92:846–849.
60. Davie IT, Slawson KB, Burt RA: A double-blind comparison of parenteral morphine, placebo, and oral fenoprofen in management of postoperative pain. Anesth Analg 1982;61:1002–1005.
61. Aho MS, Erkola OA, Scheinin H, et al: Effect of intravenously administered dexmedetomidine on pain after laparoscopic tubal ligation. Anesth Analg 1991;73:112–118.
62. Putland AJ, McCluskey A: The analgesic efficacy of tramadol versus ketorolac in day-case laparoscopic sterilisation. Anaesthesia 1999;54:382–385.
63. Cade L, Kakulas P: Ketorolac or pethidine for analgesia after elective laparoscopic sterilization. Anaesth Intensive Care 1995;23:158–161.
64. Rosenblum M, Weller RS, Conard PL, et al: Ibuprofen provides longer lasting analgesia than fentanyl after laparoscopic surgery. Anesth Analg 1991;73:255–259.
65. Salman MA, Yucebas ME, Coskun F, Aypar U: Day-case laparoscopy: A comparison of prophylactic opioid, NSAID or local anesthesia for postoperative analgesia. Acta Anaesthesiol Scand. 2000;44:536–542.
66. Crocker S, Paech M: Preoperative rectal indomethacin for analgesia after laparoscopic sterilization. Anesth Intensive Care 1992;20:337–340.
67. Hong JY, Lee IH: Suprascapular nerve block or a piroxicam patch for shoulder tip pain after day case laparoscopic surgery. Eur J Anesthesiol 2003;20:426.
68. McMahon AJ, Russell IT, Ramsay G, et al: Laparoscopic and minilaparotomy cholecystectomy: A randomized trial comparing postoperative pain and pulmonary function. Surgery 1994;115:533–539.
69. Fredman B, Olsfanger D, Jedeikin R: A comparative study of ketorolac and diclofenac on post-laparoscopic cholecystectomy pain. Eur J Anaesthesiol 1995;12:501–504.
70. Lane GE, Lathrop JC, Boysen DA, Lane RC: Effect of intramuscular intraoperative pain medication on narcotic usage after laparoscopic cholecystectomy. Am Surg 1996;62:907–910.
71. Wilson YG, Rhodes M, Ahmed R, et al: Intramuscular diclofenac sodium for postoperative analgesia after laparoscopic cholecystectomy: A randomised, controlled trial. Surg Laparosc Endosc 1994;4:340–344.
72. Forse A, El-Beheiry H, Butler PO, Pace RF: Indomethacin and ketorolac given preoperatively are equally effective in reducing early postoperative pain after laparoscopic cholecystectomy. Can J Surg 1996;39:26–30.

73. Horattas MC, Evans S, Sloan-Stakleff KD, et al: Does preoperative rofecoxib (Vioxx) decrease postoperative pain with laparoscopic cholecystectomy? Am J Surg 2004;188:271–276.
74. Gan TJ, Joshi GP, Zhao SZ, et al: Presurgical intravenous parecoxib sodium and follow-up oral valdecoxib for pain management after laparoscopic cholecystectomy surgery reduces opioid requirements and opioid-related adverse effects. Acta Anaesthesiol Scand 2004;48:1194–1207.
75. Liu J, Ding Y, White PF, et al: Effects of ketorolac on postoperative analgesia and ventilatory function after laparoscopic cholecystectomy. Anesth Analg 1993;76:1061–1066.
76. Elhakim M, Amine H, Kamel S, Saad F: Effects of intraperitoneal lidocaine combined with intravenous or intraperitoneal tenoxicam on pain relief and bowel recovery after laparoscopic cholecystectomy. Acta Anaesthesiol Scand 2000;44:929–933.
77. Nagele F, Connor HO, Davies A, et al: 2500 outpatient diagnostic hysteroscopies. Obstet Gynecol 1996;88:87–92.
78. Nagele F, Lockwood G, Magos AL: Randomised placebo controlled trial of mefenamic acid for premedication at outpatient hysteroscopy: A pilot study. Br J Obstet Gynecol 1997;104:842–844.
79. Tam WH, Yuen PM: Use of diclofenac as an analgesic in outpatient hysteroscopy: A randomized, double-blind, placebo-controlled study. Fertil Steril 2001;76:1070–1072.
80. Mercorio F, De Simone R, Landi P, et al: Oral dexketoprofen for pain treatment during diagnostic hysteroscopy in postmenopausal women. Maturitas 2002;43:277–281.
81. Ding Y, Fredman B, White PF: Use of ketorolac and fentanyl during outpatient gynecologic surgery. Anesth Analg 1993;77:205–210.
82. De Lia JE, Rodman KC, Jolles CJ: Comparative efficacy of oral flurbiprofen, intramuscular morphine sulfate, and placebo in the treatment of gynecologic postoperative pain. Am J Med 1986 24;80:60–64.
83. Jones RDM, Miles W, Prankerd R, et al: Tenoxicam IV in major gynecologic surgery—pharmacokinetic, pain relief and hematologic effects. Anesth Intensive Care 2000;28:491–500.
84. Tang J, Li S, White PF, et al: Effect of parecoxib, a novel intravenous cyclooxygenase type-2 inhibitor, on the postoperative opioid requirement and quality of pain control. Anesthesiology 2002;96:1305–1309.
85. Bloomfield SS, Mitchell J, Cissell G, Barden TP: Analgesic sensitivity of two post-partum pain models. Pain 1986;27:171–179.
86. Bloomfield SS, Cissell GB, Mitchell J, Barden TP: Codeine and aspirin analgesia in postpartum uterine cramps: Qualitative aspects of quantitative assessments. Clin Pharmacol Ther 1983;34:488–495.
87. Bloomfield SS, Barden TP, Mitchell J: Naproxen, aspirin, and codeine in postpartum uterine pain. Clin Pharmacol Ther 1977;21:414–421.
88. Sunshine A, Zighelboim I, Olson NZ, et al: A comparative oral analgesic study of indoprofen, aspirin, and placebo in postpartum pain. J Clin Pharmacol 1985;25:374–380.
89. Sunshine A, Zighelboim I, Laska E, et al: A double-blind, parallel comparison of ketoprofen, aspirin, and placebo in patients with postpartum pain. J Clin Pharmacol 1986;26:706–711.
90. Sunshine A, Roure C, Olson N, et al: Analgesic efficacy of two ibuprofen-codeine combinations for the treatment of postepisiotomy and postoperative pain. Clin Pharmacol Ther 1987;42:374–379.
91. Kitterman JA: Patent ductus arteriosus: Current clinical status. Arch Dis Child 1980;55:106–109.
92. Zukerman H, Shaler E, Gilad G, Katzuni E: Further study of the inhibition of premature labor by indomethacin—part II double blind study. J Perinat Med 1984;12:25–29.
93. Spigset O: Anesthetic agents and excretion in breast milk. Acta Anesth Scand 1994;38:94–103.
94. Code WE, Yip RW, Rooney ME, et al: Preoperative naproxen sodium reduces postoperative pain following arthroscopic knee surgery. Can J Anaesth 1994;41:98–101.
95. Ogilvie-Harris DJ, Bauer M, Corey P: Prostaglandin inhibition and the rate of recovery after arthroscopic meniscectomy: A randomised double-blind prospective study. J Bone Joint Surg Br 1985;67:567–571.
96. Nelson WE, Henderson RC, Almekinders LC, et al: An evaluation of pre- and postoperative nonsteroidal antiinflammatory drugs in patients undergoing knee arthroscopy: A prospective, randomized, double-blinded study. Am J Sports Med 1993;21:510–516.
97. Sandin R, Sternlo JE, Stam H, et al: Diclofenac for pain relief after arthroscopy: A comparison of early and delayed treatment. Acta Anaesthesiol Scand 1993;37:747–750.
98. Norris A, Un V, Chung F, et al: When should diclofenac be given in ambulatory surgery: Preoperatively or postoperatively? J Clin Anesth 2001;13:11–15.
99. Reuben SS, Bhopatkar S, Maciolek H, et al: The preemptive analgesic effect of rofecoxib after ambulatory arthroscopic knee surgery. Anesth Analg 2002;94:55–59.
100. Dennis AR, Leeson-Payne CG, Hobbs GJ: A comparison of diclofenac with ketorolac for pain relief after knee arthroscopy. Anaesthesia 1995;50:904–906.
101. Berti M, Albertin A, Casati A, et al: A prospective, randomized comparison of dexketoprofen, ketoprofen or paracetamol for postoperative analgesia after outpatient knee arthroscopy. Minerva Anestesiol 2000;66:549–554.
102. Laitinen J, Nuutinen L, Kiiskila EL, et al: Comparison of intravenous diclofenac, indomethacin and oxycodone as post-operative analgesics in patients undergoing knee surgery. Eur J Anaesthesiol 1992;9:29–34.
103. Barber FA, Gladu DE: Comparison of oral ketorolac and hydrocodone for pain relief after anterior cruciate ligament reconstruction. Arthroscopy 1998;14:605–612.
104. White PF, Joshi GP, Carpenter RL, Fragen RJ: A comparison of oral ketorolac and hydrocodone-acetaminophen for analgesia after ambulatory surgery: Arthroscopy versus laparoscopic tubal ligation. Anesth Analg 1997;85:37–43.
105. Dahl V, Dybvik T, Steen T, et al: Ibuprofen vs. acetaminophen vs. ibuprofen and acetaminophen after arthroscopically assisted anterior cruciate ligament reconstruction. Eur J Anaesthesiol. 2004;21:471–475.
106. Van Lancker P, Vandekerckhove B, Cooman F: The analgesic effect of preoperative administration of propacetamol, tenoxicam or a mixture of both in arthroscopic, outpatient knee surgery. Acta Anaesthesiol Belg 1999;50:65–69.
107. Colbert ST, Curran E, O'Hanlon DM, et al: Intra-articular tenoxicam improves postoperative analgesia in knee arthroscopy. Can J Anaesth 1999;46:653–657.
108. Elhakim M, Fathy A, Elkott M, Said MM: Intra-articular tenoxicam relieves post-arthroscopy pain. Acta Anaesthesiol Scand 1996;40:1223–1236.
109. Gupta A, Axelsson K, Allvin R, et al: Postoperative pain following knee arthroscopy: The effects of intra-articular ketorolac and/or morphine. Reg Anesth Pain Med 1999;24:225–230.
110. Izdes S, Orhun S, Turanli S, et al: The effects of preoperative inflammation on the analgesic efficacy of intraarticular piroxicam for outpatient knee arthroscopy. Anesth Analg 2003;97:1016–1019.
111. Pookarnjanamorakot C, Laohacharoensombat W, Jaovisidha S: The clinical efficacy of piroxicam fast-dissolving dosage form for postoperative pain control after simple lumbar spine surgery: A double-blinded randomized study. Spine 2002;27:447–451.
112. De Decker K, Vercauteren M, Hoffmann V, et al: Piroxicam versus tenoxicam in spine surgery: A placebo controlled study. Acta Anaesthesiol Belg 2001;52:265–269.
113. McGlew IC, Angliss DB, Gee GJ, et al: A comparison of rectal indomethacin with placebo for pain relief following spinal surgery. Anaesth Intensive Care 1991;19:40–45.
114. Nissen I, Jensen KA, Ohrstrom JK: Indomethacin in the management of postoperative pain. Br J Anaesth 1992;69:304–306.
115. Reuben SS, Connelly NR, Lurie S, et al: Dose-response of ketorolac as an adjunct to patient-controlled analgesia morphine in patients after spinal fusion surgery. Anesth Analg 1998;87:98–102.
116. Reuben SS, Connelly NR, Steinberg R: Ketorolac as an adjunct to patient-controlled morphine in postoperative spine surgery patients. Reg Anesth 1997;22:343–346.
117. Le Roux PD, Samudrala S: Postoperative pain after lumbar disc surgery: A comparison between parenteral ketorolac and narcotics. Acta Neurochir (Wien) 1999;141:261–267.
118. Bekker A, Cooper PR, Frempong-Boadu A, et al: Evaluation of preoperative administration of the cyclooxygenase -2 inhibitor rofecoxib for the treatment of postoperative pain after lumbar disc surgery. Neurosurgery 2002;50:1053–1057.
119. Karst M, Kegel T, Lukas A, et al: Effect of celecoxib and dexamethasone on postoperative pain after lumbar disc surgery. Neurosurgery 2003;53:331–336.
120. Reuben SS, Connelly NR: Postoperative analgesic effects of celecoxib

or rofecoxib after spinal fusion surgery. Anesth Analg 2000;91: 1221–1225.
121. Dahl V, Raeder JC, Drosdal S, et al: Prophylactic oral ibuprofen or ibuprofen-codeine versus placebo for postoperative pain after primary hip arthroplasty. Acta Anaesthesiol Scand 1995;39:323–326.
122. Buvanendran A, Kroin JS, Tuman KJ, et al: Effects of perioperative administration of a selective cyclooxygenase 2 inhibitor on pain management and recovery of function after knee replacement: A randomized controlled trial. JAMA 2003;290:2411–2418.
123. Reynolds LW, Hoo RK, Brill RJ, et al: The COX-2 specific inhibitor, valdecoxib, is an effective, opioid-sparing analgesic in patients undergoing total knee arthroplasty. J Pain Symptom Manag 2003;25: 133–141.
124. Malan TP Jr, Marsh G, Hakki SI, et al: Parecoxib sodium, a parenteral cyclooxygenase-2 selective inhibitor, improves morphine analgesia and is opioid-sparing following total hip arthroplasty. Anesthesiology 2003;98:950–956.
125. Rasmussen GL, Steckner K, Hogue C, et al: Intravenous parecoxib sodium for acute pain after orthopedic knee surgery. Am J Orthop 2002;31:336–343.
126. Etches RC, Warriner CB, Badner N, et al: Continuous intravenous administration of ketorolac reduces pain and morphine consumption after total hip or knee arthroplasty. Anesth Analg 1995;81:1175–1180.
127. Bugter ML, Dirksen R, Jhamandas K, et al: Prior ibuprofen exposure does not augment opioid drug potency or modify opioid requirements for pain inhibition in total hip surgery. Can J Anaesth 2003;50:445–449.
128. Hommeril JL, Bernard JM, Gouin F, Pinaud M: Ketoprofen for pain after hip and knee arthroplasty. Br J Anaesth 1994;72:383–387.
129. Iohom G, Walsh M, Higgins G, Shorten G: Effect of perioperative administration of dexketoprofen on opioid requirements and inflammatory response following elective hip arthroplasty. Br J Anaesth 2002;88:520–526.
130. Boeckstyns ME, Backer M, Petersen EM, et al: Piroxicam spares buprenorphine after total joint replacement: Controlled study of pain treatment in 81 patients. Acta Orthop Scand 1992;63:658–660.
131. Anderson SK, al Shaikh BA: Diclofenac in combination with opiate infusion after joint replacement surgery. Anaesth Intensive Care 1991;19:535–538.
132. Segstro R, Morley-Forster PK, Lu G: Indomethacin as a postoperative analgesic for total hip arthroplasty. Can J Anaesth 1991;38:578–581.
133. Schlondorff D: Renal prostaglandin synthesis: Sites of production and specific actions of prostaglandins. Am J Med 1986;81:1–10.
134. Scharschmidt L, Simonson M, Dunn MJ: Glomerular prostaglandins, angiotensin II, and nonsteroidal anti-inflammatory drugs. Am J Med 1986;81:30–42.
135. Komhoff M, Grone HJ, Klein T, et al: Localization of cyclooxygenase -1 and -2 in adult and fetal human kidney: Implication for renal function. Am J Physiol 1997;272:F460–F468.
136. Dunn MJ, Zambraski EJ: Renal effects of drugs that inhibit prostaglandin synthesis. Kidney Int 1980;18:609–622.
137. Novis BK, Roizen MF, Aronson S, Thisted RA: Association of preoperative risk factors with postoperative acute renal failure. Anesth Analg 1994;78:143–149.
138. Zipser RD, Hoefs JC, Speckart PF, et al: Prostaglandins: Modulators of renal function and pressor resistance in chronic liver disease. J Clin Endocrinol Metab 1979;48:895–909.
139. Walshe JJ, Venuto RC: Acute oliguric renal failure induced by indomethacin: Possible mechanism. Ann Intern Med 1979;91:47–49.
140. Feldman HI, Kinman JL, Berlin JA, et al: Parenteral ketorolac: The risk for acute renal failure. Ann Intern Med 1997;126:193–199.
141. Lee A, Cooper MC, Craig JC, et al: The effects of nonsteroidal anti-inflammatory drugs (NSAIDs) on postoperative renal function. Cochrane Database Syst Rev 2004;(2):CD002765.
142. Swan SK, Rudy DW, Lasseter KC, et al: Effect of cyclooxygenase-2 inhibition on renal function in elderly persons receiving a low-salt diet. Ann Intern Med 2000;133:1–9.
143. Rossat J, Maillard M, Nussberger J, et al: Renal effects of selective cyclooxygenase -2 inhibition in normotensive salt-depleted subjects. Clin Pharmacol Ther 1999;66:76–84.
144. Lichtenstein DR, Syngal S, Wolfe MM: Nonsteroidal anti-inflammatory drugs and the gastrointestinal tract. Arthritis Rheum 1995; 38:5–18.

148. Ristimaki A, Honkanen N, Jankala H, et al: Expression of cyclooxygenase -2 in human gastric carcinoma. Cancer Res 1997;57: 1276–1280.
149. Halter F, Tarnaski AS, Schmassman A, Peskar BM: Cyclooxygenase 2—implications on maintenance of gastric mucosal integrity and ulcer healing: Controversial issues and perspectives. Gut 2001;49:443–453.
150. Schoen RT, Vender RJ: Mechanisms of nonsteroidal anti-inflammatory drug induced gastric damage. Am J Med 1989;86:449–458.
151. Whittle BJR, Higgs GA, Eakins KE, et al: Selective inhibition of prostaglandin production in inflammatory exudates and gastric mucosa. Nature 1980;284:271–273.
152. Raskin JB: Gastrointestinal effects of nonsteroidal anti-inflammatory therapy. Am J Med 1999;106:3S–12S.
153. Graham DY, Smith JL, Dobbs SM: Gastric adaptation occurs with aspirin administration in man. Dig Dis Sci 1983;28:1–6.
154. O'Laughlin JC, Hoftiezer JW, Ivey KJ: Effect of aspirin on the human stomach in normals: Endoscopic comparison of damage produced on hour, 24 hours, and 2 weeks after administration. Scand J Gastroenterol Suppl 1981;67:211–214.
155. Strom BL, Berlin JA, Kinman JL, et al: Parenteral ketorolac and risk of gastrointestinal and operative site bleeding: A postmarketing surveillance study. JAMA 1996;275:376–382.
156. Forrest JB, Camu F, Greer IA, et al: Ketorolac, diclofenac, and ketoprofen are equally safe for pain relief after major surgery. Br J Anaesth 2002;88:227–233.
157. Silverstein FE, Graham DY, Senior JR, et al: Misoprostol reduces serious gastrointestinal complications in patients with rheumatoid arthritis receiving nonsteroidal anti-inflammatory drugs. Ann Intern Med 1995;123:241–249.
158. Ehsanullah RSB, Page MC, Tildesley G, Wood JR: Prevention of gastroduodenal damage induced by nonsteroidal anti-inflammatory drugs: Controlled trial of ranitidine. BMJ 1988;297:1017–1021.
159. Robinson MG, Griffin JW, Bowers J, et al: Effect of ranitidine on gastroduodenal mucosal damage induced by nonsteroidal anti-inflammatory drugs. Dig Dis Sci 1989;34:424–428.
160. Yeomans ND, Tulassay Z, Juhasz L, et al: A comparison of omeprazole with ranitidine for ulcers associated with nonsteroidal anti-inflammatory drugs. N Engl J Med 1998;338:719–726.
161. Hawkey CJ, Karrasch JA, Szczepanski L, et al: Omeprazole compared with misoprostol for ulcers associated with nonsteroidal anti-inflammatory drugs. N Engl J Med 1998;338:727–734.
162. Bombardier C, Laine L, Reicin A, et al: Comparison of upper gastrointestinal toxicity of rofecoxib and naproxen in patients with rheumatoid arthritis. VIGOR Study Group. Engl J Med 2000;343:1520–1528.
163. Silverstein FE, Faich G, Goldstein JL, et al: Gastrointestinal toxicity with celecoxib vs. nonsteroidal anti-inflammatory drugs for osteoarthritis and rheumatoid arthritis: The CLASS study: A randomized controlled trial. Celecoxib Long-term Arthritis Safety Study. JAMA 2000;284:1247–1255.
164. Stemme V, Swedenborg J, Claesson H, Hansson GK: Expression of cyclooxygenase -2 in human atherosclerotic carotid arteries. Eur J Vasc Endovasc Surg 2000;20:146–152.
165. Schonbeck U, Sukhova GK, Graber P, et al: Augmented expression of cyclooxygenase -2 in human atherosclerotic lesions. Am J Pathol 1999;155:1281–1291.
166. Belton O, Byrne D, Kerney D, et al: Cyclooxygenase-1 and -2-dependent prostacyclin formation in patients with atherosclerosis. Circulation 2000;102:840–845.
167. Fitzgerald GA: Cardiovascular pharmacology of nonselective nonsteroidal antiinflammatory drugs and coxibs: Clinical considerations. Am J Cardiol 2002;89(Suppl):26D–32D.
168. Vila L: Cyclooxygenase and 5-lipoxygenase pathways in the vessel wall: Role in atherosclerosis. Med Res Rev 2004;24:399–424.
169. Ross R: Atherosclerosis: An inflammatory disease. N Engl J Med 1999;340:115–126.
170. Smith EF, Lefer AM: Stabilization of cardiac lysosomal and cellular membranes in protection of ischemic myocardium due to coronary occlusion: Efficacy of the nonsteroidal antiinflammatory agent, naproxen. Am Heart J 1981;101:394–402.
171. Garcia Rodriguez LA, Varas C, Patrono C: Differential effects of aspirin and nonaspirin nonsteroidal antiinflammatory drugs in the primary prevention of myocardial infarction in post-menopausal

2002;162:1099–1104.
173. Ray WA, Stein C, Hall K, et al: Nonsteroidal antiinflammatory drugs and risk of serious coronary heart disease. Lancet 2002;359:118–123.
174. Rahme E, Pilote L, Lelorier J: Association between naproxen use and protection against acute myocardial infarction. Arch Intern Med 2002;162:1111–1115.
175. Watson DJ, Rhodes T, Cai HB, Guess HA: Lower risk of thromboembolic events with naproxen among patients with rheumatoid arthritis. Arch Intern Med 2002;162:1105–1110.
176. Mamdani M, Rochon P, Juurlinl DN, et al: Effect of cyclooxygenase 2 inhibitors and naproxen on short-term risk of acute myocardial infarction in the elderly. Arch Intern Med 2003;163:481–486.
177. Fitzgerald GA, Patrono C: The coxibs, selective inhibitors of cyclooxygenase-2. N Engl J Med 2001;345:433–442.
178. Verma S, Raj SR, Shewchuk L, et al: Cyclooxygenase-2 blockade does not impair endothelial vasodilator function in healthy volunteers: Randomized evaluation of rofecoxib versus naproxen on endothelium-dependent vasodilation. Circulation 2001;104:2879–2882.
179. Fitzgerald GA, Smith B, Pedersen AK, Brash AR: Increased prostacyclin biosynthesis in patients with severe atherosclerosis and platelet activation. N Engl J Med 1984;310:1065–1068.
180. Cipollone F, Prontera C, Pini B, et al: Overexpression of functionally coupled cyclooxygenase-2 and prostaglandin E synthase in symptomatic atherosclerotic plaques as a basis of prostaglandin E2-dependent plaque instability. Circulation 2001;104:921–927.
181. Hankey GJ, Eikelboom JW: Cyclooxygenase-2 inhibitors: Are they really atherothrombotic, and if not, why not? Stroke 2003;34:2736–2740.
182. Nussmeier NA, Whelton AA, Brown MT, et al: Complications of the COX-2 inhibitors parecoxib and valdecoxib after cardiac surgery. N Engl J Med 2005;352:1081–1091.
183. Mukherjee D, Nissen SE, Topol EJ: Risk of cardiovascular events associated with selective COX-2 inhibitors. JAMA 2001;286:954–959.
184. Solomon DH, Schneeweiss S, Glynn RJ, et al: Relationship between selective cyclooxygenase inhibitors and acute myocardial infarction in older adults. Circulation 2004;109:2068–2073.
185. Chenevard R, Hürlimann D, Béchir M, et al: Selective COX-2 inhibition improves endothelial function in coronary artery disease. Circulation 2003;107:415–419.
186. Altman R, Luciardi HL, Muntaner J, et al: Efficacy assessment of meloxicam, a preferential cyclooxygenase -2 inhibitor, in acute coronary syndromes without ST-segment elevation: The Nonsteroidal Anti-Inflammatory Drugs in Unstable Angina Treatment-2 (NUT-2) Study. Circulation 2002;106:191–195.
187. Konstam MA, Weir MR, Reicin A, et al: Cardiovascular thrombotic events in controlled, clinical trials of rofecoxib. Circulation 2001;104:2280–2288.
188. Jüni P, Nartey L, Reichenbach S, et al: Risk of cardiovascular events and rofecoxib: Cumulative meta-analysis. Lancet 2004;364:2021–2029.
189. Bresalier RS, Sandler RS, Quan H, et al: Cardiovascular events associated with rofecoxib in a colorectal adenoma chemoprevention trial. N Engl J Med 2005;352:1092–1102.
190. Solomon SD, McMurray JJV, Pfeffer MA, et al, Adenoma Prevention with Celecoxib (APC) Study Investigators: Cardiovascular risk associated with celecoxib in a clinical trial for colorectal adenoma prevention. N Engl J Med 2005;352:1071–1080.
191. Wennmalm A: Influence of indomethacin on the systemic and pulmonary vascular resistance in man. Clin Sci 1978;54:141–145.
192. Nowak J, Wennmalm A: Influence of indomethacin and of prostaglandin E1 on total and regional blood flow in man. Acta Physiol Scand 1978;102:484–491.
193. Safar ME, Hornych AF, Levenson JA, et al: Central hemodynamics and plasma prostaglandin E2 in borderline and sustained essential hypertensive patients before and after indomethacin. Clin Sci 1981;61:323S–325S.
194. Brown J, Dollery C, Valdes G: Interaction of nonsteroidal anti-inflammatory drugs with antihypertensive and diuretic agents: Control of vascular reactivity by endogenous prostanoids. Am J Med 1986;81:43–57.
195. Pope JE, Anderson JJ, Felson DT: A meta-analysis of the effects of nonsteroidal anti-inflammatory drugs on blood pressure. Arch Intern Med 1993;153:477–484.
196. Muscara MN, Vergnolle N, Lovren F, et al: Selective cyclooxygenase-2 inhibition with celecoxib elevates blood pressure and promotes leukocyte adhesion. Br J Pharmacol 2000;129:1423–1430.
197. FDA CLASS Advisory Committee: CLASS Advisory Committee Briefing Document. Feb 7 2001. Available at www.fda.gov/ohrms/dockets/ac/01/briefing/3677_b1_searle.pdf
198. Whelton A, White WB, Bello AE, et al: Effects of celecoxib and rofecoxib on blood pressure and edema in patients ≥65 years of age with systemic hypertension and osteoarthritis. Am J Cardiol 2002;90:959–963.
199. Collins R, Peto R, MacMahon S, et al: Blood pressure, stroke, and coronary heart disease. Part 2: Short-term reductions in blood pressure: Overview of randomized drug trials in their epidemiological context. Lancet 1990;335:827–838.
200. Bleumink GS, Feenstra J, Sturkenboom MCJM, Stricker BH: Nonsteroidal anti-inflammatory drugs and heart failure. Drugs 2003;63:525–534.
201. Page J, Henry D: Consumption of NSAIDs and the development of congestive heart failure in elderly patients. Arch Intern Med 2000;160:777–784.
202. Feenstra J, Heerdink ER, Grobbee DE, Stricker BH: Association of nonsteroidal anti-inflammatory drugs with first occurrence of heart failure and with relapsing heart failure. Arch Intern Med 2002;162:265–270.
203. Schafer AI: Effects of nonsteroidal anti-inflammatory therapy on platelets. Am J Med 1999;106:25S–36S.
204. Schafer AI: Effects of nonsteroidal anti-inflammatory drugs on platelet function and systemic hemostasis. J Clin Pharmacol 1995;35:209–219.
205. Cronberg S, Wallmark E, Soderberg I: Effect on platelet aggregation of oral administration of 10 nonsteroidal analgesics to humans. Scand J Haematol 1984;33:155–159.
206. Stuart MJ, Miller ML, Davey FR, Wold JA: The post-aspirin bleeding time: A screening test for evaluating haemostatic disorders. Br J Haematol 1979;43:649–659.
207. Barbui T, Buelli M, Cortelazzo S, et al: Aspirin and risk of bleeding in patients with thrombocythemia. Am J Med 1987;83:265–268.
208. Deykin D, Janson P, McMahon L: Ethanol potentiation of aspirin-induced prolongation of bleeding time. N Engl J Med 1982;306: 852–854.
209. Jakubowski JA, Vaillancourt R, Deykin D: Interaction of ethanol, prostacyclin, and aspirin in determining human platelet reactivity in vitro. Arteriosclerosis 1988;8:436–441.
210. James MJ, Walsh JA: Effects of aspirin and alcohol on platelet thromboxane synthesis and vascular prostacyclin synthesis. Thromb Res 1985;39:587–593.
211. Forrest JB, Camu F, Greer IA, et al: Ketorolac, diclofenac, and ketoprofen are equally safe for pain relief after major surgery. Br J Anesth 2002;88:227–233.
212. Wierod FS, Frandsen NJ, Jacobsen JD, et al: Risk of haemorrhage from transurethral prostatectomy in acetylsalicylic acid and NSAID-treated patients. Scand J Urol Nephrol 1998;32:120–122.
213. Zhu JP, Davidsen MB, Meyhoff HH: Aspirin, a silent risk factor in urology. Scand J Urol Nephrol 1994;29:369–374.
214. Marret E, Flahault A, Samama CM, Bonnet F: Effects of postoperative, nonsteroidal, anti–inflammatory drugs on bleeding risk after tonsillectomy: Meta-analysis of randomized, controlled trials. Anesthesiology 2003;98:1497–1502.
215. Moiniche S, Romsing J, Dahl JB, Tramer MR: Nonsteroidal anti-inflammatory drugs and the risk of operative site bleeding after tonsillectomy: A quantitative systematic review. Anesth Analg 2003;96:68–77.
216. Romsing J, Walther-Larsen S: Peri-operative use of nonsteroidal anti-inflammatory drugs in children: Analgesic efficacy and bleeding. Anaesthesia 1997;52:673–683.
217. Assia EI, Raskin T, Kaiserman I, et al: Effect of aspirin intake on bleeding during cataract surgery. J Cataract Refract Surg 1998; 24:1243–1246.
218. Connelly CS, Panush RS: Should nonsteroidal anti-inflammatory drugs be stopped before elective surgery? Arch Intern Med 1991;151:1963–1966.
219. Slappendel R, Weber EW, Benraad B, et al: Does ibuprofen increase perioperative blood loss during hip arthroplasty? Eur J Anaesthesiol 2002;19:829–831.
220. Amrein PC, Ellman L, Harris WH: Aspirin-induced prolongation of bleeding time and perioperative blood loss. JAMA 1981;245:1825–1828.

221. Schnitzer TJ, Donahue JR, Toomey EP, et al: Effect of nabumetone on hemostasis during arthroscopic knee surgery. Clin Ther 1998; 20:110–124.
222. Horlocker TT, Wedel DJ, Benzon H, et al: Regional anesthesia in the anticoagulated patient: Defining the risks (the second ASRA Consensus Conference on Neuraxial Anesthesia and Anticoagulation). Reg Anesth Pain Med 2003;28:172–197.
223. CLASP: A randomized trial of low-dose aspirin for the prevention and treatment of pre-eclampsia among 9364 pregnant women. CLASP (Collaborative Low-Dose Aspirin Study in Pregnancy) Collaborative Group. Lancet 1994;343:619–629.
224. Horlocker TT, Bajwa ZH, Ashraft Z, et al: Risk assessment of hemorrhagic complications associated with nonsteroidal anti-inflammatory medications in ambulatory pain clinic patients undergoing epidural steroid injection. Anesth Analg 2002;95:1691–1697.
225. Gajraj NM: The effect of cyclooxygenase -2 inhibitors on bone healing. Reg Anesth Pain Med 2003;28:456–465.
226. Kawaguchi H, Pilbeam CC, Harrison JR, Raisz LG: The role of prostaglandins in the regulation of bone metabolism. Clin Orthop 1995;313:36–46.
227. Dekel S, Lenthall G, Francis MJ: Release of prostaglandins from bone and muscle after tibial fracture: An experimental study in rabbits. J Bone Joint Surg Br 1981;63:185–189.
228. Allen HW, Wase A, Bear WT: Indomethacin and aspirin: Effect of nonsteroidal anti-inflammatory agents on the rate of fracture repair in the rat. Acta Orthop Scand 1980;51:595–600.
229. Altman RD, Latta LL, Keer R, et al: Effect of nonsteroidal anti-inflammatory drugs on fracture healing: A laboratory study in rats. J Orthop Trauma 1995;9:392–400.
230. Hogevold HE, Grogaard B, Reikeras O: Effects of short-term treatment with corticosteroids and indomethacin on bone healing. Acta Orthop Scand 1992;63:607–611.
231. Simon AM, Manigrasso MB, O' Connor JP: Cyclooxygenase 2 function is essential for bone fracture healing. J Bone Miner Res 2002; 17:963–976.
232. Zhang X, Schwarz EM, Young DA: Cyclooxygenase-2 regulates mesenchymal cell differentiation into the osteoblast lineage and is critically involved in bone repair. J. Clin Invest. 2002;109:1405–1415.
233. Giannoudis PV, MacDonald DA, Matthews SJ, et al: Nonunion of the femoral diaphysis: The influence of reaming and nonsteroidal anti-inflammatory drugs. J Bone Joint Surg Br 2000;82:655–658.
234. Smith RM: Personal communication, 2005.
235. Glassman SD, Rose SM, Dimar JR, et al: The effect of postoperative nonsteroidal anti-inflammatory drug administration on spinal fusion. Spine 1998;23:834–838.
236. Davis TRC, Ackroyd CE: Nonsteroidal anti-inflammatory agents in the management of Colles' fractures. Br J Clin Pract 1988;42:184–189.
237. Neal BC, Rodgers A, Clark T, et al: A systematic survey of 13 randomized trials of non-steroidal anti-inflammatory drugs for the prevention of heterotopic bone formation after major hip surgery. Acta Orthop Scand 2000;71:122–128.
238. Wurnig C, Schwameis E, Bitzan P, Kainberger F: Six-year results of a cementless stem with prophylaxis against heterotopic bone. Clin Orthop 1998;361:150–158.
239. Persson E, Sodemann B, Nilsson OS: Preventive effects of ibuprofen on periarticular heterotopic ossification after total hip arthroplasty. Acta Orthop Scand 1998;69:111–115.
240. Carretta A, Zannini P, Chiesa G, et al: Efficacy of ketorolac tromethamine and extrapleural intercostals nerve block on postthoracotomy pain: A prospective, randomized study. Int Surg 1996; 81:224–228.
241. Prados W, Blaylock S: The effect of ketorolac on the postoperative narcotic requirements of gynecological surgery outpatients. Anesthesiology 1991;75:A6.
242. Yeh CC, Wu CT, Lee MS, et al: Analgesic effects of preincisional administration of dextromethorphan and tenoxicam following laparoscopic cholecystectomy. Acta Anaesthesiol Scand 2004;48: 1049–1053.
243. Munro FJ, Young SJ, Broome IJ, et al: Intravenous tenoxicam for analgesia following laparoscopic cholecystectomy. Anaesth Intensive Care 1998;26:56–60.
244. Rorarius MG, Suominen P, Baer GA, et al: Diclofenac and ketoprofen for pain treatment after elective caesarean section. Br J Anaesth 1993;70:293–297.
245. Elhakim M, Nafie M: IV tenoxicam for analgesia during caesarean section. Br J Anaesth 1995;74:643–646.
246. Bush DJ, Lyons G, MacDonald R: Diclofenac for analgesia after caesarean section. Anaesthesia 1992;47:1075–1077.
247. Pavy TJ, Paech MJ, Evans SF: The effect of intravenous ketorolac on opioid requirement and pain after cesarean delivery. Anesth Analg 2001;92:1010–1014.
248. Lowder JL, Shackelford DP, Holbert D, Beste TM: A randomized, controlled trial to compare ketorolac tromethamine versus placebo after cesarean section to reduce pain and narcotic usage. Am J Obstet Gynecol. 2003;189:1559–1562.
249. Wilder-Smith CH, Hill L, Dyer RA, et al: Postoperative sensitization and pain after cesarean delivery and the effects of single IM doses of tramadol and diclofenac alone and in combination. Anesth Analg 2003;97:526–533.
250. Olofsson CI, Legeby MH, Nygards EB, Ostman KM: Diclofenac in the treatment of pain after caesarean delivery: An opioid-saving strategy. Eur J Obstet Gynecol Reprod Biol 2000;88:143–146.
251. Lim NL, Lo WK, Chong JL, Pan AX: Single dose diclofenac suppository reduces post-cesarean PCEA requirements. Can J Anaesth 2001;48:383–386.
252. Dennis AR, Leeson-Payne CG, Hobbs GJ: Analgesia after caesarean section: The use of rectal diclofenac as an adjunct to spinal morphine. Anaesthesia 1995;50:297–299.
253. Cardoso MM, Carvalho JC, Amaro AR, et al: Small doses of intrathecal morphine combined with systemic diclofenac for postoperative pain control after cesarean delivery. Anesth Analg 1998;86: 538–541.
254. Sun HL, Wu CC, Lin MS, et al: Combination of low-dose epidural morphine and intramuscular diclofenac sodium in postcesarean analgesia. Anesth Analg 1992;75:64–68.
255. Rautoma P, Santanen U, Avela R, et al: Diclofenac premedication but not intra-articular ropivacaine alleviates pain following day-case knee arthroscopy. Can J Anaesth 2000;47:220–224.
256. Hoe-Hansen C, Norlin R: The clinical effect of ketoprofen after arthroscopic subacromial decompression: A randomized double-blind prospective study. Arthroscopy 1999;15:249–252.
257. Rasmussen S, Thomsen S, Madsen SN, et al: The clinical effect of naproxen sodium after arthroscopy of the knee: A randomized, double-blind, prospective study. Arthroscopy 1993;9:375–380.
258. Smith I, Shively RA, White PF: Effects of ketorolac and bupivacaine on recovery after outpatient arthroscopy. Anesth Analg 1992;75: 208–212.
259. Arvidsson I, Eriksson E: A double blind trial of NSAID versus placebo during rehabilitation. Orthopedics 1987;10:1007–1014.
260. Pedersen P, Nielsen KD, Jensen PE: The efficacy of Na-naproxen after diagnostic and therapeutic arthroscopy of the knee joint. Arthroscopy 1993;9:170–173.
261. Morrow BC, Bunting H, Milligan KR: A comparison of diclofenac and ketorolac for postoperative analgesia following day-case arthroscopy of the knee joint. Anaesthesia 1993;48:585–587.
262. Twersky RS, Lebovits A, Williams C, Sexton TR: Ketorolac versus fentanyl for postoperative pain management in outpatients. Clin J Pain 1995;11:127–133.
263. McLoughlin C, McKinney MS, Fee JP, Boules Z: Diclofenac for day-care arthroscopy surgery: Comparison with a standard opioid therapy. Br J Anaesth 1990;65:620–623.
264. Drez D Jr, Ritter M, Rosenberg TD: Pain relief after arthroscopy: Naproxen sodium compared to propoxyphene napsylate with acetaminophen. South Med J 1987;80:440–443.
265. Morrow BC, Milligan KR, Murthy BV: Analgesia following day-case knee arthroscopy—the effect of piroxicam with or without bupivacaine infiltration. Anaesthesia 1995;50:461–463.
266. Gurkan Y, Kilickan L, Buluc L, et al: Effects of diclofenac and intra-articular morphine/bupivacaine on postarthroscopic pain control. Minerva Anestesiol 1999;65:741–745.
267. Mack PF, Hass D, Lavyne MH, et al: Postoperative narcotic requirement after microscopic lumbar discectomy is not affected by intraoperative ketorolac or bupivacaine. Spine 2001;26:658–661.
268. Rosenow DE, Albrechtsen M, Stolke D: A comparison of patient-

controlled analgesia with lornoxicam versus morphine in patients undergoing lumbar disk surgery. Anesth Analg 1998;86:1045–1050.
269. Fletcher D, Negre I, Barbin C, et al: Postoperative analgesia with IV propacetamol and ketoprofen combination after disc surgery. Can J Anaesth 1997;44:479–485.
270. Thienthong S, Jirarattanaphochai K, Krisanaprakornkit W, et al: Treatment of pain after spinal surgery in the recovery room by single dose lornoxicam: A randomized, double blind, placebo-controlled trial. J Med Assoc Thai 2004;87:650–655.
271. Silvanto M, Lappi M, Rosenberg PH: Comparison of the opioid-sparing efficacy of diclofenac and ketoprofen for 3 days after knee arthroplasty. Acta Anaesthesiol Scand 2002;46:322–328.
272. Zhou TJ, Tang J, White PF: Propacetamol versus ketorolac for treatment of acute postoperative pain after total hip or knee replacement. Anesth Analg 2001;92:1569–1575.
273. Kostamovaara PA, Hendolin H, Kokki H, Nuutinen LS: Ketorolac, diclofenac and ketoprofen are equally efficacious for pain relief after total hip replacement surgery. Br J Anaesth 1998;81:369–372.
274. Eggers KA, Jenkins BJ, Power I: Effect of oral and IV tenoxicam in postoperative pain after total knee replacement. Br J Anaesth 1999;83:876–881.
275. Beattie WS, Warriner CB, Etches R, et al: The addition of continuous intravenous infusion of ketorolac to a patient-controlled analgetic morphine regime reduced postoperative myocardial ischemia in patients undergoing elective total hip or knee arthroplasty. Anesth Analg 1997;84:715–722.
276. Fragen RJ, Stulberg SD, Wixson R, et al: Effect of ketorolac tromethamine on bleeding and on requirements for analgesia after total knee arthroplasty. J Bone Joint Surg Am 1995;77:998–1002.
277. Reuben SS, Fingeroth R, Krushell R, Maciolek H: Evaluation of the safety and efficacy of the perioperative administration of rofecoxib for total knee arthroplasty. J Arthroplasty 2002;17:26–31.
278. Cepeda MS, Carr DB, Miranda N, et al: Comparison or morphine, ketorolac, and their combination for postoperative pain. Anesthesiology 2005;103:1225–1232.

19 多模式镇痛疗法

JOSEPH PERGOLIZZI · LEONARD M. WILLS

多模式镇痛的循证依据

循证医学（EBM）有助于决策为患者选择最合适的治疗方案。本书目的是运用 EBM 的原则进行急性疼痛的治疗（有关 EBM 的一般概念已在第 1 章和第 2 章论述）。本章主要论述多模式治疗——即联合运用不同作用机制的药物或技术。多模式治疗不只局限于疼痛控制方面，其已普遍应用于全世界的临床实践。例如在另一篇文章中提到的多模式治疗指通过使用作用机制不同的几种化疗药物，同时进行放疗或手术来治疗癌症。因此，多模式疼痛治疗是一个广泛的概念，适用于治疗肿瘤、感染、高血压和许多其他情况[1]。

围术期使用多模式镇痛在节约药物方面的益处已被一个多学科专家组确认。他们召开会议研究了关于术后恶心呕吐的文献（postoperative nausea and vomiting，PONV），以提出处理 PONV 的循证指南。专家组得出的结论认为，围术期使用多模式镇痛治疗不仅能提高镇痛效果，也降低了 PONV 发生率，尤其在采用了节约阿片类药物技术后[2]。

本章描述了多模式镇痛的基本原理，包括其可能的利弊和固定剂量联合用药；应用 EBM 技术综合分析了有关多模式镇痛的文献；指出现有文献的局限性；陈述了关于这一话题系统性定性的回顾结果。

多模式镇痛的基本原理

疼痛可能源于不同的病因和机制——感受伤害性、炎症性和神经病理性（见表 19-1；图 19-1）。疼痛治疗是针对不同的受体、酶、通径和过程。由于疼痛通常是多种机制同时起作用所介导的，因此宜合理地联合几种同时针对不同靶位点的药物以达到更完全地抑制伤害性感受。联合两种或多种不同作用机制的镇痛药物，不仅可提高疗效，也可通过减少不良反应而增加安全性，甚至通过它们互补的药代动力学活性，而对镇痛时程有更大的预见性[3,4]。旁注 19-1 列出了多模式镇痛的常用药物。

多模式镇痛治疗的潜在优点

尽管单一形式的镇痛有效，但是所有镇痛药物都有不良反应。非甾体类抗炎药（NSAID）可导致胃肠道不适和出血，而阿片类可引起恶心、呕吐、镇静和便秘。多模式镇痛可减少每种药物的剂量（节约药物），因此减轻各种药物不良反应的严重程度，同时达到与单种药物相同或更好的解痛效果（图 19-2）。多模式镇痛也可减少不良反应（包括其发生率、严重性、类型），提供更好的镇痛效果（起效、持续时间和镇痛质量），而且更方便、可行（旁注 19-2）。由于每种药物可能都有叠加或协同作用[5]，因此当联合用药时，每种药物都要使用较低的初始剂量，延长用药间隔时间，减慢给药速度。

表 19-1	刺激种类和处理过程		
疼痛	刺激	机制	特性
感受伤害性	短暂性	"活化"广动力域神经元,"激惹性"	压迫感,灼热感,可逆性
炎症性	反复性	"调制",中枢和外周敏化	痛觉过敏,痛觉异常,慢性可逆
神经病理性	持久性	"修改",神经营养性变化,中枢敏化	痛觉过敏,痛觉异常,自发疼痛持久性

From Woolf CJ, Salter MW: Neuronal plasticity: Increasing the gain in pain. Science 2000;288:1765-1769.

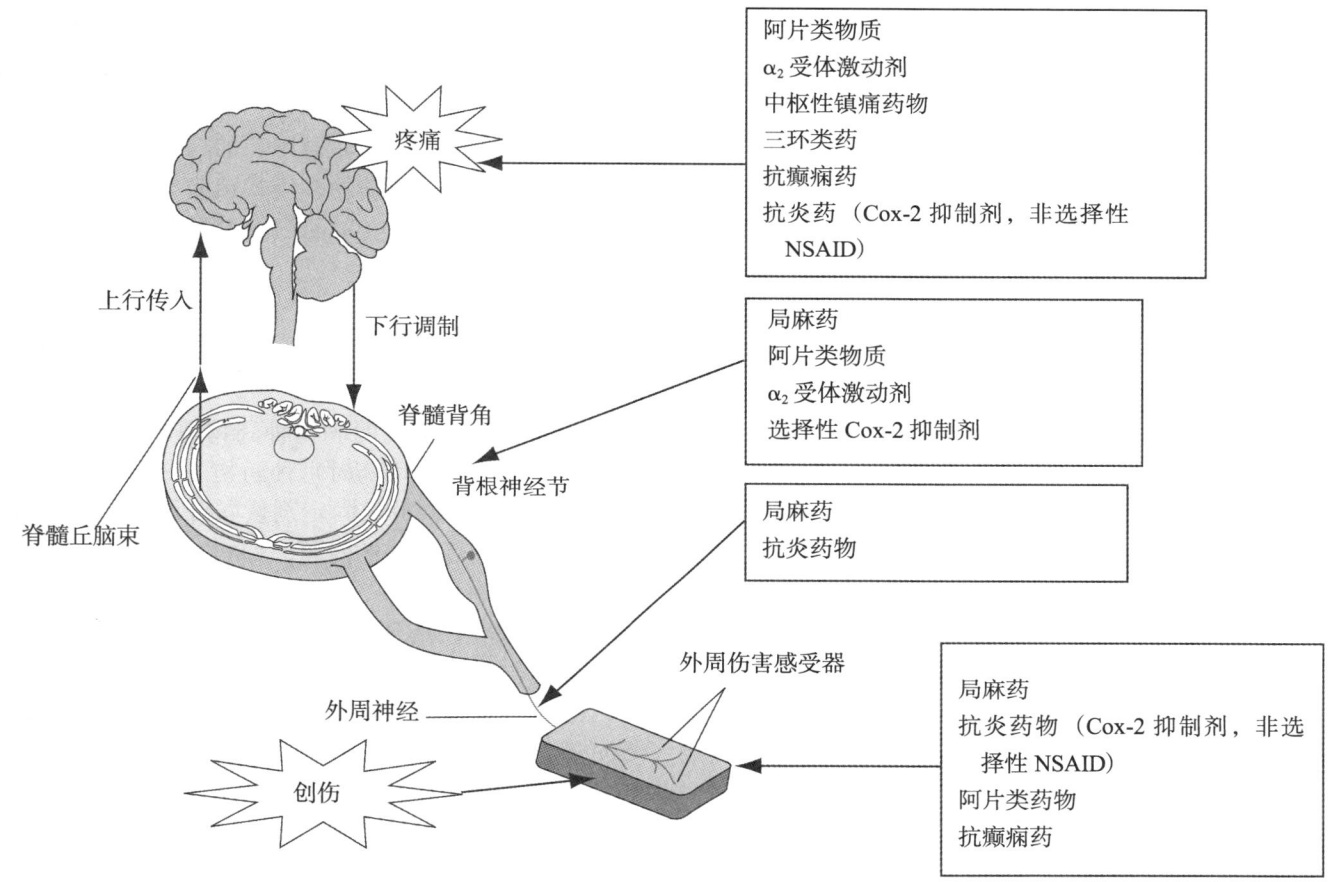

图 19-1 镇痛及疼痛通径。(Adapted from Gottschalk A. Smith DS: New concepts in acute pain therapy: Preemptive analgesia. Am Fam Physician 2001; 63:1979–1984.)

旁注 19-1	多模式镇痛的常用药物

- 局部麻醉药
- 阿片类药物
- 非选择性非甾体类抗炎药（NSAID）
- Cox-2 选择性抑制剂
- 对乙酰氨基酚
- 抗痛觉超敏药：抗 NMDA 作用（氯胺酮、右美沙芬、金刚烷胺、美金刚），加巴喷丁，腺苷，α_2 受体激动剂等
- 其他辅助治疗：补充和替代医学（CAM）、经皮电神经刺激等

旁注 19-2	多模式镇痛的潜在益处

- 协同镇痛效应：作用的起效时间与持续时间，镇痛质量等
- 预防疼痛或弱化伤害性感受
- 减轻应激反应
- 减弱敏化作用
- 改善不良反应：发生率、严重程度、类型等
- 改善依从性：方便性等
- 改善效价比

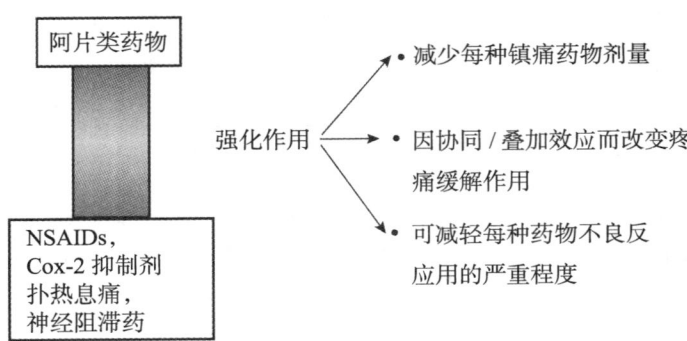

图19-2 多模式镇痛的潜在益处。(From Kehlet H, Dahl JB: The value of "multimodal" or "balanced analgesia" in postoperative pain treatment. Anesth Analg 1993;77:1048-1056.)

数项研究已表明通过联合用药可节约药物。如将在下面讨论的可少用阿片类、少用 NSAID 和少用 Cox-2 抑制剂的联合用药[3,6-8]。研究证实多模式镇痛治疗的益处，例如少用阿片类药物的联合用药方式，可以通过使用较低剂量的阿片类药物来避免镇静和呼吸抑制，减轻便秘和瘙痒，降低术后恶心呕吐的风险，而且患者也可更快恢复，更早出院[9-11]。

多模式镇痛治疗的潜在缺点

较低剂量镇痛药物的联合应用有如下主要的可能结果：

- 极好结果——不良反应发生率降低，镇痛效果更好；
- 很好结果——镇痛效果相同，不良反应发生率降低；
- 尚好结果——不良反应发生率相同，但镇痛效果更好；
- 不良结果——不良反应发生率较高，但镇痛效果更好；
- 极差结果——不良反应发生率较高，镇痛效果相同。

用药安全性是最重要的：联合用药必须最大限度地减少不良反应的发生率。即使不良反应发生率确实减少，也要求从临床角度考虑其意义。一些研究已经证实多模式镇痛并没有提供叠加或协同镇痛作用。一些联合用药模式能够增强镇痛，但也增加不良反应。在这种情况下，必须评定这种联合用药是否是真正的多模式镇痛——即这种特殊联合用药是针对多种疼痛路径，而不是针对同一疼痛路径的两种药物的简单组合？同时使用两种或多种药物并不能保证它们在临床上相互协同作用。而且，在一些特殊情况下，使用时必须考虑所用药物的药代动力学和药效动力学特性。

在某些情况下，如治疗老年患者，多模式治疗和使用多种药物可增加发生不良反应及多种疾病的风险。因为患者已经同时服用数种药物，如降脂药等。产生不同毒性的有关因素包括年龄相关的药代动力学、药效动力学和生理因素以及同时存在的疾病状态。多种药物混合服用是一个特殊问题，当医生并不清楚患者服用哪些药物时，无意间开出的处方可能会与已服用药物发生相互竞争或相互干扰。多种药物混合服用甚至可能改变镇痛效果和联合用药的药代动力学及药效动力学特性。一个成功的多模式镇痛例子就是美国常用的偏头痛三联处方，对乙酰氨基酚联合阿司匹林及咖啡因。

固定剂量与灵活剂量联合用药的比较

现有临床数据已明确每种药物等效镇痛的剂量，从而固定剂量联合用药时每种药物的剂量都应低于这个基础值（表19-2）。固定剂量联合用药能够克服灵活剂量联合用药带来的问题，如相互作用指数低、不良反应发生率增加等，还能防止患者自行调整药量。固定剂量联合用药还能增强镇痛效果、加大疗效谱、加大益处与风险比率以及患者的依从性。

表示两种药物联合时如何相互作用的一种方式是等效线图解法（isobologram），它是一种分析简单化学混合物质联合作用的常用图表性统计工具。建立一个等效线图，首先必须建立一个基点来计量单独使用一种特殊药物或两种药物以不同比例混合的结果。具有代表性的是，评价镇痛药物用于急性疼痛时，基点是

表 19-2	联合治疗
为什么联合？	建立最优联合用药比率
联合什么？	具有不同作用机制的药物
用多少剂量？	开始联合每种药物的 1/2 剂量，然后以固定比率增加/减少剂量
其他	保持一种药物剂量不变，增加其他药物剂量
哪种途径给药？	侵袭最小
变量	镇痛效果和不良反应

Material taken from the first Meeting of the Working Group on Pain Management, Dec. 14, 2005, Taplow, UK. Courtesy of Professor M. Puig.

使50%疼痛缓解。然后,描出两种药物同时使用达到同一基点的剂量。当两种药物剂量比率发生变化时,达到该同一基点所需的剂量可能低于达到同样基点时所需每种药物剂量相对应的直线。如果是这样的话,那么两种药物的相互作用就是所谓的协同作用;如果两种药物剂量的比率正好落在该直线上,那么其相互作用称为相加作用;如果高于该直线,那就称为拮抗作用。

曲马多是一种中枢性阿片类镇痛药,具有两种相互补充的作用机制:与阿片类μ受体相结合及抑制去甲肾上腺素和5-羟色胺的再摄取。对乙酰氨基酚是一种非阿片类解热镇痛药,也是较弱的前列腺素生物合成抑制剂。图19-3显示曲马多和对乙酰氨基酚联合使用的等效线图,显示了它们在每种剂量联合时都是协同作用。在实验中,老鼠先分别单独口服曲马多、对乙酰氨基酚或两种药物固定剂量混合物。30min后注射化学刺激物(乙酰胆碱),没有特定的行为反应即提示存在镇痛效果(实际上为抗伤害性感受)。在等效线图解法中,连接每种药物的平均 ED_{50} 值成一直线,ED_{50} 是由曲马多和对乙酰氨基酚单独的剂量-反应曲线得出的[(0, y) 和 (x, 0)]坐标之间仅描出了 ED_{50} 值]。连接两种药物的 ED_{50} 得出一条线,表示曲马多和对乙酰氨基酚联合使用在理论上两者是相加作用。

接着,使用两种药物的实际固定剂量混合物进行实验,从这些剂量-反应曲线中确定的 ED_{50} 值描绘为开环,每条线代表了一个特定联合用药的 ED_{50}。在相加作用直线之下的 ED_{50} 值为协同作用区域(在其上为拮抗作用区域)。该曲线是由实验确定的 ED_{50} 拟合得出的。

药物相互作用可用等效线图解法来评定,等效线图解法可以帮助决定药物联合使用时的最佳剂量比率。图19-4显示联合使用曲马多和安乃近8h时的研究范例。从图上反映产生了同样反应水平的(视觉模拟量表疼痛评分为2.4~2.7)安乃近(横坐标)和曲马多(纵坐标)平均累加剂量[平均标准差(SEM)]。对角线连接每种药物单独使用时达到同样效果时的剂量,称之为相加作用直线(零相互作用直线)。图中其他点是通过描出每个治疗组中每一对联合用药的累加量(SEM)得出的[12]。这些药物是在子宫肌瘤术后镇痛以1:1的效价联合应用。它们在镇痛和不良反应方面都呈协同作用,包括恶心、呕吐和镇静,治疗指数大约为3[12]。

联合用药的调整

目前,权威部门仅批准了有限的联合镇痛药物配

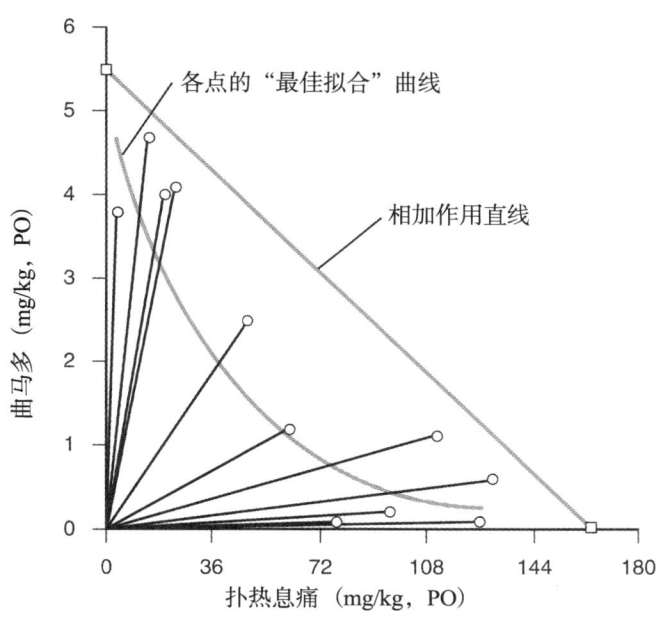

图19-3 曲马多和对乙酰氨基酚以不同剂量联合使用的等效线图解法。(From Tallarida RJ, Raffa RB. Testing for synergism over a range of fixed ratio drug combinations. Replacing the isobologram. Life Sci 1996;58:PL23—PL28.)

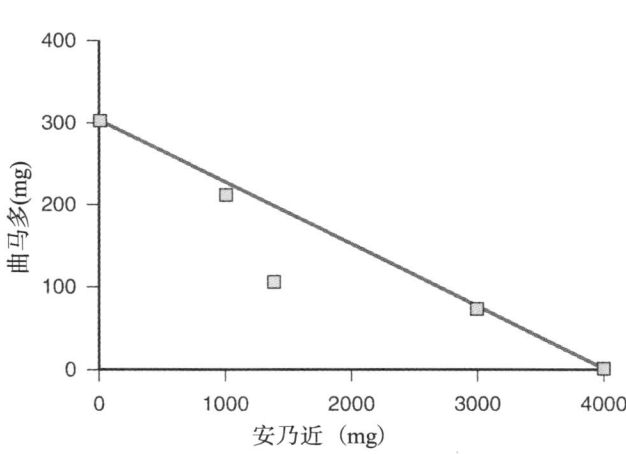

图19-4 曲马多-安乃近相互作用的等效线图解法。(From Montes A, et al: Use of intravenous patient-controlled analgesia for the documentation of synergy between tramadol and metamizol. Brit J Anaesth 2000;85:217-223.)

方来处理术后疼痛。绝大多数镇痛药物的联合都是"宽松"的联合，它们都未经正规机构如美国食品药品管理局（FDA）和欧洲药品评估机构（EMEA）的严格测试。因而，对所有患者来说，它们真正的药理学和临床效果都是未知数。

像 FDA 和 EMEA 这类的正规机构已经修订了测试和批准联合治疗方案的程序。现在 FDA 要求建立单剂量研究，从而可以将镇痛药物固定剂量联合用药与单一药物、安慰剂及标准组相比较。更重要的是，考虑将一个新的镇痛药联用方法用于所有类型的疼痛和患者时，必须要证明其比任一单药都更有益、有效。

为了解决镇痛药物应该如何联用的问题，制药公司已经介绍几种固定剂量联用制剂，而且正在计划推出更多制剂。然而，公司资助的试验越来越倾向于公布对其有利的数据，包括固定剂量联合用药。关于这一问题，De Angelis 等[13]在 2004 年《新英格兰医学杂志》中发表头条文章指出：公司资助的临床试验所得结果除非此试验首先已登记在册，否则不应在同行评审的杂志上刊出。登记处必须可电子查询，而且公众可无偿使用，对所有登记注册者公开，而且必须建立确保登记数据真实可靠的机制[13]。而且，他们提议试验组织者应该签署完整的加强报告试验标准（CONSORT）承诺和 Cochrane 数据库文件。同样重要的是，需要灵活剂量联合用药，特别是在较大范围的人群中；需要进一步评价其在特殊人群中的药代动力学与药效动力学特征和临床效果，如小儿和老年患者。

多模式镇痛/抗痛觉过敏

已用于围手术期减轻伤害性感受敏化的辅助药（见后）和局麻药（抗痛觉过敏药）包括抗 NMDA（氯胺酮、右美沙芬、金刚烷胺、美金刚）、加巴喷丁、腺苷、α_2-肾上腺素受体激动剂、利多卡因和美西律[14]。抗痛觉过敏药氯胺酮 0.5mg/kg 治疗术后疼痛患者，术后 1～7d 疼痛区域少于 25cm^2（使用安慰剂为 175～200cm^2）[15]。加巴喷丁在超前镇痛方面具有潜在的益处，从而预防与手术刺激相关的更大的神经元敏化；而且该药具有抗痛觉过敏特性，能够防止患者伤害性感受系统发生手术恶性后遗症，如慢性疼痛[16-18]。Menigaux[19]在实施关节镜前交叉韧带修复术的研究中，术后 1d 和 2d 分别使用加巴喷丁 1200mg 能达到最大活动度的 76% 和 84%（而使用安慰剂则为 63% 和

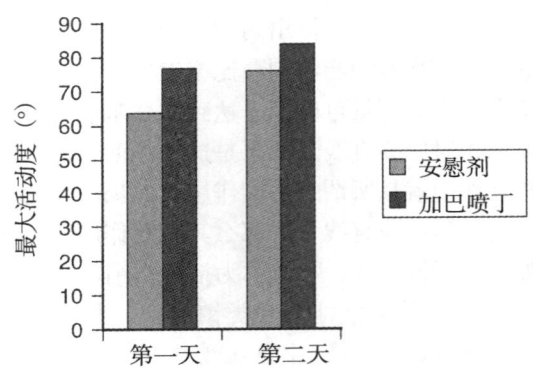

图 19-5 加巴喷丁在关节镜行前交叉韧带修复中的抗痛觉过敏特性。(From Menigaux C, Adam F, Guignard B, et al: Preoperative gabapentin decreases anxiety and improves early functional recovery from knee surgery. Anesth Analg 2005;100: 1394-1399.)

76%）（图 19-5）。理论上，联合应用其他具有不同作用机制的药物可加强加巴喷丁潜在的保护作用。

现在临床试验正在研究传统阿片类药物和抗痛觉过敏药固定剂量联合用药。例如，氯胺酮能减少已用吗啡患者手术切口周围痛觉过敏区域[15]。并进一步研究了术中使用"亚镇痛剂量"氯胺酮对术后痛觉过敏的影响[20]。

现在正在应用和研究灵活剂量联合用药，但至今仍无 IA 类数据[I 代表大型随机对照试验（RCT），每组 N≥100，A 代表支持建议的有利证据]。Panchal 等[21]报道了开胸手术患者联合应用镇痛药/抗痛觉过敏药的最新的成功范例（表 19-3）。

循证综述：急性疼痛的单一疗法和多模式镇痛

大多数药物都作为一个单独药物进行过研究；然而，正如文章所述，多模式疗法是联合应用各种不同类型的药物。这样就引出一个问题，即是否已经应用循证的方法来确定多模式镇痛的风险/益处比率，尤其当临床试验设计方法和结果报道方法存在相关问题时。

单一疗法不满意

大多数患者接受单一疗法来治疗术后疼痛[18]，而且有足够数据显示许多镇痛药物单次剂量用于该适应

表 19-3	开胸手术患者的镇痛和抗痛觉超敏治疗
术前和术中	1. 伐地考昔 40mg 口服和加巴喷丁 1200mg 口服加上 2. 切皮前经胸段硬膜外（T4-T5 或 T3-T4）注入 0.25%布比卡因 3~5ml；术中每 2 h 追加一次
术后镇痛	持续： 1. 胸段硬膜外使用 0.0625%布比卡因加 1μg/ml 舒芬太尼作为患者自控镇痛：间隔 10 分钟给予 3~5ml，基础速率 3~4ml/h 2. 每日口服 40mg 伐地考昔，服用 14 天

证的效果，但调查结果却表明患者通常对术后疼痛处理不满意[22]。近几十年来的临床统计数据说明传统治疗方法镇痛不充分，近期国家的统计和调查结果提示术后疼痛治疗一直不完善[23-24]。

镇痛不足和患者不满意的原因可能是所选用特殊治疗方法所致。例如，在这种情况下，经常会使用阿片类药物，但众所周知，正在接受一种镇痛药物治疗的术后疼痛患者更愿意接受非阿片类药物治疗（图 19-6）[25]。此时，可能优先考虑非阿片类或少用阿片类的用药方案。错误可能就是这种替代和补充方法。单一疗法只是针对可能介导疼痛刺激的许多通径之一；

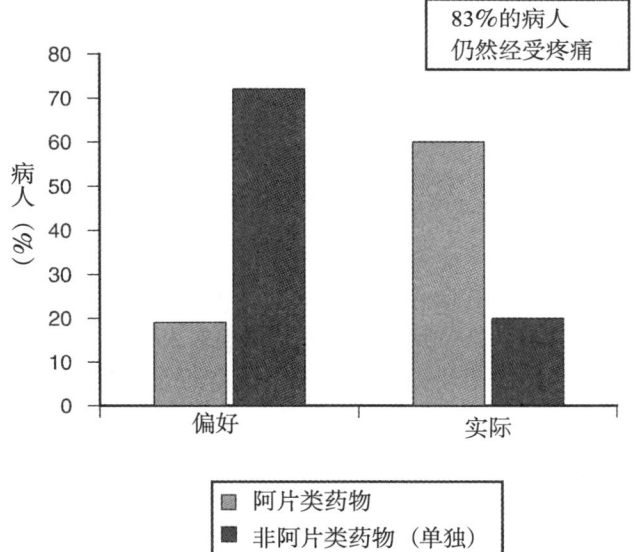

图 19-6 术后疼痛：患者偏好和实际接受的镇痛治疗。(From Apfelbaum JL: Postoperative pain experience:Results from a national survey suggest postoperative pain continues to be undermanaged. Anesth Analg 2003;97:534-540.)

多模式疗法除了可以减少剂量，还通过作用于多条疼痛通径，而可能起到更好效果。

多模式疗法结果的系统性回顾

为了系统性回顾急性疼痛的多模式镇痛结果，作者从描述疼痛多模式治疗的 10 个术语（见附录）中选择三个最常用的术语，检索 1995-2004 年的 Medline 文摘，检索出 47 项涉及"多模式疼痛治疗"或"多模式疼痛方法"的 RCT，35 项涉及"多模式镇痛"的 RCT。这些术后镇痛试验对固定剂量与灵活剂量联合用药药物、辅助用药与替代用药（alternative medicine，CAM）以及联合镇痛技术进行了评价。但是不能对这些试验进行荟萃分析，因为它们在研究人群、联合药物、剂量方案、给药途径以及结果评定和研究持续时间方面都有很大差异。

多模式疗法的阳性结果

大多数来自 Medline 的研究都报道了阳性结果。数项研究显示，阿片类物质可增强联合用药的镇痛效果，而其他研究证实多模式镇痛中阿片类药物剂量可减少或用药时间可延长。Buvanendran 等[26]研究显示，在全膝关节成形术后，多模式镇痛中使用 Cox-2 抑制剂罗非考昔可减少阿片类药物的用量（少用阿片类药物），也可缓解疼痛，减少呕吐和睡眠干扰，并改善运动范围。NSAID 和阿片类因通过不同机制起效，故二者联用可达到协同镇痛效果。Hanna 等[27]指出，使用酮洛芬可以减少吗啡用量，而且镇痛效果良好。最近一项综合性荟萃分析证实，在患者自控镇痛（PCA）吗啡中加入 NSAID 可减少阿片类药物的使用[28]。

数项研究探讨了剖宫产术后多模式镇痛中阿片类药物的应用。Cardoso 等[29]评价了鞘内低剂量吗啡联合肌注双氯芬酸，结果证实 0.025mg 吗啡剂量下镇痛效果良好，吗啡导致瘙痒的发生率低。事实上，当联合使用双氯芬酸时，较大剂量吗啡并不能增加任何益处。另一项研究结果显示：鞘内注入吗啡、切口浸润布比卡因并联合布洛芬和对乙酰氨基酚的患者，术后早期镇痛效果优于应用静脉 PCA（IV-PCA）吗啡，而后改为联合口服对乙酰氨基酚与可待因[30]。

Michaloliakou 等[10]发现，对于日间腹腔镜胆囊切除术后疼痛患者，多模式镇痛（局部麻醉药+NSAID+阿片类药物）相对于单种镇痛药物加盐水来说，可明显降低疼痛患者数量、疼痛严重程度（减轻6倍）以及恶心发生率，而且更早达到满意出院。

数项研究已经表明，减少Cox-2抑制剂的多模式镇痛方案可用于治疗病理1年以上的骨关节患者。Emhey等[31]和Silverfield等[32]报道曲马多和对乙酰氨基酚作为Cox-2抑制剂的辅助用药有效而安全。进一步分析Silverfield关于老年患者的数据得出了与总体研究一样的阳性结果[33]。

快速起效的非巴比妥类麻醉药（抗痛觉过敏药）氯胺酮已经作为多模式镇痛的辅助用药。Chia等[34]证实，大手术患者多模式硬膜外镇痛（吗啡、布比卡因和肾上腺素）中加入氯胺酮能更好地缓解术后疼痛，减少镇痛药物使用，而且会起到镇痛相加的效果。Menigaux等[35]进行的类似研究证明，膝关节镜术后，在多模式镇痛（吗啡、萘普生钠和联丙氧芬）中加入氯胺酮能提高镇痛效果，改善功能恢复。

2篇Cochrane数据库的综述结果显示，术后多模式镇痛的结论不一致。第一篇是定量分析单用羟考酮、羟考酮加对乙酰氨基酚治疗急性术后疼痛的RCT（77项报道）。大多数羟考酮剂量下以及羟考酮加对乙酰氨基酚的镇痛效能显著优于空白组。羟考酮加用或不加用对乙酰氨基酚的镇痛效能似乎与肌内注射吗啡和NSAID一样，尽管其常伴有中枢神经系统不良反应[36]。第二篇综述包括数项试验及一项荟萃分析，其比较了右丙氧芬单用与联合对乙酰氨基酚治疗中重度术后疼痛的效果。术后镇痛治疗中，65mg右丙氧芬加上650mg对乙酰氨基酚的疗效相当于单剂量的100mg曲马多，但是前者不良事件的发生率较低。然而650mg对乙酰氨基酚加上60mg可待因疗效似乎更好，不良反应相近[37]。

曲马多与对乙酰氨基酚联合用药 如本章前面所述，曲马多加对乙酰氨基酚是FDA批准的固定剂量联合用药的范例。这两种药物都是有效的镇痛药，且有不同的药代动力学特性。当联用时，它们作用于两条不同而互补的通径，能达到优于单独用药的镇痛目的，且不良反应减少。曲马多加对乙酰氨基酚的药代动力学特性产生了有益的药效动力学特征，即对乙酰氨基酚快速起效，而曲马多持续时间长，从而可用于急性和慢性疼痛治疗（图19-7）。

总之，多模式镇痛已在几种急性疼痛状态下显示其镇痛优势。联合NSAID、阿片类药物和（或）Cox-

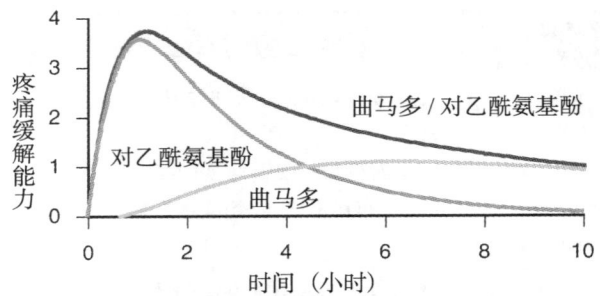

图19-7 曲马多和对乙酰氨基酚两种药物联用时有益的药代/药效动力学特性，显示随着时间的积累，曲马多和对乙酰氨基酚的疼痛缓解能力分离。

2抑制剂会产生相加或协同的镇痛效果，镇痛平稳，效果较好和（或）不良反应发生率较低，身体和心理恢复较快，制动和康复时间较短[28,38-46]。总之，现有资料综述和循证指南支持以多模式镇痛作为控制术后疼痛的默认方法[47]。

多模式超前镇痛的阳性结果

手术创伤使得患者对伤害感受敏化，从而导致术后疼痛程度放大、疼痛时间延长。使用阿片类药物多模式超前镇痛可有效地抑制这种疼痛。Rockemann等[48]指出，在腹部手术前多模式超前镇痛（双氯芬酸、安乃近、硬膜外吗啡和甲哌卡因）能显著降低术后处理疼痛的需要，切皮前用药的效果优于手术结束时用药。Rosaeg等[49]证明，在关节镜膝韧带修复术患者，多模式超前镇痛使用酮咯酸、关节内注射吗啡/罗哌卡因/肾上腺素及罗哌卡因股神经阻滞可降低疼痛评分，减少吗啡用量。

多模式镇痛的阴性或可疑结果

显然，并非所有单用时可有效镇痛的药物在多模式镇痛中同样有效。正如前面讨论的等效线图解法数据所示，联合治疗并不总是能改善患者的结果。而且，联用某些镇痛药物还能导致不良反应增加。数项多模式镇痛双盲RCT的结果混杂或呈阴性。如Choi等[50]指出，剖宫产患者硬膜外使用吗啡的基础上加口服右美沙芬并未减轻术后疼痛。Paech等[51]对240例女性患者进行的研究认为：剖宫产在蛛网膜下腔联合使用布比卡因、芬太尼、吗啡和可乐定的，疼痛缓解的效果优于单独使用吗啡或可乐定，但是增加术中嗜睡和呕吐的可能。Keita等[52]将盐水、布比卡因、吗啡分别与布比卡因加吗啡在妇科腹腔镜手术后镇痛进行比较，发现并不能显著改善术后镇痛。

多模式超前镇痛的阴性或可疑结果

Nagatsuka 等[53]报道，在下颌升支矢状劈开截骨术中，使用双氯芬酸、布托啡诺和利多卡因并无超前镇痛效果[53]。Doyle 和 Bowler[54]也指出，在后外侧开胸术前进行多模式超前镇痛（吗啡、双氯芬酸、肋间神经阻滞）对镇痛效果、镇痛药使用量和远期结果影响甚微。Reuben 等[55]的研究表明，急诊前交叉韧带修复术后患者接受多模式镇痛（包括围术期 NSAID、关节内注射布比卡因以及外敷冰块）的镇痛效果并不优于加用关节内注射吗啡[55]。

从 2005 年起，Cochrane 数据库没有对多模式镇痛在术后应用进行评价。然而，来自 Cochrane 数据库的 Bell[56]的一份报道定量分析了 4 项 RCT 和 32 项多模式镇痛/抗痛觉过敏药联合药物的研究，探讨了氯胺酮作为阿片类药物的辅助用药在治疗癌症疼痛方面的作用。研究表明氯胺酮可改善吗啡的疗效，然而，资料的合并分析并不恰当，而且一些患者在吗啡单用和与氯胺酮合用时均出现幻觉。Bell 结论认为，现有证据不足以证明氯胺酮可用作阿片类药物疗法的辅助用药。

多模式镇痛：现有选择和进退两难的窘境

几种主要镇痛药物联合应用可能导致不良反应增加，能获得相同或协同的镇痛效果。这些镇痛药包括局麻药、阿片类药物、非选择性 NSAID、Cox-2 抑制剂、α_2 激动剂和对乙酰氨基酚（表 19-4）。最常见的联合用药是阿片类药物 + NSAID±局麻药+辅助药物。辅助药物通常对于人类伤害性疼痛作用弱或几无镇痛作用，但能增强经典镇痛药对伤害性疼痛感觉的镇痛效果。一些辅助药物是治疗神经病理性疼痛的一线药物。一些用于治疗急性术后疼痛的联合用药范例如下：

- 阿片类药物 +NSAID 或 α_2 激动剂
- 吗啡 + 氯胺酮
- 对乙酰氨基酚 +NSAID

用于治疗急性术后疼痛（脊髓性疼痛）的例子是局麻药 + 阿片类药物±α_2 激动剂。

表 19-4 多模式镇痛方案中的镇痛药物 *

非甾体类抗炎药	对乙酰氨基酚
	Cox-2 抑制剂
	双氯芬酸
	布洛芬
	酮洛芬
	酮咯酸
	萘普生
阿片类药物	布托啡诺
	可待因
	芬太尼
	吗啡
	羟考酮
	曲马多
局麻药	布比卡因
	利多卡因
	甲哌卡因
	罗哌卡因
辅助药物	α_2- 受体激动剂
	抗癫痫药
	抗抑郁药
	氯胺酮

* 见正文

药物联合应用于术后疼痛的选择

镇痛药都有其各自的优缺点。多模式镇痛选择合适的药物组合是成功治疗术后疼痛的关键。表 19-5 列出了 NSAID、Cox-2 抑制剂和阿片类药物的一些优缺点。

尤其值得一提的是，NSAID 为多模式药物治疗提供了一个基础。这些药物在联合用药中可增强阿片类药物在几个 CNS 区域的镇痛作用，降低不良反应，如最常见的尿潴留、呼吸抑制和 CNS 作用。阿片类药物通常用于治疗术后疼痛是因为它们用于镇痛时没有封顶效应。然而，增加阿片类药物剂量可导致无法忍受的不良反应，因此限制了它们在急性疼痛治疗中单独使用或作为主要成分的使用[57]。NSAID 在多模式镇痛中的作用及其优点见旁注 19-3。

表 19-5　不同种类镇痛药物的比较

镇痛药物种类	优点	缺点
非选择性 NSAID	有效缓解与肌肉骨骼疼痛有关的炎症 急性术后疼痛中短期使用（<1 周）所致胃肠道或心血管风险的不良反应最小	长期使用非选择性 NSAID 可增加上、下消化道不良反应 单用非处方性非选择性 NSAID 或联合应用非选择性 NSAID 处方药可引起患者滥用或过量使用的风险 肾功能不全患者应慎用所有非选择性 NAID
Cox-2 抑制剂	有效缓解与肌肉骨骼疼痛有关的炎症	长期服用罗非考昔（>25mg/d）引起心血管危险（心肌梗死、水肿、高血压） 术后心血管危险导致 FDA 反对将任何 Cox-2 抑制剂用于术后疼痛（2005 年 4 月） 磺胺过敏患者禁用塞来昔布和伐地考昔 肾功能不全患者应慎用所有 NSAID 和 Cox-2 抑制剂
阿片类药物	对于大多数患者均有效	在一些研究中高达 38% 的患者没有反应，即使任意使用 神经病理性疼痛或伤害感受性疼痛患者的镇痛效能可能有所差异 不良反应包括便秘、镇静、恶心、神经毒性、呼吸抑制 潜在的药物滥用、成瘾性或耐药性

旁注 19-3　多模式镇痛中的 NSAID

NSAID 在多模式镇痛中的作用：
- 减少外周感受伤害性感受器的激动和敏化
- 减弱炎症反应
- 可能的中枢效应
- 可能作用于 NMDA 受体
- 无依赖性／成瘾性可能
- 与阿片类药物呈协同作用
- 减少阿片类药物用药（节约 20%～50%）
- 对睡眠无影响
- 用作多模式镇痛中"平衡镇痛"的一部分

NSAID 相比于阿片类药物的优点：
- 超前镇痛效应（减弱神经元敏化）
- 预防疼痛（减轻术后疼痛）
- 无呼吸抑制
- 比阿片类药物的恶心呕吐发生率低
- 术后肠梗阻和进食时间缩短
- 个体剂量差异小于阿片类药物
- 对一些疼痛效果优于阿片类药物（骨痛、外伤痛、呼吸痛、运动痛）
- 无瞳孔改变（神经学评价）
- 无认知损害（老年患者允许使用）

Cox-2 窘境

疼痛可反应性引起外周和中枢产生 Cox-2，抑制 Cox-2 是极其重要的镇痛靶点。疼痛性损害后使用 Cox-2 抑制剂可能阻止发生中枢敏化、痛觉过敏和持久性病理性疼痛的可能。

3 项研究表明，Cox-2 抑制剂作为多模式镇痛中的一部分与安慰剂相比，可使疼痛评分降低，呼吸抑制减轻，吗啡用量降低，而且使吗啡首次使用时间延长[8,58,59]。

在 Reuben 等[8]的一项研究中，60 例关节镜下半月板切除术患者被随机分成 3 组。切皮前 1h 或手术结束时使用罗非考昔 50mg，第三组使用安慰剂。24h 时，术前用罗非考昔组的对乙酰氨基酚／羟考酮用量（1.5±0.6 片）少于术后组（3.3±1.3 片）和对照组（5.5±1.6 片）。术前用罗非考昔组，在膝关节术后 24h 时，对乙酰氨基酚／羟考酮的需要量明显减少，而且阿片类药物首次使用时间明显延长（术前组 803min，术后组 461min，安慰剂组 318 min）。另外，术后恢复过程中，运动性疼痛评分较低。术前组不需使用阿片类药物的患者例数多于其他两组[8]。

Cox-2 抑制剂的两难窘境是，虽然其消化道和出血性不良反应较少，但是长期使用的有关不良反应值得关注——即对肾和心血管的有害作用，尤其老年人。因此，长期使用 Cox-2 抑制剂已受到 EMEA 和 FDA 质疑。一般认为，长期应用 NSAID，广义地包括 Cox-2 抑制剂的不良反应明显，不同于短时间应用的相关不良反应。然而，由于一项大型 RCT 发现在冠脉搭桥术后应用伐地考昔引起心血管并发症的发生率较高[60]，因而 Cox-2 抑制剂注射剂伐地考昔术后立即应用的安全性受到质疑。从 2005 年 6 月，FDA 药物评估和研究中心基于对可用数据的全面回顾，认为"短期使用 NSAID 治疗急性疼痛，特别是低剂量似乎并不增加严重心血管不良反应的发生风险（除外冠脉搭桥术后患者立即使用伐地考昔的情况）"[61]。2005 年早期，伐地考昔被撤出市场，但现在很可能会重新上市。如果这类药物继续用于慢性疼痛治疗，它与其他药物（如阿片类药物诸如曲马多和右丙氧芬）联用来减少不良反应的风险可能成为研究课题。

因此，多模式镇痛的应用可能会从短期治疗过渡到长期治疗，如术后恢复期间。现在，尤其是鉴于有关 NSAID 短期（<1W）用于控制大手术术后疼痛引起消化道、肾、心血管安全性的多国大量文献[62]，术后常规多模式镇痛中似宜应用更成熟的药物，而不用 Cox-2 抑制剂。

疼痛治疗中补充性和交替用药

急性疼痛的控制方法并不只限于药物治疗。最佳的疼痛治疗措施还包括非药理学方法和整体/补充方法，如神经调理、消融和减压技术及体能康复技术（锻炼、经皮神经电刺激、针灸）。心理治疗方法，包括放松和想像，可能有助于术后患者疼痛治疗。行为学方法治疗术后疼痛的试验结果不一。

根据 RCT 和系统性文献综述的证据，Astin[63]对交替治疗作出如下建议：

- 术后疼痛——术前进行精神-身体治疗（如想像、催眠、放松）能缩短恢复时间，减轻疼痛
- 侵害性操作过程中改善疼痛——精神-身体治疗可作为辅助治疗方法

Astin[63]也总结了慢性疼痛（如慢性腰背痛、类风湿性关节炎、骨关节炎和复发性头痛）时，使用这些治疗方法的证据。

少用药物方法的潜在效价值和不良反应降低

急性术后疼痛治疗不充分导致的不良临床结果包括住院时间延长、预后不佳、高发病率和死亡率及演变成慢性疼痛状态。术后疼痛带来的经济负担巨大，包括超出医疗费用的直接经济负担，以及患者功能和工作能力降低所带来的间接损失。例如，一例 30 岁患者一辈子治疗慢性术后疼痛可能要花费高达 100 万美元[25]。Macrae 等以及 Perkins 和 Kehlet[18]进行的大量流行病学研究表明，急性疼痛治疗不善似是发展成慢性疼痛的一个危险因素。慢性术后疼痛除了严重影响患者生活质量外，还可能引起患者忧郁及焦虑[2,6]。另一方面，患者更希望即使疼痛缓解较少，也要减轻阿片类药物不良反应（如恶心和呕吐）严重程度[2]。

为了解决这些问题，使用不同药物和技术的多模式镇痛方法能有效地减轻术后疼痛，但是目前所用的治疗方法限制了多模式镇痛的应用。就单一疗法而言，阿片类药物的疗效确切，但对其依赖性和不良反应有顾虑。NSAID 是多模式镇痛中有效的辅助药，但有相关不良反应。Cox-2 抑制剂，如塞来昔布、罗非考昔和伐地考昔，能保证非选择性 NSAID 疗效而减少其相关毒性，可减少术中阿片类药物的用量[6]，然而目前研究显示它们潜在的心血管不良反应事件风险较大，从而对它们未来使用产生了怀疑。联合使用这些药物能够减少每种或每类药物的用量，减轻每种或每类药物的不良反应。

未来方向

许多临床试验数据尚未报道出来，而它们的结论可能很重要。试验药物结论为阴性的 RCT 报道不足，可引导人们产生高估药物作用效能的偏见。由制药公司资助的阳性研究结果可能广为传播，如通过宣传册，这样可能会高估这些药物的优点。这些临床试验结果认识上的偏差，包括镇痛药，尤其是结果报道上的偏见可能影响荟萃分析得出的结论。

为了回应这些报道和论文报道的偏见，由临床试验专家、媒体杂志编辑和统计专家组成的一个国际组织，通过使用标准清单和流程图，建立了 CONSORT 声明书来改进报道的公正性[64]。这些专家们认为，为了获得更公正的结果，所有 RCT 应该注册在完全公开的数据库中。然而，镇痛药试验设计、入选标准以及结果评价的非均一性使得大多数发表的有关急性和其他类型疼痛的 RCT 不能结合起来进行荟萃分析，所以许多疼痛研究领域专家呼吁应更加谨慎地使用 CONSORT 来报道镇痛试验。更有利的措施是建立 Cochrane 数据库，通过提供有关治疗方法的最有用信息，包括对治疗有效性和恰当性的支持信息和反对信息，来解决发表论文内在的偏倚。目前，已经建立 Cochrane 合作综合组织用于麻醉以及疼痛、姑息疗法和支持治疗。

未来，用需要治疗的人数（number-needed-to-treat，

NNT）低值来检测药物，为根据各药物单独治疗时的效能来确定药物联合使用提供了基础。各种不同类或不同模式作用的镇痛药物联合以最低 NNT 值达到最优组合，不仅可获得相加作用，还可获得协同作用，达到最大镇痛效果，而且每种药物的剂量降低，相关不良反应减少（图 19-8）。

尽管一些镇痛药联合应用可能显示阴性结果，但是这些结论并不一定反映方法上的问题，而是表示一些药物药理学相互作用不理想，例如可能均作用于同一受体或酶。首先，应确定相互作用可能良好的镇痛药，这仍是一项挑战。随着临床前研究的深入，对疼痛传递的病理生理学更好的了解，将来镇痛药试验药物可能包括 NMDA 受体拮抗剂、缓激肽受体拮抗剂、神经元烟碱型乙酰胆碱受体激动剂、谷氨酸释放抑制剂、P 物质抑制剂、过氧化物歧化酶激动剂和一氧化氮合成酶抑制剂。对这些药物联合应用的评价，或许以固定剂量方式，可能会使多模式镇痛成为治疗许多种疼痛（尤其是急性疼痛）的金标准。

（李双双译　邓小明校）

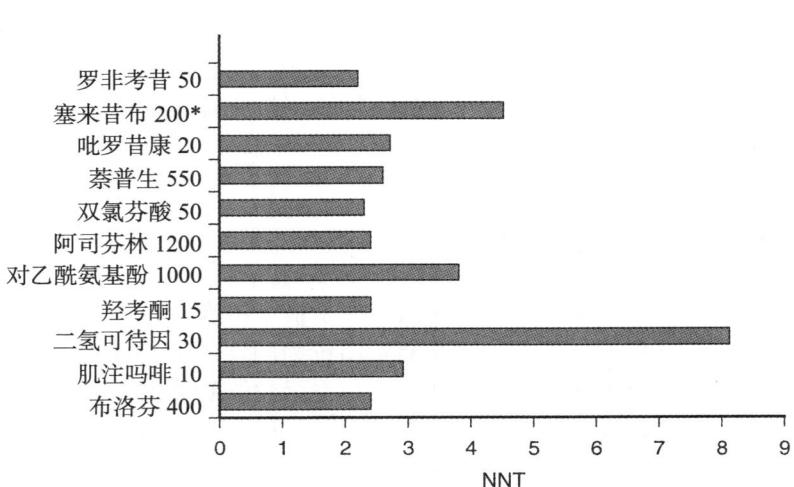

图 19-8　单一使用各种镇痛药物治疗急性术后疼痛 NNT 值的比较，所列药物除了吗啡（肌内注射）外，均为口服，以 mg 计。*建议急性疼痛时塞来昔布剂量为 400mg。注：罗非考昔于 2005 年由其生产厂家撤出市场。(Data from Barden J, Edwards J, Moore RA, McQuay HJ: Single dose oral diclofenac for postoperative pain. Cochrane Database Syst Rev 2004, Issue 2, article no. CD004768. DOI: 10.1002/14651858.CD004768; Edwards et al: Cochrane Database Syst Rev 2000, article no. CD00276; Edwards et al: The Cochrane Library 2004, Issue 2; Moore et al: Cochrane Database Syst Rev 2004, article no. CD004234; Barden et al: Cochrane Database Syst Rev 2004, Is sue 1, article no. CD004604.)

参考文献

1. Walker SM, Goudas LC, Cousins MJ, Carr DB: Combination spinal analgesic chemotherapy: A systematic review. Anesth Analg 2002; 95:674–715.
2. Gan TJ: Consensus guidelines for managing postoperative nausea and vomiting. Anesth Analg 2003;97:62–71.
3. Kehlet H, Dahl JB: The value of "multimodal" or "balanced analgesia" in postoperative pain treatment. Anesth Analg 1993;77:1048–1056.
4. Gottschalk A, Smith DS: New concepts in acute pain therapy: Preemptive analgesia. Am Fam Physician 2001;63:1979–1984.
5. Raffa RB: Pharmacology of oral combination analgesics: Rational therapy for pain. J Clin Pharm Ther 2001;26:257–264.
6. Stephens J, et al: The burden of acute postoperative pain and the potential role of the COX-2-specific inhibitors. Rheumatology 2003; (Suppl 3):iii40–iii52.
7. Siddik SM, et al: Diclofenac and/or propacetamol for postoperative pain management after cesarean delivery in patients receiving patient controlled analgesia morphine. Reg Anesth Pain Med 2001;26:310–315.
8. Reuben SS, et al: The preemptive analgesic effect of rofecoxib after ambulatory arthroscopic knee surgery. Anesth Analg 2002;94:55–59.
9. Olofsson CI, et al: Diclofenac in the treatment of pain after caesarean delivery: An opioid-saving strategy. Eur J Obstet Gynecol Reprod Biol 2000;88:143–146.
10. Michaloliakou C, et al: Preoperative multimodal analgesia facilitates recovery after ambulatory laparoscopic cholecystectomy. Anesth Analg 1996;82:44–51.
11. Scuderi P, et al: Multimodal antiemetic management prevents early postoperative vomiting after outpatient laparoscopy. Anesth Analg 2000;91:1408–1414.
12. Montes A, et al: Use of intravenous patient-controlled analgesia for the documentation of synergy between tramadol and metamizol. Brit J Anaesth 2000;85:217–223.
13. De Angelis C, et al: Clinical trial registration: A statement from the International Committee of Medical Journal Editors. N Engl J Med 2004;351:1250–1251.
14. Fassoulaki A, Patris K, Sarantopoulos C, Hogan Q: The analgesic effect of gabapentin and mexiletine after breast surgery for cancer. Anesth Analg 2002;95:985–991.
15. Stubhaug A, et al: Mapping of punctate hyperalgesia around a surgical incision demonstrates that ketamine is a powerful suppressor of central sensitization to pain following surgery. Acta Anaesthesiol Scand 1997; 41:1124–1132.
16. Pertunnen K, Tasmuth T, Kalso E: Chronic pain after thoracic surgery: A follow-up study [comment in Acta Anaesthesiol Scand 2000;44: 220]. Acta Anaesthesiol Scand 1999;43:563–567.
17. Poobalan AS, Bruce J, King PM, et al:. Chronic pain and quality of life following open inguinal hernia repair. Br J Surg 2001;88:1122–1126.
18. Perkins FM, Kehlet H: Chronic pain as an outcome of surgery: A review of predictive factors. Anesthesiology 2000;93:1123–1133.
19. Menigaux C, Adam F, Guignard B, et al: Preoperative gabapentin decreases anxiety and improves early functional recovery from knee surgery. Anesth Analg 2005;100:1394–1399.
20. De Kock M, Lavand'homme P, Waterloos H: 'Balanced analgesia' in the perioperative period: Is there a place for ketamine? Pain 2001;92: 373–380.

21. Panchel SJ: Personal communication, January 2005.
22. Carr DB, Jacox AK, Chapman CR, et al: 1992 Acute pain management in infants, children, and adolescents: Operative and medical procedures: Quick reference guide for clinicians (AHCPR Publication No. 92-0020). Rockville, MD: Agency for Health Care Policy and Research. September 2002. Available at http://www.ahcpr.gov/gils/00000052.htm/
23. Dolin SJ, Cashman JN, Bland JM: Effectiveness of acute postoperative pain management. I: Evidence from published data. Br J Anaesth 2002;89:409–423.
24. Powell AE, Davies HT, Bannister J, Macrae WA: Rhetoric and reality on acute pain services in the UK: A national postal questionnaire survey. Br J Anaesth 2004;92:689–693.
25. Apfelbaum JL: Postoperative pain experience: Results from a national survey suggest postoperative pain continues to be undermanaged. Anesth Analg 2003;97:534–540.
26. Buvanendran A, et al: Effects of perioperative administration of a selective cyclooxygenase 2 inhibitor on pain management and recovery of function after knee replacement: A randomized controlled trial. JAMA 2003;290:2411–2418.
27. Hanna MH, et al: Comparative study of analgesic efficacy and morphine-sparing effect of intramuscular dexketoprofen trometamol with ketoprofen or placebo after major orthopaedic surgery. Br J Clin Pharmacol 2003;55:126–133.
28. Marret E, Kurdi O, Zufferey P, Bonnet F: Effects of nonsteroidal antiinflammatory drugs on patient-controlled analgesia morphine side effects: Meta-analysis of randomized controlled trials. Anesthesiology 2005;102:1249–1260.
29. Cardoso MM, et al: Small doses of intrathecal morphine combined with systemic diclofenac for postoperative pain control after cesarean delivery. Anesth Analg 1998;86:538–541.
30. Rosaeg OP, et al: Peri-operative multimodal pain therapy for caesarean section: Analgesia and fitness for discharge. Can J Anaesth 1997;44:803–809.
31. Emkey R, et al: Efficacy and safety of tramadol/acetaminophen tablets (Ultracet) as add-on therapy for osteoarthritis pain in subjects receiving a COX-2 nonsteroidal antiinflammatory drug: A multicenter, randomized, double-blind, placebo-controlled trial. J Rheumatol 2004;31:150–156.
32. Silverfield JC, et al: Tramadol/acetaminophen combination tablets for the treatment of osteoarthritis flare pain: A multicenter, outpatient, randomized, double-blind, placebo-controlled, parallel-group, add-on study. Clin Ther 2002;24:282–297.
33. Rosenthal NR, et al: Tramadol/acetaminophen combination tablets for the treatment of pain associated with osteoarthritis flare in an elderly patient population. J Am Geriatr Soc 2004;52:374–380.
34. Chia YY, et al: Adding ketamine in a multimodal patient-controlled epidural regimen reduces postoperative pain and analgesic consumption. Anesth Analg 1998;86:1245–1249.
35. Menigaux C, et al: Intraoperative small-dose ketamine enhances analgesia after outpatient knee arthroscopy. Anesth Analg 2001;93:606–612.
36. Edwards JE, Moore RA, McQuay HJ: Single dose oxycodone and oxycodone plus paracetamol (acetaminophen) for acute postoperative pain (Cochrane Review). In The Cochrane Library, Issue 4. Chichester, UK, John Wiley & Sons, Ltd., 2004.
37. Collins SL, Edwards JE, Moore RA, McQuay HJ: Single dose dextropropoxyphene, alone and with paracetamol (acetaminophen), for postoperative pain (Cochrane Review). In The Cochrane Library, Issue 4. Chichester, UK:, John Wiley & Sons, Ltd., 2004.
38. Lauretti GR, et al: Tramadol and beta-cyclodextrin piroxicam: Effective multimodal balanced analgesia for the intra- and postoperative period. Reg Anesth 1997;22:243–248.
39. Anderson AD, et al: Randomized clinical trial of multimodal optimization and standard perioperative surgical care. Br J Surg 2003;90:1497–1504.
40. Barratt SM, et al: Multimodal analgesia and intravenous nutrition preserves total body protein following major upper gastrointestinal surgery. Reg Anesth Pain Med 2002;27:15–22.
41. Bisgaard T, et al: Multi-regional local anesthetic infiltration during laparoscopic cholecystectomy in patients receiving prophylactic multimodal analgesia: A randomized, double-blinded, placebo-controlled study. Anesth Analg 1999;89:1017–1024.
42. Liu SS, et al: Effects of perioperative analgesic technique on rate of recovery after colon surgery. Anesthesiology 1995;83:757–765.
43. Mulroy MF, et al: Femoral nerve block with 0.25% or 0.5% bupivacaine improves postoperative analgesia following outpatient arthroscopic anterior cruciate ligament repair. Reg Anesth Pain Med 2001;26:24–29.
44. Rasmussen S, et al: Intra-articular glucocorticoid, bupivacaine and morphine reduces pain, inflammatory response and convalescence after arthroscopic meniscectomy. Pain 1998;78:131–134.
45. Van Ee R, et al: Effects of ketoprofen and mesosalpinx infiltration on postoperative pain after laparoscopic sterilization. Obstet Gynecol 1996;88:568–572.
46. Schumann R, et al: A comparison of multimodal perioperative analgesia to epidural pain management after gastric bypass surgery. Anesth Analg 2003;96:469–474.
47. Australian and New Zealand College of Anaesthetists and Faculty of Pain Medicine: Acute Pain Management: Scientific Evidence, 2nd ed (Publication No. CP104). Canberra, National Health and Medical Research Council, 2005. Available at http://www.nhmrc.gov.au/publications/_files/cp104.pdf/
48. Rockemann MG, et al: Prophylactic use of epidural mepivacaine/morphine, systemic diclofenac, and metamizole reduces postoperative morphine consumption after major abdominal surgery. Anesthesiology 1996;84:1027–1034.
49. Rosaeg OP, et al: Effect of preemptive multimodal analgesia for arthroscopic knee ligament repair. Reg Anesth Pain Med 2001;26:125–130.
50. Choi DM, et al: Dextromethorphan and intrathecal morphine for analgesia after Caesarean section under spinal anaesthesia. Br J Anaesth 2003;90:653–658.
51. Paech MJ, et al: Postcesarean analgesia with spinal morphine, clonidine, or their combination. Anesth Analg 2004;98:1460–1466.
52. Keita H, et al: Prophylactic IP injection of bupivacaine and/or morphine does not improve postoperative analgesia after laparoscopic gynecologic surgery. Can J Anaesth 2003;50:362–367.
53. Nagatsuka C, et al: Preemptive effects of a combination of preoperative diclofenac, butorphanol, and lidocaine on postoperative pain management following orthognathic surgery. Anesth Prog 2000;47:119–124.
54. Doyle E, Bowler GM: Pre-emptive effect of multimodal analgesia in thoracic surgery. Br J Anaesth 1998;80:147–151.
55. Reuben SS, et al: Intraarticular morphine in the multimodal analgesic management of postoperative pain after ambulatory anterior cruciate ligament repair. Anesth Analg 1998;86:374–378.
56. Bell R: Ketamine as an adjuvant to opioids for cancer pain (Cochrane Review). The Cochrane Library, Issue 4. Chichester, UK, Wiley & Sons, 2004.
57. Cashman JN, Dolin SJ: Respiratory and haemodynamic effects of acute postoperative pain management: Evidence from published data. Br J Anaesth 2004;93:212–223.
58. Sinatra RS, et al: Preoperative rofecoxib oral suspension as an analgesic adjunct after lower abdominal surgery: The effects on effort-dependent pain and pulmonary function. Anesth Analg 2004;98:135–140.
59. Camu F, et al: Valdecoxib, a COX-2-specific inhibitor, is an efficacious, opioid-sparing analgesic in patients undergoing hip arthroplasty. Am J Ther 2002;9:43–51.
60. Nussmeier NA, Whelton AA, Brown MT, et al: Complications of the COX-2 inhibitors parecoxib and valdecoxib after cardiac surgery. N Engl J Med 2005;352:1081–1091.
61. U.S. Food and Drug Administration, Office of New Drugs and Office of Pharmacoepidemiology and Statistical Science: Analysis and recommendation for Agency action regarding non-steroidal anti-inflammatory drugs and cardiovascular risk. Memorandum, April 6, 2005. Available at http://www.fda.gov/cder/drug/infopage/COX2/NSAIDdecisionMemo.pdf/
62. Forrest JB, Camu F, Greer IA, et al: Ketorolac, diclofenac, and ketoprofen are equally safe for pain relief after major surgery. Br J Anaesth 2002;88:2227–2233.
63. Astin JA: Mind-body therapies for the management of pain. Clin J Pain 2004;20:27–32.
64. Moher D, et al: The CONSORT statement: Revised recommendations for improving the quality of reports of parallel-group randomised trials. Lancet 2001;357:1191–1194.

附录：1995—2005年间多模式镇痛治疗Medline检索结果

以下为本章引用的Medline检索文献，随后列出符合前三个检索的参考文献。

1995—2005年间多模式镇痛治疗Medline检索结果

检索年限（1995—2005）	相符的文献数量	临床试验数量	RCT
Multimodal treatment pain*	217	55	47
Multimodal therapy pain*	210	55	47
Multimodal analgesia*	123	38	35
Multidisciplinary intervention pain	109		
Multimodal pain management	98		
Multidisciplinary approach pain	77		
Multimodal perioperative analgesia	29		
Multimodal pain relief	8		
Multimodal preemptive approach pain	3		
Multimodal optimization pain	2		

*所附参考文献列出了符合此检索词的文献

前三个检索词的参考文献

"MULTIMODAL TREATMENT PAIN"

1. Atlantis E, Chow CM, Kirby A, Singh MF: An effective exercise-based intervention for improving mental health and quality of life measures: a randomized controlled trial. Prev Med 2004;39:424–434.
2. Paech MJ, Pavy TJ, Orlikowski CE, et al: Postcesarean analgesia with spinal morphine, clonidine, or their combination. Anesth Analg 2004; 98:1460–1466.
3. Brown DR, Hofer RE, Patterson DE, et al: Intrathecal anesthesia and recovery from radical prostatectomy: A prospective, randomized, controlled trial. Anesthesiology 2004;100:926–934.
4. Ma H, Tang J, White PF, et al: Perioperative rofecoxib improves early recovery after outpatient herniorrhaphy. Anesth Analg 2004;98:970–975.
5. Anderson AD, McNaught CE, MacFie J, et al: Randomized clinical trial of multimodal optimization and standard perioperative surgical care. Br J Surg 2003;90:1497–1504.
6. Buvanendran A, Kroin JS, Tuman KJ, et al: Effects of perioperative administration of a selective cyclooxygenase 2 inhibitor on pain management and recovery of function after knee replacement: A randomized controlled trial. JAMA 2003;290:2411–2418.
7. Bisgaard T, Klarskov B, Kehlet H, Rosenberg J: Preoperative dexamethasone improves surgical outcome after laparoscopic cholecystectomy: A randomized double-blind placebo-controlled trial. Ann Surg 2003;238:651–660.
8. Choi DM, Kliffer AP, Douglas MJ: Dextromethorphan and intrathecal morphine for analgesia after Caesarean section under spinal anaesthesia. Br J Anaesth 2003;90:653–658.
9. Keita H, Benifla JL, Le Bouar V, et al: Prophylactic IP injection of bupivacaine and/or morphine does not improve postoperative analgesia after laparoscopic gynecologic surgery. Can J Anaesth 2003;50: 362–367.
10. Hanna MH, Elliott KM, Stuart-Taylor ME, et al: Comparative study of analgesic efficacy and morphine-sparing effect of intramuscular dexketoprofen trometamol with ketoprofen or placebo after major orthopaedic surgery. Br J Clin Pharmacol 2003;55:126–133.
11. Schumann R, Shikora S, Weiss JM, et al: A comparison of multimodal perioperative analgesia to epidural pain management after gastric bypass surgery. Anesth Analg 2003;96:469–474.
12. Issioui T, Klein KW, White PF, et al: Cost-efficacy of rofecoxib versus acetaminophen for preventing pain after ambulatory surgery. Anesthesiology 2002;97:931–937.
13. Carli F, Mayo N, Klubien K, et al: Epidural analgesia enhances functional exercise capacity and health-related quality of life after colonic surgery: Results of a randomized trial. Anesthesiology 2002;97:540–549.
14. Ekman EF, Fiechtner JJ, Levy S, Fort JG: Efficacy of celecoxib versus ibuprofen in the treatment of acute pain: A multicenter, double-blind, randomized controlled trial in acute ankle sprain. Am J Orthop 2002; 31:445–451.
15. Hammas B, Thorn SE, Wattwil M: Superior prolonged antiemetic prophylaxis with a four-drug multimodal regimen—comparison with propofol or placebo. Acta Anaesthesiol Scand 2002;46:232–237.
16. Boisseau N, Rabary O, Padovani B, et al: Improvement of 'dynamic analgesia' does not decrease atelectasis after thoracotomy. Br J Anaesth 2001;87:564–569.
17. Henriksen MG, Jensen MB, Hansen HV, et al: Enforced mobilization, early oral feeding, and balanced analgesia improve convalescence after colorectal surgery. Nutrition 2002;18:147–152.
18. Barratt SM, Smith RC, Kee AJ, et al: Multimodal analgesia and intravenous nutrition preserves total body protein following major upper gastrointestinal surgery. Reg Anesth Pain Med 2002;27:15–22.
19. Camu F, Beecher T, Recker DP, Verburg KM: Valdecoxib, a COX-2-specific inhibitor, is an efficacious, opioid-sparing analgesic in patients undergoing hip arthroplasty. Am J Ther 2002;9:43–51.
20. Menigaux C, Guignard B, Fletcher D, et al: Intraoperative small-dose ketamine enhances analgesia after outpatient knee arthroscopy. Anesth Analg 2001;93:606–612.
21. Siddik SM, Aouad MT, Jalbout MI, et al: Diclofenac and/or propacetamol for postoperative pain management after cesarean delivery in patients receiving patient controlled analgesia morphine. Reg Anesth Pain Med 2001;26:310–315.
22. Nagatsuka C, Ichinohe T, Kaneko Y: Preemptive effects of a combination of preoperative diclofenac, butorphanol, and lidocaine on postoperative pain management following orthognathic surgery. Anesth Prog 2000; 47:119–124.
23. Brodner G, Van Aken H, Hertle L, et al: Multimodal perioperative management—combining thoracic epidural analgesia, forced mobilization, and oral nutrition—reduces hormonal and metabolic stress and improves convalescence after major urologic surgery. Anesth Analg 2001;92:1594–1600.

24. Rosaeg OP, Krepski B, Cicutti N, et al: Effect of preemptive multimodal analgesia for arthroscopic knee ligament repair. Reg Anesth Pain Med 2001;26:125–130.
25. Taylor D: More than personal change: Effective elements of symptom management. Nurse Pract Forum 2000;11:79–86.
26. Mulroy MF, Larkin KL, Batra MS, et al: Femoral nerve block with 0.25% or 0.5% bupivacaine improves postoperative analgesia following outpatient arthroscopic anterior cruciate ligament repair. Reg Anesth Pain Med 2001;26:24–29.
27. Scuderi PE, James RL, Harris L, Mims GR 3rd: Multimodal antiemetic management prevents early postoperative vomiting after outpatient laparoscopy. Anesth Analg 2000;91:1408–1414.
28. Reuben SS, Connelly NR: Postoperative analgesic effects of celecoxib or rofecoxib after spinal fusion surgery. Anesth Analg 2000;91:1221–1225.
29. Bisgaard T, Klarskov B, Trap R, et al: Pain after microlaparoscopic cholecystectomy: A randomized double-blind controlled study. Surg Endosc 2000;14:340–344.
30. Taimela S, Takala EP, Asklof T, et al: Active treatment of chronic neck pain: A prospective randomized intervention. Spine 2000;25:1021–1027.
31. Olofsson CI, Legeby MH, Nygards EB, Ostman KM: Diclofenac in the treatment of pain after vaginal delivery: An opioid-saving strategy. Eur J Obstet Gynecol Reprod Biol 2000;88:143–146.
32. Bisgaard T, Klarskov B, Kristiansen VB, et al: Multi-regional local anesthetic infiltration during laparoscopic cholecystectomy in patients receiving prophylactic multi-modal analgesia: A randomized, double-blinded, placebo-controlled study. Anesth Analg 1999;89:1017–1024.
33. Petersen-Felix S, Luginbuhl M, Schnider TW, et al: Comparison of the analgesic potency of xenon and nitrous oxide in humans evaluated by experimental pain. Br J Anaesth 1998;81:742–747.
34. Rasmussen S, Larsen AS, Thomsen ST, Kehlet H: Intra-articular glucocorticoid, bupivacaine and morphine reduces pain, inflammatory response and convalescence after arthroscopic meniscectomy. Pain 1998;78:131–134.
35. Lauretti GR, Mattos AL, Reis MP, Pereira NL: Combined intrathecal fentanyl and neostigmine: Therapy for postoperative abdominal hysterectomy pain relief. J Clin Anesth 1998;10:291–296.
36. Chia YY, Liu K, Liu YC, et al: Adding ketamine in a multimodal patient-controlled epidural regimen reduces postoperative pain and analgesic consumption. Anesth Analg 1998;86:1245–1249.
37. Doyle E, Bowler GM: Pre-emptive effect of multimodal analgesia in thoracic surgery. Br J Anaesth 1998;80:147–151.
38. Haldorsen EM, Kronholm K, Skouen JS, Ursin H: Multimodal cognitive behavioral treatment of patients sicklisted for musculoskeletal pain: A randomized controlled study. Scand J Rheumatol 1998;27:16–25.
39. Reuben SS, Steinberg RB, Cohen MA, et al: Intraarticular morphine in the multimodal analgesic management of postoperative pain after ambulatory anterior cruciate ligament repair. Anesth Analg 1998;86:374–378.
40. Rosaeg OP, Lui AC, Cicutti NJ, et al: Peri-operative multimodal pain therapy for caesarean section: Analgesia and fitness for discharge. Can J Anaesth 1997;44:803–809.
41. Lauretti GR, Mattos AL, Lima IC: Tramadol and beta-cyclodextrin piroxicam: Effective multimodal balanced analgesia for the intra- and postoperative period. Reg Anesth 1997;22:243–248.
42. Van Ee R, Hemrika DJ, De Blok S, et al: Effects of ketoprofen and mesosalpinx infiltration on postoperative pain after laparoscopic sterilization. Obstet Gynecol 1996;88:568–572.
43. Provinciali L, Baroni M, Illuminati L, Ceravolo MG: Multimodal treatment to prevent the late whiplash syndrome. Scand J Rehabil Med 1996;28:105–111.
44. Rockemann MG, Seeling W, Bischof C, et al: Prophylactic use of epidural mepivacaine/morphine, systemic diclofenac, and metamizole reduces postoperative morphine consumption after major abdominal surgery. Anesthesiology 1996;84:1027–1034.
45. Katz J, Jackson M, Kavanagh BP, Sandler AN: Acute pain after thoracic surgery predicts long-term post-thoracotomy pain. Clin J Pain 1996;12:50–55.
46. Michaloliakou C, Chung F, Sharma S: Preoperative multimodal analgesia facilitates recovery after ambulatory laparoscopic cholecystectomy. Anesth Analg 1996;82:44–51.
47. Jensen I, Nygren A, Gamberale F, et al: The role of the psychologist in multidisciplinary treatments for chronic neck and shoulder pain: A controlled cost-effectiveness study. Scand J Rehabil Med 1995;27:19–26.

"MULTIMODAL THERAPY PAIN"

1. Atlantis E, Chow CM, Kirby A, Singh MF: An effective exercise-based intervention for improving mental health and quality of life measures: A randomized controlled trial. Prev Med 2004;39:424–434.
2. Paech MJ, Pavy TJ, Orlikowski CE, et al: Postcesarean analgesia with spinal morphine, clonidine, or their combination. Anesth Analg 2004;98:1460–1466.
3. Brown DR, Hofer RE, Patterson DE, et al: Intrathecal anesthesia and recovery from radical prostatectomy: A prospective, randomized, controlled trial. Anesthesiology 2004;100:926–934.
4. Ma H, Tang J, White PF, et al: Perioperative rofecoxib improves early recovery after outpatient herniorrhaphy. Anesth Analg 2004;98:970–975.
5. Anderson AD, McNaught CE, MacFie J, et al: Randomized clinical trial of multimodal optimization and standard perioperative surgical care. Br J Surg 2003;90:1497–1504.
6. Buvanendran A, Kroin JS, Tuman KJ, et al: Effects of perioperative administration of a selective cyclooxygenase 2 inhibitor on pain management and recovery of function after knee replacement: A randomized controlled trial. JAMA 2003;290:2411–2418.
7. Bisgaard T, Klarskov B, Kehlet H, Rosenberg J: Preoperative dexamethasone improves surgical outcome after laparoscopic cholecystectomy: A randomized double-blind placebo-controlled trial. Ann Surg 2003;238:651–660.
8. Choi DM, Kliffer AP, Douglas MJ: Dextromethorphan and intrathecal morphine for analgesia after Caesarean section under spinal anaesthesia. Br J Anaesth 2003;90:653–658.
9. Keita H, Benifla JL, Le Bouar V, et al: Prophylactic IP injection of bupivacaine and/or morphine does not improve postoperative analgesia after laparoscopic gynecologic surgery. Can J Anaesth 2003;50:362–367.
10. Hanna MH, Elliott KM, Stuart-Taylor ME, et al: Comparative study of analgesic efficacy and morphine-sparing effect of intramuscular dexketoprofen trometamol with ketoprofen or placebo after major orthopaedic surgery. Br J Clin Pharmacol 2003;55:126–133.
11. Schumann R, Shikora S, Weiss JM, et al: A comparison of multimodal perioperative analgesia to epidural pain management after gastric bypass surgery. Anesth Analg 2003;96:469–474.
12. Issioui T, Klein KW, White PF, et al: Cost-efficacy of rofecoxib versus acetaminophen for preventing pain after ambulatory surgery. Anesthesiology 2002;97:931–937.
13. Carli F, Mayo N, Klubien K, et al: Epidural analgesia enhances functional exercise capacity and health-related quality of life after colonic surgery: Results of a randomized trial. Anesthesiology 2002;97:540–549.
14. Ekman EF, Fiechtner JJ, Levy S, Fort JG: Efficacy of celecoxib versus ibuprofen in the treatment of acute pain: A multicenter, double-blind, randomized controlled trial in acute ankle sprain. Am J Orthop 2002;31:445–451.
15. Hammas B, Thorn SE, Wattwil M: Superior prolonged antiemetic prophylaxis with a four-drug multimodal regimen—comparison with propofol or placebo. Acta Anaesthesiol Scand 2002;46:232–237.
16. Boisseau N, Rabary O, Padovani B, et al: Improvement of 'dynamic analgesia' does not decrease atelectasis after thoracotomy. Br J Anaesth 2001;87:564–569.
17. Henriksen MG, Jensen MB, Hansen HV, et al: Enforced mobilization, early oral feeding, and balanced analgesia improve convalescence after colorectal surgery. Nutrition 2002;18:147–152.
18. Barratt SM, Smith RC, Kee AJ, et al: Multimodal analgesia and intravenous nutrition preserves total body protein following major upper gastrointestinal surgery. Reg Anesth Pain Med 2002;27:15–22.
19. Camu F, Beecher T, Recker DP, Verburg KM: Valdecoxib, a COX-2-specific inhibitor, is an efficacious, opioid-sparing analgesic in patients undergoing hip arthroplasty. Am J Ther 2002;9:43–51.
20. Menigaux C, Guignard B, Fletcher D, et al: Intraoperative small-dose ketamine enhances analgesia after outpatient knee arthroscopy. Anesth Analg 2001;93:606–612.
21. Siddik SM, Aouad MT, Jalbout MI, et al: Diclofenac and/or propacetamol for postoperative pain management after cesarean delivery in patients receiving patient controlled analgesia morphine. Reg Anesth Pain Med 2001;26:310–315.
22. Nagatsuka C, Ichinohe T, Kaneko Y: Preemptive effects of a combination of preoperative diclofenac, butorphanol, and lidocaine on postoperative pain management following orthognathic surgery. Anesth Prog 2000;

47:119–124.
23. Brodner G, Van Aken H, Hertle L, et al: Multimodal perioperative management—combining thoracic epidural analgesia, forced mobilization, and oral nutrition—reduces hormonal and metabolic stress and improves convalescence after major urologic surgery. Anesth Analg 2001;92:1594–1600.
24. Rosaeg OP, Krepski B, Cicutti N, et al: Effect of preemptive multimodal analgesia for arthroscopic knee ligament repair. Reg Anesth Pain Med 2001;26:125–130.
25. Taylor D: More than personal change: Effective elements of symptom management. Nurse Pract Forum 2000;11:79–86.
26. Mulroy MF, Larkin KL, Batra MS, et al: Femoral nerve block with 0.25% or 0.5% bupivacaine improves postoperative analgesia following outpatient arthroscopic anterior cruciate ligament repair. Reg Anesth Pain Med 2001;26:24–29.
27. Scuderi PE, James RL, Harris L, Mims GR 3rd: Multimodal antiemetic management prevents early postoperative vomiting after outpatient laparoscopy. Anesth Analg 2000;91:1408–1414.
28. Reuben SS, Connelly NR: Postoperative analgesic effects of celecoxib or rofecoxib after spinal fusion surgery. Anesth Analg 2000;91:1221–1225.
29. Bisgaard T, Klarskov B, Trap R, et al: Pain after microlaparoscopic cholecystectomy: A randomized double-blind controlled study. Surg Endosc 2000;14:340–344.
30. Taimela S, Takala EP, Asklof T, et al: Active treatment of chronic neck pain: A prospective randomized intervention. Spine 2000;25:1021–1027.
31. Olofsson CI, Legeby MH, Nygards EB, Ostman KM: Diclofenac in the treatment of pain after caesarean delivery: An opioid-saving strategy. Eur J Obstet Gynecol Reprod Biol 2000;88:143–146.
32. Bisgaard T, Klarskov B, Kristiansen VB, et al: Multi-regional local anesthetic infiltration during laparoscopic cholecystectomy in patients receiving prophylactic multi-modal analgesia: A randomized, double-blinded, placebo-controlled study. Anesth Analg 1999;89:1017–1024.
33. Petersen-Felix S, Luginbuhl M, Schnider TW, et al: Comparison of the analgesic potency of xenon and nitrous oxide in humans evaluated by experimental pain. Br J Anaesth 1998;81:742–747.
34. Rasmussen S, Larsen AS, Thomsen ST, Kehlet H: Intra-articular glucocorticoid, bupivacaine and morphine reduces pain, inflammatory response and convalescence after arthroscopic meniscectomy. Pain 1998;78:131–134.
35. Lauretti GR, Mattos AL, Reis MP, Pereira NL: Combined intrathecal fentanyl and neostigmine: Therapy for postoperative abdominal hysterectomy pain relief. J Clin Anesth 1998;10:291–296.
36. Chia YY, Liu K, Liu YC, et al: Adding ketamine in a multimodal patient-controlled epidural regimen reduces postoperative pain and analgesic consumption. Anesth Analg 1998;86:1245–1249.
37. Doyle E, Bowler GM: Pre-emptive effect of multimodal analgesia in thoracic surgery. Br J Anaesth 1998;80:147–151.
38. Haldorsen EM, Kronholm K, Skouen JS, Ursin H: Multimodal cognitive behavioral treatment of patients sicklisted for musculoskeletal pain: A randomized controlled study. Scand J Rheumatol 1998;27:16–25.
39. Reuben SS, Steinberg RB, Cohen MA, et al: Intraarticular morphine in the multimodal analgesic management of postoperative pain after ambulatory anterior cruciate ligament repair. Anesth Analg 1998;86:374–378.
40. Rosaeg OP, Lui AC, Cicutti NJ, et al: Peri-operative multimodal pain therapy for caesarean section: Analgesia and fitness for discharge. Can J Anaesth 1997;44:803–809.
41. Lauretti GR, Mattos AL, Lima IC: Tramadol and beta-cyclodextrin piroxicam: Effective multimodal balanced analgesia for the intra- and postoperative period. Reg Anesth 1997;22:243–248.
42. Van Ee R, Hemrika DJ, De Blok S, et al: Effects of ketoprofen and mesosalpinx infiltration on postoperative pain after laparoscopic sterilization. Obstet Gynecol 1996;88:568–572.
43. Provinciali L, Baroni M, Illuminati L, Ceravolo MG: Multimodal treatment to prevent the late whiplash syndrome. Scand J Rehabil Med 1996;28:105–111.
44. Rockemann MG, Seeling W, Bischof C, et al: Prophylactic use of epidural mepivacaine/morphine, systemic diclofenac, and metamizole reduces postoperative morphine consumption after major abdominal surgery. Anesthesiology 1996;84:1027–1034.
45. Katz J, Jackson M, Kavanagh BP, Sandler AN: Acute pain after thoracic surgery predicts long-term post-thoracotomy pain. Clin J Pain 1996;12:50–55.
46. Michaloliakou C, Chung F, Sharma S: Preoperative multimodal analgesia
47. Jensen I, Nygren A, Gamberale F, et al: The role of the psychologist in multidisciplinary treatments for chronic neck and shoulder pain: A controlled cost-effectiveness study. Scand J Rehabil Med 1995;27:19–26.

"MULTIMODAL ANALGESIA"

1. Paech MJ, Pavy TJ, Orlikowski CE, et al: Postcesarean analgesia with spinal morphine, clonidine, or their combination. Anesth Analg 2004;98:1460–1466.
2. Brown DR, Hofer RE, Patterson DE, et al: Intrathecal anesthesia and recovery from radical prostatectomy: A prospective, randomized, controlled trial. Anesthesiology 2004;100:926–934.
3. Buvanendran A, Kroin JS, Tuman KJ, et al: Effects of perioperative administration of a selective cyclooxygenase 2 inhibitor on pain management and recovery of function after knee replacement: A randomized controlled trial. JAMA 2003;290:2411–2418.
4. Basse L, Madsen JL, Billesbolle P, et al: Gastrointestinal transit after laparoscopic versus open colonic resection. Surg Endosc 2003;17:1919–1922.
5. Choi DM, Kliffer AP, Douglas MJ: Dextromethorphan and intrathecal morphine for analgesia after Caesarean section under spinal anaesthesia. Br J Anaesth 2003;90:653–658.
6. Keita H, Benifla JL, Le Bouar V, et al: Prophylactic IP injection of bupivacaine and/or morphine does not improve postoperative analgesia after laparoscopic gynecologic surgery. Can J Anaesth 2003;50:362–367.
7. Hanna MH, Elliott KM, Stuart-Taylor ME, et al: Comparative study of analgesic efficacy and morphine-sparing effect of intramuscular dexketoprofen trometamol with ketoprofen or placebo after major orthopaedic surgery. Br J Clin Pharmacol 2003;55:126–133.
8. Schumann R, Shikora S, Weiss JM, et al: A comparison of multimodal perioperative analgesia to epidural pain management after gastric bypass surgery. Anesth Analg 2003;96:469–474.
9. Issioui T, Klein KW, White PF, et al: Cost-efficacy of rofecoxib versus acetaminophen for preventing pain after ambulatory surgery. Anesthesiology 2002;97:931–937.
10. Carli F, Mayo N, Klubien K, et al: Epidural analgesia enhances functional exercise capacity and health-related quality of life after colonic surgery: Results of a randomized trial. Anesthesiology 2002;97:540–549.
11. Boisseau N, Rabary O, Padovani B, et al: Improvement of 'dynamic analgesia' does not decrease atelectasis after thoracotomy. Br J Anaesth 2001;87:564–569.
12. Henriksen MG, Jensen MB, Hansen HV, et al: Enforced mobilization, early oral feeding, and balanced analgesia improve convalescence after colorectal surgery. Nutrition 2002;18:147–152.
13. Barratt SM, Smith RC, Kee AJ, et al: Multimodal analgesia and intravenous nutrition preserves total body protein following major upper gastrointestinal surgery. Reg Anesth Pain Med 2002;27:15–22.
14. Camu F, Beecher T, Recker DP, Verburg KM: Valdecoxib, a COX-2-specific inhibitor, is an efficacious opioid-sparing analgesic in patients undergoing hip arthroplasty. Am J Ther 2002;9:43–51.
15. Menigaux C, Guignard B, Fletcher D, et al: Intraoperative small-dose ketamine enhances analgesia after outpatient knee arthroscopy. Anesth Analg 2001;93:606–612.
16. Siddik SM, Aouad MT, Jalbout MI, et al: Diclofenac and/or propacetamol for postoperative pain management after cesarean delivery in patients receiving patient controlled analgesia morphine. Reg Anesth Pain Med 2001;26:310–315.
17. Nagatsuka C, Ichinohe T, Kaneko Y: Preemptive effects of a combination of preoperative diclofenac, butorphanol, and lidocaine on postoperative pain management following orthognathic surgery. Anesth Prog 2000;47:119–124.
18. Brodner G, Van Aken H, Hertle L, et al: Multimodal perioperative management—combining thoracic epidural analgesia, forced mobilization, and oral nutrition—reduces hormonal and metabolic stress and improves convalescence after major urologic surgery. Anesth Analg 2001;92:1594–1600.
19. Rosaeg OP, Krepski B, Cicutti N, et al: Effect of preemptive multimodal analgesia for arthroscopic knee ligament repair. Reg Anesth Pain Med 2001;26:125–130.
20. Mulroy MF, Larkin KL, Batra MS, et al: Femoral nerve block with 0.25% or 0.5% bupivacaine improves postoperative analgesia following outpatient arthroscopic anterior cruciate ligament repair. Reg Anesth Pain Med 2001:26:24–29.

21. Reuben SS, Connelly NR: Postoperative analgesic effects of celecoxib or rofecoxib after spinal fusion surgery. Anesth Analg 2000;91:1221–1225.
22. Olofsson CI, Legeby MH, Nygards EB, Ostman KM: Diclofenac in the treatment of pain after caesarean delivery: An opioid-saving strategy. Eur J Obstet Gynecol Reprod Biol 2000;88:143–146.
23. Bisgaard T, Klarskov B, Kristiansen VB, et al: Multi-regional local anesthetic infiltration during laparoscopic cholecystectomy in patients receiving prophylactic multi-modal analgesia: A randomized, double-blinded, placebo-controlled study. Anesth Analg 1999;89:1017–1024.
24. Petersen-Felix S, Luginbuhl M, Schnider TW, et al: Comparison of the analgesic potency of xenon and nitrous oxide in humans evaluated by experimental pain. Br J Anaesth 1998;81:742–747.
25. Lauretti GR, Mattos AL, Reis MP, Pereira NL: Combined intrathecal fentanyl and neostigmine: Therapy for postoperative abdominal hysterectomy pain relief. J Clin Anesth 1998;10:291–296.
26. Chia YY, Liu K, Liu YC, et al: Adding ketamine in a multimodal patient-controlled epidural regimen reduces postoperative pain and analgesic consumption. Anesth Analg 1998;86:1245–1249.
27. Doyle E, Bowler GM: Pre-emptive effect of multimodal analgesia in thoracic surgery. Br J Anaesth 1998;80:147–151.
28. Cardoso MM, Carvalho JC, Amaro AR, et al: Small doses of intrathecal morphine combined with systemic diclofenac for postoperative pain control after cesarean delivery. Anesth Analg 1998;86:538–541.
29. Reuben SS, Steinberg RB, Cohen MA, et al: Intraarticular morphine in the multimodal analgesic management of postoperative pain after ambulatory anterior cruciate ligament repair. Anesth Analg 1998;86:374–378.
30. Rosaeg OP, Lui AC, Cicutti NJ, et al: Peri-operative multimodal pain therapy for caesarean section: Analgesia and fitness for discharge. Can J Anaesth 1997;44:803–809.
31. Lauretti GR, Mattos AL, Lima IC: Tramadol and beta-cyclodextrin piroxicam: Effective multimodal balanced analgesia for the intra- and postoperative period. Reg Anesth 1997;22:243–248.
32. Rockemann MG, Seeling W, Bischof C, et al: Prophylactic use of epidural mepivacaine/morphine, systemic diclofenac, and metamizole reduces postoperative morphine consumption after major abdominal surgery. Anesthesiology 1996;84:1027–1034.
33. Katz J, Jackson M, Kavanagh BP, Sandler AN: Acute pain after thoracic surgery predicts long-term post-thoracotomy pain. Clin J Pain 1996;12:50–55.
34. Michaloliakou C, Chung F, Sharma S: Preoperative multimodal analgesia facilitates recovery after ambulatory laparoscopic cholecystectomy. Anesth Analg 1996;82:44–51.
35. Liu SS, Carpenter RL, Mackey DC, et al: Effects of perioperative analgesic technique on rate of recovery after colon surgery. Anesthesiology 1995;83:757–765.

20 非常规及辅助镇痛

KATE FITZGERALD · DONAL BUGGY

术后镇痛需要达到缓解疼痛和避免不必要的不良反应之间的平衡。这种平衡在非住院（门诊）手术中尤为重要，目前这种手术正在为越来越多的患者所接受。理想的术后镇痛药应可提供完全镇痛而没有任何不良反应。尽管这样的镇痛药尚未面世，然而试图寻找镇痛药或镇痛药的组合以达到良好镇痛且尽可能减少其不良反应的努力从未停止。一些常规疗法，如世界卫生组织镇痛阶梯疗法，历史悠久且被广泛接受，从而成为惯例。然而，常规镇痛有局限性，主要是全身给予阿片类药物的不良反应（恶心、呕吐、过度镇静、呼吸抑制）和非甾体类抗炎药（NSAID）的不良反应（胃肠黏膜出血、肾功能损伤、血栓栓塞风险增大）。

患者经常恐惧术后疼痛，而后者往往并未得到良好控制。这一现状增加了患者对非传统镇痛治疗的需求和接受程度。其他可供选择的疗法包括一些尚未被医学界广泛认可的镇痛药及镇痛技术。1998年发表的一项研究表明，42%的美国成人使用过某种形式的非传统镇痛疗法[1]。已报道过很多非传统形式的镇痛药物或疗法，包括物理镇痛、药物镇痛及心理学形式的镇痛（表20-1）。本章我们将阐述其中部分疗法用于术后镇痛的依据。

非药物镇痛

经皮电神经刺激

经皮电神经刺激（transcutaneous electrical nerve stimulation，TENS）的理论依据是 Melzack 和 Wall 提出的疼痛门控理论[2]。TENS 是由微小电流所产生的震动感觉，这一电流由放置于镇痛部位的两个塑胶垫之间产生一个低电压电场（图20-1）。电流可以有不同的频率和振幅。TENS 的作用机制是激活 Aβ 周围神经纤维细胞，从而降低中枢伤害性神经细胞的活性[3]。一项系统性回顾表明 TENS 在术后镇痛方面并无作用[4]。事实可能如此，但也可能是由于研究所使用的频率低于最适频率导致疗效不佳。

随后的一项随机对照试验（randomized controlled trials，RCT）荟萃分析研究了 TENS 和类似针灸样经皮电神经刺激疗法（acupuncture-like transcutaneous electrical nerve stimulation，ALTENS）[5]疗效。进行了充分治疗的亚组分析，包括切口区域电极的放置。所有试验表明：在 TENS 或 ALTENS 之后镇痛药的消耗量平均减少 26.5%（范围：-6%～+51%），优于安慰剂。该研究包括 21 项试验，共 1350 例腹部或整形外科手术后患者。其中 11 项研究接受了足够强度、低伤害及恰当频率的神经电刺激的 964 例患者中，镇痛药的消耗量减少了 36%（范围：14%～51%），同样优于安慰剂。此外，9 项研究未经证实使用了足够的电流强度及合适频率，为达到积极治疗，镇痛剂的消耗量增加了 4%（范围：-10%～29%）。在研究中发现 TENS 最佳频率的中位数为 85 Hz，而 ALTENS 为 2Hz[6]。该项荟萃分析研究表明 TENS 可以显著降低术后疼痛的镇痛药消耗。使用这项技术不良反应很小，只在电极接触部位略有不适。

表 20-1	非传统形式的术后止痛药物和方法
药物	腺苷
	抗惊厥剂
	抗组胺类
	巴氯芬
	咖啡因
	大麻素类
	辣椒素
	可乐定
	丹曲林
	右苯丙胺
	氯胺酮
	利诺卡因（静脉）
	咪达唑仑
	新斯的明
	昂丹司琼
	奥芬那君
非药物治疗	针灸
	行为疗法
	冷疗法和热疗法
	催眠术
	电离子透入疗法
	音乐
	经皮电神经刺激

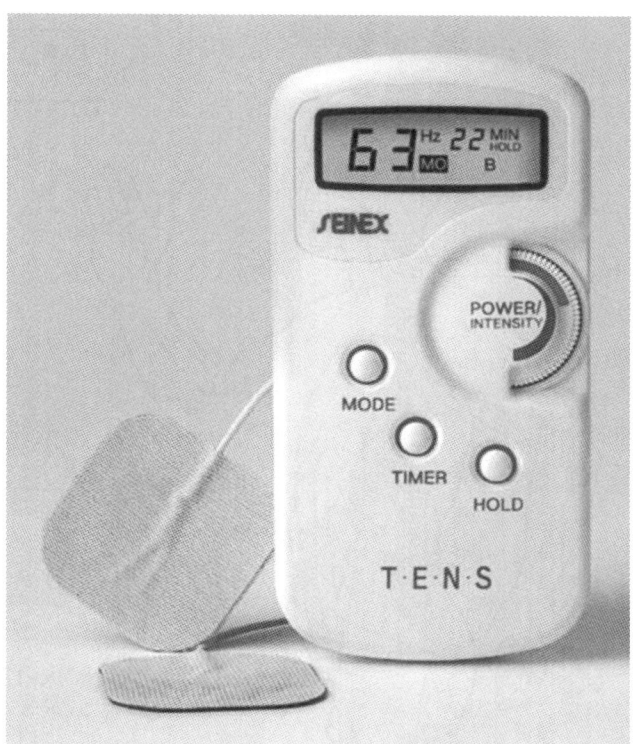

图 20-1　经皮电刺激神经治疗仪及电极片示意图——Seinex SE33 TENS。(Source:http://www.medisave.co.uk/popup_image.php/pID/761/)

因此，有可靠的证据表明 TENS 可能有利于患者的术后镇痛。然而，在将 TENS 技术广泛推广作为术中镇痛的辅助措施之前，还需要在不同手术条件下做更多的临床研究。

针灸

针灸是中医的一项传统技术，它的历史长达 3000 年之久。它是将很细的针插入身体特定的穴位（图 20-2），通过这些针可以加手动刺激、热刺激或电刺激。在最为广泛接受的针灸模型中，针灸肌肉神经纤维将使冲动传递到脊髓。3 个神经中枢被激活——脊髓、中脑及下丘脑-垂体系统。疼痛抑制是由内啡肽、单胺类神经递质所介导的。如果由有经验的医师进行操作，针灸很少有并发症。

美国国家卫生研究所于 1997 年发表了关于针灸共识的声明。结论表明：有充足的证据证明针灸疗法对牙科术后急性疼痛有效[7]。很多已出版的关于针灸的文献都是病例报道，关于针灸疗法的随机对照试验（RCT）较少，并且缺乏双盲对照研究。

在 2002 年一项综述中，Akca 等[8]调查了 4 项评估术中应用针灸疗法是否可以减少麻醉药用量，同时维持合适麻醉深度的 RCT。其中 3 项研究未证明麻醉药用量减少。然而，Kotani 等[9]证明至少有些针灸疗法为腹部手术提供了实质性术后镇痛，并使阿片类药物的用量减少。对于在上腹部或下腹部手术时使用全麻复合硬膜外麻醉的患者，术前使用皮内针灸疗法可以减轻切口痛及内脏痛。

尽管针灸疗法应用于术中可以提供一些益处，但是仅有一项 RCT 证明术前应用针灸有益于术后镇痛，且能减少阿片类药物的用量。观察和判断针灸是否适用于各种手术值得进一步探讨。目前尚不能推荐针灸疗法应用于术中。

催眠术

催眠术是一种诱导患者进入注意力高度集中的状态，从而使其更容易接受暗示并改变其知觉的技术。已经发现催眠可以作用于疼痛三级控制系统并使其作用减弱：伤害反射（脊髓及下行控制系统）、对疼痛强

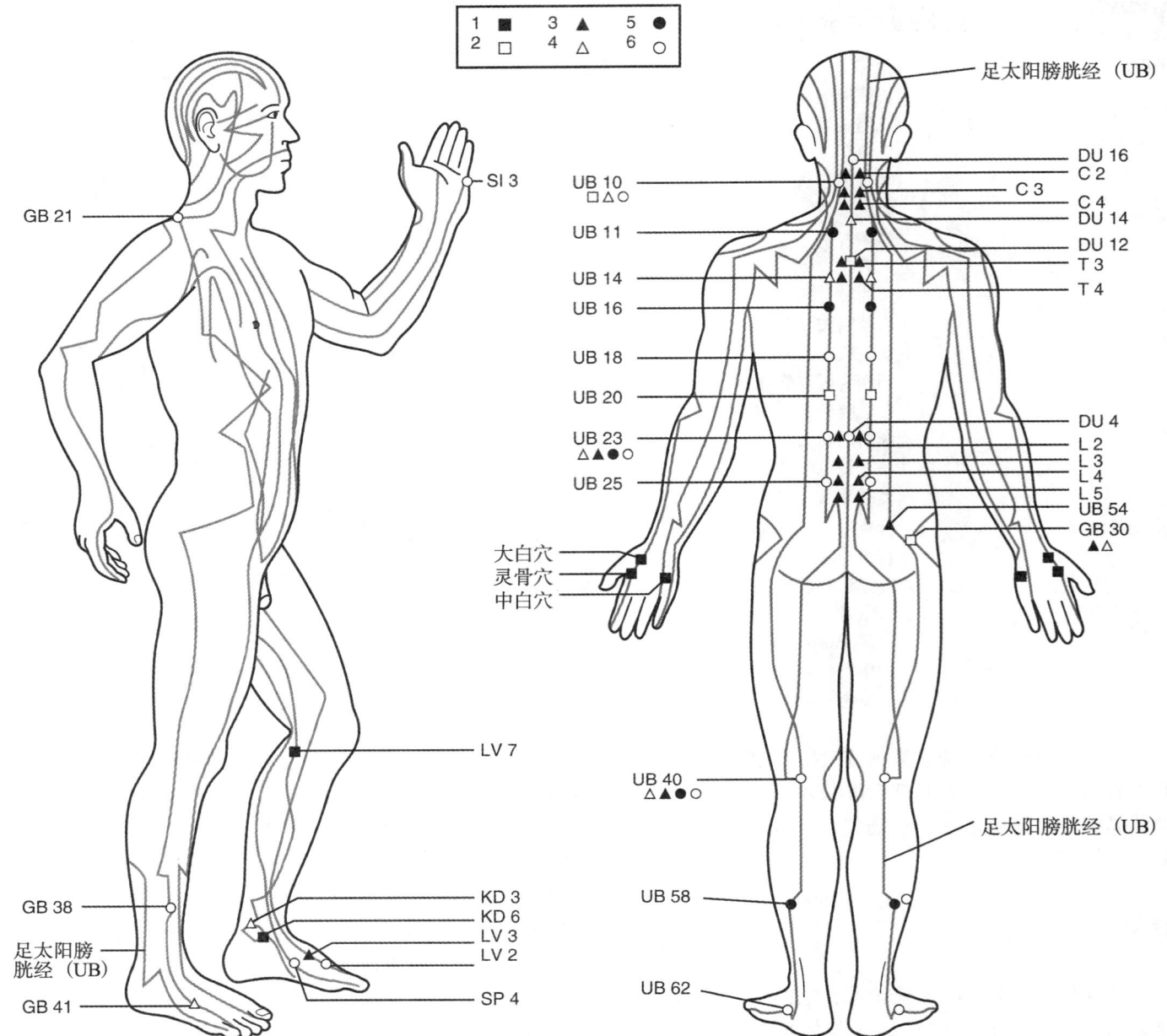

图 20-2 中医的穴位位置与相应各重要脏器的刺激点示意图。(Source: http://www.medscape.com/content/2001/00/41/07/410779/art-smj9405.08.fig.jpg/)

度的感知（脊髓及上行抑制系统）和不愉快的痛觉体验（感觉及情感抑制系统）[10]。

文献证实催眠术辅助术后镇痛有效。最初的证据来源于一些病例报告或系列病例报告，提示对成人和小儿实施手矫形术、椎板切除术[11]、口腔手术及颈部内分泌手术[12]有一定作用。一项回顾研究评估了 337 例整形外科手术中催眠术作为局部麻醉患者静脉清醒镇静的辅助措施，利用催眠术辅助镇痛组术中阿芬太尼及咪达唑仑的用量较少，镇痛较完善，且患者的满意度更高[13]。

当应用于合适的患者、合适的手术时，催眠术似乎在与镇痛联合应用中可能起到一定的作用。在更充分地评价联合常规平衡镇痛中催眠术的可能作用之前，仍需要进行临床RCT。

电离子透入疗法

电离子透入疗法是一项通过外在电场将药物电离成电荷分子贯穿皮肤,从而使其在真皮层吸收的技术。转移过程由两块电极之间形成的微小电流完成,给药速度与该电流强度成正比。该技术可以将药物输送到特定的靶点。因此,局部麻醉药及类固醇等药物可以通过该技术导入组织中。

已应用吗啡经皮给药,可以使血浆吗啡浓度达到20～50 ng/ml,而同时减少术后经静脉给予阿片类药物的用量。1992 年发表的一项前瞻性单盲随机对照试验阐述了吗啡通过电离子透入疗法给药的可行性[14]。38 例接受过关节置换术的患者被随机分组,术后 6 h 内在使用吗啡患者自控镇痛(patient-controlled analgesia,PCA)的基础上,一组通过电离子透入疗法给吗啡,另一组给予安慰剂。在吗啡电离子透入疗法组中,PCA 吗啡的需要量大大降低。在广泛推广该项技术应用于围手术期之前,还需要进一步的评估。

冷疗法和热疗法

物理疗法如冷疗法和热疗法在术后镇痛中可能起到一定作用。冷疗法常用于急性损伤后降低肿胀及疼痛,因为冷疗法可以使血管收缩,并且降低神经传导速度。一项研究显示,前十字韧带重建术后前 4 天接受手术侧膝部放置冷却装置的患者阿片类药物的用量减少[15]。

热疗法可以通过传导、对流或其他热能传导方式如红外线治疗、短波透热疗法及超声疗法来实施。这些对于治疗软组织损伤及慢性疼痛有一定作用。但是,还未有证据证明热疗法对术后急性镇痛有效。

音乐疗法

音乐疗法是一项可能减轻患者在麻醉后监护病房中疼痛感知的护理措施。研究表明,该方法可以减少焦虑,提高患者的满意度[16]。此外,一项 RCT 的结论认为,术中使用全身麻醉的同时运用音乐疗法可能有益于术后康复[17,18]。该 RCT 的另一篇论文结果表明[19],术中使用音乐疗法有减轻疼痛的短期效果[20]。

心身疗法

相当一部分非药物疗法可以归类为心身疗法。绝大多数心身疗法旨在促使患者平静及全面的康复,而非仅仅减轻术后疼痛。在 2004 年的一项综述中,Astin 指出一些证据表明心身疗法可能会对术后疼痛有作用[21]。研究发现该法对于术后疼痛的影响可分为两类,术前教授放松疗法和在全身麻醉当中播放对患者有积极建议的录音带。

放松训练

1984 年,Scott 和 Clum 研究了在术前对患者进行放松训练的作用[22],发现结果取决于患者个体对疼痛的应对方式,对于"易感"的患者是有作用的,而对逃避患者则不会减轻其术后疼痛。Mogan 等发现在 72 例实施腹部外科手术的患者中[23],放松训练对术后疼痛及对镇痛剂的需要量无明显改变;Daltroy 等发现在 222 例实施髋关节或膝关节置换术的患者中,术前是否进行心理辅导并无影响[24]。

然而,一种特殊的放松训练——引导想像却是有益的。在 Cleveland 诊所,随机选择患者进行引导想像训练,结果显示,与对照组相比,经过训练的患者术后疼痛评分降低(是对照组的 59%),吗啡的需要量也减少(是对照组的 58%)(两者 $P<0.001$)[25]。同样,Halpin 等[26]研究发现该疗法减少了心脏术后镇痛药的需要量。Laurion 和 Fetzer 研究表明引导想像疗法减轻了腹腔镜检查的疼痛[27]。尽管如此,放松训练充其量仅仅能减少术前的焦虑,由此减少这些焦虑患者术后镇痛药的需要量。

术中暗示

在全身麻醉时为患者播放有积极暗示作用的音乐,似乎对术后疼痛有一定影响。在 1990 年,McLintock 等[28]进行的一项有 60 例参与者的试验显示,接受了术中积极暗示的患者在经腹子宫切除术后对吗啡的需求量略有减少($P=0.028$),但是这些患者术后疼痛评分与对照组相同。后来的一些研究表明,对于实施了全身麻醉及妇科操作的患者,术中运用积极的暗示对减轻术后疼痛没有任何积极意义[29-31]。

药物镇痛

腺苷

腺苷是一种普遍存在的内源性嘌呤物质。最初发现其对心血管有益，同时，腺苷也有神经调节作用——通过作用于突触前受体和脊髓 A_1 及 A_3 受体[32-33]，抑制 G 蛋白，从而下调环磷酸腺苷（cyclic adenosine monophosphate，cAMP）[34]。鼠动物模型显示[35]，鞘内注射腺苷可以起到术后镇痛作用。然而，在 Rane 等对 48 名行腹部子宫切除术女性患者进行的一项随机对照试验中[36]，鞘内注射腺苷对术后疼痛没有作用。Apan 等将 60 例在臂丛神经阻滞下接受手术的患者随机分为两组，一组鞘内注射腺苷，而另一组给予安慰剂，发现腺苷组可以延长臂丛阻滞时间，然而两组的临床结果评价（要求首次追加麻醉药的时间、麻醉剂的需要量、视觉模拟评分）很相近，且腺苷组中有 2 名患者出现不良反应——胸痛和心悸[37]。

表 20-2　术后镇痛药物的剂量范围及不良反应

药物	剂量或剂量范围	不良反应	章节参考文献
腺苷	鞘内注射：500μg 静脉输注：50～500μg	胸痛、心悸、面红、支气管痉挛	36-40
抗惊厥剂		肝功能障碍	
普加巴林	50～300 mg	镇静	132
抗组胺类药物		镇静	
苯托沙敏	60 mg		149
大麻素类		潜在的依赖性、增加知晓	
δ-9-四氢大麻酚	5 mg		152
辣椒素	0.025%～0.075%（外用）	初次使用灼热感	146，147
可乐定	全身用药：0.3～5μg/kg 关节内给药：150μg 局部给药：1μg/kg 硬膜外给药：3μg/kg 鞘内给药：15～150μg	低血压、心动过缓、镇静	43-63，159-166
丹曲林	1.5 mg/kg，50～150 mg	肌无力、变态反应	124-126
右苯丙胺	5～10 mg	潜在的依赖性	153
氯胺酮	一次性给药：300μg/kg 输注：1～14μg/kg 骶管给药：250～500μg/kg 肌内注射：0.5～1mg/kg	心血管兴奋、脊髓毒性	89，90，105，167
利诺卡因	静脉给药：1.5mg/(kg·h)	心力衰竭、心律失常	123
咪达唑仑	肌内给药：5mg（一次给药） 骶管给药：50μg/kg 硬膜外给药：150μg/kg	镇静、低血压	116，119，121
新斯的明	鞘内给药：1～50μg/kg 关节内给药：500μg	恶心、呕吐	68-73，79
奈福泮	0.4 mg/kg，15～30 mg	出汗、心动过速	110-113，168
昂丹司琼	—	与曲马多合用于镇痛	157，158
奥芬那君	25～30 mg	恶心、呕吐	128，129

在 2 项随机对照临床试验中，Segerdahl 等[38,39]给接受乳房手术及经腹子宫切除术的患者外周输注腺苷[80μg/（kg·min）]可减少麻醉药及术后吗啡的需要量。Fukunaga 等[40]将 62 名实施重大手术的患者随机分为两组，术中及全身麻醉过程中分别输注瑞芬太尼[0.05～0.5μg/（kg·min），总剂量 2.5mg]或腺苷[50～500μg/（kg·min），总剂量 2500mg]，根据心血管反应滴定剂量。研究者发现两组术后疼痛和吗啡需要量有显著不同，腺苷组表现得更好，而腺苷组第一个 48 h 吗啡的累积需要量显著少于瑞芬太尼组（53±26mg vs 92±35mg，$P=0.001$）。

人工合成的腺苷受体激动剂已研制成功，但是随机临床试验显示其对术后疼痛无效[41]。

总之，随机临床试验证明全身麻醉中应用腺苷可以改善术后镇痛并减少阿片类药物的需要量，然而心血管方面的不良反应可能会限制其广泛应用[38-40]，如 Apan 等的研究报道[37]。

可乐定

可乐定是一种 α_2 肾上腺素能受体激动剂，该药物最初作为抗高血压药物应用于临床，而由于其具有镇痛、镇静、抗焦虑、交感神经阻滞、轻度麻醉和稳定血流动力学作用，目前被广泛应用于临床麻醉。可乐定、右旋美托咪啶以及盐酸替扎尼定等药物对中枢和外周均有作用。通过分子遗传技术已鉴定有 4 个受体亚型：2A、2B、2C 和 2D。2A 亚型介导 α_2 受体激动剂的抗伤害性作用。

可乐定已被广泛证明可以通过静脉、硬膜外、骶管[42,43]、肌内、口服[44,45]、经皮、外周、关节内注射[46]等方式给药，均可加强术后急性疼痛的镇痛作用。

尽管 α 受体激动剂和阿片类药物对镇痛有协同或相加作用，但值得庆幸的是，它们在呼吸抑制方面并没有协同或相加作用。这使 α 受体激动药可作为镇痛辅助用药，提高镇痛作用并且减少不良反应。α 受体激动剂的主要不良反应——低血压、心动过缓及镇静作用呈剂量相关。术前口服可乐定和术中经皮给予可乐定贴剂可以减少术后吗啡的需要量[47-49]。

由于可乐定的药代动力学特点及半衰期较短，因此静脉给予可乐定时，在一次性给药后需持续输注，以 $45μg/（kg·h）$ 的速率持续给药，剂量过大会导致镇静和低血压[43]。

目前已对可乐定与局麻药和阿片类复合硬膜外输注进行了研究[50]。硬膜外复合给予可乐定和吗啡可以提供更持久和更有效的镇痛[51-53]。然而，一项荟萃分析试图寻找硬膜外给予可乐定的最佳剂量，却未能成功[54]。

在腹股沟修复术中鞘内给予 15～30μg 可乐定复合布比卡因可以降低术后疼痛[55]。鞘内复合给予可乐定和吗啡对于心脏外科手术也是有意义的[56]。对于将要进行剖宫产的临产妇，鞘内复合给予布比卡因、阿片类及可乐定可以提供最佳术后镇痛[57]。

关节内给予可乐定可以达到麻醉效果，甚至与关节内给予吗啡效果一样好[58]。对于进行膝关节镜检查的非住院患者，膝关节内复合给予可乐定和局部麻醉药可以改善术后疼痛[59]。

可乐定和局麻药联合用于周围神经阻滞，可以短时间内减少局麻药剂量。在周围神经阻滞中，可乐定仅在与局部麻醉药联合应用时才有效[60,61]。可乐定已被用于胸部术后肌间神经阻滞及足部手术中[62,63]。

作为静脉局部麻醉的辅助用药，可乐定在 1μg/kg 剂量时可以改善术后镇痛[64]，但其益处有限[65]。

总之，可乐定被证明在局部麻醉和全身麻醉中作为麻醉辅助用药是有益的，值得广泛推广应用于平衡麻醉中。

新斯的明

新斯的明作为 M 胆碱酯酶抑制剂广泛应用于麻醉过程中，可以拮抗非去极化肌松药作用，同时，新斯的明也可用于镇痛。研究表明新斯的明可以经鞘内、硬膜外、骶管和关节内给药。

研究表明，新斯的明经椎管内给药具有良好的镇痛效果，但其不良反应如恶心、呕吐、镇静和低血压等限制了其应用[66,67]。

关于新斯的明经硬膜外或骶管给药辅助用于小儿手术的局部麻醉有一个很好的实例。在给予局麻药基础上，单次经骶管给予接受泌尿生殖器手术的患儿新斯的明 2μg/kg 可以降低疼痛评分（$P<0.005$），并可延长首次镇痛需要时间（$P<0.05$）[68]。另一项研究表明，在布比卡因骶管麻醉的同时加用新斯的明 2μg/kg 可以提供良好的镇痛，延长术后镇痛时间，减少镇痛药的追加量，但同时呕吐的发生率也有所增加[69]。第三项研究显示，骶管注入新斯的明 20～50μg/kg

可产生剂量相关的镇痛作用,而当剂量大于 30μg/kg 时恶心和呕吐的发生率增加[70]。

在成人妇产科手术中,新斯的明的镇痛作用有限。鞘内注入新斯的明 25～75μg 可以减少成人妇产科术后的吗啡需要量[71]。在妇科手术后,鞘内注射布比卡因和吗啡的基础上加用新斯的明 1～5μg 可以使镇痛时间延长一倍,并可减少术后第一个 24 h 内的镇痛药需要量,却不增加术后恶心呕吐的发生率[72]。此外,剖宫产术中鞘内复合给予新斯的明和吗啡可以显著减少术后 PCA 的需要量,两者联合应用的镇痛效果优于单用其中任何一种,同时,单独使用新斯的明可以增加恶心的发生率[73]。

全膝置换术患者鞘内注射新斯的明运动阻滞时间较吗啡更长,而且产生的术后瘙痒更多,术后疼痛的发生延迟,镇痛时间延长[74]。

因此,硬膜外给予新斯的明不管是单独应用还是和局麻药联合运用,均可延长术后镇痛时间,且可以减少局麻药的用量[74-76]。鞘内给予新斯的明在与局麻药联合使用的时候效果较好,但单用时术后常常出现无法接受的恶心、呕吐[77]。

在半月板修复手术后,膝关节内注入新斯的明 500μg 比注入吗啡 2 mg 的镇痛效果更好,且不良反应方面无差别[78]。

总之,新斯的明可以改善术后镇痛。硬膜外给予新斯的明最好与局麻药一起联合应用。鞘内注射新斯的明同样可以减少局麻药的用量,其主要缺点为术后恶心呕吐,但是可以通过和局麻药联合应用使该不良反应降至最小。全身应用新斯的明没有作用,但新斯的明关节腔内给药有良好的前景。

氯胺酮

氯胺酮是一种全身麻醉的诱导药,为 N-甲基-D-天冬氨酸(N-methyl-d-aspartate,NMDA)受体的非竞争性拮抗剂。NMDA 受体作用机制与术后疼痛及超敏反应相关。氯胺酮具有镇痛作用,但其导致的精神症状和心血管刺激作用限制了其应用。然而,关于 NMDA 受体在伤害性疼痛传入过程中作用的阐述,重新引起了人们对于氯胺酮作为镇痛药的兴趣[79]。一个假说认为[80],氯胺酮的镇痛作用是非阿片类机制介导的,可能包含苯环利定受体介导的 NMDA 受体离子通道阻断作用。氯胺酮阻断分布于外周和中枢神经系统中的钠离子通道。氯胺酮同样可以作用于 u、δ 及 κ 受体[81],以及单胺能敏感和电压敏感的钙离子通道[82,83]、烟碱受体和毒蕈碱受体[81]。

氯胺酮是一种消旋混合物,包含两种异构体——S^+ 氯胺酮及 R^- 氯胺酮;而纯 S^+ 氯胺酮的镇痛作用是 R^- 氯胺酮的 3～4 倍。目前有证据表明,小剂量氯胺酮在术后镇痛中发挥重要作用,它可以作为局麻药、阿片类药和其他镇痛药物的辅助用药,同时可以减轻阿片类药物的不良反应。

迄今为止,关于氯胺酮经口服、胃肠道外、皮下[84]、椎管内、关节内及经皮[85]给药的临床试验均已进行。一项系统回顾表明,术前预先给予氯胺酮可以起到改善术后镇痛的作用[86]。

基于亚麻醉剂量的氯胺酮具有镇痛及对抗术后痛觉过敏的假说,研究者在术中给予患者小剂量氯胺酮[87]。研究可根据氯胺酮的给药方式分为几类:一次性给药、给予负荷剂量后连续输注、连续输注、PCA。氯胺酮的镇痛效果取决于给药速度、负荷剂量和是否同时给予阿片类药物。一次性快速给予氯胺酮大于 300μg/kg 可以产生短效镇痛作用。小剂量输注氯胺酮低于 4μg/kg 且不给予负荷剂量时,对于术后镇痛没有影响。有证据表明,在给予负荷剂量基础上,以 1～6μg/(kg·min) 的速度输注氯胺酮有镇痛作用。氯胺酮的镇痛效能目前仍未明确。当在给予负荷剂量基础上,以 1～14μg/(kg·min) 的速度输注氯胺酮同时复合应用阿片类药物,可以使阿片类药物剂量减少 50%。在复合局部麻醉[88,89]时,一次性给药后连续输注氯胺酮也可减少术后阿片类药物的需要量[90,91],且可促进早期活动[92]。

在和吗啡联合应用于 PCA 时,氯胺酮可以提供术后镇痛并减少吗啡的需要量[93]。这种影响可一直延续至术后 48 h;在一组对照试验中,剖腹术后以 2.5μg/(kg·min) 的速度输注氯胺酮的一组患者术后 48 h 吗啡的累积需要量明显降低(28 mg vs 54 mg,$P=0.0003$)[94]。有些研究发现氯胺酮和吗啡联合应用于 PCA 没有益处[95],这可能与氯胺酮的剂量不恰当有关。

通过硬膜外给予吗啡和不含防腐剂的氯胺酮可以减轻疼痛、延长镇痛时间并减少吗啡用量[96-100]。对于行上腹部手术的患者,经硬膜外给予布比卡因、氯胺酮和吗啡可以有效减轻术后疼痛,并显著减少吗啡需要量——从 12.5 mg(范围:3～42 mg)减至 6.0 mg(范围:1～200 mg)($P=0.005$)。关于氯胺酮用于硬膜外患者自控镇痛（patient-controlled epidural analgesia, PECA）的研究已经进行[101]，且结果令人振奋。在儿科脐以下手术时，局麻药中加入氯胺酮 0.25 mg/kg 行骶管麻醉可以延长阻滞时间[102-106]。

由于氯胺酮对脊髓的毒性作用，鞘内给药是不可行的，无论对于不含防腐剂的氯胺酮和含防腐剂的氯胺酮均如是[107]。对接受关节镜手术的患者，关节腔内给予氯胺酮的镇痛效果比肌内注射差[108]。总之，术中，尤其是预先给药时，经静脉给予氯胺酮可以用作镇痛剂。氯胺酮经硬膜外或骶管给药可以减少局部麻醉药的用量。值得注意的是，氯胺酮在术中作为镇痛剂的作用还未得到充分发挥。

奈福泮

奈福泮作为一个非阿片类中枢作用的镇痛剂，与其他药物无明显相关性，其作用机制目前尚未明确。奈福泮的作用并不是影响前列腺素的合成，而是抑制神经细胞对 5-羟色胺、多巴胺和去甲肾上腺素等神经递质的重摄取。已发表许多关于奈福泮的临床随机试验。Tigerstedt 等[109]在 100 例腹部术后患者中比较了奈福泮和哌替啶的镇痛效果，发现奈福泮 15 mg 或 30mg 的镇痛效果介于哌替啶 50 mg 和 100 mg 之间。McLintock 等[110]研究发现，49 例行腹部手术的患者，给予奈福泮 20 mg 可以减少吗啡需要量。同样，Moffat 等[111]在 42 例腹部术后接受 PCA 的患者中证实奈福泮可以减少吗啡的需要量，尤其是和双氯芬酸联合应用时。一项包括 201 例全髋置换术患者的临床安慰剂对照 RCT 试验，证实奈福泮（口服 20 mg）可以减少吗啡的需要量。确定奈福泮和吗啡等效剂量研究表明，奈福泮 0.4 mg/kg 等效于吗啡 0.1 mg/kg，奈福泮 18 mg 等效于吗啡 5 mg[112]。尽管目前还未开始广泛应用，但奈福泮作为术后平衡镇痛的辅助用药可减少阿片类药物的用量，因此应受到应有的重视。

咪达唑仑

咪达唑仑是一种中效的苯二氮䓬类药物，最初主要用于镇静，同时也具有抗伤害刺激的作用。它有助于改善急性疼痛造成的情感变化。

咪达唑仑全身用药，如在术前 30 分钟肌内注射，可减少门诊手术患者的术后疼痛（$P=0.035$）[113]。在拔除第三磨牙的手术中，在局部麻醉基础上辅用咪达唑仑镇静可大大减轻术后疼痛（$P<0.005$），并减少镇痛剂用量（$P<0.001$）[114]。在女性经腹子宫切除术术前和术中给予咪达唑仑可以降低疼痛评分并减少吗啡的需要量（$P<0.002$）[115]。同样，椎管内给予咪达唑仑也已被研究。在膝关节镜检查术和剖宫产术后，椎管内联合给予咪达唑仑和布比卡因较单独使用布比卡因术后镇痛效果更好（$P<0.05$）[116,117]。同样，在小儿骶管阻滞中，布比卡因中加入咪达唑仑可使术后镇痛时间延长一倍（$P<0.001$）[118]。单独经骶管给予咪达唑仑也是有效的，可以减少疝切开术后镇痛剂的需要量（$P<0.05$）[119]。Nishiyama[120]发表的一系列文献表明，咪达唑仑经硬膜外单次给药或持续输注均可以用于腹部手术术后的镇痛[121]。

咪达唑仑经蛛网膜下腔或硬膜外给药均有明确的术后镇痛作用[122]。然而，由于担心可能存在的神经毒性，因此需要进一步研究以确定咪达唑仑用于术后镇痛的最适剂量和用药时限，但是其在平衡镇痛中有广泛的应用前景是不容忽视的。

利诺卡因

利诺卡因是一种临床普遍应用的局部麻醉剂，具有很多的临床使用价值。目前引起关注的是，静脉注射利诺卡因可能有止痛效果。阻滞外周机械敏感性伤害感受器的钠离子通道可抑制中枢疼痛致敏。对于行腹部重大手术的患者，在切皮之前给予利诺卡因 1.5mg/kg，推注，随后以 1.5 mg/(kg·h) 的速度持续泵注，可使术后 72 h 内吗啡的累积需要量大大减少（103±72 mg vs 159±73.3 mg，$P=0.5$）[123]。显然，还需要进一步地研究，但初步研究结果是令人振奋的。

丹曲林

已知丹曲林钠有肌松作用，这是由于其可部分抑制肌细胞的肌浆网侧囊释放钙离子。它禁用于急性肝脏疾病患者。大量研究已经证明丹曲林可以减轻术后肌肉疼痛。

在一项随机临床试验中，48 例患者术前 2 h 口服单次剂量丹曲林（100～150 mg）可使氯化琥珀胆碱导致的肌痛发生率从 56% 降至 4%，而不影响氯化琥珀胆碱的作用持续时间[124]。由于目前氯化琥珀胆碱已很少使用，因此该作用的重要性也随之减小了。113 例扁桃腺切除术患者，在术后前 5 天，分别口服丹曲林 [每日 4 次，每日剂量 1.5 mg/(kg·d)]和安慰剂，结果发现丹曲林对减轻扁桃腺切除术后疼痛有一定效果[125]。然而一项包括 40 名行直肠脱垂手术患者的双盲对照试验显示，口服丹曲林与安慰剂在控制术后疼痛方面没有明显差异[126]。

综上所述，丹曲林有减轻氯化琥珀胆碱导致的肌痛作用[124]，但对临床术后镇痛无效。

奥芬那君

奥芬那君是一种中枢性抗胆碱能肌松药，其在术后应用的文献报道极少。1979 年，Fry[127] 报道了关于阿片全碱-奥芬那君复合用药的预试验。他主张在手术即将结束时给予奥芬那君，可以延长阿片全碱的镇痛效果，从而推迟术后加用止痛剂的时间。然而，随后的文献未见发表。同年，Winter 和 Post 进行了一项双盲试验[128]，在 200 例行口腔外科手术的患者中，分别给予奥芬那君（25 mg）、对乙酰氨基酚（325mg）、两药合用和安慰剂。结果显示联合用药组的镇痛效果最好，单独使用奥芬那君的镇痛效果也优于安慰剂。随后在捷克共和国[128]，Malek 等[29]在门诊关节镜术后患者中随机静脉注射吡罗昔康、安慰剂及联合给予双氯芬酸 75 mg 和奥芬那君 30 mg。结果双氯芬酸、奥芬那君联合用药组术后镇痛效果最好，不良反应也最少。总之，这 2 项相隔 25 年发表的试验，显示奥芬那君可能是有益的。然而，在其被推荐为镇痛辅助药之前，可能还需要更多进一步的试验验证。

抗惊厥药

抗惊厥剂是一种膜稳定剂，目前已明确该类药可通过阻滞神经自主放电，从而治疗神经痛，但是关于其术后应用的研究却很少[130]。由于大多数抗惊厥药都有比较显著的不良反应，因此在处理慢性疼痛时，抗惊厥药往往从小剂量开始逐渐增量，直到产生预期效果。这一原因限制了其在术后镇痛中的应用。然而，Field 等[131]在小鼠后肢模型上证明加巴喷丁和 S-+3-isobutylgaba 有术后镇痛作用。临床研究表明，拔牙后 γ-氨基丁酸（GABA）的前体普瑞巴林的镇痛作用优于布洛芬和安慰剂[132]。虽然经一步研究表明术中使用普瑞巴林可能有镇痛作用，但目前抗惊厥剂尚未用于控制术后疼痛。

三环类和四环类抗抑郁药

三环类和四环类抗抑郁药主要作为治疗精神类疾病的药物，由于其具有调节大脑和脊髓中 5-羟色胺和去甲肾上腺素水平的作用而被认为具有镇痛作用[133]。动物实验研究支持这一观点，认为抗抑郁药有特殊的生物化学镇痛作用，而非仅仅通过改善情绪以减轻疼痛导致的抑郁[134,135]。关于术后的临床研究较少。Iacono 等[136]发现，三环类抗抑郁药对于预防和治疗下肢截肢术后的幻肢痛有效。

抗抑郁药是目前已经确定的一线慢性疼痛治疗药物，而大多数研究者均聚焦于此。一般认为，服用抗抑郁药数周后才会起到镇痛作用，这是限制其用于术后镇痛的主要原因。三环类和四环类抗抑郁药的镇痛作用仍主要体现于治疗慢性神经性疼痛。

咖啡因

咖啡因长期来用作各种镇痛药的辅助用药。最佳证据来源于 1984 包括 30 个试验 10 000 例患者的一项荟萃分析，结果证明镇痛剂复合应用咖啡因所产生的镇痛效果为其单独应用的 1.4 倍[137]。一组关于牙科后给予布洛芬和阿司匹林加用或不加用咖啡因的随机试验显示[138,139]，加用咖啡因效果更好。随后的系统回顾质疑了小剂量咖啡因和对乙酰氨基酚或阿司匹林联合应用的益处[140,141]，并提出了对镇痛药性肾病和咖啡因增强镇痛之间相关性的担忧。尽管被 IA（I 指大型 RCT[142]，每组 N≥100；A 表示推荐具有充分证据支持）证据所支持[137]，咖啡因仍不能广泛用于平衡镇痛疗法。需要进行进一步的研究以确定咖啡因的最佳剂量和外科适用范围，从而评估其是否存在作为镇痛剂应用的价值。

辣椒素

红辣椒中提取出的辣椒素常用于治疗各种疼痛[143]。它通过减少神经递质 P 物质及降钙素基因相关肽（calcitonin gene-related peptide，CGRP）的储存，从而使无鞘 C 神经纤维和纤细的有鞘 $A_δ$ 神经纤维的伤害性感受器脱敏[144,145]。虽然辣椒素初期应用于局部会导致灼痛，但是通过反复应用可以达到脱敏作用，这是一个钙依赖性的可逆脱敏作用。应用高剂量辣椒素可以产生神经毒性。一项关于23例患有乳房切除术后疼痛综合征的随机对照试验证明，局部运用辣椒素（0.075%）的有效率是62%，而安慰剂为30%[146]。由于辣椒素治疗时产生灼热感，从而使该项研究很难达到"双盲"的要求，这一问题解释了为何绝大多数辣椒素研究缺乏对照组。例如，Dini等[147]研究发现，给予一组21例患有乳房切除术后疼痛综合征的女性患者2个月辣椒辣素乳剂（0.025%）治疗，结果其中13例（62%）对治疗有反应，11例（52%）在疗程结束后3个月仍未感到疼痛。尽管单独看待该研究显示了令人振奋的结果，然而可惜的是在其他研究中显示安慰剂也有18%~30%的有效率[143,146-148]。因此，辣椒素不太可能用于术后疼痛的临床治疗。

抗组胺类药物

大多数抗组胺类药物被用作镇静剂、止吐剂和抗毒蕈碱剂，然而其也具有镇痛作用，可能较传统镇痛剂更为有效。大多数抗组胺类药物的镇痛作用可以部分通过它的镇静作用来解释。一组包括200例妇科住院患者的RCT发现，复合使用苯甲苯氧胺60 mg和对乙酰氨基酚650 mg对减轻外阴切开术后疼痛方面优于单独使用对乙酰氨基酚[149]。然而，这项单中心的研究还不足以充分证明抗组胺类药在控制术后疼痛中的作用。

巴氯芬

巴氯芬是一种肌肉松弛剂，激动$GABA_\beta$受体。它作用于突触前受体，通过阻止钙离子内流和抑制神经递质释放发挥作用。巴氯芬通常用于治疗神经性疼痛，但该药的临床应用受到其不良反应的限制，如镇静和谵妄。它也用作脊柱外科术后的解痉剂，但与镇痛无关。一项单中心试验发现，手术前给予巴氯芬和吗啡有协同的镇痛作用，但未发现和喷他佐辛有协同作用。单独使用巴氯芬和安慰剂没有差别，甚至在减轻牙科术后疼痛的效果比对乙酰氨基酚差[150]。巴氯芬没有减轻术后急性疼痛的作用。

大麻素类

大麻素类为大麻的活性成分，推测其可能具有抗焦虑和止痛的作用。大麻素类作用于大麻素受体CB_1和CB_2，从而抑制腺苷酸环化酶和N型钙电流。大麻素类在脊髓和神经轴索水平均可能产生抵抗伤害性刺激的作用。CB_1受体在脑和脊髓占优势，因此可能在镇痛中起主要作用。CB_1受体激动剂很有可能作为止痛药，对控制慢性疼痛有作用，尤其对于晚期病症[151]。在最近的一项关于大麻素类术后镇痛的随机对照试验中，在经腹行子宫切除术后2天内给予δ-9-四氢大麻酚酸与安慰剂相比在镇痛方面无明显差异[152]。

右苯丙胺

右苯丙胺是一种精神兴奋剂，1977年的一组随机对照试验试图研究其是否具有术后镇痛作用。10 mg右苯丙胺和吗啡复合应用可以使吗啡产生2倍的镇痛效果，同时可以减少阿片类药物的常见过度镇静和嗜睡不良反应[153]。然而，目前已知苯异丙胺有成瘾的不良反应，因此不可能作为术后镇痛剂应用于临床。

昂丹司琼

昂丹司琼为$5-HT_3$受体拮抗剂，是有效的止吐剂[154]。一些研究者根据5-羟色胺路径推测昂丹司琼可能具有止痛作用。有两篇临床随机双盲对照试验文献。Doenicke等[155]随机对100位接受小手术的患者静脉注射昂丹司琼或安慰剂，发现昂丹司琼无止痛作用。Broome等[156]在拔牙手术后给患者口服昂丹司琼或甲氧氯普胺联合双氯芬酸或曲马多，发现在镇痛方面无差异。此外，昂丹司琼和曲马多竞争$5-HT_3$受体，从而可以降低曲马多的镇痛效果[157,158]。该文献证明昂丹司琼不仅在镇痛方面没有有益的作用，反而会干扰曲马多的镇痛效果。

总结

历年来文献报道了多种用于术后镇痛的药物和方法，其中一些基于有力证据已进入常规疗法的行列，如氯胺酮、可乐定和新斯的明；一些被证明无效或有不良反应而被废弃，如右苯丙胺；还有一些由于证据不足或存在争论仍被常规使用，此类包括本章所讨论的其余大多数药物和方法。很多时候，由于缺少合理的随机对照试验所提供的结果，我们很难获得最终的证据。很明显，对于某些药物或技术，通过严格监管的试验获得证据存在技术上的局限性，但即使这一问题得以解决，这些疗法是否有效仍不应由临床执业医师来评判。

本文讨论了很多已被用于改善术后镇痛的药物和方法。循证医学表明，其中大多数应得到更为广泛的应用。催眠、针灸和TENS对于某些患者，尤其是那些先前曾使用过且奏效的患者是很有效的。

有证据表明，很多还未被广泛认知的具有镇痛作用的药物，应有更好的应用前景。经硬膜外给予小剂量新斯的明和可乐定可以减少局部麻醉药的用量，而且在推荐剂量范围内所产生的不良反应在可接受范围内。静脉给予 0.2 mg/kg 剂量的氯胺酮是有效的，并且不良反应最小；临床镇痛研究同样推荐应用咪达唑仑、奥芬那君和腺苷。阿片类药物、NSAID和对乙酰氨基酚可能依然是治疗急性疼痛的首选，但仍有很多药物可以加强术后镇痛，且不良反应较小。

在进一步进行临床研究以确定药物剂量和给药途径的同时，提高麻醉医师、手术护士、药剂师和外科医师对这些药物的认识也是需要克服的挑战之一。

(孟　岩　水恒兵译　朱科明　熊源长校)

参考文献

1. Eisenberg DM, Davis RB, Ettner SL: Trends in alternative medicine use in the United States, 1990–1997: Results of a follow-up national survey. JAMA 1998;280:246–252.
2. Melzack R, Wall PD: Pain mechanisms: A new theory. Science 1965;150:971–979.
3. Garrison DW, Foreman RD: Decreased activity of spontaneous and noxiously evoked dorsal horn cells during transcutaneous electrical nerve stimulation (TENS). Pain 1994;58:309–315.
4. Carroll D, Tramer M, McQuay H, et al: Randomization is important in studies with pain outcomes: Systematic review of transcutaneous electrical nerve stimulation in acute postoperative pain. Br J Anaesth 1996;77:798–803.
4a. http://www.jr2ox.ac.uk/bandolier/booth/booths/ebmstor.html
5. Bjordal JM, Johnson MI, Ljunggreen AE: Transcutaneous electrical nerve stimulation (TENS) can reduce postoperative analgesic consumption: A meta-analysis with assessment of optimal treatment parameters for postoperative pain. Eur J Pain 2003;7:181–188.
6. Hamza MA, White PF, Ahmed HE, Ghoname EA: Effect of the frequency of transcutaneous electrical nerve stimulation on the postoperative analgesic requirement and recovery profile. Anesthesiology 1999; 91:1232–1328.
7. Acupuncture. MH Consensus Statement. 1997, Nov. 3–5;15(5):1–34.
8. Akca O, Sessler DI: Acupuncture: A useful complement of anesthesia? Minerva Anestesiol 2002;68:147–151.
9. Kotani N, Hashimoto H, Sato Y, et al: Preoperative intradermal acupuncture reduces postoperative pain, nausea and vomiting, analgesic requirement, and sympathoadrenal responses. Anesthesiology 2001; 95:349–356.
10. Gracely RH: Hypnosis and hierarchical pain control systems. Pain 1995;60:1–2.
11. Snow BR: The use of hypnosis in the management of preoperative anxiety and postoperative pain in a patient undergoing laminectomy. Bull Hosp Jt Dis Orthop Inst 1985;45:143–149.
12. Meurisse M: [Thyroid and parathyroid surgery under hypnosis: from fiction to clinical application.] Bull Mem Acad R Med Belg 1999; 154:142–150.
13. Faymonville ME, Fissette J, Mambourg PH, et al: Hypnosis as adjunct therapy in conscious sedation for plastic surgery. Reg Anesth 1995; 20:145–151.
14. Ashburn MA, Stephen RL, Ackerman E, et al: Iontophoretic delivery of morphine for postoperative analgesia. J Pain Symptom Manag 1992;7:27–33.
15. Cohn BT, Draeger RI, Jackson DW: The effects of cold therapy in the postoperative management of pain in patients undergoing anterior cruciate ligament reconstruction. Am J Sports Med 1989;17:344–349.
16. Heitz L, Symreng T, Scamman FL: Effect of music therapy in the postanesthesia care unit: A nursing intervention. J Post Anesth Nurs 1992;7:22–31.
17. Good M, Anderson GC, Stanton-Hicks M, et al: Relaxation and music reduce pain after gynecologic surgery. Pain Manage Nursing 2002; 3:61–70.
18. Koch ME, Kain ZN, Ayoub C, Rosenbaum SH: The sedative and analgesic sparing effect of music. Anesthesiology 1998;89:300–306.
19. Nilsson U, Rawal N, Unestahl LE, et al: Improved recovery after music and therapeutic suggestions during general anaesthesia: A double-blind randomised controlled trial. Acta Anaesth Scand 2001;45:812–817.
20. Nilsson U, Rawal N, Unosson M: A comparison of intra-operative or postoperative exposure to music—a controlled trial of the effects on postoperative pain. Anaesthesia 2003;58:699–703.
21. Astin JA: Mind-body therapies for the management of pain. Clin J Pain 2004;20:27–32.
22. Scott LE, Clum GA: Examining the interaction effects of coping style and brief interventions in the treatment of postsurgical pain. Pain 1984;20:279–291.
23. Mogan J, Wells N, Robertson E: Effects of preoperative teaching on postoperative pain: A replication and expansion. Int J Nurs Stud 1985;22:267–280.
24. Daltroy LH, Morlino CI, Eaton HM, et al: Preoperative education for total hip and knee replacement patients. Arthritis Care Res 1998;11:469–478.
25. Tusek DL, Church JM, Strong SA, et al: Guided imagery: A significant advance in the care of patients undergoing elective colorectal surgery. Dis Colon Rectum 1997;40:172–178.
26. Halpin LS, Speir AM, CapoBianco P, Barnett SD: Guided imagery in cardiac surgery. Outcomes Manag 2002;6:132–137.
27. Laurion S, Fetzer SJ: The effect of two nursing interventions on the postoperative outcomes of gynecologic laparoscopic patients. J Perianesth Nurs 2003;18:254–261.
28. McLintock TT, Aitken H, Downie CF, Kenny GN: Postoperative analgesic requirements in patients exposed to positive intraoperative suggestions. BMJ 1990;301:788–790.
29. Block RI, Ghoneim MM, Sum Ping ST, Ali MA: Efficacy of therapeutic suggestions for improved postoperative recovery presented during general anesthesia. Anesthesiology 1991;75:746–755.
30. Lebovits AH, Twersky R, McEwan B: Intraoperative therapeutic suggestions in day-case surgery: Are there benefits for postoperative

outcome? Br J Anaesth 1999;82:861–866.
31. Dawson P, Van Hamel C, Wilkinson D, et al: Patient-controlled analgesia and intra-operative suggestion. Anaesthesia 2001;56:65–69.
32. Sawynok J: Adenosine receptor activation and nociception. Eur J Pharmacol 1998;347:1–11.
33. Sollevi A: Adenosine for pain control. Acta Anaesthesiol Scand Suppl 1997;110:135–136.
34. Gordh T, Karlsten R, Kristensen J: Intervention with spinal NMDA, adenosine, and NO systems for pain modulation. Ann Med 1995;27:229–234.
35. Chiari AI, Eisenach JC: Intrathecal adenosine: Interactions with spinal clonidine and neostigmine in rat models of acute nociception and postoperative hypersensitivity. Anesthesiology 1999;90:1413–1421.
36. Rane K, Sollevi A, Segerdahl M: Intrathecal adenosine administration in abdominal hysterectomy lacks analgesic effect. Acta Anaesthesiol Scand 2000;44:868–872.
37. Apan A, Ozcan S, Buyukkocak U, et al: Perioperative intravenous adenosine infusion to extend postoperative analgesia in brachial plexus block. Eur J Anaesthesiol 2003;20:916–919.
38. Segerdahl M, Ekblom A, Sandelin K, et al: Perioperative adenosine infusion reduces the requirements for isoflurane and postoperative analgesics. Anesth Analg 1995;80:1145–1149.
39. Segerdahl M, Irestedt L, Sollevi A: Antinociceptive effect of perioperative adenosine infusion in abdominal hysterectomy. Acta Anaesthesiol Scand 1997;41:473–479.
40. Fukunaga AF, Alexander GE, Stark CW: Characterization of the analgesic actions of adenosine: Comparison of adenosine and remifentanil infusions in patients undergoing major surgical procedures. Pain 2003;101:129–138.
41. Seymour RA, Hawkesford JE, Hill CM, et al: The efficacy of a novel adenosine agonist (WAG 994) in postoperative dental pain. Br J Clin Pharmacol 1999;47:675–680.
42. Bernard JM, Hommeril JL, Passuti N, Pinaud M: Postoperative analgesia by intravenous clonidine. Anesthesiology 1991;75:577–582.
43. Marinangeli F, Ciccozzi A, Donatelli F, et al: Clonidine for treatment of postoperative pain: A dose-finding study. Eur J Pain 2002;6:35–42.
44. Van Elstraete AC, Pastureau F, Lebrun T, Mehdaoui H: Caudal clonidine for postoperative analgesia in adults. Br J Anaesth 2000;84:401–402.
45. Constant I, Gall O, Gouyet L, et al: Addition of clonidine or fentanyl to local anaesthetics prolongs the duration of surgical analgesia after single shot caudal block in children. Br J Anaesth 1998;80:294–298.
46. De Kock M, Wiederkher P, Laghmiche A, Scholtes JL: Epidural clonidine used as the sole analgesic agent during and after abdominal surgery: A dose-response study. Anesthesiology 1997;86:285–292.
47. Park J, Forrest J, Kolesar R, et al: Oral clonidine reduces postoperative PCA morphine requirements. Can J Anaesth 1996;43:900–906.
48. Goyagi T, Tanaka M, Nishikawa T: Oral clonidine premedication enhances postoperative analgesia by epidural morphine. Anesth Analg 1999;89:1487–1491.
49. Yu HP, Hseu SS, Yien HW, et al: Oral clonidine premedication preserves heart rate variability for patients undergoing laparoscopic cholecystectomy. Acta Anaesthesiol Scand 2003;47:185–190.
50. Milligan KR, Convery PN, Weir P, et al: The efficacy and safety of epidural infusions of levobupivacaine with and without clonidine for postoperative pain relief in patients undergoing total hip replacement. Anesth Analg 2000;91:393–397.
51. Anzai Y, Nishikawa T: Thoracic epidural clonidine and morphine for postoperative pain relief. Can J Anaesth 1995;42:292–297.
52. Capogna G, Celleno D, Zangrillo A, et al: Addition of clonidine to epidural morphine enhances postoperative analgesia after cesarean delivery. Reg Anesth 1995;20:57–61.
53. Carabine UA, Milligan KR, Mulholland D, Moore J: Extradural clonidine infusions for analgesia after total hip replacement. Br J Anaesth 1992;68:338–343.
54. Armand S, Langlade A, Boutros A, et al: Meta-analysis of the efficacy of extradural clonidine to relieve postoperative pain: An impossible task. Br J Anaesth 1998;81:126–134.
55. Dobrydnjov I, Axelsson K, Thorn SE, et al: Clonidine combined with small-dose bupivacaine during spinal anesthesia for inguinal herniorrhaphy: A randomized double-blinded study. Anesth Analg 2003;96:1496–1503.
56. Lena P, Balarac N, Arnulf JJ, et al: Intrathecal morphine and clonidine for coronary artery bypass grafting. Br J Anaesth 2003;90:300–303.
57. Paech MJ, Pavy TJ, Orlikowski CE, et al: Postcesarean analgesia with spinal morphine, clonidine, or their combination. Anesth Analg 2004;98:1460–1466.
58. Joshi W, Reuben SS, Kilaru PR, et al: Postoperative analgesia for outpatient arthroscopic knee surgery with intraarticular clonidine and/or morphine. Anesth Analg 2000;90:1102–1106.
59. Reuben SS, Connelly NR: Postoperative analgesia for outpatient arthroscopic knee surgery with intraarticular clonidine. Anesth Analg 1999;88:729–733.
60. Sia S, Lepri A: Clonidine administered as an axillary block does not affect postoperative pain when given as the sole analgesic. Anesth Analg 1999;88:1109–1112.
61. Singelyn FJ, Gouverneur JM, Robert A: A minimum dose of clonidine added to mepivacaine prolongs the duration of anesthesia and analgesia after axillary brachial plexus block. Anesth Analg 1996;83:1046–1050.
62. Tschernko EM, Klepetko H, Gruber E, et al: Clonidine added to the anesthetic solution enhances analgesia and improves oxygenation after intercostal nerve block for thoracotomy. Anesth Analg 1998;87:107–111.
63. Reinhart DJ, Wang W, Stagg KS, et al: Postoperative analgesia after peripheral nerve block for podiatric surgery: Clinical efficacy and chemical stability of lidocaine alone versus lidocaine plus clonidine. Anesth Analg 1996;83:760–765.
64. Reuben SS, Steinberg RB, Klatt JL, Klatt ML: Intravenous regional anesthesia using lidocaine and clonidine. Anesthesiology 1999;91:654–658.
65. Kleinschmidt S, Stockl W, Wilhelm W, Larsen R: The addition of clonidine to prilocaine for intravenous regional anaesthesia. Eur J Anaesthesiol 1997;14:40–46.
66. Klamt JG, Slullitel A, Garcia IV, Prado WA: Postoperative analgesic effect of intrathecal neostigmine and its influence on spinal anaesthesia. Anaesthesia 1997;52:547–551.
67. Lauretti GR, Mattos AL, Gomes JM, Pereira NL: Postoperative analgesia and antiemetic efficacy after intrathecal neostigmine in patients undergoing abdominal hysterectomy during spinal anesthesia. Reg Anesth 1997;22:527–533.
68. Turan A, Memis D, Basaran UN, et al: Caudal ropivacaine and neostigmine in pediatric surgery. Anesthesiology 2003;98:719–722.
69. Abdulatif M, El Sanabary M: Caudal neostigmine, bupivacaine, and their combination for postoperative pain management after hypospadias surgery in children. Anesth Analg 2002;95:1215–1218.
70. Batra YK, Arya VK, Mahajan R, Chari P: Dose response study of caudal neostigmine for postoperative analgesia in paediatric patients undergoing genitourinary surgery. Paediatr Anaesth 2003;13:515–521.
71. Lauretti GR, Hood DD, Eisenach JC, Pfeifer BL: A multi-center study of intrathecal neostigmine for analgesia following vaginal hysterectomy. Anesthesiology 1998;89:913–918.
72. Almeida RA, Lauretti GR, Mattos AL: Antinociceptive effect of low-dose intrathecal neostigmine combined with intrathecal morphine following gynecologic surgery. Anesthesiology 2003;98:495–498.
73. Chung CJ, Kim JS, Park HS, Chin YJ: The efficacy of intrathecal neostigmine, intrathecal morphine, and their combination for post-cesarean section analgesia. Anesth Analg 1998;87:341–346.
74. Kaya FN, Sahin S, Owen MD, Eisenach JC: Epidural neostigmine produces analgesia but also sedation in women after cesarean delivery. Anesthesiology 2004;100:381–385.
75. Omais M, Lauretti GR, Paccola CA: Epidural morphine and neostigmine for postoperative analgesia after orthopedic surgery. Anesth Analg 2002;95:1698–1701.
76. Nakayama M, Ichinose H, Nakabayashi K, et al: Analgesic effect of epidural neostigmine after abdominal hysterectomy. J Clin Anesth 2001;13:86–89.
77. Lauretti GR, de Oliveira R, Reis MP, et al: Study of three different doses of epidural neostigmine coadministered with lidocaine for postoperative analgesia. Anesthesiology 1999;90:1534–1538.
78. Yang LC, Chen LM, Wang CJ, Buerkle H: Postoperative analgesia by intra-articular neostigmine in patients undergoing knee arthroscopy. Anesthesiology 1998;88:334–339.
79. Ilkjaer S, Petersen KL, Brennum J, et al: Effect of systemic NMDA receptor antagonist (ketamine) on primary and secondary hyperalgesia in humans. Br J Anaesth 1996;76:829–834.
80. Willets J, Balster RL, Leander P: The behavioural pharmacology of NMDA receptor antagonists. Trends Pharmacol Sci 1990;11:423–428.
81. Scheller M, Bufler J, Hertle I, et al: Ketamine blocks currents through

mammalian nicotinic acetylcholine receptor channels by interaction with both the open and the closed state. Anesth Analg 1996; 83:830–836.
82. Hustveit O, Maurset A, Oye I: Interaction of the chiral forms of ketamine with opioid, phencyclidine, sigma and muscarinic receptors. Pharmacol Toxicol 1995;77:355–359.
83. Smith DJ, Pekoe GM, Martin LL, Coalgate B: The interaction of ketamine with the opiate receptor. Life Sci 1980;26:789–795.
84. Dich-Nielsen JO, Svendsen LB, Berthelsen P: Intramuscular low-dose ketamine versus pethidine for postoperative pain treatment after thoracic surgery. Acta Anaesthesiol Scand 1992;36:583–587.
85. Azevedo VM, Lauretti GR, Pereira NL, Reis MP: Transdermal ketamine as an adjuvant for postoperative analgesia after abdominal gynecological surgery using lidocaine epidural blockade. Anesth Analg 2000; 91:1479–1482.
86. Schmid RL, Sandler AN, Katz J: Use and efficacy of low-dose ketamine in the management of acute postoperative pain: A review of current techniques and outcomes. Pain 1999;82:111–125.
87. De Kock M, Lavand'homme P, Waterloos H: 'Balanced analgesia' in the perioperative period: Is there a place for ketamine? Pain 2001;92:373–380.
88. Argiriadou H, Himmelseher S, Papagiannopoulou P, et al: Improvement of pain treatment after major abdominal surgery by intravenous S+-ketamine. Anesth Analg 2004;98:1413–14'8.
89. Aida S, Yamakura T, Baba H, et al: Preemptive analgesia by intravenous low-dose ketamine and epidural morphine in gastrectomy: A randomized double-blind study. Anesthesiology 2000; 92:1624–1630.
90. Guignard B, Coste C, Costes H, et al: Supplementing desflurane-remifentanil anesthesia with small-dose ketamine reduces perioperative opioid analgesic requirements. Anesth Analg 2002;95:103–108.
91. Kararmaz A, Kaya S, Karaman H, et al: Intraoperative intravenous ketamine in combination with epidural analgesia: Postoperative analgesia after renal surgery. Anesth Analg 2003;97:1092–1096.
92. Menigaux C, Fletcher D, Dupont X, et al: The benefits of intraoperative small-dose ketamine on postoperative pain after anterior cruciate ligament repair. Anesth Analg 2000;90:129–135.
93. Sveticic G, Gentilini A, Eichenberger U, et al: Combinations of morphine with ketamine for patient-controlled analgesia: a new optimization method. Anesthesiology 2003;98:1195–1205.
94. Adriaenssens G, Vermeyen KM, Hoffmann VL, et al: Postoperative analgesia with i.v. patient-controlled morphine: Effect of adding ketamine. Br J Anaesth 1999;83:393–396.
95. Reeves M, Lindholm DE, Myles PS, et al: Adding ketamine to morphine for patient-controlled analgesia after major abdominal surgery: A double-blinded, randomized controlled trial. Anesth Analg 2001; 93:116–120.
96. Subramaniam K, Subramaniam B, Pawar DK, Kumar L: Evaluation of the safety and efficacy of epidural ketamine combined with morphine for postoperative analgesia after major upper abdominal surgery. J Clin Anesth 2001;13:339–344.
97. Himmelseher S, Ziegler-Pithamitsis D, Argiriadou H, et al: Small-dose S(+)-ketamine reduces postoperative pain when applied with ropivacaine in epidural anesthesia for total knee arthroplasty. Anesth Analg 2001;92:1290–1295.
98. Wong CS, Lu CC, Cherng CH, Ho ST: Pre-emptive analgesia with ketamine, morphine and epidural lidocaine prior to total knee replacement. Can J Anaesth 1997;44:31–37.
99. Xie H, Wang X, Liu G, Wang G: Analgesic effects and pharmacokinetics of a low dose of ketamine preoperatively administered epidurally or intravenously. Clin J Pain 2003;19:317–322.
100. Taura P, Fuster J, Blasi A, et al: Postoperative pain relief after hepatic resection in cirrhotic patients: The efficacy of a single small dose of ketamine plus morphine epidurally. Anesth Analg 2003;96:475–480.
101. Wu CT, Yeh CC, Yu JC, et al: Pre-incisional epidural ketamine, morphine and bupivacaine combined with epidural and general anaesthesia provides pre-emptive analgesia for upper abdominal surgery. Acta Anaesthesiol Scand 2000;44:63–68.
102. Tan PH, Kuo MC, Kao PF, et al: Patient-controlled epidural analgesia with morphine or morphine plus ketamine for post-operative pain relief. Eur J Anaesthesiol 1999;16:820–825.
103. Chia YY, Liu K, Liu YC, et al: Adding ketamine in a multimodal patient-controlled epidural regimen reduces postoperative pain and analgesic consumption. Anesth Analg 1998;86:1245–1249.
104. Marhofer P, Krenn CG, Plochl W, et al: S(+)-ketamine for caudal block in paediatric anaesthesia. Br J Anaesth 2000;84:341–345.
105. De Negri P, Ivani G, Visconti C, De Vivo P: How to prolong postoperative analgesia after caudal anaesthesia with ropivacaine in children: S-ketamine versus clonidine. Paediatr Anaesth 2001;11:679–683.
106. Lee HM, Sanders GM: Caudal ropivacaine and ketamine for postoperative analgesia in children. Anaesthesia 2000;55:806–810.
107. Malinovsky JM, Lepage JY, Cozian A, et al: Is ketamine or its preservative responsible for neurotoxicity in the rabbit. Anesthesiology 1993;78:109–115.
108. Rosseland LA, Stubhaug A, Sandberg L, Breivik H: Intra-articular (IA) catheter administration of postoperative analgesics: A new trial design allows evaluation of baseline pain, demonstrates large variation in need of analgesics, and finds no analgesic effect of IA ketamine compared with IA saline. Pain 2003;104:25–34.
109. Tigerstedt I, Sipponen J, Tammisto T, Turunen M: Comparison of nefopam and pethidine in postoperative pain. Br J Anaesth 1977; 49:1133–1138.
110. McLintock TT, Kenny GN, Howie JC, et al: Assessment of the analgesic efficacy of nefopam hydrochloride after upper abdominal surgery: A study using patient controlled analgesia. Br J Surg 1988;75:779–781.
111. Moffat AC, Kenny GN, Prentice JW: Postoperative nefopam and diclofenac: Evaluation of their morphine-sparing effect after upper abdominal surgery. Anaesthesia 1990;45:302–305.
112. Beloeil H, Delage N, Negre I, et al: The median effective dose of nefopam and morphine administered intravenously for postoperative pain after minor surgery: A prospective randomized double-blinded isobolographic study of their analgesic action. Anesth Analg 2004; 98:395–400.
113. Kain ZN, Sevarino F, Pincus S, et al: Attenuation of the preoperative stress response with midazolam: Effects on postoperative outcomes. Anesthesiology 2000;93:141–147.
114. Ong CK, Seymour RA, Tan JM: Sedation with midazolam leads to reduced pain after dental surgery. Anesth Analg 2004;98:1289–1293.
115. Gilliland HE, Prasad BK, Mirakhur RK, Fee JP: An investigation of the potential morphine sparing effect of midazolam. Anaesthesia 1996;51:808–811.
116. Batra YK, Jain K, Chari P, et al: Addition of intrathecal midazolam to bupivacaine produces better post-operative analgesia without prolonging recovery. Int J Clin Pharmacol Ther 1999;37:519–523.
117. Shah FR, Halbe AR, Panchal ID, Goodchild CS: Improvement in postoperative pain relief by the addition of midazolam to an intrathecal injection of buprenorphine and bupivacaine. Eur J Anaesthesiol 2003;20:904–910.
118. Bano F, Haider S, Sultan ST: Comparison of caudal bupivacaine and bupivacaine-midazolam for peri and postoperative analgesia in children. J Coll Physicians Surg Pak 2004;14:65–68.
119. Naguib M, el Gammal M, Elhattab YS, Seraj M: Midazolam for caudal analgesia in children: Comparison with caudal bupivacaine. Can J Anaesth 1995;42:758–764.
120. Nishiyama T: The post-operative analgesic action of midazolam following epidural administration. Eur J Anaesthesiol 1995; 12:369–374.
121. Nishiyama T, Matsukawa T, Hanaoka K: Effects of adding midazolam on the postoperative epidural analgesia with two different doses of bupivacaine. J Clin Anesth 2002;14:92–97.
122. Murphy TM: Psychoactive drugs for pain control. Pain Reviews 1994;1:9–14.
123. Koppert W, Weigand M, Neumann F, et al: Perioperative intravenous lidocaine has preventive effects on postoperative pain and morphine consumption after major abdominal surgery. Anesth Analg 2004; 98:1050–1055.
124. Collier CB: Dantrolene and suxamethonium: The effect of pre-operative dantrolene on the action of suxamethonium. Anaesthesia 1979; 34:152–158.
125. Salassa JR, Seaman SL, Ruff T, et al: Oral dantrolene sodium for tonsillectomy pain: A double-blind study. Otolaryngol Head Neck Surg 1988;98:26–33.
126. Morganti I: [Evaluation of the mechanism determining the painful symptomatology after proctological interventions.] Minerva Med 1988;79:463–466.

127. Fry EN: Postoperative analgesia using papaveretum and orphenadrine: A preliminary trial. Anaesthesia 1979;34:281–283.
128. Winter LJ., Post A: Analgesic combinations with orphenadrine in oral post-surgical pain. J Int Med Res 1979;7:240–246.
129. Malek J, Nedelova I, Lopourova M, et al: [Diclofenac 75mg. and 30 mg. orfenadine (Neodolpasse) versus placebo and piroxicam in postoperative analgesia after arthroscopy.] Acta Chir Orthop Traumatol Cech 2004;71:80–83.
130. Hays H, Woodroffe MA: Using gabapentin to treat neuropathic pain. Can Fam Physician 1999;45:2109–2112.
131. Field MJ, Holloman EF, McCleary S, et al: Evaluation of gabapentin and S-(+)-3-isobutylGABA in a rat model of postoperative pain. J Pharmacol Exp Ther 1997;282:1242–1246.
132. Hill CM, Balkenohl M, Thomas DW, et al: Pregabalin in patients with postoperative dental pain. Eur J Pain 2001;5:119–124.
133. Onghena P, Van Houdenhove B: Antidepressant-induced analgesia in chronic non-malignant pain: A meta-analysis of 39 placebo-controlled studies. Pain 1992;49:205–219.
134. Archid D, Eschalier A, Lavarenne J: Evidence for a central but not peripheral analgesic effect of clomipramine in rats. Pain 1991;45:100.
135. Archid D, Guilbaud G: Antinociceptive effects of acute and chronic injections of tricyclic antidepressant drugs in a new model of mononeuropathy in rats. Pain 1992;49:279–287.
136. Iacono RP, Linford J, Sandyk R: Pain management after lower extremity amputation. Neurosurgery 1987;20:496–500.
137. Laska EM, Sunshine A, Mueller F, et al: Caffeine as an analgesic adjuvant. JAMA 1984;251:1711–1718.
138. Forbes JA, Beaver WT, Jones KF, et al: Effect of caffeine on ibuprofen analgesia in postoperative oral surgery pain. Clin Pharmacol Ther 1991;49:674–684.
139. Forbes JA, Jones KF, Kehm CJ, et al: Evaluation of aspirin, caffeine, and their combination in postoperative oral surgery pain. Pharmacotherapy 1990;10:387–393.
140. Zhang WY, Li Wan PA: Analgesic efficacy of paracetamol and its combination with codeine and caffeine in surgical pain—a meta-analysis. J Clin Pharm Ther 1996;21:261–282.
141. Zhang WY, Po AL: Do codeine and caffeine enhance the analgesic effect of aspirin? A systematic overview. J Clin Pharm Ther 1997;22:79–97.
142. Zhang WY: A benefit-risk assessment of caffeine as an analgesic adjuvant. Drug Saf 2001;24:1127–1142.
143. Watson CP: Topical capsaicin as an adjuvant analgesic [review; 69 refs]. J Pain Symptom Manag 1994;9:425–433.
144. Dubner R: Pain and hyperalgesia following tissue injury: New mechanisms and new treatments. Pain 1991;44:213–214.
145. Jagger SI, Rice ASC: Novel vistas in analgesic pharmacology for the treatment of chronic pain. Anaesth Pharmacol Physiol Rev 1996;4:66–73.
146. Watson CP, Evans RJ: The postmastectomy pain syndrome and topical capsaicin: A randomized trial. Pain 1992;51:375–379.
147. Dini D, Bertelli G, Gozza A, Forno GG: Treatment of the postmastectomy pain syndrome with topical capsaicin. Pain 1993;54:223–226.
148. Ellison N, Loprinzi CL, Kugler J, et al: Phase III placebo-controlled trial of capsaicin cream in the management of surgical neuropathic pain in cancer patients. J Clin Oncol 1997;15:2974–2980.
149. Sunshine A, Zighelboim I, De Castro A, et al: Augmentation of acetaminophen analgesia by the antihistamine phenyltoloxamine. J Clin Pharmacol 1989;29:660–664.
150. Terrence CF, Potter DM, Fromm GH: Is baclofen an analgesic? Clin Neuropharmacol 1983;6:241–245.
151. Hirst RA, Lambert DG, Notcutt WG: Pharmacology and the potential therapeutic uses of cannabis. Br J Anaesth 1998;81:77–84.
152. Buggy DJ, Toogood L, Maric S, et al: Lack of analgesic efficacy of oral delta-9-tetrahydrocannabinol in postoperative pain. Pain 2003;106:169–172.
153. Forrest WH Jr, Brown BW Jr, Brown CR, et al: Dextroamphetamine with morphine for the treatment of postoperative pain. N Engl J Med 1977;296:712–715.
154. Sung YF, Wetchler BV, Duncalf D, Joslyn AF: A double-blind, placebo-controlled pilot study examining the effectiveness of intravenous ondansetron in the prevention of postoperative nausea and emesis. J Clin Anesth 1993;5:22–29.
155. Doenicke A, Mayer M, Vogginger T: [Postoperative pain therapy: The efficacy of a serotonin antagonist (GR 38032F;ondansetron) and the prostaglandin synthesis inhibitor lysin acetylsalicylate (Aspisol).] Anaesthesist 1993;42:800–806.
156. Broome IJ, Robb HM, Raj N, et al: The use of tramadol following day—case oral surgery. Anaesthesia 1999;54:289–292.
157. De Witte JL, Schoenmaekers B, Sessler DI, Deloof T: The analgesic efficacy of tramadol is impaired by concurrent administration of ondansetron. Anesth Analg 2001;92:1319–1321.
158. Arcioni R, della RM, Romano S, et al: Ondansetron inhibits the analgesic effects of tramadol: A possible 5-HT(3) spinal receptor involvement in acute pain in humans. Anesth Analg 2002;94:1553–1557.
159. Alayurt S, Memis D, Pamukcu Z: The addition of sufentanil, tramadol or clonidine to lignocaine for intravenous regional anaesthesia. Anaesth Intensive Care 2004;32:22–27.
160. Buerkle H, Huge V, Wolfgart M, et al: Intra-articular clonidine analgesia after knee arthroscopy. Eur J Anaesthesiol 2000;17:295–299.
161. Casati A, Magistris L, Beccaria P, et al: Improving postoperative analgesia after axillary brachial plexus anesthesia with 0.75% ropivacaine: A double-blind evaluation of adding clonidine. Minerva Anestesiol 2001;67:407–412.
162. Casati A, Magistris L, Fanelli G, et al: Small-dose clonidine prolongs postoperative analgesia after sciatic-femoral nerve block with 0.75% ropivacaine for foot surgery. Anesth Analg 2000;91:388–392.
163. Gentili M, Houssel P, Osman M, et al: Intra-articular morphine and clonidine produce comparable analgesia but the combination is not more effective. Br J Anaesth 1997;79:660–661.
164. Gentili M, Juhel A, Bonnet F: Peripheral analgesic effect of intra-articular clonidine. Pain 1996;64:593–596.
165. Gentili M, Enel D, Szymskiewicz O, et al: Postoperative analgesia by intraarticular clonidine and neostigmine in patients undergoing knee arthroscopy. Reg Anesth Pain Med 2001;26:342–347.
166. Sung CS, Lin SH, Chan KH, et al: Effect of oral clonidine premedication on perioperative hemodynamic response and postoperative analgesic requirement for patients undergoing laparoscopic cholecystectomy. Acta Anaesthesiol Sin 2000;38:23–29.
167. Hagelin A, Lundberg D: Ketamine for postoperative analgesia after upper abdominal surgery. Clin Ther 1981;4:229–233.
168. Phillips G, Vickers MD: Nefopam in postoperative pain. Br J Anaesth 1979;51:961–965.

第 4 部分 临床特殊人群的术后疼痛管理

21 婴儿与儿童术后疼痛管理

YUAN-CHI LIN

疼痛是生存所必需的一种保护机制。疼痛在小儿所导致的痛苦和生理改变与成人相似。即使是小儿，疼痛和应激也能引起明显的生理和行为改变。监护人错误的观念和知识的缺乏，以及镇痛知识应用的不足导致不能有效进行疼痛管理。

疼痛是术后、疾病及诊断操作时最常见的不良刺激之一，常给患儿和家人带来焦虑和压力。患儿应当接受的镇痛治疗总是不能得到满足[1,2]。对疼痛生理、发展、环境因素的透彻理解，包括对患儿和家属的心理准备，可为患儿围手术期提供最佳的治疗。小儿及家属也应了解术后镇痛的详细情况。使更多患者得到治疗及已有更经济的方法已成为小儿疼痛管理的发展动力。在过去几年中，小儿术后疼痛的管理质量已得到明显改善[3]。

2002年瑞典在全国范围内进行了一项小儿术后急性疼痛的流行病学调查，大多数是门诊手术。尽管进行了镇痛治疗，但仍有23%的患儿出现了中重度疼痛，31%的患儿疼痛由其他原因所致。在与成人接受同样治疗的部门及小儿患者较少的部门，术后镇痛的问题更大。镇痛不满意常常与药物剂量不足、患儿及家属的焦虑有关，当然也与治疗方法无效有关[4]。

疼痛是门诊手术最常见的并发症。小儿返家后，父母就有责任对疼痛进行评估及治疗。在189例行门诊手术的2～12岁小儿的一项调查中，每位父母均记录了3天小儿疼痛日志及缓解方法。结果发现，手术类型不同，疼痛报告亦明显不同。扁桃体切除术、包皮环切术、斜视纠正术的术后患儿中有50%出现了明显疼痛。68%的患儿父母已被告知在"必要时"给予对乙酰氨基酚，13%的父母被告知规律服用对乙酰氨基酚，8%的父母未被告知。有些"小手术"也会导致剧烈疼痛。即使父母知道患儿疼痛，大多数人也不能给予足够剂量的药物以减轻疼痛[5]。

在一项对100例门诊手术患儿的调查中，调查者在患儿术后24h内与其父母保持电话联系。如果其父母接受镇痛指导，他们就能够在家中正确处理患儿的疼痛[6]。

新发现帮助我们理解疼痛机制并找到应用于治疗小儿术后疼痛的更好方法。安全有效的术后疼痛管理应具备合适的镇痛技术和药物、剂量个体化及合适的环境[7]。实施小儿疼痛管理需要足够的创造性和主动性。在小儿疼痛治疗上尚缺乏随机对照试验（randomized controlled trial，RCT）。现行小儿疼痛治疗的推荐方案并非基于最佳证据。本文以批判的眼光回顾文献，希望能为小儿疼痛治疗提供循证医学证据。

感受疼痛的神经发育

感受伤害的传入系统与生俱有。新生儿未成熟的神经系统对疼痛的感受反应也能引起应激。新生儿脊髓内对感觉的处理尚未成熟，引起兴奋和敏化的阈值较低，从而可能放大组织损害性传入的中枢效应。新生儿期外周和中枢感受连接的可塑性意味着婴儿期早期受损能引起疼痛传导径路结构与功能的长期改变，并持续到成年[8]。与成年人相比，新生儿屈肌反射较为亢进，反射的阈值较低，参与反射肌群的收缩更加同步、持久[9]。反复刺激皮肤会导致明显的兴奋过度或中枢性敏化。早产儿的屈肌反射阈值特别低下，但随着后天神经系统的发育而提高[10]。出生时皮肤神经分布包括有髓鞘A型粗纤维和无髓鞘C型细纤维[11]。神经系统发育过程中，70%~80%的C型细纤维伤害感受器表达神经生长因子[12]。

疼痛系统在围生期经历了重要的重组。新生儿期轻度或重度疼痛刺激可能影响未成熟疼痛系统的结构与功能。基本的兴奋过程发育较早，然而抑制过程发育延迟。新生儿对疼痛刺激的行为反应有时难以预测。由于缺乏适当的抑制机制，机体对所有感觉传入都可能表现为放大和泛化反应。出生后早期新生儿外周神经、脊髓和脊髓上疼痛传入系统发育显著地渐趋成熟，但是在该期间仍能对组织损伤作出反应，包括特异性行为和应激与痛苦状态下自主神经、内分泌及代谢的反应。出生后小儿对吗啡敏感性的变化可能与初级传入神经突触的结构与功能重组、神经递质/受体的表达与功能以及较高级大脑中枢兴奋与抑制的调制有关[13]。了解神经传递的发育将明显有助于理解新生儿疼痛药理学治疗特殊方法的重要性[14]。

疼痛评估

对新生儿与儿童难以进行疼痛评估，但是定期评定疼痛的存在和严重程度以及小儿对治疗的反应是小儿疼痛管理的基础[15]。根据小儿的年龄和交流能力，可通过心理方法、生理检查或行为观察来评估疼痛。合适的术后疼痛评估需要综合考虑小儿疼痛感觉以及心理与发育因素。处理小儿患者的疼痛必须采用与年龄相符的疼痛评估方法。根据患者年龄与临床状态，可应用主观与客观评估方法。

由于疼痛是一种主观感受，因此往往首先倾听个体自己表述。3~7岁的患儿能够描述疼痛的部位、性质、强度和耐受程度。行为观察应该作为患儿陈述的补充，在不能清楚表达的患儿疼痛评估中更加重要。应在术前或疼痛出现前告知疼痛评估方法。每个机构对小儿患者的疼痛评估必须采取统一方法。

改良六脸谱面部表情疼痛评分方法可用于4岁及以上患儿急性疼痛强度的评估。该方法的优点在于可与广泛应用的计量评分系统（0~10）联合使用，并确定具有密切的线性关系[16]。Baxt等对276例儿童的研究证实小儿损伤后应用Bieri面部表情疼痛评分与颜色模拟评分来评价疼痛的可行性，也证实当小儿不能自述时，其父母所述疼痛的重要性[17]。

术后在家中对疼痛进行评估对父母来说是一项特别困难的任务。Chambers等[18]的研究证明15项父母术后疼痛测定（Parents' Postoperative Pain Measure, PPPM）作为评估2~12岁儿童术后疼痛评估的可靠性与有效性。Koh等[19]比较了152例认知障碍患儿与138例无认知障碍患儿。结果显示手术的认知障碍患儿围手术期所需的阿片类药物少于无认知障碍的患儿。面部表情-腿-活动-哭泣-可安慰性（Face, Legs, Activity, Cry, Consolability：FLACC）的疼痛评价方法可能有助于可靠、有效地评价认知障碍患儿的疼痛[20]。

疼痛治疗

对乙酰氨基酚和非甾体类抗炎药

对乙酰氨基酚和非甾体类抗炎药布洛芬是市售的最普遍用于缓解疼痛的药物，常用于轻中度术后疼痛。单次剂量布洛芬（4~10 mg/kg）和对乙酰氨基酚（7~15 mg/kg）对于缓解中重度疼痛的功效相似，作为止痛药或退热药的安全性相似。给药2 h、4 h、6 h后，布洛芬（5~10 mg/kg）的退热效果优于对乙酰氨基酚（10~15 mg/kg）[21]。布洛芬的不良反应包括胃炎、可能的胃肠出血、血小板与肾功能损害。非甾体类抗炎药作用机制是通过抑制环氧合酶（cyclooxygenase, Cox）来抑制前列腺素合成。不建议将阿司匹林用于小儿患者，因为其与Reye综合征有关。选择性Cox-2抑制剂如塞来昔布也能用于儿童。

酮咯酸（ketorolac）是一种经胃肠外给药的NSAID，常用作小儿急性疼痛治疗的辅助用药[22]。建议小儿经静脉应用酮咯酸（0.3~0.5 mg/kg）。小儿静脉应用酮咯酸（0.5 mg/kg，每 4~6 h 1 次，可用 5 d 或少于 5 d）耐受性良好，能减少阿片类药物的不良反应[23]。该药在儿童、年轻人和成人的维持剂量相近[24]。

全身阿片类药物镇痛

阿片类药物常用于小儿术后疼痛治疗。除了新生儿期外，婴儿与儿童阿片类药物的药代动力学和药效动力学与成人并无明显差别，相关危险并不更高。吗啡是阿片类药物的代表，用于小儿的药理学研究很多。新生儿吗啡的分布容积似小于成人，但是稍大儿童的数值即达到成人水平。所研究过的所有阿片类药物在新生儿的清除均慢于成人。其清除率在 1 岁以内一般即可达到，甚至超过成人水平。药物代谢速度快则要求药物剂量更大。婴儿和儿童对阿片类药物作用的敏感程度似乎并不大于成人[25]。

患者自控镇痛（patient-controlled analgesia，PCA）可安全用于 6 岁以上的儿童。吗啡、氢吗啡酮和芬太尼同样有效（表 21.1）。对于不能使用 PCA 的太小小儿，常由护士控制镇痛，其更为灵活。PCA 每次追加量加上基础速率持续输注模式能改善儿童夜间睡眠。一些患者可能需要负荷量，以建立镇痛。锁定间隔时间（激活 PCA 装置时，该期间不给予任何药物）可短至 5 min。

对于不适用 PCA 的患者，可使用单次注射和持续输注的方法给药。吗啡以 10~30 μg/(kg·h) 输注可达血清浓度 10~22 ng/ml，具有足够的镇痛作用[26]。

如果患儿能耐受口服给药，应优先考虑口服。应根据药物的口服生物利用度来调整用量。并将剂量调整到适当的镇痛效果。口服阿片类药物制剂（可待因、羟考酮、吗啡）以及阿片类药物与 NSAID 联用广泛而有效地用于儿童术后疼痛治疗。曲马多通过作用于 μ 受体产生镇痛效应，4~7 岁儿童口服曲马多 1.5 mg/kg 可达到 7 h 的有效镇痛[27]。

区域麻醉

婴儿与儿童区域镇痛技术优于全身镇痛技术[28]。在围手术期疼痛治疗中最成功的是区域滴注镇痛。儿童区域麻醉的总体病死率低下。合理选择局麻药、穿刺途径、阻滞程序并适当小心监测应该能够防止严重不良作用，并使区域麻醉成为儿童耐受良好的有效镇痛方法[29]。

骶管硬膜外阻滞

骶管硬膜外阻滞是小儿脐部以下门诊手术最常用的区域麻醉技术之一。该技术适于下胸部、臀部、骨盆、泌尿生殖／肛周区域以及下肢的手术。该技术也能为骨髓采集术后患儿提供有效的镇痛。

骶管阻滞易于实施。小儿门诊者单次注射就有长时间术后镇痛作用。此外通过标准的静脉导管置入硬膜外导管，以达到长时间术后镇痛的作用。Conroy 等[30]比较了 35 例腹股沟疝修补术后儿童骶管硬膜外阻滞与伤口浸润作为术后镇痛的效果。结果骶管硬膜外阻滞麻醉恢复时间较短，疼痛相关性行为较少，且术后阿片类药物的需求量较小。骶管硬膜外阻滞的一般禁忌证包括未纠正的凝血障碍和穿刺点局部感染。特殊禁忌证包括脊柱畸形如脊髓脊膜突出以及骶管解剖结构异常。

一般情况下，骶管硬膜外阻滞很安全。罕见并发症包括药物注入皮下、硬膜穿破、药物注入蛛网膜下腔、药物注入血管、药物注入骨髓内、血肿、感染以及尿潴留。Broadman 报道连续 1154 例小儿手术中使用骶管阻滞，无 1 例严重并发症。有 1 例硬膜穿破，但在注入局麻药前通过抽吸得以确认[31]。Fisher 等[32]在 82 例行腹股沟疝修补术和睾丸固定术的儿童证实，术后排尿时间与是否应用骶管硬膜外阻滞或髂腹股沟神经阻滞无关。骶管麻醉似乎是一种经济、简单、有效的技术，不仅可作为术后镇痛的一种方法，而且还可

药物	负荷量	背景量	PCA 追加量
吗啡（1 mg/ml 或 5 mg/ml）	0.03 mg/kg	0.01 mg/(kg·h)	0.02~0.03 mg/kg
氢吗啡酮（100 μg/ml）	5 μg/kg	1 μg/(kg·h)	2 μg/(kg·h)
芬太尼（50 μg/ml）	0.3 μg/kg	0.1 μg/(kg·h)	0.2~0.3 μg/(kg·h)

表 21-1 儿童 PCA 中所用的药物

作为独特的麻醉方法[33]。

腰段硬膜外阻滞

腰段硬膜外阻滞适用于臀部、骨盆以及下肢的手术。对于以往有直肠和骶骨区域手术或骶骨区域解剖结构异常者，可用腰段硬膜外阻滞替代骶管硬膜外阻滞。硬膜外麻醉可减少全麻需求量，并缓解术后疼痛[34]。大多数患儿在阻滞前需要镇静或全身麻醉。硬膜外间隙的深度可由修正的 Dohi 公式来推测：

深度（mm）= 18+[1.5 × 年龄（岁）]。

注射局麻药前，回抽血液和脑脊液（cerebrospinal fluid，CSF）必须是阴性结果。可通过硬膜外导管单次给药或持续给药来维持硬膜外麻醉。其并发症包括硬脊膜意外穿破、脊髓直接创伤、硬膜外穿刺时造成的空气栓塞以及持续注入布比卡因引起的癫痫发作。

硬膜外镇痛药可有效减轻局部剧痛、躯体痛和内脏痛。与胃肠外镇痛相比，硬膜外镇痛药在较低剂量下镇痛效果更好，镇静作用更弱。儿童硬膜外技术的心血管系统安全性高，镇痛作用强[35]，可减轻婴儿腹部手术的应激反应[36]，改善动脉导管结扎术后患儿的预后[37]。目前建议用持续硬膜外滴注作为硬膜外镇痛用于婴儿[38]、儿童、青少年[39,40]。患者自控硬膜外镇痛（Patient-controlled epidural analgesia，PCEA）也能用于一些患者[41]。该技术可防止周期性疼痛，更便于麻醉和护理的管理。

硬膜外镇痛最常见的穿刺入路：①小于 12 个月患儿的骶部入路；②大于 12 个月患儿的腰部入路；③特殊适应证患儿的胸部入路，如胸部或上腹部手术。另外，单次骶管阻滞非常适用于短小手术。

最好避免使用充盈空气的注射器检测阻力消失感，以定位硬膜外腔。这种方法可导致某些患儿空气栓塞。使用电刺激定位引导硬膜外导管从骶管置入胸段。这种简易评价方法可很好地确定硬膜外导管尖端的位置，以达到有效控制疼痛[42]。

对于较小的婴儿，硬膜外阻滞使用的 0.1% 布比卡因中可加入 3μg/ml 的氢吗啡酮，给药速度为 0.2～0.4 ml/(kg·h)，建议新生儿硬膜外持续输注布比卡因的速率为 0.2～0.3 mg/(kg·h)[43-45]。持续胸段硬膜外输注镇痛可有效地用于胸廓畸形术后，可减少静脉阿片类药物的需求量；一项研究表明，没有导管相关性并发症[46]。持续性区域技术包括硬膜外输注可有效用于小儿患者。由于存在可能的并发症，因此这些阻滞技术需由经过培训的有经验的人员来实施、监测和管理[47]。

外周神经阻滞

腋路臂丛神经阻滞

腋路臂丛神经阻滞适用于上臂和手部的手术，能安全用于儿童。该技术与成人相似，只是儿童通常需要镇静或麻醉，以发挥神经刺激定位的优势。腋动脉可作为定位腋鞘的标志，腋鞘包含腋动脉与静脉、正中神经、桡神经和尺神经。使用 23k 号或 25 号针头直对着腋动脉搏动点穿刺。缓慢进针，直到小于 0.5 mA 的电流刺激神经引出远端肌肉收缩。穿刺针近端平行腋鞘所产生的镇痛平面高于穿刺针垂直于腋鞘。回抽无血和脑脊液后方可注入所有的局麻药。另外，也可用两次注入法，半量局麻药向动脉头端对向正中神经，半量向动脉尾端对向尺神经。

常用局麻药包括利多卡因、甲哌卡因和布比卡因，均可给予 0.5～0.75 ml/kg。此外，也可使用 1% 利多卡因（起效迅速）加 0.1% 丁卡因（作用时间长）的混合液，总量为 0.5 ml/kg。将 20 mg 的丁卡因晶体溶于 1% 利多卡因 20 ml 中可得到该混合液。Ivani 和 Tonnetti[48]报道的方法是单次给予 0.5～1 ml/kg 的 0.2% 罗哌卡因或 0.25% 左旋丁哌卡因加可乐定 2μg/kg，随后续滴注 0.1～0.3 ml/(kg·h) 的 0.2% 罗哌卡因或 0.25% 左布比卡因，加上 3 μg/(kg·24h) 可乐定，持续 48～72 h。腋路臂丛神经阻滞的并发症包括血管内注射、直接损伤神经或动脉、血肿和感染[49]。

斜角肌间阻滞

斜角肌间阻滞适用于锁骨、肩部和上臂的手术。患者仰卧位。嘱患者抬头以显露肌间沟，并在全麻诱导前做好标记。因为需要患者的配合，所以该阻滞技术可能不适于较小患儿。在环状软骨水平，使用 22～25 号针进入肌间沟，向内、向下、向后朝着 C6 横突方向穿刺。神经刺激能帮助正确确定针的位置。肌间沟阻滞可使用 1% 利多卡因 0.5 ml/kg 与 0.1% 丁卡因混合液，或 0.25%～0.5% 布比卡因 0.5 ml/kg。也可留置导管持续输注[50]。

肌间沟阻滞的并发症包括局麻药误入血管、血肿、感染。也有报道发生膈神经阻滞，造成一侧膈肌麻痹、注入蛛网膜下腔导致全脊麻以及误入基底动脉。

股神经阻滞和"三合一"阻滞（腹股沟血管旁技术）

股神经阻滞和"三合一"阻滞（腹股沟血管旁技术）适于股骨手术、股四头肌和股外侧肌活检以及股前取皮。这两种阻滞技术都可减轻股骨干骨折后的肌肉痉挛。

股动脉可用作解剖标志，其位于股神经的内侧。股神经阻滞时，使用短斜面针在腹股沟韧带上，股动脉搏动外侧垂直刺入皮肤。并不一定要求有异感。神经刺激可帮助定位该神经[51]。回抽无血和脑脊液后，将局麻药以扇形方式注入股动脉的外侧与深部，以阻滞股后皮神经。"三合一"阻滞方法与股神经阻滞非常相似。穿刺针朝头侧与股前平面呈30°角刺入。按压穿刺针远端的股管，然后注入局麻药。

建议股神经阻滞应用0.25%~0.5%布比卡因0.2~0.3 ml/kg，"三合一"阻滞应用0.25%~0.5%布比卡因0.5~0.7 ml/kg（最大剂量2.5 mg/kg）。两种阻滞镇痛作用时间为3~6 h。并发症包括交感神经阻滞、邻近血管损伤以及血肿。交感神经阻滞为暂时性，可改善下肢外周循环[52-54]。

股外侧皮神经阻滞

股外侧皮神经阻滞适用于大腿肌肉活检、皮肤移植取皮和大腿外侧手术[55,56]。股外侧皮神经没有运动成分，这种阻滞不会影响下肢运动功能。股骨外侧皮神经（L_2~L_3）走行于髂筋膜下，在腹股沟韧带下方、髂前上棘内侧进入股深部。在腹股沟韧带水平，髂前上棘内侧相当于患者1~2个手指宽度处使用22号短斜面针穿刺。可感到针有阻力地依次穿过腹外斜肌腱膜、腹内斜肌和髂筋膜。

髂筋膜室阻滞

髂筋膜室阻滞适于股骨切开术、股骨骨折修复术、髋部手术、膝关节镜检查以及肌肉活检。患者仰卧位，定位标志包括髂前上棘、耻骨结节和腹股沟韧带。穿刺点位于腹股沟韧带中外1/3点偏下侧0.5 cm处，垂直皮肤进针。当针尖穿破髂筋膜和阔筋膜时可感觉到明显的阻力消失。然后，注射局麻药的同时向穿刺针下方加压。这样可使局麻药在髂筋膜间隙内向头侧扩散。Dalens等[57]比较了60例儿童髂筋膜间隙阻滞与60例儿童"三合一"阻滞的效果。前者90%镇痛效果良好，而后者只有20%镇痛效果良好。一种有效的局部麻醉药组合为1%利多卡因与0.5%布比卡因1∶1混合，再加入1∶200 000的肾上腺素。局麻药容量取决于患者体重：小于20 kg—0.7 ml/kg；20~30 kg—15ml；30~40 kg—20 ml；40~50 kg—25 ml；大于50kg—27.5 ml。髂筋膜室阻滞作用可持续12~15 h。

腘窝神经阻滞

腘窝神经阻滞可麻痹坐骨神经及其两个分支：胫神经和腓神经。这种阻滞方法适用于膝以下的手术，如姆趾外翻手术、肌腱手术、跖关节滑膜切除术、截趾术、异物取出和肿瘤切除。腘窝呈菱形，其上界为股二头肌、半腱肌、半膜肌构成，下界由腓肠肌的内侧头与外侧头构成。坐骨神经在腘窝顶端分叉，发出内侧的胫神经及外侧的腓总神经。神经刺激可帮助精确定位[58]。患者俯卧位或侧卧位，膝关节微屈，使更易触及腘窝上界。患者俯卧位时，针进入腘窝顶端，可阻滞坐骨神经，结果除了内踝周围皮肤外，小腿和足被完全麻醉。单独阻滞胫骨神经和腓骨神经易实施。当针尖穿破腘窝筋膜时，有阻力消失感，随后针尖再进入5 mm。这种技术是膝以下手术更常用麻醉方法的安全可靠的替代方法[58,59]。

阴茎神经阻滞

阴茎接受来自阴茎背神经、生殖股神经和髂腹下神经的神经分布。双侧阴茎背神经在1点和11点钟处，自耻骨联合下方发出，沿阴茎体Buck筋膜下走行，支配阴茎远端2/3的感觉。阴茎神经阻滞适用于包皮环切割术或远端尿道下裂修复术。一项包皮环切割术的比较研究显示，阴茎神经阻滞与骶管阻滞同样有效，且前者无运动神经阻滞[60,61]。

阴茎神经阻滞有3种方法。第一，使用22号短斜面针在耻骨联合下缘中线垂直进针，阻力消失表示穿破Buck筋膜，回抽无血和CSF后注入局麻药。第二，在1点钟和11点钟深达Buck筋膜处注入局麻药。第三，在阴茎根部皮下环形浸润阻滞。最有效的方法是联合1点钟与11点钟阴茎背神经阻滞和阴茎根部背侧3点钟至9点钟处皮下浸润[62]。绝对禁用含肾上腺素的液体。阴茎神经阻滞的并发症包括血管内注射、血肿、感染和缺血。

髂腹股沟和髂腹下神经阻滞

髂腹股沟和髂腹下神经阻滞常用于腹股沟疝修补

术和睾丸固定术。这种阻滞可提供有效的手术和术后镇痛。Cross 和 Barrett[63]比较了 0.25% 布比卡因加 1：200 000 的肾上腺素行髂腹下神经和髂腹股沟神经阻滞与 0.25% 布比卡因行骶管阻滞在儿童疝修补术和睾丸固定术中的应用。结果这两种方法在镇痛作用持续时间与效果、呕吐发生率或首次排尿时间均无差异。主要解剖标志是髂前上棘。在髂前上棘内侧患者一横指处用 22～25 号短斜口针垂直皮肤进针。针尖穿破腹外斜肌腱膜和腹内斜肌筋膜时可有微弱的突破感。回抽无血和 CSF 后注入局麻药。单纯髂腹股沟与髂腹下神经阻滞可为儿童疝修补术提供满意的镇痛效果[64]。

不良反应的处理和术后监测

预先印妥有关 PCA、持续输注镇痛药、硬膜外镇痛、PCEA 的程序单，包括不良反应的处理及标准监测，将有助于处理儿童术后疼痛[65]。推荐在开始输注或增快输注速率的第一个 24 h 应用脉搏氧饱和度监测。恶心呕吐可用甲氧氯普胺治疗，每次 0.1～0.2 mg/kg（最大剂量 10 mg）静脉注射，必要时每 6 h 1 次，或昂丹司琼每次 0.1 mg/kg（最大剂量 2 mg）静脉注射，必要时每 4～8 h 1 次。瘙痒可用纳布啡治疗，每次 0.01～0.02 mg/kg（最大剂量 1.5 mg）静脉注射，必要时每 6 h 1 次；或苯海拉明每次 0.25～0.5 mg/kg（最大剂量 25 mg）静脉注射，必要时每 6 h 1 次。呼吸抑制应该立即处理，必要时静脉注射纳洛酮 1 μg/kg（最大剂量 80 μg）。

小儿术后硬膜外导管留置时间短，罕见硬膜外感染[66]。Kost-Byery 等[67]研究了儿童持续硬膜外导管的细菌定植和感染率。结果显示，留置骶管硬膜外导管的 3 岁或 3 岁以上儿童发生硬膜外导管细菌定植的可能性小于 3 岁以下儿童。年龄并不影响穿刺点发生蜂窝织炎的可能性。尽管骶部与腰部硬膜外导管可能出现细菌定植，但是调查显示短时间硬膜外镇痛不会出现严重的全身与局部感染[67]。Seth 等[68]研究了连续 100 例 1 天至 15 岁患儿的术后硬膜外镇痛。结果显示，小儿硬膜外持续输注期间常见炎症和感染的轻微局部体征。硬膜外导管尖端培养也常呈现阳性，无论患儿有无局部体征，都不会出现感染的进一步体征或症状[68]。

其他疼痛治疗方法

任何时候如有可能，应该考虑应用术中区域阻滞或局部浸润作为小儿术后镇痛的方法[69]。非药物治疗也是有益的辅助方法，如催眠、放松、生物反馈、经皮神经电刺激（transcutaneous electrical nerve stimulation，TENS）、艺术疗法及针灸可能缓解小儿和青少年的疼痛[70,71]。协调综合治疗有利于处理小儿和青少年急性疼痛。处理小儿患者围手术期疼痛的麻醉医师应该熟悉这些群体的特征，并采用合理的药物与非药物治疗方案。

术后小儿疼痛管理服务

急性疼痛服务的大多数患者是经历手术的住院患者。理想的小儿疼痛管理团队应该包括小儿麻醉医师以及护理、小儿心理与小儿理疗的专职人员。应建立各科室之间的协作，包括小儿内科、小儿普外科、小儿泌尿外科、小儿矫形外科、小儿整形外科、小儿心脏外科、小儿神经外科、小儿耳鼻喉科及其他辅助科室，以优化医疗服务[72]。美国麻醉医师学会（American Society of Anesthesiologists，ASA）已经出版了围手术期急性疼痛管理的实践指南[73]。已经建立了小儿急性疼痛管理的标准方案，以便正确处理患儿，同时也有助于继续教育和培训，从而确保医务人员能够了解并熟练运用安全有效的治疗措施进行疼痛管理。考虑到有关小儿疼痛的感情与社会因素，患儿疼痛的最优处理需要可靠的评估手段，并对疼痛和不良反应进行积极处理[74]。

尽管目前人们已了解了安全有效的小儿疼痛管理方法，但是这些共识尚未广泛应用于临床常规工作中。幼年时的疼痛可能产生长期的行为学后果。经历围手术期疼痛的儿童与婴儿的长期后果可能主要取决于疼痛的时间、损伤程度以及镇痛药治疗及其性质。负责需要手术儿童的医务人员面临重大挑战，既要评估和处理这种疼痛，还要理解这种疼痛所带来的功能性后果[75]。

（倪丽亚译　王晓琳　邓小明校）

参考文献

1. Anand K, Hickey P: Pain and its effects on the human neonates and fetus. N Engl J Med 1987;317:1321–1329.
2. Anand KJ, Hickey P: Halothane-morphine compared with high dose sufentanil for anesthesia and postoperative analgesia in neonatal cardiac surgery. N Engl J Med 1992;326:1–9.
3. Lloyd-Thomas AR: Modern concepts of paediatric analgesia. Pharmacol Ther 1999;83:1–20.
4. Karling M, Renstrom M, Ljungman G: Acute and postoperative pain in children: A Swedish nationwide survey. Acta Paediatr 2002;91:660–666.
5. Finley GA, McGrath PJ, Forward SP, et al: Parents' management of children's pain following 'minor' surgery. Pain 1996;64:83–87.
6. Jonas DA: Parent's management of their child's pain in the home following day surgery. J Child Health Care 2003;7:150–162.
7. Berde CB, Sethna NF: Analgesics for the treatment of pain in children. N Engl J Med 2002;347:1094–1103.
8. Fitzgerald M, Beggs S: The neurobiology of pain: developmental aspects. Neuroscientist 2001;7:246–257.
9. Andrews K, Fitzgerald M: Cutaneous flexion reflex in human neonates: A quantitative study of threshold and stimulus-response characteristics after single and repeated stimuli. Dev Med Child Neurol 1999;41:696–703.
10. Fitzgerald M: A physiological study of the prenatal development of cutaneous sensory inputs to dorsal horn cells in the rat. J Physiol 1991;432:473–482.
11. Jackman A, Fitzgerald M: Development of peripheral hindlimb and central spinal cord innervation by subpopulations of dorsal root ganglion cells in the embryonic rat. J Comp Neurol 2000;418:281–298.
12. Ruit KG, Elliott JL, Osborne PA, et al: Selective dependence of mammalian dorsal root ganglion neurons on nerve growth factor during embryonic development. Neuron 1992;8:573–587.
13. Nandi R, Fitzgerald M: Opioid analgesia in the newborn. Eur J Pain 2005;9:105–108.
14. Pattinson D, Fitzgerald M: The neurobiology of infant pain: Development of excitatory and inhibitory neurotransmission in the spinal dorsal horn. Reg Anesth Pain Med 2004;29:36–44.
15. Bulloch B, Tenenbein M: Assessment of clinically significant changes in acute pain in children. Acad Emerg Med 2002;9:199–202.
16. Hicks CL, von Baeyer CL, Spafford PA, et al: The Faces Pain Scale–Revised: Toward a common metric in pediatric pain measurement. Pain 2001;93:173–183.
17. Baxt C, Kassam-Adams N, Nance ML, et al: Assessment of pain after injury in the pediatric patient: Child and parent perceptions. J Pediatr Surg 2004;39:979–983.
18. Chambers CT, Finley GA, McGrath PJ, Walsh TM: The parents' postoperative pain measure: Replication and extension to 2-6-year-old children. Pain 2003;105:437–443.
19. Koh JL, Fanurik D, Harrison RD, et al: Analgesia following surgery in children with and without cognitive impairment. Pain 2004;111:239–244.
20. Voepel-Lewis T, Merkel S, Tait AR, et al: The reliability and validity of the Face, Legs, Activity, Cry, Consolability observational tool as a measure of pain in children with cognitive impairment. Anesth Analg 2002;95:1224–1229.
21. Perrott DA, Piira T, Goodenough B, Champion GD: Efficacy and safety of acetaminophen vs ibuprofen for treating children's pain or fever: A meta-analysis. Arch Pediatr Adolesc Med 2004;158:521–526.
22. Vetter T, Heiner E: Intravenous ketorolac as an adjuvant to pediatric patient-controlled analgesia with morphine. J Clin Anesth 1994;6:110–113.
23. Rusy L, Houck C, Sullivan L, et al: A double-blind evaluation of ketorolac tromethamine versus acetaminophen in pediatric tonsillectomy: Analgesia and bleeding. Anesth Analg 1995;80:226–229.
24. Hamunen K, Maunuksela EL, Sarvela J, et al: Stereoselective pharmacokinetics of ketorolac in children, adolescents and adults. Acta Anaesthesiol Scand 1999;43:1041–1046.
25. Olkkola KT, Hamunen K, Maunuksela EL: Clinical pharmacokinetics and pharmacodynamics of opioid analgesics in infants and children. Clin Pharmacokinet 1995;28:385–404.
26. Lynn A, Opheim, Tyler D: Morphine infusion after pediatric cardiac surgery. Crit Care Medi 1984;12:863–866.
27. Payne KA, Roelofse JA, Shipton EA: Pharmacokinetics of oral tramadol drops for postoperative pain relief in children aged 4 to 7 years—a pilot study. Anesth Prog 2002;49:109–112.
28. Bösenberg AT, Handley GP, Murray W: Epidural analgesia reduces postoperative ventilation requirements following esophageal atresia repair. J Pain Symptom Manag 1991;6:209A.
29. Dalens BJ, Mazoit JX: Adverse effects of regional anaesthesia in children. Drug Saf 1998;19:251–268.
30. Conroy JM, Othersen HB Jr, Dorman BH, et al: A comparison of wound instillation and caudal block for analgesia following pediatric inguinal herniorrhaphy. J Pediatr Surg 1993;28:565–567.
31. Broadman LM: Blocks and other techniques pediatric surgeons can employ to reduce postoperative pain in pediatric patients. Semin Pediatr Surg 1999;8:30–33.
32. Fisher QA, McComiskey CM, Hill JL, et al: Postoperative voiding interval and duration of analgesia following peripheral or caudal nerve blocks in children. Anesth Analg 1993;76:173–177.
33. Uguralp S, Mutus M, Koroglu A, et al: Regional anesthesia is a good alternative to general anesthesia in pediatric surgery: Experience in 1,554 children. J Pediatr Surg 2002;37:610–613.
34. Dalens B, Tanguy A, Haberer JP: Lumbar epidural anesthesia for operative and postoperative pain relief in infants and young children. Anesth Analg 1986;65:1069–1073.
35. Murat I, Delleur MM, Esteve C, et al: Continuous extradural anaesthesia in children: Clinical and haemodynamic implications. Br J Anaesth 1987;59:1441–1450.
36. Wolf AR, Eyres RL, Laussen PC, et al: Effect of extradural analgesia on stress responses to abdominal surgery in infants. Br J Anaesth 1993;70:654–660.
37. Lin YC, Sentivany-Collins SK, Peterson KL, et al: Outcomes after single injection caudal epidural versus continuous infusion epidural via caudal approach for postoperative analgesia in infants and children undergoing patent ductus arteriosus ligation. Paediatr Anaesth 1999;9:139–143.
38. Murrell D, Gibson P, Cohen R: Continuous epidural analgesia in newborn infants undergoing major surgery. J Pediatr Surg 2 1993;28:548–552.
39. Desparmet J, Meistelman C, Bare J: Continuous epidural infusion of bupivacaine for postoperative pain relief in children. Anesthesiology 1987;67:108–110.
40. Ecoffey D, Dubousset A, Samii K: Lumbar and thoracic epidural anesthesia for urologic and upper abdominal surgery in infants and children. Anesthesiology 1986;65:87–90.
41. Caudle C, Freid E, Baley A, et al: Epidural fentanyl infusion with patient-controlled epidural analgesia for postoperative analgesia in children. J Pediatr Surg 1993;28:554–558.
42. Tsui BC, Seal R, Koller J, et al: Thoracic epidural analgesia via the caudal approach in pediatric patients undergoing fundoplication using nerve stimulation guidance. Anesth Analg 2001;93:1152–1155.
43. Berde CB: Convulsions associated with pediatric regional anesthesia. Anesth Analg 1992;75:164–166.
44. Lin Y, Krane E: Comparison of continuous epidural infusion using low dose bupivacaine with or without morphine for postoperative analgesia in neonates. Anesth Analg 1997;84:S441.
45. McCloskey J, Haun S, Deshpande J: Bupivacaine toxicity secondary to continuous caudal infusion in children. Anesth Analg 1992;75:287–290.
46. McBride WJ, Dicker R, Abajian JC, Vane DW: Continuous thoracic epidural infusions for postoperative analgesia after pectus deformity repair. J Pediatr Surg 1996;31:105–108.
47. Williams DG, Howard RF: Epidural analgesia in children: A survey of current opinions and practices amongst UK paediatric anaesthetists. Paediatr Anaesth 2003;13:769–776.
48. Ivani G, Tonetti F: Postoperative analgesia in infants and children: New developments. Minerva Anestesiol 2004;70:399–403.
49. Fisher WJ, Bingham RM, Hall R: Axillary brachial plexus block for perioperative analgesia in 250 children. Paediatr Anaesth 1999;9:435–438.
50. Ilfeld BM, Morey TE, Wright TW, et al: Interscalene perineural ropivacaine infusion: A comparison of two dosing regimens for postoperative analgesia. Reg Anesth Pain Med 2004;29:9–16.
51. Bosenberg AT: Lower limb nerve blocks in children using unsheathed needles and a nerve stimulator. Anaesthesia 1995;50:206–210.
52. Grossbard GD, Love BR: Femoral nerve block: A simple and safe method of instant analgesia for femoral shaft fractures in children. Aust N Z J Surg 1979;49:592–594.

53. Denton JS, Manning MP: Femoral nerve block for femoral shaft fractures in children: Brief report. J Bone Joint Surg Br 1988;70:84.
54. Ronchi L, Rosenbaum D, Athouel A, et al: Femoral nerve blockade in children using bupivacaine. Anesthesiology 1989;70:622–624.
55. Maccani RM, Wedel DJ, Melton A, Gronert GA: Femoral and lateral femoral cutaneous nerve block for muscle biopsies in children. Paediatr Anaesth 1995;5:223–227.
56. Khan ML, Hossain MM, Chowdhury AY, et al: Lateral femoral cutaneous nerve block for split skin grafting. Bangladesh Med Res Counc Bull 1998;24:32–34.
57. Dalens B, Vanneuville G, Tanguy A: Comparison of the fascia iliaca compartment block with the 3-in-1 block in children. Anesth Analg 1989;69:705–713.
58. Singelyn FJ, Gouverneur JM, Gribomont BF: Popliteal sciatic nerve block aided by a nerve stimulator: A reliable technique for foot and ankle surgery. Reg Anesth 1991;16:278–281.
59. Tobias JD, Mencio GA: Popliteal fossa block for postoperative analgesia after foot surgery in infants and children. J Pediatr Orthop 1999;19:511–514.
60. Vater M, Wandless J: Caudal or dorsal nerve block? A comparison of two local anaesthetic techniques for postoperative analgesia following day case circumcision. Acta Anaesthesiol Scand 1985;29:175–179.
61. Yeoman P, Cooke R, Hain W; Penile block for circumcision? A comparison with caudal blockade. Anaesthesia 1983;38:862–866.
62. Dalens B, Vanneuville G, Dechelotte P: Penile block via the subpubic space in 100 children. Anesth Analg 1989;69:41–45.
63. Cross GD, Barrett RF: Comparison of two regional techniques for postoperative analgesia in children following herniotomy and orchidopexy. Anaesthesia 1987;42:845–849.
64. Lim SL, Ng Sb A, Tan GM: Ilioinguinal and iliohypogastric nerve block revisited: Single shot versus double shot technique for hernia repair in children. Paediatr Anaesth 2002;12:255–260.
65. Brenn B, Rose J: Pediatric pain services: Monitoring for epidural analgesia in the non-intensive care unit setting. Anesthesiology 1995;83:432.
66. Strafford MA, Wilder RT, Berde CB: The risk of infection from epidural analgesia in children: A review of 1620 cases. Anesth Analg 1995;80:234–238.
67. Kost-Byerly S, Tobin J, Greenberg R, et al: Bacterial colonization and infection rate of continuous epidural catheters in children. Anesth Analg 1998;86:712–716.
68. Seth N, Macqueen S, Howard RF: Clinical signs of infection during continuous postoperative epidural analgesia in children: The value of catheter tip culture. Paediatr Anaesth 2004;14:996–1000.
69. Lin Y, Krane EJ: Regional anesthesia for the pediatric outpatient. Refesher Courses in Anesthesiology 1996;24:163–175.
70. Chambliss CR, Heggen J, Copelan DN, Pettignano R: The assessment and management of chronic pain in children. Paediatr Drugs 2002;4:737–746.
71. Hobbie C: Relaxation techniques for children and young people. J Pediatr Health Care 1989;3:83–87.
72. Cohen MH, Kemper KJ: Complementary therapies in pediatrics: A legal perspective. Pediatrics 2005;115:774–780.
73. Ready L, Ashburn M, Caplan R, et al: Practice guidelines for acute pain management in the peri-operative setting. Anesthesiology 1995;82:1071–1081.
74. Lin Y: Analgesics and sedatives for critical ill infants and children. J Intensive Care Med 1992;7:221–222.
75. Howard RF: Current status of pain management in children [erratum appears in JAMA 2004;291:695]. JAMA 2003;290:2464–2469.

22 老年患者术后疼痛管理

DIARMUID MCCOY · DOMINIC HARMON

不完善的术后镇痛可导致患者康复延迟且术后并发症增加，老年患者尤其如此[1]。围手术期疼痛的严重程度能影响手术后慢性疼痛的发生。这种可能性对于那些饱受慢性疼痛折磨的老年患者具有重要意义[2]。老年患者术后疼痛管理复杂，这不仅与手术种类有关，还受到合并疾病、合并用药和疼痛评估困难的影响。

老年患者占手术人群中的比例逐渐增加，据报道所有住院手术患者中约1/3为老年患者[3]。同样，针对这些老年患者施行的手术也越来越复杂。2000年发表的一篇文章预计澳大利亚65岁以上（含65岁）老年人所占总人口比例将由2000年的12%升到2020年的18%和2050年的25%[4]。欧洲和北美洲的趋势与此相近。

随着外科技术和麻醉管理水平的进步，越来越多的老年患者接受越来越大的手术[5]，从而产生急性疼痛处理的问题。除了这种手术后急性疼痛外，老年人常见一些疼痛，如关节炎急性恶化、骨质疏松继发性骨折以及间歇性急性疼痛（如心绞痛）。除了上述复杂因素外，生理以及药效学与药代学方面的变化、疼痛感知和疼痛过程的改变以及如何精确评估疼痛程度的问题都使得老年患者术后急性疼痛处理具有挑战性。

妨碍老年患者术后镇痛的因素与其他人群基本相同。这些因素包括：①认为疼痛只是一种症状，而其本身无害；②不了解镇痛药的药理学；③对阿片类药物成瘾的恐惧；④与患者就镇痛需求方面进行交流困难。老年患者特殊障碍可能是由于患者因素，如对不熟悉设备的担忧或不适，如患者自控镇痛（patient-controlled analgesia，PCA）装置。医务人员认为老年患者不能耐受阿片类药物以及随年龄增长痛感会降低，也是障碍。患者家庭和医务人员常见的其他障碍因素包括：担心药物不良反应以及认为疼痛是老龄患者必有的症状。非常遗憾，疼痛文献中普遍存在急性疼痛治疗不理想，患者正遭受着不必要的痛苦；这也许仍然是实情，但必须承认已取得一定成就，而且我们正朝着理想的疼痛管理大踏步前进，尤其对于老年患者。

老年患者疼痛感知的生理

目前人们已经认识到，中枢神经系统随着年龄的增长发生了很大变化。这些包括伴随着阿片类系统某些退化而产生的神经化学、解剖学和功能的变化。疼痛抑制系统受损，导致疼痛过程发生显著变化[6]。与C纤维相比，Aδ纤维受损更明显，导致早期疼痛感知的变化。传导速度减慢、神经递质浓度降低（包括P物质）以及外周神经纤维减少，这均可改变疼痛的性质及感觉。诱发疼痛的实验证明，老年患者热刺激产生疼痛的阈值升高；然而，机械刺激产生疼痛的阈值改变尚不明确，电刺激产生疼痛的阈值不变[7]。各种实验性疼痛刺激的研究提示，老年患者耐受疼痛的能力下降意味着剧烈疼痛对其影响可能更大。

老年患者药理学改变

老年患者生理学变化使其对药物代谢也发生改变（表22-1）。心排出量和脑、肾、肝血流量随着年龄增长而下降。肝功能，尤其是1相氧化酶功能可能下降25%，肾小球滤过率和肌酐清除率可能下降30%～50%，从而使药物或活性代谢产物的清除降低[8]。脂肪含量的改变使药物分布容积增大，白蛋白浓度下降使游离药物浓度增高，这些因素使单次静脉用药时个体差异增加。

有一项研究测定了应用芬太尼时脑电图值的变化，证实随着年龄的增长，芬太尼药代动力学几乎无变化，但是脑对芬太尼的敏感性增加了50%[9]。这种敏感性的增加可能是由于阿片类受体敏感性改变、游离药物浓度增高或者两者兼而有之。动物实验结果显示，随着年龄增长，一些阿片类受体数量减少[10]。

老年患者疼痛的评价

除了那些感觉缺失的个别患者，几乎每个人都经历过急性疼痛。正常情况下，疼痛是一种非常明确、相当强烈的感觉（伤害感受性疼痛）或者是定位模糊的钝痛（内脏痛）。疼痛描述与测定的问题涉及疼痛的诊断与治疗以及对疼痛产生的研究。大多数学者使用100 mm视觉模拟疼痛评分（visual analogue pain score，VAPS）作为标准测量工具。然而，疼痛是一种多维感受，这种伤害感受性体验受环境、疾病、合并内科或精神疾病以及认知能力所调节。据估计，15%老年人可能存在认知障碍，其以记忆力、注意力、立体感、语言以及行为能力衰退为特征[11]。认知障碍患者的急性疼痛更可能未被治疗或者治疗不足[12]。谵妄是老年人群认知障碍的常见表现形式；其发生的危险因素包括：高龄、发热和感染、已有痴呆、抑郁、

表22-1 老年患者生理参数的改变及其对药代动力学的影响

生理过程	改变的方向及幅度（%）	药物用量对策
全身：		
心排出量	↓0～20	减少首剂量
脂肪	↑10～50	减慢注射速度
肌肉质量/血流量	↓20	↓维持量
血浆容量	几乎不变	↓维持量
体液总量	↓10	
血浆白蛋白	↓20	对单次注射剂量产生不同影响
$α_1$-糖蛋白	↑30～50	对维持量几乎没有影响
药物结合	↑（不定）	
肝：		
肝血流量	↓25～40	↓维持量
肝酶		
Ⅰ相	↓25	
Ⅱ相	几乎不变	
肾：		
肾血流量	↓10（每10岁）	↓经肾排泄药物的维持量
肾小球滤过率	↓50	监测活性代谢产物的蓄积
肌酐清除率	↓50～70	
中枢神经系统：		
脑血流量	↓20	对剂量几乎没有影响
脑容量	↓20	

Adapted from Macintyre PE, Upton RN, Ludbrook GL: Acute pain management in the elderly: In Rowbotham D, Macintyre PE, Breivik H, et al (eds):Clinical Pain Management: Acute Pain. London, Arnold, 2002.

贫血、药物治疗或停药（包括乙醇）、水与电解质紊乱、低氧以及未能缓解的疼痛[13]。

老年患者的疼痛评估应该与年轻患者一样（旁注22-1）。可能有必要根据患者的认知水平适当修改评估方法。应该进行基本的术前疼痛评估，包括体格检查、疼痛病史、既往疼痛经历和知识、用药史以及疼痛自诉能力。

许多老年患者由于慢性疾病以及其他原因而患有疼痛，这种疼痛必须与手术引起的疼痛相区别。既往疼痛的经历及知识均能指导术后疼痛处理，包括以前镇痛药物的使用及其效果与不良反应以及用于缓解疼痛的非药物方法。必须重视患者对疼痛的态度和认识以及对成瘾和镇痛药不良反应的担忧。药物治疗史对于发现镇痛治疗方案中可能影响镇痛药物作用的用药具有重要意义。

疼痛自诉是疼痛是否存在及其强度的最可靠指标[14]。为了获得老年患者的疼痛自诉，可能有必要改变评估疼痛的方法。重要的是不能想当然地认为感知障碍患者不能自诉疼痛。大多数老年患者包括轻至中度感知障碍的患者能够使用一些疼痛分级评分来描述疼痛的强度[15]。没有任何一种疼痛评估方法适用于所有老年患者。一旦选定某种适合于某位老年患者喜好和认知/机能状态的评估方法，就应在整个住院期间一直使用这种方法。

疼痛治疗小组应该考虑各种方法，使得疼痛评估方法在老年患者中的应用更加成功。只要患者有合适的眼镜或者助听器，就能弥补听觉或视觉障碍。医护人员应该除了语言指令外，还可减慢语速、降低外界噪声或提供书面文字，也可改变评估方法以使评估变得更加简明易懂。

一项研究比较了常用于老年急性疼痛患者的5种疼痛评分方法，结果发现词语描述量表（verbal descriptor scale，VDS）最可靠、最敏感，尽管其在患者喜好方面不如数字等级评分法而排名第二[16]。一般认为VDS最适合老年患者，包括轻度认知障碍的患者[16]。通过观察严重痴呆患者面部的痛苦表情和声音可准确发现疼痛的存在，但不能评估其疼痛程度[16]。无论静息还是活动时，必须观察患者的行为指标[17]。认知障碍患者可能更少表现兴奋和攻击等明显的行为指标。

患者教育

患者教育是术后疼痛管理的一个重要组成部分。患者及其家属需要知道未缓解的疼痛产生有害作用的相关信息。应该告知他们疼痛是如何被处理的、报告疼痛的重要性以及疼痛控制有利于恢复。应该解释镇痛药和非药物方法的不良作用。重要的是应避免使用可引起患者担忧药物成瘾的词汇，如麻醉性镇痛药[18]。

老年患者术后镇痛药物

人们总是将物理和心理方法与药物治疗相结合来治疗所有术后患者的疼痛，包括老年患者。镇痛药剂量个体化是老年患者有效术后疼痛管理的重要观念。术后早期推荐持续输注镇痛药。这可提高镇痛效果，降低不良反应，并可避免老年患者不愿提出对镇痛药物的要求。还必须考虑老年患者既往复杂用药史。已经证实多模式镇痛有利于老年患者术后疼痛管理[19]。急性疼痛治疗的推荐方法包括轻中度疼痛应用简单的镇痛药，中重度疼痛加用阿片类药物[20]。

阿片类药物

老年患者术后阿片类药物的需求量少于年轻人，但是个体间差异很大。剂量必须依个体有效量而定。阿片类药物需求量的下降，远远超过预测的年龄相关性生理变化[8]。吗啡和芬太尼需求量总体下降2~4倍，与疼痛自诉增加无关[21]。曲马多不是严格意义上的纯阿片类药物，其消除半衰期稍有延长，因此需求量较少。肾功能损害能引起阿片类药物活性代谢产物（去甲基哌替啶、吗啡-3-葡萄糖苷酸、吗啡-6-葡萄糖苷酸、去甲基曲马多）蓄积。

阿片类药物镇痛不足的最常见原因是担心老年患

旁注 22-1　老年患者的术后疼痛评估

1. 考虑疼痛的各种病因，不仅仅考虑手术伤口
2. 如有必要，可使用合适的方法获得患者对疼痛的自诉
3. 如患者对疼痛不能自诉，应用行为观察方法
4. 获取护理人员关于患者行为学改变的意见
5. 定时间断记录和评估疼痛
6. 整个过程使用相同的疼痛评分方法

者呼吸抑制，尤其是已有呼吸系统疾病的患者。与其他患者一样，适当监测镇静在很大程度上就能避免这个问题。术后恶心、呕吐和瘙痒发生率随着年龄的增长而下降[22]。芬太尼的认知功能抑制和意识错乱可能少于吗啡。必须记住，一些镇吐药物在老年患者更易产生不良反应。

局麻药

老年患者对局部麻醉药的作用更敏感。老年人内在神经元敏感的药效学与药代学变化可解释这种差异[23]。随着年龄的增长，单次硬膜外腔给药后，利多卡因与布比卡因终末半衰期延长，而其血浆总清除率下降[24]。持续应用局部麻醉药时，老年患者清除率降低可导致血浆浓度增高。

对乙酰氨基酚

尚无证据表明必须调整老年患者对乙酰氨基酚的剂量，并且这种药物在多模式镇痛中起到有益作用。但是在虚弱老年患者以及肝或肾功能损害的患者，其每日剂量应减少（50%）。

非甾体类抗炎药

老年患者服用非甾体类抗炎药后更易发生胃炎、胃溃疡和肾功能障碍。部分患者还可能出现认知障碍[25]。已有肾功能损害者，要特别小心肾衰竭。这种情况可能因为合并肝硬化、心功能衰竭、使用利尿药和降压药而加重。NSAID与华法林、口服降糖药、苯妥英及氨基糖苷类药物之间的药物不良相互作用可进一步危害老年患者的肾功能。

选择性环氧合酶-2（cyclooxygenase-2，Cox-2）抑制剂用于老年人群的不良作用明显下降。然而，有明确证据表明，Cox-2抑制剂的不良作用与传统NSAID没有任何差别。研究证实，老年患者最好避免使用Cox-2抑制剂，即使是术后短时间应用。

氯胺酮

尚无任何证据提示老年患者氯胺酮剂量需要改变。然而，氯胺酮是NMDA受体拮抗剂，老年人NMDA受体结构发生变化，结合位点减少，因此所需氯胺酮剂量较低。

患者自控镇痛

PCA是老年患者术后镇痛的有效方式（表22-2）[26]。认知功能障碍是PCA的相对禁忌证。老年患者应用PCA的疼痛评分明显低于皮下间断注射吗啡。听力、视力和运动功能损害可能妨碍老年患者术后成功使用PCA；但是，术前反复清晰指导可克服这些障碍。如果患者手因手术或关节炎而活动受限，一些设备可改装成由脚来控制。研究表明，与肌内注射吗啡

表22-2 各年龄组的PCA评分及每日满意度

	年轻患者（39±9）(n=45)	老年患者（67±8）(n=44)	P*
第1日满意度（cm）†	8.2±1.9	8.4±1.8	无显著差异
第2日满意度（cm）†	8.0±2.0	8.2±2.1	无显著差异
PCA调查（%）：			
对PCA满意度	81±9	82±11	无显著差异
对疼痛缓解的满意度	49±16	43±11	无显著差异
对控制程度的满意度	32±12	32±9	无显著差异
对成瘾性及不良反应的担心	47±12	46±11	无显著差异
对仪器使用或故障的担心	40±11	38±10	无显著差异

* 数值以均数±标准差表示
† 0~10cm模拟评分：0=完全不满意；10=完全满意

Adapted from Gagliese L Jackson M, Ritvo P, et al: Age is not an impediment to effective use of patient controlled analgesia by surgical patients. Anaesthesiology 2000;93:601-610.

相比，应用 PCA 的老年男性患者肺部并发症和谵妄发生率较低，镇痛效果较好[27]。有些患者可能正在口服阿片类药物控制慢性疼痛，在术后疼痛管理中必须考虑该因素。对于这些患者，背景输注剂量必须包括每日口服阿片类药物的相当剂量。对未使用过阿片类药物的患者，PCA 应避免联合应用背景输注阿片类药物。

区域麻醉技术

研究结果提示，大多数患者人群全身麻醉与区域麻醉技术的死亡率或重要发病率方面无任何差异[28]。常推荐区域麻醉用于老年患者，因为临床研究表明，最小镇静下患者可较好地保持定向力，并能更快地恢复正常功能[29]。老年患者区域麻醉下髋关节术后血栓溶解性事件[30]、失血量[31]以及深静脉血栓[32]的发生率均低于全身麻醉。区域麻醉可提供良好的术后镇痛，并可降低术后心血管不良事件的发生率[33]。区域麻醉其他优点还包括术后肠道功能恢复更快[34]，免疫系统功能完整[35]。为了使老年患者获得上述有利作用，必须慎重考虑年龄相关生理变化。

脊髓麻醉尽管技术简单且效果确切，但是并非没有风险，尤其在老年患者。老年患者摆放体位和穿刺更加困难。老年患者骨性标志更易识别，但是脊柱韧带钙化使得穿刺针不易进入硬膜外腔和蛛网膜下腔。因此建议采用旁入法[36]。必须考虑脊柱和神经组织的改变及其对局麻药吸收、分布和持续时间的影响。老年患者脑脊液总容量减少，其比重增高[24]。脊髓麻醉后年龄与镇痛扩散平面相关的研究结果尚不一致[24]。老年患者围手术期相关不良事件的风险更高，因此必须严密监护。高位脊髓阻滞对老年人的影响更加明显。

随着年龄增加，椎间孔的密度增加，故老年人硬膜外腔容积较小。这使得局麻药注射后更易向头侧扩散[38]。动脉硬化和糖尿病可加剧这种作用[38]。由于老年人硬脊膜通透性增高和蛛网膜绒毛体积增大，因此硬膜外麻醉起效迅速[39]。由于心血管事件的风险较高，所以减少局麻药剂量也很重要。椎管狭窄在老年患者中更常见。因此，大剂量局麻药加长时间硬膜外麻醉与老年患者马尾综合征的发生有关[40]。不管是静息还是活动的老年患者，硬膜外腔给予布比卡因与舒芬太尼的疼痛评分低于静脉 PCA 应用阿片类药物。另外，硬膜外镇痛的患者满意度较高，胃肠道功能恢复较快

[41]。随着年龄增加，硬膜外阿片类药物需求量减少（表22-3）。

表22-3	腰椎硬膜外镇痛依年龄给予 0.1% 布比卡因和 5μg/ml 芬太尼 * 混合液的输注速率	
	年轻患者（≤40岁）	老年患者（>70岁）
持续输注速率（ml/h）	7～14	4～8
必要时单次注射量（ml）	4～7	2 或 3

* 所有患者的剂量均个体化

各种外周神经阻滞适用于老年患者[42]。如上所述，老年患者骨性标志更明显，但是关节炎改变可能妨碍患者最佳体位的摆放。年龄相关的神经及神经周围组织的变化能改变外周神经阻滞的特点。随着年龄增长，髓鞘神经纤维变细、变少[37]。随着年龄增长，髓鞘神经纤维内 Schwann 细胞之间的距离缩短，因此局麻药作用的钠通道增多[37]。结缔组织鞘上的黏多糖减少，使局麻药更易渗入神经鞘内[37]。随着年龄增长，神经对局麻药越来越敏感；这种变化与神经元数目减少以及外周神经传导速率降低有关[43]。由于药物清除率下降，老年患者更易发生药物蓄积毒性反应。因此，应避免使用大剂量局麻药，并且追加剂量要小心谨慎。

尽管区域麻醉优点诸多，但是区域麻醉或全麻哪个结果更好仍有争议。这个临床问题受许多因素的影响，包括手术类型与时间、并存基础疾病以及麻醉医师和外科医师的技术和经验。对于老年患者，失败的区域麻醉所带来的危害大于成功的全麻[36]。最重要的是麻醉质量，而不是麻醉类型。

老年患者的非药物镇痛技术

人们已经研究过多种非药物技术用于术后疼痛处理[44]。这些技术可分为经皮刺激干预和认知-行为干预两类。经皮刺激干预是刺激皮肤和皮下组织来减弱疼痛的传导[45]。认知-行为干预可改变加剧疼痛或妨碍心理应对能力的想法和行为[45]。患者必须有良好的精神和身体状态来参与这些干预措施。必须应用镇痛药物良好地控制疼痛，才能使患者集中精力参加认知-行为干预措施。

总结

接受外科手术的老年患者数量将会持续增加。生理变化、多种合并疾病及认知障碍使得老年患者术后急性疼痛管理更具有挑战性。视力、听力、语言和认知功能障碍可能使疼痛评估、测定及治疗更为困难。手术前就应计划术后疼痛管理。区域麻醉是适合老年患者的麻醉技术。在保证同样麻醉效果的前提下，需要改进区域麻醉技术，并减少局麻药剂量，以确保老年患者区域麻醉的安全。术后良好镇痛结合多学科康复治疗将有助于老年患者的恢复。

（张　杰　赵晓虹译　邹毅清　李金宝　邓小明校）

参考文献

1. Feldt KS, Oh HL: Pain and hip fracture outcomes for older adults. Orthop Nurs 2000;19:35–44.
2. Katz J, Jackson M, Kavanagh BP, et al: Acute pain after thoracic surgery predicts long-term post-thoracotomy pain. Clin J Pain 1996;12:50–55.
3. Hall MJ, Owings MF: 2000 National Hospital Discharge Survey, vol 329. Hyattsville, MD, National Cancer Center for Health Statistics, 2002.
4. Australian Bureau of Statistics: Population Deaths 2000. Published ABS. Canberra, Australia.
5. Richardson J, Bresland K: The management of post surgical pain in the elderly population. Drugs Aging 1998;13:17–31.
6. Gibson SJ, Farrell M: A review of age differences in neurophysiology of nociception and the perceptual experience of pain. Clin J Pain 2004;20:227–239.
7. Gibson SJ: Pain and ageing the pain experience over the adult life span. In Proceedings of the 10th World Congress in Pain. Seattle, IASP Press, 2003, pp 767–790.
8. Macintyre PE, Upton R, Ludbrook GL: Pain in the elderly. In Rowbotham DJ, Macintyre PE, Breivik H, et al (eds): Clinical Pain Management: Acute Pain. London, Arnold, 2002.
9. Scott JC, Stanski DR: Decreased fentanyl and alfentanyl requirements with age: A simultaneous pharmacokinetic and pharmacodynamic evaluation. J Pharmacol Exp Ther 1987;240:159–166.
10. Vuyk J: Pharmacodynamics in the elderly. Best Pract Res Clin Anaesthesiol 2003;17:207–218.
11. Ferrell B, Ferrell B (eds): Pain in the Elderly: Task Force on Pain in the Elderly. Seattle, IASP Press, 1996.
12. Morrison RS, Siu AL: A comparison of pain and its treatment in advanced dementia and cognitively intact patients with hip fracture. J Pain Symptom Manag 2000;19:240–248.
13. Bekker AY, Weeks EJ: Cognitive function after anaesthesia in the elderly. Best Pract Res Clin Anaesthesiol 2003;17:259–272.
14. American Geriatrics Society Panel on Persistent Pain in Older Persons: Clinical Practice Guidelines: The management of chronic pain in older persons. J Am Geriatr Soc 2002;50:S205–S224.
15. Chibnall J, Tait R: Pain assessment in cognitively and non cognitively impaired older adults: A comparison of four scales. Pain 2001;92:173–186.
16. Herr KA, Spratt K, Mobily PR, Richardson G: Pain intensity in older adults: Use of experimental pain to compare psychometric properties and usability of selected pain scales with younger adults. Clin J Pain 2004;20:207–219.
17. Feldt K: The Checklist of Nonverbal Pain Indicators (CNPI). Pain Manage Nurs 2000;1:13–21.
18. Herr KA, Titler MG, Soroform BA, et al: Acute Pain Management in the Elderly. Iowa City, IA, University of Iowa Gerontological Nursing Interventions Resource Center, 2000.
19. Adrienssens G, Vermeyen KM, Hoffman VL, et al: Postoperative analgesia with I.V. patient-controlled morphine: Effect of adding ketamine. Br J Anaesth 1999;83:393–396.
20. American Pain Society: Principles of Analgesic Use in the Treatment of Acute Pain And Cancer Pain. Glenview, IL, American Pain Society, 2003.
21. Macintyre PE, Jarvis DA: Age is the best predictor of postoperative morphine requirement. Pain 1996;64:357–364.
22. Quinn AC, Brown JH, Wallace PG, et al: Studies in postoperative sequelae: Nausea and vomiting still a problem. Anaesthesia 1994;49:62–65.
23. Sadean MR, Glass PSA: Pharmacokinetics in the elderly. Best Pract Res Clin Anaesthesiol 2003;17:191–205.
24. Veering BT: The role of aging in regional anaesthesia. Pain Rev 1999;6:167–173.
25. Phillips AC, Polisson RP, Simon LS: NSAIDS and the elderly: Toxicity and economic implications. Drugs Aging 1997;10:119–130.
26. Gagliese L Jackson M, Ritvo P, et al: Age is not an impediment to effective use of patient controlled analgesia by surgical patients. Anaesthesiology 2000;93:601-610.
27. Egbert AM, Parks LH, Short LM, et al: Randomized trial of postoperative patient controlled analgesia vs intramuscular narcotics in elderly frail men. Arch Intern Med 1990;150:1897–1903.
28. Roy RC: Choosing general versus regional anesthesia for the elderly. Anesthesiol Clin North Am 2000;18:91:104.
29. Chung F, Meier R, Lautenslager E, et al: General or spinal anesthesia: Which is better in the elderly? Anesthesiology 1987;67:422–427.
30. Modig J, Borg T, Karlstrom G, et al: Thromboembolism after total hip replacement: Role of epidural and general anesthesia. Anesth Analg 1983;62:174–180.
31. Keith J: Anesthesia and blood loss in total hip replacement. Anesthesia 1977;32:444–450.
32. Sorensen RM, Pace NL: Anesthetic techniques during surgical repair of femoral neck fractures. Anesthesiology 1992;77:1095–1104.
33. Matot I, Oppenheim-Eden A, Ratrot R, et al: Preoperative cardiac events in elderly patients with hip fracture randomized to epidural or conventional analgesia. Anesthesiology 2003;98:156–163.
34. Breen P, Park KW: General anesthesia versus regional anesthesia. Int Anesthesiol Clin 2002;40:61–71.
35. Nielson KC, Steele SM: Outcome after regional anaesthesia in the ambulatory setting: Is it really worth it? Best Prac Res Clin Anaesthesiol 2002;16:145–157.
36. Mulroy MF: Modification of regional anesthetic techniques. In McLesky CH (ed): Geriatric Anesthesiology. Baltimore, Williams & Wilkins, 1997, pp 381–388.
37. Bromage PR: Epidural Analgesia. Philadelphia, WB Saunders, 1978, pp 40–42.
38. Bromage PR: Exaggerated spread of epidural analgesia in arteriosclerotic patients: Dosage in relation to biological and chronological ageing. BMJ 1962;5320:1634–1638.
39. Veering BT, Braun AG, van Kleef JW, et al: Epidural anesthesia with bupivacaine: Effects of age on neural blockade and pharmacokinetics. Anesth Analg 1987;66:589–593.
40. Faccenda KA, Finucane BT: Complications of regional anaesthesia: Incidence and prevention. Drug Saf 2001;24:13–42.
41. Mann C, Pouzeratte Y, Boccara G: Comparison of intravenous or epidural patient-controlled analgesia in the elderly after major abdominal surgery. Anaesthesiology 2000;92:433–441.
42. Raj PP: Conduction blocks. In Textbook of Regional Anesthesia. Philadelphia, Churchill Livingstone, 2002, pp 285–306.
43. Dorfman LJ, Bosley TM: Age-related changes in peripheral and central nerve conduction in man. Neurology 1979;29:38–44.
44. Agency for Healthcare Research and Quality: System to Rate the Strength of Scientific Evidence, Rockville, MD, U.S. Department of Health and Human Services, 2003.
45. Herr KA, Kwekkeboom KL: Assisting older clients with pain management in the home. Home Health Care Manage Pract 2003;15:237–250.

23 剖宫产术后疼痛的处理

RACHEL A. FARRAGHER · JOHN G. LAFFEY

剖宫产是美国最常见的手术[1]，每年有100万例以上。人们能预计这种重大手术后存在显著不适与疼痛。提供有效的术后镇痛对于促进产妇早期下床活动、婴儿健康包括母乳喂养、母婴亲密关系以及防止术后不良事件（肺炎、血栓形成等）具有非常重要的作用。此外，必须考虑药物转移到乳汁的可能性。镇痛方法必须达到以下目标：镇痛安全、有效且对母婴不良反应最小。最好是促进，至少不干扰早期母婴亲密关系。最可能达到这些目的的镇痛方法是多种方法联用。

剖宫产所用的麻醉方法可影响术后镇痛方法的选择。区域麻醉是最常用的方法，在英国占剖宫产麻醉的78%[2]。这项技术有利于椎管内给药作为术后镇痛方法的主要组成部分。静脉患者自控镇痛（intravenous patient-controlled analgesia，IV-PCA）广泛用作一项单独的技术或联合椎管内阻滞，并且是全麻剖宫产术后主要的镇痛方法。常以上述各种方法联用各种辅助药如非甾体类抗炎药及单纯麻醉性镇痛药，并且已经明确证实这些方法可降低阿片类需要量及阿片类药物引起的不良反应。

有关剖宫产术后疼痛处理的进展非常迅速，这已经使临床医师不能明确哪些进展能真正用于临床实践。本章通过分析当前综合性信息，探讨根据现有证据，哪些临床实践是（或不是）不合理的。

硬膜外镇痛技术

对于分娩和剖宫产术后镇痛，经硬膜外途径给予药物，尤其阿片类药物，是术后疼痛缓解的有效方法[1]（旁注23-1）。

硬膜外给予阿片类药物

硬膜外给予麻醉性镇痛药能提供高质量镇痛，剖宫产术后单次给予吗啡即可提供有效且长效的镇痛作用。随机对照试验显示，硬膜外单次给予吗啡比肌内注射吗啡能提供更有效的镇痛，而不良反应相近[3]。通过患者自控硬膜外镇痛（patient-controlled epidural analgesia，PCEA）装置给予哌替啶的镇痛效果优于肌内注射给药[4]。Negre等[5]证实硬膜外给予5mg吗啡可改善术后镇痛作用，明显减少剖宫产术后3d内IV-PCA阿片类药物的用量（图23-1）。Duale等[6]的研究表明，与鞘内（intrathecal，IT）给予75 μg吗啡相比，硬膜外给予2 mg吗啡在术后最初24 h期间所提

旁注 23-1 椎管内阿片类药物镇痛的优点

- "效能增益作用"——镇痛强度大于胃肠外给予同等剂量的药物，水溶性药物更为明显。允许应用极小剂量，并且阿片类药物用药总量减少。
- 与胃肠外应用阿片类药物相比，较低剂量实际上意味着没有胎盘转移、母乳蓄积最少以及镇静较轻。
- 选择性镇痛——与局麻药相比，没有运动或交感阻滞。
- 促进患者行走，同时低血压风险最小。
- 用脂溶性药物可改善患者术中舒适度。
- 术后镇痛效果极佳，时间长。

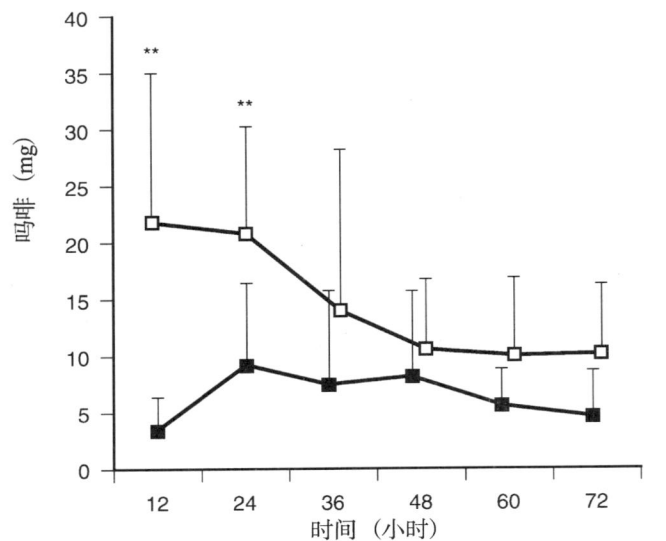

图 23-1 术后 3 天经静脉患者自控镇痛（IV-PCA）吗啡的消耗量。虚框表示对照组，实框表示硬膜外吗啡组。$P<0.01$。(From Negre I, Gueneron JP, Jamali SJ, et al: Preoperative analgesia with epidural morphine. Anesth Analg 1994;79:298-302.)

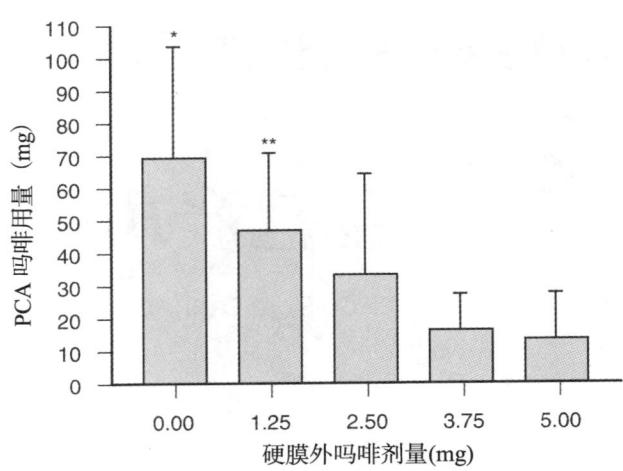

图 23-2 硬膜外吗啡多种剂量下 PCA 吗啡 24 h 总用量。组间有明显差异；$P<0.001$。*0 mg 组与 2.5 mg，3.75mg 和 5.0 mg 组有显著差异。**1.25 mg 组与 3.75 mg 和 5.0 mg 组有显著差异。(From Palmer CM, Nogami WM, Van Maren G, Alves DM: Postcesarean epidural morphine: A dose-response study. Anesth Analg 2000;90:887–891.)

供的镇痛效果较强，需要追加的阿片类药物量减少，而不良反应相同。

留置硬膜外导管有利于婴儿娩出后经硬膜外给予阿片类药物，排除药物通过胎盘的任何风险。研究显示切皮前硬膜外给予舒芬太尼确实能引起新生儿轻度短暂性神经行为抑制，所以宜强调婴儿娩出后给药的重要性[7]。

吗啡

吗啡是第一个获得美国食品药品管理局（Food and Drug Administration，FDA）批准用于椎管内的阿片类药物，在临床上已经被广泛深入地研究和应用。硬膜外吗啡的最佳剂量范围是 2.5～3.75 mg（图 23-2）[8,9]。吗啡作用的高峰在硬膜外给药后 60～90 min，能维持长达 24 h 的镇痛效果（表 23-1）。剖宫产术后连续硬膜外输注吗啡并不优于单次注射吗啡[10]。

用于硬膜外麻醉的局麻药可能影响随后硬膜外所用吗啡的效能。2-氯普鲁卡因可降低硬膜外吗啡所产生的镇痛质量与持续时间[11,12]。其机制尚未明了，但研究提示可能与氯普鲁卡因及其代谢产物的抗阿片类受体-特异性拮抗剂作用有关[13]。

美国 FDA 已经批准一种新型单次剂量缓释吗啡制剂。三期试验显示，与单次剂量非包裹的硫酸吗啡相比，硬膜外单次应用 10 mg 和 15 mg DepoDur 可明显改善择期剖宫产术后 48 h 内的镇痛效果和功能性能力[14]。

表 23-1　剖宫产硬膜外应用阿片类药物的特点

阿片类药物	剂量	起效（min）	最大效应（min）	持续时间（h）
吗啡	2～4 mg	45～60	60～120	12～24
芬太尼	50～100 μg	5	20	2～3
舒芬太尼	25～50 μg	5	15～20	2～4
哌替啶	50 mg	15	30	4～6
吗啡/芬太尼	3 mg/50μg	10	15	12～24

短效脂溶性阿片类药物

并未批准芬太尼用于椎管内给药，但是一些研究已经证实椎管内给予芬太尼能提供有效的镇痛，但作用时间有限[15-22]。硬膜外芬太尼和舒芬太尼的镇痛作用是由脊髓直接作用所介导的，而不是由于全身吸收入血而产生的间接作用[15-17]。硬膜外舒芬太尼与芬太尼的相对镇痛效能之比为5∶1。Grass等[19]报道芬太尼和舒芬太尼提供剖宫产术后镇痛作用的硬膜外最佳剂量分别是 100 µg 和 20 µg。在等效镇痛剂量下，这两种阿片类药物在镇痛作用的起效时间与作用时间方面无差异。然而，PCEA 舒芬太尼的呕吐发生率高于 PCEA 芬太尼，因此并不优于硬膜外芬太尼[20]。稀释溶液的容量可影响脂溶性阿片类药物所产生的镇痛质量，容量稀释到 10 ml 或更多，则起效更快，作用时间更长。总之，虽然硬膜外芬太尼和舒芬太尼产生的有效镇痛作用起效迅速，但是作用时间短（平均 117～138 min），使其不能单次用药用于术后疼痛处理（图 23-3；表 23-1）[19,21,22]。

其他阿片类药物

硬膜外哌替啶术后有效镇痛作用时间较短（25mg 时中间值为 165 min）。单次剂量哌替啶 25mg 的镇痛作用优于 12.5 mg，但 50 mg 或更大剂量并不能改善

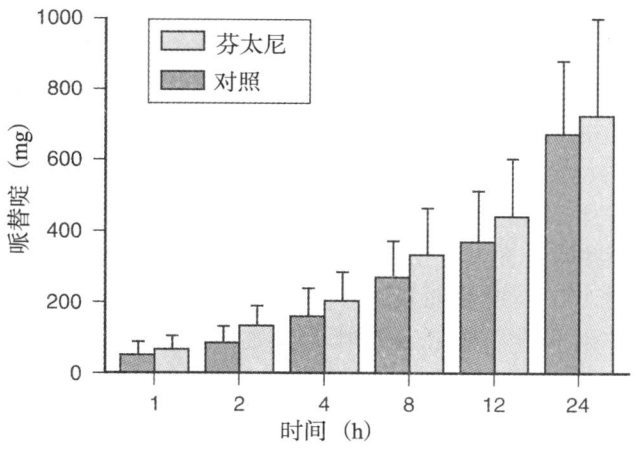

图 23-3 硬膜外注射芬太尼或生理盐水后哌替啶的总需要量。硬膜外芬太尼产生的镇痛作用时间有限，并不影响剖宫产术后 IV-PCA 的需要量。(From Sevarino FB, McFarlane C, Sinatra RS: Epidural fentanyl does not influence intravenous PCA requirements in the post-caesarean patient. Can J Anaesth 1991;39:450-453.)

镇痛质量或镇痛作用时间[23]。

氢吗啡酮为吗啡的羟化衍生物，其脂溶性较强，镇痛作用起效较快，持续时间较短。硬膜外吗啡与氢吗啡酮的镇痛效能比为5∶1。然而，在等效镇痛剂量下，硬膜外氢吗啡酮用于临床剖宫产术后镇痛时的镇痛作用和不良反应严重程度方面并不优于吗啡[24]。

与安慰剂相比，硬膜外曲马多可延长第一次需要追加镇痛的时间，减少术后阿片类药物和 NSAID 消耗量[25]。100 mg 和 200 mg 曲马多的效能无差别。

二醋吗啡是吗啡的一个脂溶性衍生物。其硬膜外镇痛作用产生迅速而有效，但是全身吸收率高，作用持续时间只有6～8 h。硬膜外二醋吗啡加入肾上腺素能改善8 h时的镇痛质量，但并不减少吗啡的追加剂量[26]。二醋吗啡的镇痛作用强于氢吗啡酮[27]。

硬膜外腔给予混合性阿片类激动剂-拮抗剂药物在理论上有两个优点。首先，它们可能选择性兴奋调理内脏伤害感受的 κ 阿片类受体。其次，可能产生呼吸抑制的封顶效应；即使药物分子向头侧扩散到脑干，这种作用也应该可限制呼吸驱动力的降低。然而，Camann 等[28]并不能证实临床上硬膜外给予布托啡诺优于静脉给药[28]。Abboud 等[29]报道硬膜外布托啡诺的镇痛效果相当于硬膜外吗啡，但前者瘙痒和呼吸抑制较少；作者应用了大剂量吗啡，这有可能影响不良反应的发生率。

阿片类药物的联合应用

吗啡与脂溶性阿片类药物联合应用可能具有某些优点。脂溶性阿片类药物镇痛作用起效迅速，可能弥补吗啡的起效潜伏期，从而联合应用可提供更好的术中镇痛作用和区域麻醉消退时镇痛作用的平稳过渡。硬膜外吗啡（2～4 mg）与芬太尼（100 µg）或舒芬太尼（20～30 µg）联合应用所产生的有效镇痛作用起效迅速，持续时间延长，而不增加其不良反应[30-32]。与单独应用氢吗啡酮相比，纳布啡和氢吗啡酮联合应用可产生有效的镇痛作用，而恶心较少[33]。硬膜外吗啡中加入布托啡诺可明显减少瘙痒和恶心，并且似乎可在镇痛作用不变的情况下降低呼吸抑制的发生率[34]。

非阿片类药物

妇女剖宫产分娩后硬膜外给予新斯的明可产生适度的剂量依赖性镇痛作用[35]。新斯的明也可产生数小

时的轻度镇静作用，从而使其在剖宫产分娩后单次给药的应用价值有限。

可乐定联合舒芬太尼可减少阿片类药物的需要量，并倾向于改善术后镇痛作用[36]。

剖宫产术后硬膜外单次剂量阿片类药物中加入1:200 000的肾上腺素能加快镇痛起效，并延长其作用时间[37,38]。然而，PCEA哌替啶中加入肾上腺素并不能改善镇痛作用，反而确能增加其不良反应[39]。

患者自控硬膜外镇痛

吗啡起效潜伏期长，有迟发性呼吸抑制的危险，这使其不太适合用于PCEA。因此，人们已经评价了较多的脂溶性阿片类药物用于PCEA。PCEA应用哌替啶可产生有效的镇痛作用，并且优于IV-PCA哌替啶、硬膜外吗啡和PCEA芬太尼[40-42]。一项研究显示，PCEA芬太尼的镇痛效果优于IV-PCA吗啡，且术后恶心与嗜睡较少，但是瘙痒的发生较早[43]。相反，PCEA单独应用芬太尼的镇痛效果并不优于硬膜外单次注射3 mg吗啡[44]。PCEA中增加背景剂量输注并无临床意义，药物消耗量增加而镇痛效果并无改善（表23-2）[45-47]。

PCEA中单纯应用局麻药可产生明显的运动阻滞作用[48,49]。相反，PCEA中联合应用芬太尼、布比卡因和肾上腺素所产生的镇痛作用强于PCEA单用芬太尼，且前者不良反应较少[50]。研究表明，PCEA中应用布比卡因与舒芬太尼的镇痛质量优于鞘内应用吗啡，且前者恶心和呕吐较少[51]。这些结论证实，椎管内多种药物联合应用镇痛效果与不良反应方面均优于单纯应用吗啡。然而，这些技术较昂贵，主要因为PCEA所需装置较贵[51]。

表23-2	患者自控硬膜外镇痛的优点
通过硬膜外单次注射或持续输注阿片类药物	患者控制，具有自主性 患者满意度较高 焦虑较少 阿片类药物需求量减少 镇痛效能增加
静脉PCA	患者满意度较高 镇静较轻 阿片类药物需求量减少

鞘内镇痛药

脊麻是紧急情况下剖宫产首选的麻醉技术[2]，这使鞘内给予阿片类药物成为缓解术后疼痛的理想方法（见旁注23-1）。鞘内与硬膜外单纯给予局麻药的患者中，有50%的患者存在内脏痛，这更加促进了鞘内阿片类药物的应用[52]。

鞘内阿片类药物的应用

吗啡

鞘内吗啡可产生高质量的镇痛作用，起效时间为30 min，镇痛作用的高峰时间在45~60 min，作用持续时间为18~24 h（表23-3；图23-4）[53-55]。不良反应与硬膜外吗啡类似，但所需吗啡量较少，这反映起效潜伏期时间长与蛛网膜下腔注射药物有关。此特征特别有利于关注乳汁中阿片类药物积聚的产妇。

多项研究和一项荟萃分析指出鞘内100 μg吗啡能产生非常满意的镇痛作用，而且不良反应最小（图23-5）[54-59]。增加吗啡剂量高于100 μg并不能增强镇痛作用（见图23-4）[55-58]，反而可能增加其不良反应的发生率，尤其是瘙痒（图23-6）[55,56,58]。很少有鞘内注射100 μg吗啡而发生呼吸抑制的报道[54]。相反，鞘内注射吗啡后恶心与呕吐的发生率似乎与剂量无关

表23-3	剖宫产鞘内应用阿片类药物的特点			
阿片类药物	剂量	起效（min）	最大效应（min）	持续时间（h）
吗啡	0.1~0.3 mg	30	60	18~24
芬太尼	10~20 μg	5	10	2~4
舒芬太尼	5~10 μg	5	10	2~4
哌替啶	10 mg	10	15	4~5

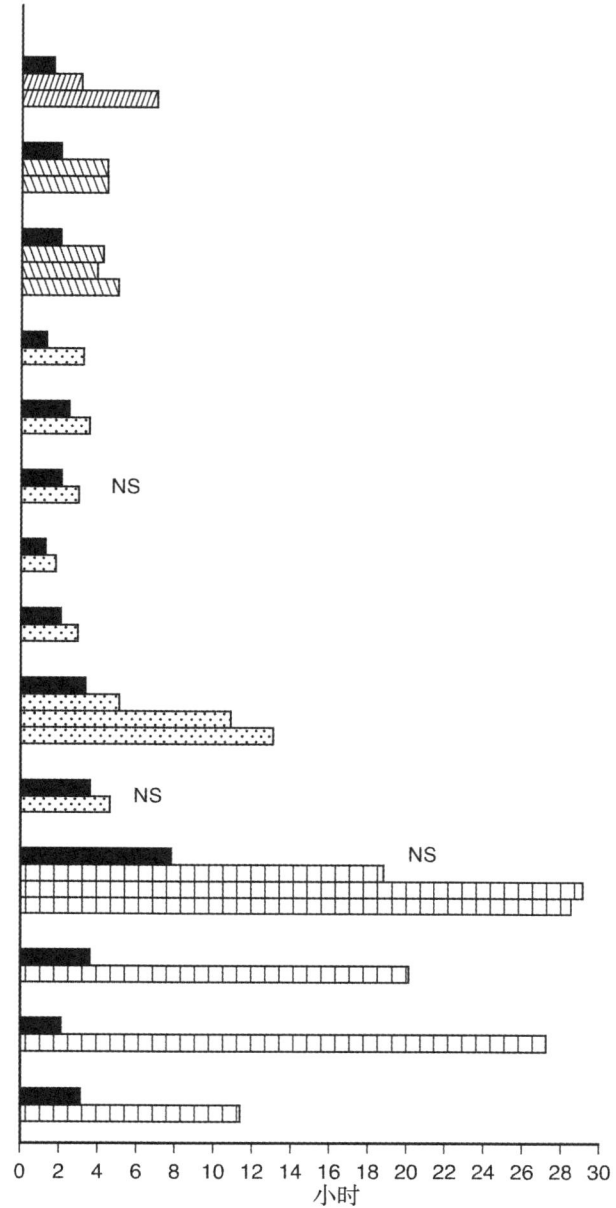

图 23-4 单纯应用不同剂量局麻药（实柱）或者联合应用不同剂量局麻药与不同剂量丁丙诺啡、舒芬太尼、芬太尼或吗啡（图形条）进行脊麻的患者术后首次追加镇痛药的时间（h）。NS，与对照组相比，无显著统计学差异。(From Dahl JB, Jeppesen IS, Jorgensen H, et-al: Intraoperative and postoperative analgesic efficacy and adverse effects of intrathecal opioids in patients undergoing cesarean section with spinal anesthesia: A qualitative and quantitative systematic review of randomized controlled trials. Anesthesiology 1999;91:1919-1927.)

[55,56]，尽管一些研究结论并不这么认为[57,58]。鞘内吗啡的用量小于 100 μg 似乎没有优点。虽然鞘内注射吗啡 75 μg 确实能产生明显的镇痛作用，但是 50 μg 似乎并不能产生临床意义的相关镇痛作用（图 23-4）[55,56]。在这组患者中，为达到最佳镇痛作用，似乎需要在脊髓与脊髓以上部位应用阿片类激动剂。因此，为了达到阿片类药物介导的最大镇痛作用，必须通过 IV-PCA 应用吗啡来增强脊髓以上阿片类激动作用[56]。

二醋吗啡

二醋吗啡是吗啡的脂溶性衍生物，英国常用。该药镇痛作用起效迅速，持续时间长，是由于其活性代谢产物 6-单醋酸吗啡和吗啡的作用所致。二醋吗啡在脊髓的作用持续时间类似于吗啡，并且两者起效潜伏期也相近[60]。二醋吗啡的脂溶性使其作用起效减慢，使其向头侧扩散引起呼吸抑制的可能性下降。鞘内注射 200 μg 二醋吗啡所产生的镇痛作用相当于 200 μg 吗啡，但前者发生瘙痒和嗜睡较少[60]。一项剂量相关性研究显示，鞘内注射二醋吗啡 250 μg 和 375 μg 的镇痛作用均强于 125 μg。瘙痒与呕吐的发生率和严重性呈剂量相关性，但是没有发生呼吸抑制[61]。已有应用 0.5 mg 和 1 mg 二醋吗啡作为单一术后阿片类药物鞘内

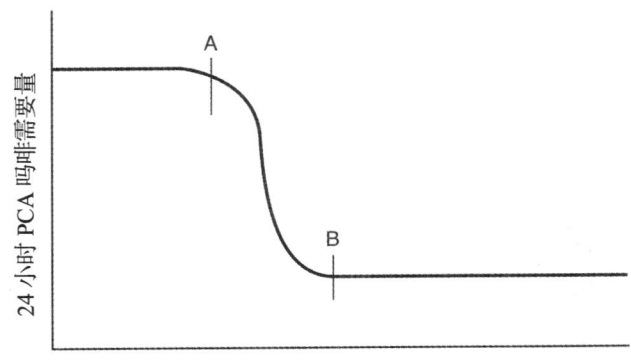

图23-5 鞘内吗啡剂量对应PCA吗啡用量的剂量-反应曲线推测图形。A，0.075 mg吗啡；B，0.1 mg吗啡。(From Palmer CM, Emerson S, Volgoropolous D, Alves D: Doseresponse relationship of intrathecal morphine for postcesarean analgesia. Anesthesiology 1999;90:437-444.)

镇痛药联合直肠应用双氯芬酸的报道[62]。

短效脂溶性阿片类物质

脊髓给予脂溶性阿片类药物如芬太尼和舒芬太尼的主要优点是其能够改善剖宫产术中的镇痛作用，因为其术后镇痛作用的持续时间有限（图23-4）[55]。Dahl等[55]的一项荟萃分析发现，虽然鞘内芬太尼剂量大于6.25 μg确实能延长需要追加镇痛药的时间，但是鞘内芬太尼或舒芬太尼都不具有临床意义的术后镇痛作用[55]。鞘内注射25 μg芬太尼的术后镇痛质量不如100 μg吗啡，且与安慰剂组无差异[63]。芬太尼在40 μg和60 μg的剂量下可能产生有意义的镇痛作用，但在较高剂量范围内镇静和瘙痒较多见[64]。研究证实鞘内注射舒芬太尼2.5 μg和5 μg可减少术后最初6 h追加镇痛药的剂量，但是此后没有影响[65]。

哌替啶

剖宫产术后鞘内注射10 mg哌替啶具有有效的术后镇痛作用，持续时间中等（4~5 h）[66]。虽然资料有限，但是鞘内注射20 mg哌替啶似乎并不优于10 mg[67]。

其他阿片类药物

研究证实鞘内注射布托啡诺对绵羊具有神经毒性作用，这限制了其临床应用[68]。就我们所知，尚无剖宫产术后患者鞘内应用美沙酮的报道。

阿片类药物联合用药

与鞘内吗啡联合应用高脂溶性药物能发挥脂溶性药物起效时间短和水溶性药物作用时间较长的优点[69]。但是这尚有争论，鞘内联合应用这些阿片类药物可能增加不良反应的发生率，而对镇痛作用几无影响[63]。此外，吗啡与芬太尼联合用药的术后镇痛作用似乎并不优于单用吗啡[69]。相反，鞘内联合注射吗啡150 μg和起效较快的哌替啶10 mg可能产生稳定的镇痛作用，在局麻药阻滞消退与吗啡镇痛作用起效期间不会出现疼痛缓解不足[66]。

非阿片类药物

鞘内给予新斯的明可抑制脊髓释放的乙酰胆碱的代谢，产生镇痛作用，而无瘙痒或呼吸抑制。一项标签公开的剂量结果研究显示，鞘内给予新斯的明10 μg、30 μg和100 μg可引起术后10 h剂量非依赖性吗啡用量减少[70]。未发现任何胎儿不良影响[70]。另一项研究表明，鞘内给予新斯的明25 μg的镇痛作用与100 μg吗啡相似[71]。有趣的是，联合应用新斯的明

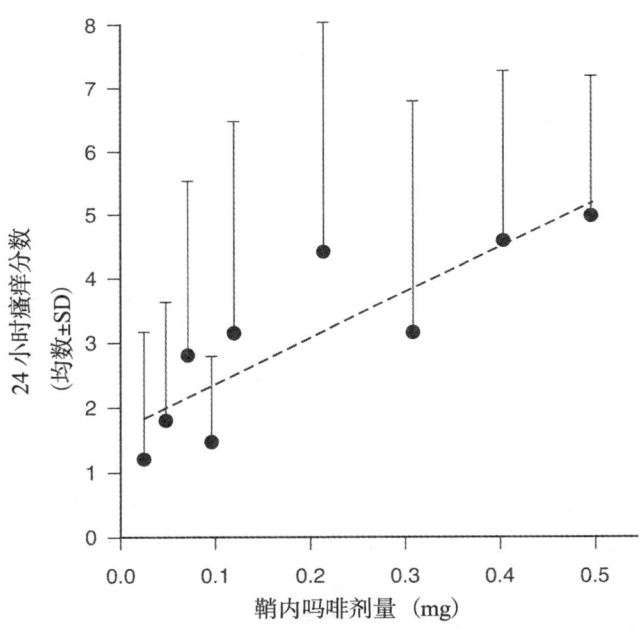

图23-6 鞘内不同剂量吗啡下24 h瘙痒评分（均数±SD）。组间有显著差异；$P = 0.003$。破折线表示随着鞘内吗啡剂量的增加，瘙痒评分趋势增高。（线性回归分析；$P = 0.001$）。(From Palmer CM, Emerson S, Volgoropolous D, Alves D: Dose-response relationship of intrathecal morphine for postcesarean analgesia. Anesthesiology 1999;90:437-444.)

12.5 μg 和吗啡 50 μg 似乎能产生最好的疼痛缓解作用，同时不良反应最少[71]。遗憾的是，术后恶心与呕吐的总体发生率和严重程度大大限制了鞘内新斯的明的临床应用[70-72]。

研究证实，在含有 200 μg 吗啡的重比重布比卡因中加入 0.2 mg 肾上腺素能增强术中及术后的镇痛作用[73]。肾上腺素的作用机制不明，但是似乎与血管收缩引起蛛网膜下腔吸收布比卡因减少无关[73]。

鞘内给予可乐定通过抑制 P 物质的释放而产生镇痛作用，这可减弱伤害性刺激对伤害性感受神经元的激活作用。可乐定单独应用[74]或联合应用鞘内阿片类药物[75]或新斯的明都能提供有效的镇痛作用[76]。单独用药时，75 μg 可乐定并无术后镇痛作用[77]，而 150 μg 可产生数小时的有效镇痛作用[74]。但是，鞘内注射可乐定的不良反应包括低血压、术后恶心与呕吐以及镇静，较大剂量时更易发生[74]。联合应用吗啡 100 μg 和可乐定 60 μg 的术后镇痛效果明显优于单独应用吗啡 100 μg 或可乐定 150 μg[75]，但是前者可能增加术中镇静与呕吐[75]。联合应用可乐定 150 μg 和新斯的明 50 μg 的术后镇痛效果优于二者单独用药[76]。

椎管内应用阿片类药物的不良影响

硬膜外和鞘内注射阿片类药物的患者瘙痒、恶心和呕吐发生率增加。瘙痒在产科患者中比其他任何科患者都更为常见，也是椎管内应用阿片类药物后患者不满意的最常见原因。鞘内注入吗啡后瘙痒的发生率和严重程度与用药剂量相关，剂量大于 100 μg 更易发生[55,56]。恶心可能是由于药物在脑脊液中向头侧扩散至脑干或血管吸收进入呕吐中枢和化学感受器触发区域所致。其剂量-反应关系尚不明确。每 100 例女性接受 0.1 mg 鞘内吗啡加入脊髓麻醉药中，结果 43 例瘙痒，10 例恶心，术后有 12 例恶心[55]。

呼吸抑制是椎管内应用阿片类药物后最顾虑的并发症。迟发性呼吸抑制是由于亲水性吗啡通过脑脊液向头侧扩散到脑干所致，可能发生于鞘内给药后 6~10 h 时。早发型呼吸抑制发生在 30 min 内，是由于血管吸收脂溶性阿片类药物所引起，通常意义较小，因为更可能发生人多的场所（手术室，麻醉后恢复室）。

幸运的是，呼吸抑制在剖宫产术后是一种罕见的事件。临产妇具有较高水平的呼吸刺激剂——孕酮，且通常为健康个体。Dahl 等[55]的荟萃分析结果显示，鞘内应用阿片类药物的 458 例患者中有 1 例出现呼吸抑制。结果，由鞘内注射阿片类药物引起 1 例呼吸抑制所诊治的患者数即伤害需要病例数（numbers-needed-to-harm，NNH）的集合数字是 476，这与对照组相比无显著差异[55]。另一项研究报道呼吸抑制仅发生在显著肥胖患者睡眠时[78]。Aboud 等[54]报道鞘内给予 100 μg 吗啡后无 1 例出现呼吸抑制[54]。相反，该研究中胃肠外给予吗啡观察到显著的呼吸抑制[54]。虽然有这些令人安慰的数据，但是所有椎管内应用阿片类药物的患者在术后期间必须进行适当监护（旁注 23-2）。

经静脉患者自控镇痛

IV-PCA 可作为单一技术，也可联合椎管内用药。IV-PCA 是胃肠外应用阿片类药物的首选方法，是全麻下剖宫产术后的主要镇痛技术。

有效性

人们已经明确证实，与传统肌内注射吗啡相比，IV-PCA 使用吗啡术后镇痛效果更好，患者满意度更高，患者活动得以改善，镇静程度减轻[74-82]。虽然 IV-PCA 术后镇痛质量可能不如椎管内技术[81-83]，但是应用 IV-PCA 患者的满意度似乎较高。一项 IV-PCA 和 PCEA 应用二醋吗啡的比较研究结果显示，PCEA 组疼痛评分降低较快，IV-PCA 组患者术后第 1 d 的镇静程度较轻，但是总体满意评分较高[84]。实际上，所有镇痛方案中，应用 IV-PCA 的患者满意水平似乎最高。大多数接受剖宫产分娩的产妇应用 IV-PCA 可达到足够但不完全的镇痛效果。产妇似乎更愿意接受较低程度的镇痛，以便保持更清醒，恶心程度较轻，感觉更

旁注 23-2 椎管内应用阿片类药物后呼吸功能的监测

- 尚无广泛公认的方法。
- 推荐数项无创监测，如脉搏血氧饱和度、呼气末二氧化碳分压（pressure carbon dioxide，PCO_2）和呼吸暂停监测器。
- 每小时评估呼吸频率是最常用的监测方式[48]。
- 呼吸抑制发作多呈缓慢进行性，典型发生在嗜睡后。
- 病态肥胖和接受硫酸镁治疗的产妇需要更严密的监护。
- 加强观察和记录呼吸力不足、呼吸频率缓慢或异常嗜睡可能是最好的监测手段。

能与其婴儿互动交流。IV-PCA 另一重要好处是阿片类药物介导的不良反应发生率较低，如瘙痒[81-83]，并且患者控制这些不良反应的程度更大[84]。

区域麻醉下行剖宫产后接受 IV-PCA 的患者在椎管内阻滞作用消退后可能很快出现明显的疼痛[85]。应该给这些患者一个阿片类药物的"负荷量"，以使患者具有基本的有效的血浆阿片类药物浓度。通过自控 IV-PCA 单次给药方式，随后的血浆药物水平能维持在一个狭窄的治疗范围内。否则，单独应用 IV-PCA 的患者可能不具有足够的血浆阿片类药物水平来控制其疼痛，因此可能不能产生镇痛作用（表 23-4）。

阿片类药物的选择

研究已经明确证实，吗啡是 IV-PCA 首选的阿片类药物，其较哌替啶[86,87]或芬太尼[88]更有效（表 23-5）。一项剖宫产术后 IV-PCA 和肌内注射吗啡与哌替啶镇痛方案的非随机化研究结果显示，不管何种给药途径，吗啡的镇痛作用均比哌替啶更有效。所用吗啡方案的疼痛缓解效果更好，与乳汁喂养和婴儿室内时间正相关[86]。IV-PCA 芬太尼的术后镇痛效果不如 IV-PCA 吗啡，因此不推荐前者常规 PCA 用于剖宫产术后[88]。

一项剖宫产术后应用吗啡、哌替啶或羟吗啡酮 IV-PCA 的随机试验结果显示，IV-PCA 吗啡患者术后 8 h 以上的疼痛评分最低，但是母体镇静较强[87]。羟吗啡酮的镇痛作用迅速，但恶心和呕吐的发生率较高。患者运动时疼痛最严重的是哌替啶。一项 IV-PCA 丁丙诺啡和吗啡的小样本研究证实，丁丙诺啡的镇痛作用类似于吗啡，而且镇静作用较轻[89]。因此，在不愿意应用吗啡的情况下，可用羟吗啡酮和丁丙诺啡替代。

基本背景输注

剖宫产术后应用基本背景输注联合标准 IV-PCA 单次追加的方案似乎是安全的，但是并无任何特殊优点[90]。一项接受吗啡或氢吗啡酮的患者比较了单用 IV-PCA 单次追加用法与基本背景输注加单次追加用法，结果显示应用背景输注可降低疼痛评分，但是并不影响患者满意度或减少自控追加阿片类药物的需要量[90]。

表 23-4　使用 IV-PCA 治疗的问题

问题	可能原因	解决办法	备注
未能产生满意的镇痛效果	不能达到血浆阿片类药物的治疗浓度	在开始 IV-PCA 前或同时给予一个负荷剂量 使用辅助药物以减少麻醉药的用药总量	一般来说单用 IV-PCA 在合理的时间窗内不足以达到麻醉性镇痛药治疗浓度，尤其在术中未用麻醉性镇痛药的情况下[85]
	未能维持血浆阿片类药物的治疗浓度	应用阿片类药物背景输注 预计减少药物用量（如睡眠）时，使用辅助药物（如 NSAID）	已证实可降低疼痛评分，但是不能改善总体满意评分[90] 已明确证实剖宫产术后该方法有效，如经直肠给予双氯芬酸[96]
因不能耐受药物不良反应而停用	严重 PONV	术中给予止吐药 术中及术后常规使用止吐药，而非在术后有必要时才使用 PCA 麻醉性镇痛药中添加止吐剂 应用辅助药物来减少阿片类药物用药总量	可产生良好的 PONV 预防作用
	严重瘙痒	术后常规使用止痒药，而非在必要时才使用 应用辅助药物来减少阿片类药物用药总量	

IV，经静脉；NSAID，非甾体类抗炎药；PCA，患者自控镇痛；PONV，术后恶心呕吐。

表 23-5 不同阿片类药物用于静脉患者自控镇痛的优缺点

药物	优点	缺点	备注*
吗啡	镇痛质量高[86,117] 吗啡或其活性代谢产物 吗啡-6-葡糖苷酸在母乳中几乎 无蓄积作用[94] 对新生儿神经行为无或几乎无 损害作用[91]	对母体的镇静作用强于哌替啶或羟 吗啡酮[87]	为最常用的药物 有效的镇痛作用 母体镇静是其缺点 已明确母乳喂养新生儿的 安全性
丁丙诺啡	镇痛作用相当于吗啡[7]	镇静轻于吗啡	为替代吗啡的一种药物 具有镇静较轻的优点
哌替啶	在某些研究中,母体镇痛效果 及总体满意度与吗啡相同[93]	另一些研究中有效镇痛作用不如吗 啡或羟吗啡酮 必须关注去甲哌替啶蓄积导致的新 生儿神经学行为短暂性损害	应避免用于母乳喂养的母亲

与椎管内阿片类药物的联合应用

剖宫产应用椎管内阿片类药物后,应用 IV-PCA 是一种常用的镇痛方案;该方案似乎安全,患者耐受性良好,并且对母乳喂养的新生儿影响最小[91]。

安全问题

母亲

IV-PCA 技术引起呼吸抑制的可能性显而易见。Brose 等[92]研究了剖宫产术后最初 24 h 接受硬膜外吗啡、IV-PCA 哌替啶或肌内注射哌替啶镇痛患者的氧合血红蛋白饱和度。接受 IV-PCA 哌替啶患者脉搏血氧饱和度(pulse oximetry oxygen saturation,SpO_2)水平在 91%~95% 之间以及 86%~90% 之间的累积时间最长。然而,将 SpO_2 低于或等于 85% 的时间大于 30 s 定义为严重氧去饱和事件,其发生率在 IV-PCA 组最低,而在硬膜外吗啡组最高[92]。

新生儿

如果采取母乳喂养,那么母体全身应用的阿片类药物可能对胎儿带来不良影响,最重要的是呼吸抑制。在这方面,IV-PCA 吗啡似乎优于哌替啶[93]。接受 IV-PCA 吗啡的母体初乳中吗啡及其活性代谢产物吗啡-6-葡萄糖苷酸的浓度极低[94]。一项比较剖宫产术后 IV-PCA 吗啡与 IV-PCA 哌替啶的随机对照临床试验结果表明,母体接受哌替啶的哺乳婴儿在其出生第 3 d 时警觉性显著低下、人类定向反应较差[93]。以前推测这是由于去甲哌替啶蓄积所致,这对于癫痫易发作的出生低体重儿可能具有重要意义。一项随访研究表明,与阴道分娩后没有应用任何药物的正常婴儿神经行为相比较,IV-PCA 吗啡联合应用硬膜外吗啡对新生儿神经行为并没有损害作用(图 23-7)[91]。哌替啶对新生儿神经行为的影响呈短暂性,但是 IV-PCA 吗啡对于母乳喂养的母亲来说可能是一种更好的选择。

非甾体类抗炎药

应用 NSAID 是剖宫产术后患者的一种有效镇痛方案。这些药物在切口部位具有抗炎作用,通过对子宫收缩的抑制效应来减轻子宫痉挛性疼痛。剖宫产术后各种给药途径应用多种 NSAID 的大量研究证实 NSAID 能有效减轻术后疼痛(图 23-8),减少其他麻醉性镇痛药尤其是阿片类药物的用量(图 23-9),并减少阿片类药物诱发的不良反应。

双氯芬酸是剖宫产术后研究最透彻的 NSAID,大量证据支持其具有镇痛效能。双氯芬酸剂量依赖性减轻剖宫产术后伤口疼痛和子宫痉挛性疼痛[95]。常规直肠给予双氯芬酸(如每日 150 mg,分次)是最有效的方案;研究证实其在剖宫产术后最初 24 h 内可缓解术后疼痛,减少吗啡用量(减少 39%~46%,取决于剂量),减轻阿片类药物诱发的不良反应[96-98]。术后立即经直肠给予单剂量双氯芬酸有益于患者,但效果较差;

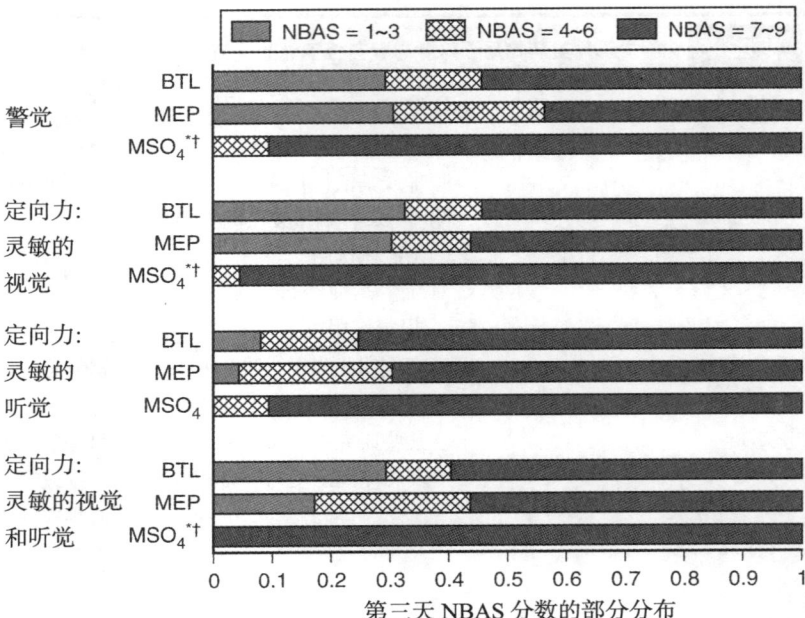

图 23-7 三组新生儿间四项神经行为结果（警觉；定向：灵敏的视觉；定向：灵敏的听觉；定向：灵敏的视觉与听觉）。BTL，人工喂养；MEP，接受含哌替啶的母乳；MSO_4，接受含吗啡的母乳。灰色条表示各组达到 Brazelton 新生儿行为评估量表（Neonatal Behavioral Assessment Scale, NBAS）1～3 分的新生儿比例；叉线条表示各组达到 Brazelton 新生儿行为评估量表（NBAS）评分 4～6 分的新生儿比例；黑色条表示各组达到 Brazelton 新生儿行为评估量表（NBAS）评分 7～9 分的新生儿比例。*$P<0.05$，与哌替啶组相比；†$P<0.05$，与人工喂养组相比。(From Wittels B, Glosten B, Faure EA, et al: Postcesarean analgesia with both epidural morphine and intravenous patient-controlled analgesia: Neurobehavioral outcomes among nursing neonates. Anesth Analg 1997;85:600-606.)

在术后最初 24 h 内，该药可将麻醉性镇痛药的追加量减少 33%，但是并不能改善术后疼痛或患者满意度[99,100]。相反，一项研究发现术前直肠单次给予双氯芬酸 100 mg 可使剖宫产术后最初 24 h 内伤口疼痛减轻、子宫痉挛性疼痛减轻、阿片类药物的追加量减少[95]。另一项研究表明，术后肌内注射 75 mg 双氯芬

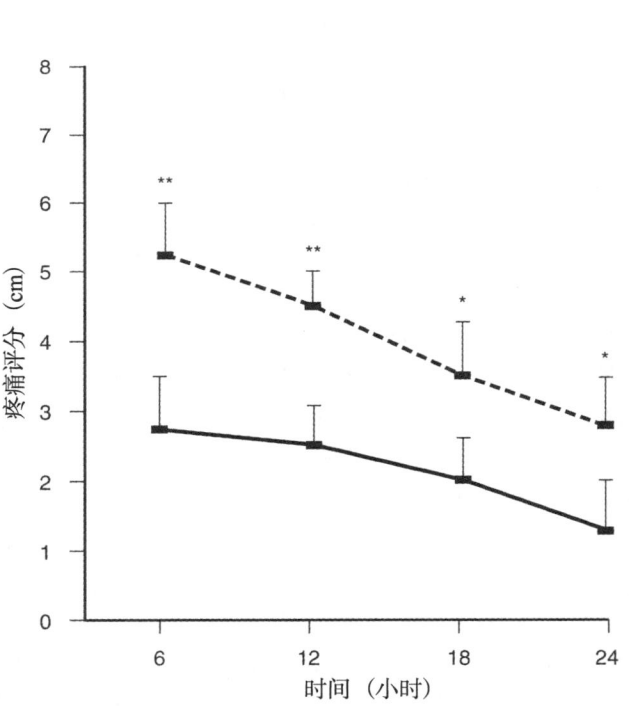

图 23-8 替诺昔康（实线）组与对照（虚线）组患者的疼痛评分均数（±SD）。*$P<0.05$；**$P<0.001$。(From Elhakim M, Nafie M: I.V. tenoxicam for analgesia during caesarean section. Br J Anaesth 1995;74:643-646.)

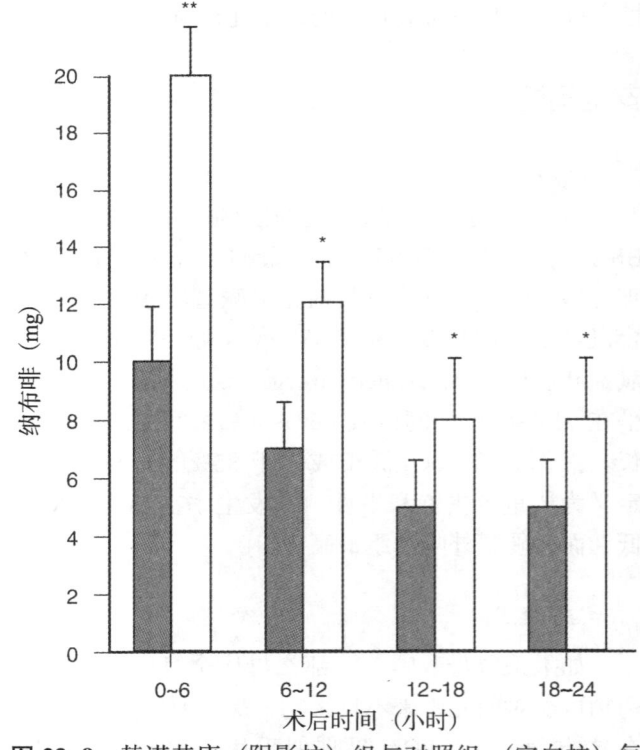

图 23-9 替诺昔康（阴影柱）组与对照组（空白柱）每小时纳布啡用量均数（±SD）。*$P<0.05$；**$P<0.01$。(From Elhakim M, Nafie M: I.V. tenoxicam for analgesia during caesarean section. Br J Anaesth 1995;74:643-646.)

酸可缓解术后最初 18 h 内的疼痛，减轻镇静，阿片类药物用量减少 33%[101]。联合肌内注射曲马多 100 mg 和双氯芬酸 75 mg 能防止剖宫产术后原发性和继发性痛觉过敏，似乎可起到协同作用[102]。

酮咯酸可通过静脉或肌内注射给药，24 h 剂量可达 120 mg。剖宫产术后最初 24 h 内，该药可减轻术后疼痛，并将麻醉性镇痛药的用量减少 30%~50%，这取决于剂量和具体研究（图 23-10）[103,104]。Gin 等[105] 发现全麻下剖宫产术后在 PACU 中肌内注射 30 mg 酮咯酸的镇痛作用时间和镇痛质量相当于肌内注射 75 mg 哌替啶，但不良反应（恶心、头晕）较少[105]。酮咯酸（蛛网膜下腔注射 1 h 后静注 60 mg，随后每 6 h 静注 30 mg，共 3 次）的术后镇痛作用相当于蛛网膜下腔应用吗啡 0.1 mg，但是前者阿片类药物诱发的不良反应较少[106]。

直肠给予吲哚美辛（术后立即给予 200 mg，以后每 12 h 给予 100 mg，共 6 次）可使脊麻下剖宫产分娩后第 1 d 术后疼痛缓解改善，第一次要求追加镇痛药的时间延长，镇痛药的追加量减少[107]。一项回顾性研究发现，直肠吲哚美辛可将区域麻醉下剖宫产分娩后麻醉性镇痛药的用量减少 28%[108]。

静脉替诺昔康（钳夹脐带后立即给予 20 mg）能降低 24 h 吗啡用量约 30%，减轻子宫痉挛性疼痛强度，但是并不减轻休息或运动时切口疼痛[109]。但是术前应用替诺昔康可使剖宫产术后最初 24 h 内术后镇痛效果改善，第一次要求追加镇痛的时间延长，阿片类药物用量减少 50%，并且镇静程度减轻[110]（图 23-8 和 23-9）

研究已证实口服酮洛芬（术后 100 mg，可长达 7 d）的镇痛效果优于联合应用 650 mg 对乙酰氨基酚和 10 mg 盐酸羟考酮，并且前者不良反应较少[111]。研究还证实酮洛芬 50 mg 对剖宫产后患者也具有有效的镇痛作用[112]。一项研究证明选择性剖宫产术后酮洛芬（24 h 以上应用 200 mg）的有效镇痛作用与双氯芬酸（24 h 以上应用 150 mg）一样[113]。研究还表明吲哚洛芬[114]和奈普生[115]对剖宫产后患者具有有效的镇痛作用。

总之，NSAID 作为多模式镇痛方案的一部分，其有效性显而易见。双氯芬酸和酮咯酸在剖宫产后患者镇痛方面的研究最多。遗憾的是，由于缺乏不同药物的比较性研究，所以尚不明确剖宫产后不同 NSAID 的相对镇痛效能。现有证据明确支持在没有禁忌证的情况下，所有剖宫产术的患者宜常规应用 NSAID。然而，必须牢记 NSAID 有促进子宫无力和出血的可能，尤其是已经存在重要危险因素时（如双胞胎妊娠或行子宫肌瘤切除术）[110,113,116]。因此，给予 NSAID 前最好是确认子宫已经持续收缩，术中已安全止血。

其他口服辅助药

对乙酰氨基酚广泛用作术后疼痛缓解的一种辅助药物，对剖宫产术后患者可能有益，尽管几乎没有这类应用研究。一项小型研究并不能证实剖宫产术后应用对乙酰氨基酚可减少吗啡的用量[96]。然而，一项对随机对照试验的全面综述证实，对乙酰氨基酚可将术后患者阿片类药物的用量减少 30%[117]。择期经腹妇科手术患者联合应用对乙酰氨基酚和一种 NSAID 的镇痛效果强于单独给予其中一种药物[118]。

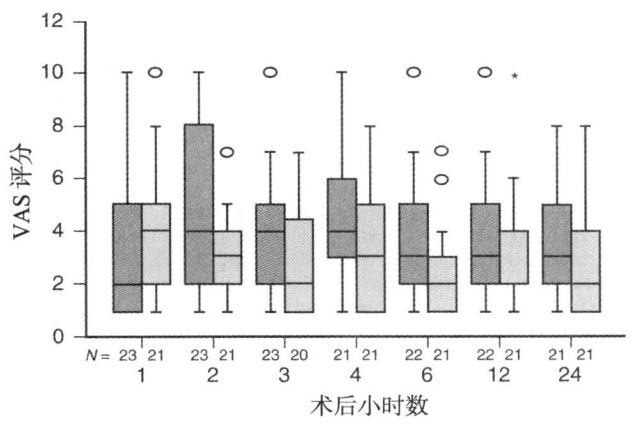

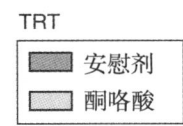

图 23-10 术后视觉模拟评分（VAS）盒状图显示每个个体数据收集点上评分。每个顶框和底框是四分位数的上限与下限值。框顶与框底之间的黑线位于中位数上。面积表示自框顶到框底 50% 受试者的分数范围。延伸到末端的垂线描记个别的极值。(From Lowder JL, Shackelford DP, Holbert D, Beste TM: A randomized, controlledtrial to compare ketorolac tromethamine versus placebo after cesarean section to reduce pain and narcotic usage. Am J Obstet Gynecol 2003;189:1559-1562.)

结论

大量研究集中在剖宫产术后疼痛治疗的最佳方案上。应用椎管内单次注射吗啡、氢吗啡酮或二醋吗啡以及PCEA阿片类药物均可产生有效的镇痛作用。然而，这些技术不良反应的发生率较高，尤其是恶心、呕吐和瘙痒，从而使患者总体满意度下降。IV-PCA吗啡产生的镇痛作用不全，但是阿片类药物诱导的不良反应发生率较低，患者控制IV-PCA的程度较高，从而患者满意水平高。术后镇痛的最佳手段是采用多模式平衡方案。应用小剂量和（或）联合应用短效与长效椎管内阿片类药物，利用或不利用IV-PCA技术，再追加NSAID和简单的镇痛药，可能是提供高质量镇痛的最好方法，同时不良反应发生率低。

（傅　冬译　王天舒　邓小明校）

参考文献

1. Gaiser RR: Changes in the provision of anesthesia for the parturient undergoing cesarean section. Clin Obstet Gynecol 2003;46:646–656.
2. Shibli KU, Russell IF: A survey of anaesthetic techniques used for caesarean section in the UK in 1997. Int J Obstet Anesth 2000;9:160–167.
3. Daley MD, Sandler AN, Turner KE, et al: A comparison of epidural and intramuscular morphine in patients following cesarean section. Anesthesiology 1990;72:289–294.
4. Yarnell RW, Polis T, Reid GN, et al: Patient-controlled analgesia with epidural meperidine after elective cesarean section. Reg Anesth 1992;17:329–333.
5. Negre I, Gueneron JP, Jamali SJ, et al: Preoperative analgesia with epidural morphine. Anesth Analg 1994;79:298–302.
6. Duale C, Frey C, Bolandard F, et al: Epidural versus intrathecal morphine for postoperative analgesia after Caesarean section. Br J Anaesth 2003;91:690–694.
7. Capogna G, Celleno D, Tomassetti M: Maternal analgesia and neonatal effects of epidural sufentanil for cesarean section. Reg Anesth 1989;14:282–287.
8. Palmer CM, Nogami WM, Van Maren G, Alves DM: Postcesarean epidural morphine: A dose-response study. Anesth Analg 2000;90:887–891.
9. Chumpathong S, Santawat U, Saunya P, et al: Comparison of different doses of epidural morphine for pain relief following cesarean section. J Med Assoc Thai 2002;(Suppl 3):S956–S962.
10. Sharar SR, Ready LB, Ross BK, et al: A comparison of postcesarean epidural morphine analgesia by single injection and by continuous infusion. Reg Anesth 1991;16:232–235.
11. Eisenach JC, Schlairet TJ, Dobson CE 2nd, Hood DH: Effect of prior anesthetic solution on epidural morphine analgesia. Anesth Analg 1991;73:119–123.
12. Karambelkar DJ, Ramanathan S: 2-Chloroprocaine antagonism of epidural morphine analgesia. Acta Anaesthesiol Scand 1997;41:774–778.
13. Camann WR, Hartigan PM, Gilbertson LI, et al: Chloroprocaine antagonism of epidural opioid analgesia: A receptor-specific phenomenon? Anesthesiology 1990;73:860–863.
14. Carvalho B, Riley E, Manvelian G, Gambling D: Management of postoperative pain following cesarean section with epidural sustained-release morphine (SKY0401). Anesthesiology 2003;99:A1165.
15. Cooper DW, Ryall DM, Desira WR: Extradural fentanyl for postoperative analgesia: Predominant spinal or systemic action? Br J Anaesth 1995;74:184–187.
16. Cohen S, Pantuck CB, Amar D, et al: The primary action of epidural fentanyl after cesarean delivery is via a spinal mechanism. Anesth Analg 2002;94:674–679.
17. Joris JL, Jacob EA, Sessler DI, et al: Spinal mechanisms contribute to analgesia produced by epidural sufentanil combined with bupivacaine for postoperative analgesia. Anesth Analg 2003;97:1446–1451.
18. Birnbach DJ, Johnson MD, Arcario T, et al: Effect of diluent volume on analgesia produced by epidural fentanyl. Anesth Analg 1989;68:808–810.
19. Grass JA, Sakima NT, Schmidt R, et al: A randomized, double-blind, dose-response comparison of epidural fentanyl versus sufentanil analgesia after cesarean section. Anesth Analg 1997;85:365–371.
20. Cohen S, Amar D, Pantuck CB, et al: Postcesarean delivery epidural patient-controlled analgesia: Fentanyl or sufentanil? Anesthesiology 1993;78:486–491.
21. Sevarino FB, McFarlane C, Sinatra RS: Epidural fentanyl does not influence intravenous PCA requirements in the post-caesarean patient. Can J Anaesth 1991;39:450–453.
22. Paech MJ: Epidural pethidine or fentanyl during caesarean section: A double-blind comparison. Anaesth Intensive Care 1989;17:157–165.
23. Ngan Kee WD, Lam KK, Chen PP, Gin T: Epidural meperidine after cesarean section: A dose-response study. Anesthesiology 1996;85:289–294.
24. Halpern SH, Arellano R, Preston R, et al: Epidural morphine vs hydromorphone in post-caesarean section patients. Can J Anaesth 1996;43:595–598.
25. Siddik-Sayyid S, Aouad-Maroun M, Sleiman D, et al: Epidural tramadol for postoperative pain after Cesarean section. Can J Anaesth 1999;46:731–735.
26. Roulson CJ, Bennett J, Shaw M, Carli F: Effect of extradural diamorphine on analgesia after caesarean section under subarachnoid block. Br J Anaesth 1993;71:810–813.
27. Haynes SR, Davidson I, Allsop JR, Dutton DA: Comparison of epidural methadone with epidural diamorphine for analgesia following caesarean section. Acta Anaesthesiol Scand 1993;37:375–380.
28. Camann WR, Loferski BL, Fanciullo GJ, et al: Does epidural administration of butorphanol offer any clinical advantage over the intravenous route? A double-blind, placebo-controlled trial. Anesthesiology 1992;76:216–220.
29. Abboud TK, Moore M, Zhu J, et al: Epidural butorphanol or morphine for the relief of post-cesarean section pain: Ventilatory responses to carbon dioxide. Anesth Analg 1987;66:887–893.
30. Tanaka M, Watanabe S, Endo T, et al: Combination of epidural morphine and fentanyl for postoperative analgesia. Reg Anesth 1991;16:214–217.
31. Dottrens M, Rifat K, Morel DR: Comparison of extradural administration of sufentanil, morphine and sufentanil-morphine combination after caesarean section. Br J Anaesth 1992;69:9–12.
32. Sinatra RS, Goldstein R, Sevarino FB: The clinical effectiveness of epidural bupivacaine, bupivacaine with lidocaine, and bupivacaine with fentanyl for labor analgesia. J Clin Anesth 1991;3:219–225.
33. Parker RK, Holtmann B, White PF: Patient-controlled epidural analgesia: Interactions between nalbuphine and hydromorphone. Anesth Analg 1997;84:757–763.
34. Lawhorn CD, McNitt JD, Fibuch EE, et al: Epidural morphine with butorphanol for postoperative analgesia after cesarean delivery. Anesth Analg 1991;72:53–57.
35. Kaya FN, Sahin S, Owen MD, Eisenach JC: Epidural neostigmine produces analgesia but also sedation in women after cesarean delivery. Anesthesiology 2004;100:381–385.
36. Vercauteren MP, Saldien V, Bosschaerts P, Adriaensen HA: Potentiation of sufentanil by clonidine in PCEA with or without basal infusion. Eur J Anaesthesiol 1996;13:571–576.
37. Dougherty TB, Baysinger CL, Henenberger JC, Gooding DJ: Epidural hydromorphone with and without epinephrine for post-operative analgesia after cesarean delivery. Anesth Analg 1989;68:318–322.
38. Ngan Kee WD, Ma ML, Khaw KS: Addition of adrenaline to pethidine for epidural analgesia after caesarean section. Anaesthesia 1997;52:853–857.
39. Ngan Kee WD, Khaw KS, Ma ML: The effect of the addition of adrenaline to pethidine for patient-controlled epidural analgesia after caesarean section. Anaesthesia 1998;53:1012–1016.
40. Goh JL, Evans SF, Pavy TJ: Patient-controlled epidural analgesia following

caesarean delivery: A comparison of pethidine and fentanyl. Anaesth Intensive Care 1996;24:45–50.
41. Fanshawe MP: A comparison of patient controlled epidural pethidine versus single dose epidural morphine for analgesia after caesarean section. Anaesth Intensive Care 1999;27:610–614.
42. Paech MJ, Moore JS, Evans SF: Meperidine for patient-controlled analgesia after cesarean section: Intravenous versus epidural administration. Anesthesiology 1994;80:1268–1276.
43. Cooper DW, Saleh U, Taylor M, et al: Patient-controlled analgesia: Epidural fentanyl and i.v. morphine compared after caesarean section. Br J Anaesth 1999;82:366–370.
44. Yu PY, Gambling DR: A comparative study of patient-controlled epidural fentanyl and single dose epidural morphine for post-caesarean analgesia. Can J Anaesth 1993;40:416–420.
45. Ngan Kee WD, Khaw KS, Ma ML: Patient-controlled epidural analgesia after caesarean section using meperidine. Can J Anaesth 1997;44:702–706.
46. Vercauteren MP, Coppejans HC, ten Broecke PW, et al: Epidural sufentanil for postoperative patient-controlled analgesia (PCA) with or without background infusion: A double-blind comparison. Anesth Analg 1995;80:76–80.
47. Parker RK, Sawaki Y, White PF: Epidural patient-controlled analgesia: Influence of bupivacaine and hydromorphone basal infusion on pain control after cesarean delivery. Anesth Analg 1992;75:740–746.
48. Buggy DJ, Hall NA, Shah J, et al: Motor block during patient-controlled epidural analgesia with ropivacaine or ropivacaine/fentanyl after intrathecal bupivacaine for caesarean section. Br J Anaesth 2000;85:468–470.
49. Cooper DW, Ryall DM, McHardy FE, et al: Patient-controlled extradural analgesia with bupivacaine, fentanyl, or a mixture of both, after Caesarean section. Br J Anaesth 1996;76:611–615.
50. Cohen S, Lowenwirt I, Pantuck CB, et al: Bupivacaine 0.01% and/or epinephrine 0.5 microg/ml improve epidural fentanyl analgesia after cesarean section. Anesthesiology 1998;89:1354–1361.
51. Vercauteren M, Vereecken K, La Malfa M, et al: Cost-effectiveness of analgesia after Caesarean section: A comparison of intrathecal morphine and epidural PCA. Acta Anaesthesiol Scand 2002;46:85–89.
52. Alahuhta S, Kangas-Saarela T, Hollmen AI, Edstrom HH: Visceral pain during caesarean section under spinal and epidural anaesthesia with bupivacaine. Acta Anaesthesiol Scand 1990;34:95–98.
53. Abouleish E, Rawal N, Rashad MN: The addition of 0.2 mg subarachnoid morphine to hyperbaric bupivacaine for cesarean delivery: A prospective study of 856 cases. Reg Anesth 1991;16:137–140.
54. Abboud TK, Dror A, Mosaad P, et al: Mini-dose intrathecal morphine for the relief of post-cesarean section pain: Safety, efficacy, and ventilatory responses to carbon dioxide. Anesth Analg 1988;67:137–143.
55. Dahl JB, Jeppesen IS, Jorgensen H, et al: Intraoperative and postoperative analgesic efficacy and adverse effects of intrathecal opioids in patients undergoing cesarean section with spinal anesthesia: A qualitative and quantitative systematic review of randomized controlled trials. Anesthesiology 1999;91:1919–1927.
56. Palmer CM, Emerson S, Volgoropolous D, Alves D: Dose-response relationship of intrathecal morphine for postcesarean analgesia. Anesthesiology 1999;90:437–444.
57. Milner AR, Bogod DG, Harwood RJ: Intrathecal administration of morphine for elective Caesarean section: A comparison between 0.1 mg and 0.2 mg. Anaesthesia 1996;51:871–873.
58. Uchiyama A, Nakano S, Ueyama H, et al: Low dose intrathecal morphine and pain relief following caesarean section. Int J Obstet Anesth 1994;3:87–91.
59. Jiang CJ, Liu CC, Wu TJ, et al: Mini-dose intrathecal morphine for post-cesarean section analgesia. Ma Zui Xue Za Zhi 1991;29:683–689.
60. Husaini SW, Russell IF: Intrathecal diamorphine compared with morphine for postoperative analgesia after caesarean section under spinal anaesthesia. Br J Anaesth 1998;81:135–139.
61. Kelly MC, Carabine UA, Mirakhur RK: Intrathecal diamorphine for analgesia after caesarean section: A dose finding study and assessment of side-effects. Anaesthesia 1998;53:231–237.
62. Stacey R, Jones R, Kar G, Poon A: High-dose intrathecal diamorphine for analgesia after Caesarean section. Anaesthesia 2001;56:54–60.
63. Sibilla C, Albertazz P, Zatelli R, Martinello R: Perioperative analgesia for caesarean section: Comparison of intrathecal morphine and fentanyl alone or in combination. Int J Obstet Anesth 1997;6:43–48.
64. Belzarena SD: Clinical effects of intrathecally administered fentanyl in patients undergoing cesarean section. Anesth Analg 1992;74:653–657.
65. Dahlgren G, Hultstrand C, Jakobsson J, et al: Intrathecal sufentanil, fentanyl, or placebo added to bupivacaine for cesarean section. Anesth Analg 1997;85:1288–1293.
66. Chung JH, Sinatra RS, Sevarino FB, Fermo L: Subarachnoid meperidine-morphine combination: An effective perioperative analgesic adjunct for cesarean delivery. Reg Anesth 1997;22:119–124.
67. Feldman JM, Griffin F, Fermo L, Raessler K: Intrathecal meperidine for pain after cesarean delivery: Efficacy and dose-response. Anesthesiology 1992;77:A1011.
68. Rawal N, Nuutinen L, Raj PP, et al: Behavioral and histopathologic effects following intrathecal administration of butorphanol, sufentanil, and nalbuphine in sheep. Anesthesiology 1991;75:1025–1034.
69. Connelly NR, Dunn SM, Ingold V, Villa EA: The use of fentanyl added to morphine-lidocaine-epinephrine spinal solution in patients undergoing cesarean section. Anesth Analg 1994;78:918–920.
70. Krukowski JA, Hood DD, Eisenach JC, et al: Intrathecal neostigmine for post-cesarean section analgesia: Dose response. Anesth Analg 1997;84:1269–1275.
71. Chung CJ, Kim JS, Park HS, Chin YJ: The efficacy of intrathecal neostigmine, intrathecal morphine, and their combination for post-cesarean section analgesia. Anesth Analg 1998;87:341–346.
72. Klamt JG, Garcia LV, Prado WA: Analgesic and adverse effects of a low dose of intrathecally administered hyperbaric neostigmine alone or combined with morphine in patients submitted to spinal anaesthesia: Pilot studies. Anaesthesia 1999;54:27–31.
73. Abouleish E, Rawal N, Tobon-Randall B, et al: A clinical and laboratory study to compare the addition of 0.2 mg of morphine, 0.2 mg of epinephrine, or their combination to hyperbaric bupivacaine for spinal anesthesia in cesarean section. Anesth Analg 1993;77:457–462.
74. Filos KS, Goudas LC, Patroni O, Polyzou V: Intrathecal clonidine as a sole analgesic for pain relief after cesarean section. Anesthesiology 1992;77:267–274.
75. Paech MJ, Pavy TJ, Orlikowski CE, et al: Postcesarean analgesia with spinal morphine, clonidine, or their combination. Anesth Analg 2004;98:1460–1466.
76. Pan PM, Huang CT, Wei TT, Mok MS: Enhancement of analgesic effect of intrathecal neostigmine and clonidine on bupivacaine spinal anesthesia. Reg Anesth Pain Med 1998;23:49–56.
77. Benhamou D, Thorin D, Brichant JF, et al: Intrathecal clonidine and fentanyl with hyperbaric bupivacaine improves analgesia during cesarean section. Anesth Analg 1998;87:609–613.
78. Baraka A, Noueihid R, Hajj S: Intrathecal injection of morphine for obstetric analgesia. Anesthesiology 1981;54:136–140.
79. Perez-Woods R, Grohar JC, Skaredoff M, et al: Pain control after cesarean birth: Efficacy of patient-controlled analgesia vs traditional therapy (IM morphine). J Perinatol 1991;11:174–181.
80. Cade L, Ashley J, Ross AW: Comparison of epidural and intravenous opioid analgesia after elective caesarean section. Anaesth Intensive Care 1992;20:41–45.
81. Eisenach JC, Grice SC, Dewan DM: Patient-controlled analgesia following cesarean section: A comparison with epidural and intramuscular narcotics. Anesthesiology 1988;68:444–448.
82. Harrison DM, Sinatra R, Morgese L, Chung JH: Epidural narcotic and patient-controlled analgesia for post-cesarean section pain relief. Anesthesiology 1988;68:454–457.
83. Cade L, Ashley J: Towards optimal analgesia after caesarean section: Comparison of epidural and intravenous patient-controlled opioid analgesia. Anaesth Intensive Care 1993;21:696–699.
84. Stoddart PA, Cooper A, Russell R, Reynolds F: A comparison of epidural diamorphine with intravenous patient-controlled analgesia using the Baxter infusor following caesarean section. Anaesthesia 1993;48:1086–1090.
85. Anwari JS, Butt A, Alkhunein S: PCA after subarachnoid block for cesarean section. Middle East J Anesthesiol 2004;17:913–926.
86. Yost NP, Bloom SL, Sibley MK, et al: A hospital-sponsored quality improvement study of pain management after cesarean delivery. Am J Obstet Gynecol 2004;190:1341–1346.
87. Sinatra RS, Lodge K, Sibert K, et al: A comparison of morphine,

meperidine, and oxymorphone as utilized in patient-controlled analgesia following cesarean delivery. Anesthesiology 1989;70:585–590.
88. Howell PR, Gambling DR, Pavy T, et al: Patient-controlled analgesia following caesarean section under general anaesthesia: A comparison of fentanyl with morphine. Can J Anaesth 1995;42:41–45.
89. Capogna G, Celleno D, Sebastiani M, et al: [Continuous intravenous infusion with patient-controlled anesthesia for postoperative analgesia in cesarean section: morphine versus buprenorphine.] Minerva Anestesiol 1989;55:33–38.
90. Sinatra R, Chung KS, Silverman DG, et al: An evaluation of morphine and oxymorphone administered via patient-controlled analgesia (PCA) or PCA plus basal infusion in postcesarean-delivery patients. Anesthesiology 1989;71:502–507.
91. Wittels B, Glosten B, Faure EA, et al: Postcesarean analgesia with both epidural morphine and intravenous patient-controlled analgesia: Neurobehavioral outcomes among nursing neonates. Anesth Analg 1997;85:600–606.
92. Brose WG, Cohen SE: Oxyhemoglobin saturation following cesarean section in patients receiving epidural morphine, PCA, or IM meperidine analgesia. Anesthesiology 1989;70:948–953.
93. Wittels B, Scott DT, Sinatra RS: Exogenous opioids in human breast milk and acute neonatal neurobehavior: A preliminary study. Anesthesiology 1990;73:864–869.
94. Baka NE, Bayoumeu F, Boutroy MJ, Laxenaire MC: Colostrum morphine concentrations during postcesarean intravenous patient-controlled analgesia. Anesth Analg 2002;94:184–187.
95. Sia AT, Thomas E, Chong JL, Loo CC: Combination of suppository diclofenac and intravenous morphine infusion in post-caesarean section pain relief—a step towards balanced analgesia? Singapore Med J 1997;38:68–70.
96. Siddik SM, Aouad MT, Jalbout MI, et al: Diclofenac and/or propacetamol for postoperative pain management after cesarean delivery in patients receiving patient controlled analgesia morphine. Reg Anesth Pain Med 2001;26:310–315.
97. Rashid M, Jaruidi HM: The use of rectal diclofenac for post-cesarean analgesia. Saudi Med J 2000;21:145–149.
98. Olofsson CI, Legeby MH, Nygards EB, Ostman KM: Diclofenac in the treatment of pain after caesarean delivery: An opioid-saving strategy. Eur J Obstet Gynecol Reprod Biol 2000;88:143–146.
99. Lim NL, Lo WK, Chong JL, Pan AX: Single dose diclofenac suppository reduces post-Cesarean PCEA requirements. Can J Anaesth 2001;48:383–386.
100. Dennis AR, Leeson-Payne CG, Hobbs GJ: Analgesia after caesarean section: The use of rectal diclofenac as an adjunct to spinal morphine. Anaesthesia 1995;50:297–299.
101. Bush DJ, Lyons G, MacDonald R: Diclofenac for analgesia after caesarean section. Anaesthesia 1992;47:1075–1077.
102. Wilder-Smith CH, Hill L, Dyer RA, et al: Postoperative sensitization and pain after cesarean delivery and the effects of single IM doses of tramadol and diclofenac alone and in combination. Anesth Analg 2003;97:526–533.
103. Lowder JL, Shackelford DP, Holbert D, Beste TM: A randomized, controlled trial to compare ketorolac tromethamine versus placebo after cesarean section to reduce pain and narcotic usage. Am J Obstet Gynecol 2003;189:1559–1562.
104. Pavy TJ, Paech MJ, Evans SF: The effect of intravenous ketorolac on opioid requirement and pain after cesarean delivery. Anesth Analg 2001;92:1010–1014.
105. Gin T, Kan AF, Lam KK, O'Meara ME: Analgesia after caesarean section with intramuscular ketorolac or pethidine. Anaesth Intensive Care 1993;21:420–423.
106. Cohen SE, Desai JB, Ratner EF, et al: Ketorolac and spinal morphine for postcesarean analgesia. Int J Obstet Anesth 1996;5:14–18.
107. Pavy TJ, Gambling DR, Merrick PM, Douglas MJ: Rectal indomethacin potentiates spinal morphine analgesia after caesarean delivery. Anaesth Intensive Care 1995;23:555–559.
108. Ambrose FP: A retrospective study of the effect of postoperative indomethacin rectal suppositories on the need for narcotic analgesia in patients who had a cesarean delivery while they were under regional anesthesia. Am J Obstet Gynecol 2001;184:1544–1547.
109. Hsu HW, Cheng YJ, Chen LK, et al: Differential analgesic effect of tenoxicam on the wound pain and uterine cramping pain after cesarean section. Clin J Pain 2003;19:55–58.
110. Elhakim M, Nafie M. I.V. tenoxicam for analgesia during caesarean section. Br J Anaesth 1995;74:643–646.
111. Sunshine A, Olson NZ, Zighelboim I, De Castro A: Ketoprofen, acetaminophen plus oxycodone, and acetaminophen in the relief of postoperative pain. Clin Pharmacol Ther 1993;54:546–555.
112. Sunshine A, Zighelboim I, Laska E, et al: A double-blind, parallel comparison of ketoprofen, aspirin, and placebo in patients with postpartum pain. J Clin Pharmacol 1986;26:706–711.
113. Rorarius MG, Suominen P, Baer GA, et al: Diclofenac and ketoprofen for pain treatment after elective caesarean section. Br J Anaesth 1993;70:293–297.
114. Sunshine A, Zighelboim I, Olson NZ, et al: A comparative oral analgesic study of indoprofen, aspirin, and placebo in postpartum pain. J Clin Pharmacol 1985;25:374–380.
115. Angle PJ, Halpern SH, Leighton BL, et al: A randomized controlled trial examining the effect of naproxen on analgesia during the second day after cesarean delivery. Anesth Analg 2002;95:741–745.
116. Diemunsch P, Alt M, Diemunsch AM, Treisser A: Post cesarean analgesia with ketorolac tromethamine and uterine atonia. Eur J Obstet Gynecol Reprod Biol 1997;72:205–206.
117. Moore A, Collins S, Carroll D, McQuay H: Paracetamol with and without codeine in acute pain: A quantitative systematic review. Pain 1997;70:193–201.
118. Montgomery JE, Sutherland CJ, Kestin IG, Sneyd JR: Morphine consumption in patients receiving rectal paracetamol and diclofenac alone and in combination. Br J Anaesth 1996;77:445–447.

24 药物依赖性患者的术后疼痛管理

SRDJAN S. NEDELJKOVIĆ · AJAY D. WASAN

术后疼痛最难处理的患者是那些已给予最高剂量阿片类药物的患者,这使医师处于两难境地。然而,长期应用阿片类药物可增加疼痛的敏感性[1],研究表明长期使用美沙酮和海洛因的患者可出现痛觉过敏[2,3]。因此,长时间使用阿片类药物患者对手术疼痛的反应更强烈就不足为奇了。近20年来,随着处方使用阿片类药物治疗慢性疼痛的病例不断增加,术前已经服用大剂量阿片类药物的患者接受手术的几率也随之增加[4,5]。一些慢性疼痛患者在接受手术前具有阿片类药物使用剂量逐步增加的病史。偶尔,接受手术的患者属于非法使用药品。药物依赖患者术后疼痛的处理是一项重大挑战。

从广义上说,药物依赖性患者术后疼痛处理不当有以下两种情况:①使用过量镇痛药进行过度治疗;或②治疗不足,导致疼痛缓解不全,患者感觉疼痛。除控制疼痛外,术后疼痛处理的目的包括:将镇痛治疗的不良反应降至最低的同时,使机体功能最快恢复,胃肠道功能快速恢复。药物依赖患者过度使用镇痛类药物能引起不良反应如镇静过度,并延缓手术恢复。慢性疼痛患者过度使用镇痛治疗后可能使患者出院时所需镇痛药用量大于入院时用量,可能会使慢性疼痛综合征门诊者的处理更为棘手。更常见的是,有时因为担心药物成瘾,药物依赖患者在术后镇痛治疗不足,从而增加了这些患者发生过度疼痛和精神痛苦的可能性。

为了完善药物依赖患者的疼痛处理,必须了解依赖性、耐药性和成瘾的概念和定义。必须了解药物滥用的基础以及这种疾病的症状与体征。必须理解所用药物的药理学作用,如阿片类药物、苯二氮䓬类、乙醇、可卡因和其他药物。必须考虑与药物滥用有关的医学问题,包括肝炎、人类免疫缺陷病毒感染和有关精神障碍。最后,医师必须为如何处理术后疼痛制定出合理的围手术期方案,以满足患者的身心需要。应该在术前与患者及其他医护人员共同讨论该方案。总之,处理这些具有挑战性的患者,围手术期所有医护人员均应该制订一套完整的治疗方案。

药物成瘾和药物滥用的概念和定义

因为慢性疼痛、精神病治疗或肿瘤综合征等合法的医疗需求,接受手术的患者可能是药物依赖者。引起药物依赖的常见处方药物是阿片类镇痛药和苯二氮䓬类药物。患者可能为药物滥用者,违法使用处方药或非法药物,如海洛因、可卡因、大麻。对于药物依赖患者,术后疼痛处理的关键在于明确该患者的药物依赖类型:患者药物依赖仅仅是生理依赖,还是药物成瘾。因此,有必要理解这两个不同的概念。

躯体依赖性是一种神经生理适应,发生于患者应用各种药物(包括阿片类药物、苯二氮䓬类药物、特定抗高血压药物以及三环类抗抑郁药)时。这是通过药效学上的底物-受体相互关系所产生的一种生理反应。对这些药物依赖患者停用这些药物时会出现戒断综合征。突然停用阿片类药物时,戒断综合征的症状和体征包括高血压、心动过速、腹泻、失眠和其他一些精神过激行为。研究表明，停用阿片类药物的患者脑内去甲肾上腺素水平较高[6]。许多长期使用阿片类药物或苯二氮䓬类药物的患者依赖于这些药物，如果停用这些药物即可出现戒断症状。研究显示，停药后数月多巴胺受体水平下降[7]，该结果可解释为何某些患者在药物代谢清除后很长时间内仍渴望药物。半衰期长的药物（如美沙酮）停药后戒断时间可达6～8周[8]。

药物成瘾是指患者通过间断或持续应用药物以获得欣快感或满足感。其显著标志是强迫性使用合法和（或）非法的药物。成瘾患者常常使用一种药物，而忽视该药物的有害作用后果，并且会不遗余力地获取该药物。患者在使用该药物时失去控制，自己不能调节其何时用或用多少。一般认为药物成瘾是一种长期、易复发、使人逐渐衰弱的一种精神疾病。两次药瘾发作间隙，患者能有数年不使用或节制使用该药物，如果再次接触滥用药物，患者易于成瘾。有药物成瘾病史的患者易于复发，使其为严格戒毒付出的所有努力付之东流。神经机制改变的研究结果认为，药物成瘾是一种终生易感性疾病，即使长时间停止应用滥用药物后，也能再次激发这种易感性[9,10]。

研究证实成瘾是一种大脑疾病，其主要是神经生物功能紊乱。对于易感患者来说，接触所滥用药物可能引起其脑内"开关"开启，使患者行为逐渐从自主用药转变为强迫用药[11,12]。接触并反复使用药物后，患者可能失去自我调节用药行为的能力。这些患者中，药物能使患者自我控制理念丧失，变成永久性强迫用药（图24-1）。在脑内多巴胺介导的反馈系统（如大

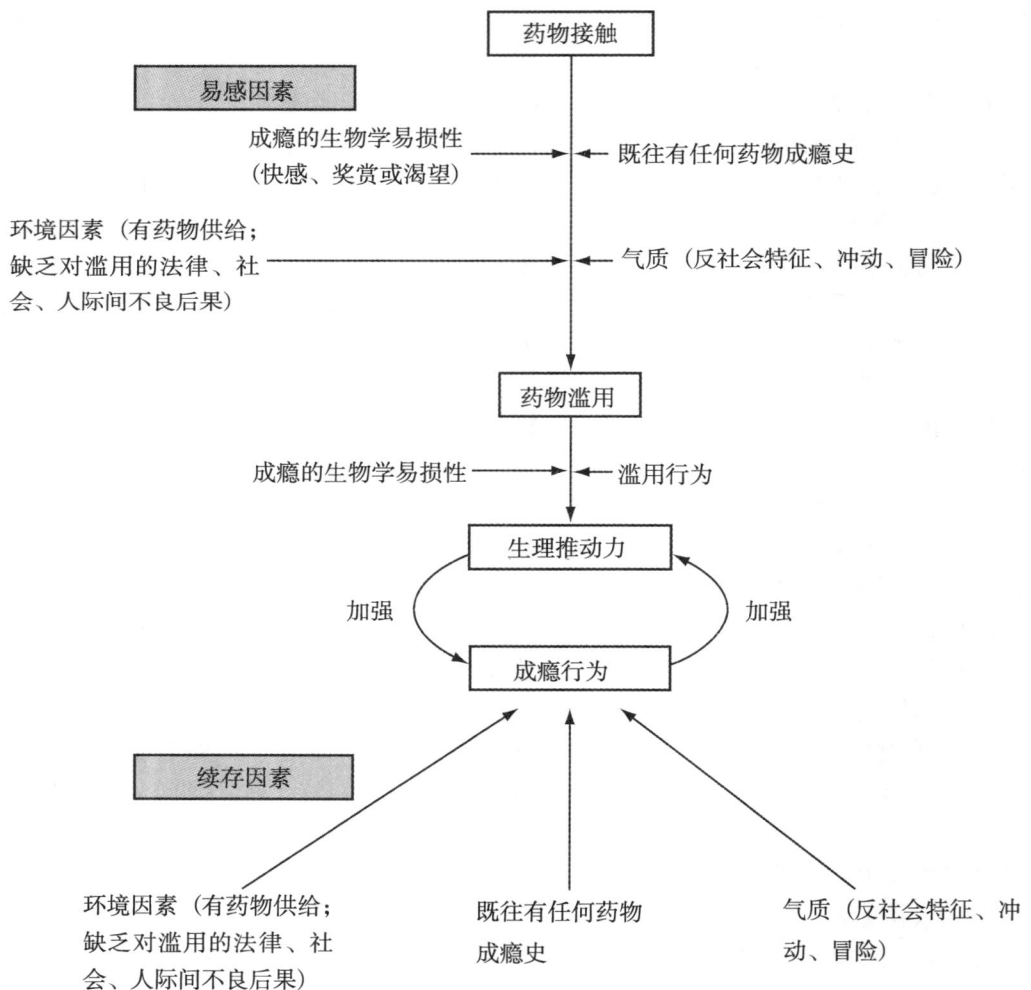

图24-1 成瘾的途径。(Adapted from Nedeljkovic' SS, Wasan A, Jamison RN: Assessment of efficacy of longterm opioid therapy in pain patients with substance abuse potential. Clin J Pain 2002;18:S39-S51.)

脑左侧前额皮质和听神经核）中可观察到功能性变化[13]。研究表明，与服用可卡因或哌醋甲酯有关的愉悦与欣快感是脑内多巴胺水平增高所致[7]。研究显示，一些使人本能愉快的活动，如吃饭、喝酒和性爱，可刺激多巴胺的释放，这类似于成瘾药物引起欣快感并导致多巴胺释放一样[14]。当戒断阿片类药物、兴奋剂、乙醇时，听神经核内多巴胺水平降低[15]。因此，多巴胺系统是维持药物成瘾奖赏强化机制的一个重要因素。

药物反复接触能引起大脑改变和神经适应。大多数患者一般需要反复用药才能引起成瘾者所见的大脑功能改变。然而，某些易感患者即使短暂接触药物也可能足以引起永久性成瘾疾病。成瘾可能是一种可以遗传的疾病，因为研究发现易成瘾动物神经系统中的内源性阿片肽和阿片类受体具有遗传差异[12]。阿片成瘾者脑内改变也见于苯丙胺、可卡因、尼古丁和乙醇所引起的改变，这称为交叉成瘾。假如患者依赖于某一种药物，那么他对其他药物产生成瘾的机会增加[16]。此外，成瘾药物的使用与其他寻求奖赏的行为如吸烟、赌博、冲动、身体多处创伤病史之间密切相关[12]。除遗传和生物因素外，社会和环境因素如缺乏精神社会支持以及有药物来源等也对药物易成瘾发挥一定作用。

耐受是指患者需要不断增大药物用量来达到同样药理学效应的一种现象。在耐药的患者中，要达到预期效果就必须使用较大剂量的止痛药或精神类药物。耐药可能有遗传基础，并与阿片类受体脱敏有关[17]。这是一种正常的生理事件，但并不意味着患者失去控制调节药物使用的能力。阿片类药物的大多数作用可发生耐受，瞳孔缩小和便秘除外。对阿片类药物的某些不良反应耐受可能有利，因为耐受患者追加阿片类药物时发生瘙痒、镇静或呼吸抑制的可能较小。但是，长时间使用阿片类药物的患者也可能耐受其镇痛作用，并耐受用于术后疼痛控制时阿片类药物标准剂量的作用。虽然对于阿片类药物镇痛作用耐受的形式及发生时间尚不确定，但是一些研究显示，即使短时间应用即可发生耐受[18]。用药时间较长、用量较大情况下，更可能发生耐受。更强效的药物（高效价）如舒芬太尼的耐受要慢于弱效的药物，如吗啡（低效价）[19]。解决药物耐受问题对药物依赖患者术后疼痛处理方面具有重要的作用，尤其是阿片类药物镇痛作用耐受的患者。

药物依赖患者术后疼痛评估与处理中，重要的是理解依赖、成瘾和耐受的差别和含义。耐受和戒断反应均能增加药物的使用量和引发成瘾行为。为了避免围手术期出现戒断综合征，应该继续使用能引起戒断反应的药物。应该提供给所有患者相关的药物或等效药物，无论患者是否滥用该药物或正当需求用药。对阿片类药物作用耐受的患者可能需要较大剂量的阿片类药物，以达到镇痛作用。由于不同阿片类药物之间存在不完全性交叉耐受，应用一种新型阿片类药物可能对一些患者有利。应该询问患者药物成瘾病史。不应该盲目增大有药物滥用病史患者的药物剂量，处理的目标在于一旦典型的术后期过去，就应该恢复至术前用于慢性疼痛或成瘾维持的药物剂量。关于药物依赖患者处理，"药物依赖患者的围手术期计划"中有更详细的建议。

药物依赖患者的药理学问题

遇到要实施手术的药物依赖患者的机会确实很大。总体来说，估计美国人口中一生乙醇滥用的发生率约为14%，其中50%以上长期戒酒[20,21]。其他药物成瘾中，一生发生率为7%，其中约30%~50%长期戒瘾[20,21]。接受手术的患者可能依赖于不同类型的药物，包括阿片类药物、乙醇、镇静药（苯二氮䓬类和巴比妥类）和兴奋剂；患者也可能对大麻成瘾。不同药物可能表现方式不一，这对术后管理医师提出了挑战。因此，重要的是了解每种药物引起的症状及其药理学知识。

乙醇

乙醇滥用或者长期使用是最可能遇到的药物依赖问题。据估计，美国有800万以上的人对乙醇依赖，而相比较而言，约有350万人使用非法药品（主要是海洛因和兴奋剂）[22]。住院或处于医疗监护的患者中约15%~20%有乙醇滥用病史[23]。小剂量乙醇可能具有兴奋作用，可抑制中枢神经系统中的抑制系统。较大剂量乙醇能导致较强的镇静作用和运动共济失调。乙醇戒断的常见症状和体征有恶心、颤抖、失眠、易激怒和体温轻微升高。乙醇戒断的罕见后果是震颤性谵妄，能引起癫痫发作、幻觉和致命性高血压。乙醇滥用患者也可能出现肝功能障碍，可能引起镇痛药物代谢的改变以及造成贫血与血小板减少。

乙醇能增强N-甲基-D-天冬氨酸盐（N-methyl-d-aspartate，NMDA）受体的功能，因此NMDA拮抗剂可能有助于乙醇戒断症状的治疗[24]。研究发现乙醇戒断可促进兴奋性谷氨酸途径的神经传递[25]。可兴奋γ-氨基丁酸（gamma-aminobutyric acid，GABA）受体的苯二氮䓬类药物以及卡马西平和丙戊酸能减轻乙醇戒断症状[26]。当使用这些药物时，发生癫痫发作和谵妄的风险降低[27]。β-肾上腺素类药物和可乐定可能减轻戒断导致的某些自主神经症状。戒酒期以后以及作为成瘾治疗的方法之一，使用阿片类药物拮抗剂如纳曲酮能减少乙醇消耗量[28]。未经治疗的患者乙醇戒断症状在72h时达到高峰，但患者的症状如失眠可能持续数周[29]。乙醇戒断的药物治疗很少需要超过1周。

镇静药（苯二氮䓬类和巴比妥类）

苯二氮䓬类药物能增强抑制性神经递质GABA的作用，产生抗焦虑和镇静作用。一直应用较大剂量药物、应用半衰期短的该类药物或较长时间应用该类药物治疗的患者，停止使用苯二氮䓬类药物时更可能出现戒断症状。有焦虑、抑郁、个人精神障碍、惊恐性障碍的患者可能更难戒断该类药物[30]。较长时间用药后如果突然停药能导致癫痫发作。患者在戒断苯二氮䓬类药物时常出现失眠、易怒、头痛和震颤，也可能出现知觉障碍和严重焦虑。苯二氮䓬类药物戒断的严重临床表现为抽搐、精神错乱以及精神疾病。

一般建议苯二氮䓬类药物的戒断治疗应该逐渐进行。2~4周能够逐渐递减剂量的50%，但是剩下50%的剂量可能需要更长时间来减少[30]。苯二氮䓬类药物戒断症状通常出现在停药后2~10d[29]。一些专家建议患者改用长效苯二氮䓬类药物，如地西泮或氯硝西泮，这样在减少剂量过程中戒断症状较少。较短效苯二氮䓬类药物的滥用可能大于较长效苯二氮䓬类药物[31]。苯二氮䓬类药物的戒断可能需要长达1年时间[30]。应用抗抑郁药（如曲唑酮和丙咪嗪）以及抗惊厥药（如卡马西平和丙戊酸）可能有助于苯二氮䓬类药物戒断治疗方案的实施。采用心理疗法而不使用药物治疗焦虑也可能有益。

阿片类药物

2003年，美国开出的长效阿片类药物处方有15 780 000张以上[32]。据估计，约750 000人依赖于海洛因[22]。最常滥用的是快速起效的药物，这些药物可产生欣快感（羟考酮、氢吗啡酮、美沙酮、芬太尼）。能被捻碎、吸入或注射（加快起效速度和增强作用效能的所有方法）的药物更可能被滥用[33]。对于某些患者，可能难于鉴别因慢性疼痛症状加重而加大阿片类药物用量的患者与专心觅药的成瘾者。

反复给予阿片类药物可引起躯体依赖与耐受。阿片类药物戒断常常表现为弥散性身体疼痛、腹部痛性痉挛、食欲缺乏、腹泻和失眠。患者可能哈欠连天。患者可能表现出对所滥用药物的渴望，可能出现交感与副交感兴奋症状，可能表现为瞳孔散大、流鼻涕、结节性红斑、躁动以及心动过速。与乙醇戒断不同，阿片类药物戒断不会引起癫痫发作。

与阿片类药物依赖有关的戒断症状可应用地芬诺酯阿托品（止泻宁）等控制腹泻，苯二氮䓬类药物控制焦虑和躁动，α_2受体激动剂和β受体阻断剂控制拟交感症状。戒断症状出现时间取决于所用药物的药理学。应用海洛因的患者在停止用药后36~72h时戒断症状可能最严重，戒断症状可能持续7~10d。使用美沙酮患者戒断症状的高峰在72~96h时，持续时间大于2周[29]，甚至长达6~7周。

处理阿片类药物成瘾的药理学方法如应用美沙酮、丁丙诺啡和其他药物详见"药物依赖与成瘾的治疗"。可应用α_2激动剂（盐酸替扎尼定、可乐定）和其他药物如β受体阻断剂来阻断戒断的肾上腺素能反应。

兴奋剂（安非他命和可卡因）

有人常服用安非他命来产生欣快感，有人服用安非他命来增强警觉性与注意力。据估计美国约有100万人依赖于安非他命。这类药物能导致心率加快、血压升高、皮质醇释放增加。长期服用这类药物能导致侵略性和妄想狂行为。如果兴奋性药物快速戒断，患者除失眠和食欲减退外，可能感到抑郁。这种抑郁一般持续长达48h，但是较轻症状可能持续约2周[29]。

可卡因也可作为一种兴奋剂，能导致患者妄想并感到皮肤下虫爬感。可卡因可阻断多巴胺、去甲肾上腺素和5-羟色胺的摄取，能引起心律失常、高血压以及侵略性行为。另外一种安非他明类药物是3,4-亚甲基去氧麻黄碱（3,4-methylenedioxymethamphetamine，MDMA），常称为摇头丸，能引起欣快、幻觉以及一种欲仙欲死的快感。过量能导致脱水、热休克、颅内出血和5-羟色胺综合征，甚至死亡。该药物的戒断能引起抑郁。该药物对5-羟色胺性神经元具有神经毒性[34]，而且研究证实长期服用该药物可能出现长时间认知功能损害[35]。

动物研究表明，氟西汀可阻断神经元摄取MDMA，可能具有神经保护作用。但是目前尚无任何一种药物对于治疗兴奋剂戒断症状具有可靠效果。β受体阻断剂可减轻戒断的血流动力学症状[36]。哌甲酯和金刚烷胺等药物为间接性多巴胺激动剂，能减少可卡因成瘾者复发的发生率[37,38]。

大麻

来自印度瓜紫麻植物的大麻是一种能被吸食的非法药物。吸食该药可产生一种幸福感；但是较大剂量能引起情绪抑郁、惊恐和神经质。大麻的戒断并不产生躯体戒断综合征，但是患者可能心理上渴望该药物。这些患者停用大麻后可能表现为不安、焦虑和失眠。长期应用该药能导致记忆障碍[39]。

小结

一般认为成瘾是一种慢性持久性疾病，对药物已经成瘾的患者易于复发成瘾行为，所以围手术期间接触所滥用的药物可能再次燃起患者潜在的成瘾状态。以前滥用药物的患者脑内多巴胺能神经元相关神经环路可能已经发生变化。由于存在交叉成瘾的可能性，所以接触苯二氮䓬类或阿片类药物也可能激发患者的渴望以及其他成瘾行为，即使曾滥用非阿片类药物（如乙醇和可卡因）的患者也如此。

维持滥用毒品的戒断是一个复杂过程，这不仅取决于躯体戒断症状的克服，而且取决于避免复发的社会与应对机制的发展[10]。心理和行为修正方式可能在这方面有所帮助，包括匿名戒酒者协会和匿名戒毒者协会。参加这些活动者以及已经戒断药物者可以理解其对围手术期是否接触所滥用药物有焦虑。某些患者拒绝使用抗焦虑药或阿片类药物，尤其在手术前清醒状态下，这些患者更倾向于通过认知和行为方法来缓解术前焦虑。然而，已有患者围手术期接触阿片类药物后成瘾复发的报道[10,40]。应激反应较强、焦虑较明显以及疼痛处理不充分均能导致患者术后阿片类药物的需求量较大[41]，即使在成瘾状态减轻的患者也如此。

对易成瘾患者的围手术期处理，必须认识到患者可能正在服用某些药物，以防止成瘾复发。这些药物包括酗酒者服用的双硫仑、减轻对乙醇依赖的阿坎酸、纳曲酮（阿片类药物拮抗剂，也用于乙醇成瘾者）以及美沙酮或丁丙诺啡（替代μ受体激动剂的药物）。还必须认识到，一直有药物滥用病史的患者精神疾病的发病率较高，包括焦虑、抑郁、精神病；并且这些患者在麻醉或术后期间可能应用各种药物治疗[10]。

药物依赖和成瘾的治疗

人们提出许多药理、心理和行为治疗方法来处理药物滥用性疾病和药物成瘾的患者。戒断的处理取决于所依赖的药物。由于多巴胺在神经生物奖赏系统中似乎起到重要的作用，因此人们一直努力地开发可修饰多巴胺能系统的药物。例如，可增加突触间隙中多巴胺和去甲肾上腺素水平的安非他酮，已发现其对于治疗尼古丁成瘾有效[42]。

酗酒

人们一直应用双硫仑来治疗乙醇中毒者，该药可抑制醛脱氢酶，使患者在摄取乙醇后发生乙醛蓄积。这种乙醛蓄积可引起患者严重不适感。双硫仑也抑制多巴胺β-羟化酶，可能导致麻醉期间心血管反应减弱[10]。双硫仑能抑制经肝系统代谢的药物，如巴比妥酸盐、三环类抗忧郁药物以及华法林[43]。

应用μ受体拮抗剂如纳曲酮和纳美芬能治疗长期乙醇滥用患者。这些药物可减轻患者对乙醇的渴望感；当应用阿片类药物时，使产生欣快感所需阿片类药物剂量增加[44]。为了便于术后管理，手术前应该停用阿片类药物拮抗剂。如果围手术期继续使用这些药物，患者可能需要较高剂量阿片类药物才能达到镇痛作用[45-47]。一直用于减轻患者对乙醇渴望感的其他药物有阿坎酸和抗惊厥药，如卡马西平、丙戊酸钠、加巴喷丁[45-47]。乙醇停用时，NMDA功能增强；阿坎酸可拮抗NMDA受体，研究证实其可使乙醇戒断成功率提高一倍[35]。选择性5-羟色胺再摄取抑制剂中的抗抑郁药如氟西汀以及抗焦虑药（如丁螺环酮）能减少抑郁或焦虑患者的乙醇饮用量[48,49]。

阿片类药物的滥用

μ 受体亚型在介导阿片类药物滥用中渴望感与奖赏机制方面似乎起到关键性作用。缺乏这种受体的小鼠没有不断摄入吗啡的强制行为[50]。人们一直应用作用于该受体的拮抗剂（如纳曲酮）来治疗阿片类药物滥用。抑制 NMDA 受体的药物（如氯胺酮和美金刚）其作用可能减轻阿片类药物诱发的耐受。

阿片类药物的戒断反应伴有交感神经系统的兴奋。停用阿片类药物后，可观察到脑内蓝斑神经元肾上腺素能神经元激活[51]。α_2 受体激动剂（如可乐定、洛非西定和替扎尼定）能减轻去甲肾上腺素能活性增强。研究显示，这些药物可调整戒断症状，减轻戒断的拟交感性反应。但是，这些药物也可能引起低血压、镇静和心动过缓，但这些不良反应在洛非西定和替扎尼定较少见。

由于应用短效阿片类药物时患者对阿片类药物的渴望感更强烈，因此人们越来越多地应用半衰期长的美沙酮和丁丙诺啡来治疗阿片类药物成瘾者。美沙酮是 μ 受体完全性激动剂，但也具有 NMDA 受体拮抗作用。丁丙诺啡（Subutex）是 μ 受体部分激动剂和 κ 受体拮抗剂。研究显示兴奋 κ 受体可降低多巴胺水平，产生厌恶反应[13]。丁丙诺啡也可与 μ 受体拮抗剂纳洛酮联合应用；这两种药物的合剂称为 Suboxone。丁丙诺啡的峰作用在 100 min，48 h 时作用回到基线水平，半衰期为 37 h。通常建议每日一次舌下含服 16 mg。由于丁丙诺啡为 μ 受体部分激动剂，因此该药物在受体最大结合后产生的反应较低下，表现出"封顶效应"。然而，因为丁丙诺啡具有镇痛作用，所以一些医师将其作为镇痛药使用。研究显示丁丙诺啡与美沙酮在治疗阿片类药物成瘾方面的效果相似。美沙酮戒断过程常常需要减少其剂量，每周减少 3% 至最多每日减少 5% 不等。L-乙酰-α-美沙醇（1-acetyl-α-methadol，LAAM）是一种可选用的长效 μ 受体激动剂。

使用任何 μ 受体激动剂的患者应该在术后继续使用通常剂量。否则，可能出现停药戒断症状，疼痛可能增强。围手术期应用其他阿片类药物取代这些药物只会使成瘾控制和镇痛处理变得更加复杂。同样，使用治疗成瘾的药物作为镇痛药，并增加其药物剂量，这将使术后康复的患者更难以撤药。简单的处理方法是维持用于成瘾的激动剂药物标准剂量，另外用静脉或短期口服镇痛药来处理术后急性疼痛。

其他成瘾

发现在大脑内源性大麻素系统中存在 CB-1 受体，而内源性大麻素系统在各种药物、尼古丁和食物的奖赏与渴望机制方面可能起到重要作用。研究发现，长期使用烟草可刺激 CB-1 受体，而缺乏 CB-1 受体的小鼠对吗啡的奖赏反应减弱。研究显示各种大麻素可增加听神经核内多巴胺的外流[52]。利莫那班可阻滞 CB-1 受体，研究表明其可减少患者对食物和烟碱的渴望感；这类药物有望在治疗阿片类药物成瘾方面起到一定作用。

从心理学角度看，成瘾药物能产生欣快感，这种欣快感起到积极的增强作用，进一步诱使患者使用。同样，摄入成瘾药物能减轻烦躁或戒断症状，这是负面的增强刺激，也增强患者获取药物的动机。环境因素能刺激条件反应，如渴望感，这会进一步促进患者用药[13]。因此，脑部的奖赏系统对环境刺激变得敏感，这种刺激不同于躯体戒断症状，并能引起药物用量增加。有冒险行为和心理异常的患者特别容易发生药物滥用行为[53,54]。所以，认知行为疗法着眼于这种异常行为，对确定药物依赖患者围手术期治疗方案可能起到重要作用。

药物依赖患者围手术期处理方案

围手术期药物依赖患者的处理中，最常见的挑战之一是对阿片类药物耐受的患者制定一项治疗方案。阿片类药物耐受的患者可能正在使用处方阿片类药物来治疗慢性或癌性疼痛，或者可能正在滥用处方阿片类药物或其他阿片类药物。尽管与处理耐受阿片类药物的患者有相似之处，无论其成瘾状态如何，但是对于生理上依赖阿片类药物，并且有药物滥用问题的患者处理时还需格外注意。总之，围手术期需要考虑阿片类药物耐受问题。一个良好的治疗方案宜重点注意解决术后急性疼痛、持续慢性疼痛以及可能影响患者心理的问题。

治疗方案的制定

只要有可能，手术前对阿片类药物依赖患者制定疼痛处理方案尤为重要。术前应该明确哪个服务小组主要负责处理疼痛，小组所有成员应该就治疗方案达成一致。这可能需要手术小组在术前咨询疼痛治疗专家。医疗小组成员应该意识到，如果不加以警惕，患者阿片类药物依赖更加可能使患者术后疼痛处理不完善。部分医护人员态度消极、缺乏宣教以及简单勉强地给"再次"成瘾者处方用药可能导致疼痛控制不良。此外，疼痛控制不好能导致患者焦虑加重、自信心减弱以及抑郁。应该使患者相信，其药物滥用史并不妨碍其获得适当的手术后疼痛处理[10]。对这些药物成瘾的患者，治疗方案中增加适当的心理健康指导将会获得更好的疗效。

有的患者可能在术后接受不恰当的大剂量阿片类药物，并且患者可能有获取过量阿片类药物的动机行为，但这种可能较小。医疗小组成员应该熟悉所计划的手术过程以及预计可能的疼痛程度。术后应根据患者的临床表现来决定是否继续使用阿片类药物。术前应准备疼痛处理方案，特别是可能需要何种方法来处理疼痛控制不良；应该与患者讨论术后阿片类药物用量减少的方案。

术前阶段

手术前应明确掌握患者是否规律服用阿片类药物；针对阿片类药物依赖或耐受的患者，应制定特殊的围手术期处理方案。对所有患者均应了解他们是否服用过或正在服用乙醇制品、烟草制品、阿片类药物、苯二氮䓬类药物或其他能导致药物依赖的处方或违法药物。与患者交谈中应特别注意了解患者正在服用阿片类药物的剂量以及服用时间。对于诚信度低的患者，尿液毒素检测可能起一定作用。应该了解既往手术及术后恢复的病史，重点在于患者疼痛控制如何。应该鉴别患者不能耐受特定阿片类药物的不良反应或该不良反应的表现，如果患者有慢性疼痛综合征，那么应该记录疼痛描述以及该疼痛对目前阿片类药物治疗的反应。

一旦获得患者疼痛治疗史，应与患者交流讨论术后疼痛控制方案。了解患者对于术后疼痛控制的期望值，并告知患者有关手术及术后恢复的预计过程，这尤为重要。围手术期的医护人员应该注意患者原有的慢性疼痛。术前描述疼痛剧烈的患者将可能报告术前和术后疼痛更为剧烈（视觉模拟评分，VAS，visual analogue scale）。医护人员可能需要应用另一种检测方法来准确地描述这些患者术后疼痛的严重程度。

手术当天

手术当天患者照常服用阿片类药物的维持剂量。大多数这些药物的作用时间持续 8~24 h，其中，经皮芬太尼甚至可达到 72 h。因此，只在术前服用这样一种药物能够维持手术期间及术后早期基础镇痛水平。对于术前忘记服用常规剂量阿片类药物的患者，可在术中静脉补充给药。

对于阿片类药物耐受的患者，疼痛处理可能更具有挑战性，因此应适当告知这些患者，存在其疼痛可能较难控制的可能性。纠正患者不合理的期望，如大手术后完全无痛，可能减轻某些患者术后焦虑程度，减少可能因错误期望而产生的不满。医师应指导患者术后采取各种方法来控制疼痛，包括应用患者自控镇痛（patient-controlled analgesia，PCA）、硬膜外和区域麻醉技术以及辅助药物，如抗焦虑药、抗炎药等。根据手术类型以及期望的恢复情况，患者可能不能口服用药来治疗其慢性疼痛，应该考虑并准备其他用药途径。应该允许患者应用常规的麻醉性镇痛药，直到手术时，常饮用一小口水与其他术前药一起服用。

术中问题

阿片类药物依赖或耐受的患者术中麻醉处理时可能需要更高剂量的麻醉性镇痛药[16,55]。通过观察患者对疼痛的心血管反应可以测定患者的反应；对于有自主呼吸的患者，应注意呼吸频率的改变。术中呼吸频率加快的患者可能需要补充阿片类药物。此外，硬膜外或区域麻醉可减少手术部位伤害性疼痛的传入冲动，可能对患者有益。患者较少发生大剂量阿片类药物产生的不良反应，如呼吸抑制史。麻醉医疗小组应该与术后医疗小组人员交流该患者术中阿片类药物的需要量以及术前阿片类药物用药史，术后医疗小组人员可能是麻醉后监护病房、普通病房或加强医疗病房的医务人员。这种交流对于阿片类药物依赖患者的治疗很重要，特别是对需要保留气管插管或药物保持肌松的患者至关重要。

术后管理

对阿片类药物产生依赖的患者术后有可能出现较剧烈的疼痛。这可能是由于以往使用麻醉性镇痛药而引起术后药物需求量增加、对阿片类药物耐受及治疗效果可能下降所致。医护人员未能对一些患者进行充分的镇痛治疗[56]。Rapp等研究显示[55]，6.6%的患者在术前有长期使用阿片类药物的病史。研究发现，术前有阿片类药物使用史的患者在术后通过PCA所消耗的阿片类药物剂量（24 h用量为135.8 mg吗啡等效剂量）大于术前未使用阿片类药物的患者（24 h用量为42.8 mg吗啡等效剂量）。长期应用阿片类药物组患者，尽管阿片类药物的用量较大，但是其疼痛评分（VAS 0~10）高于术前未使用阿片类药物的患者，无论是静止状态（VAS分别为5和3）还是运动状态（VAS分别为8和6）。长期服用阿片类药物组患者术后有18.7%需要药物治疗焦虑，而无阿片类药物使用史的患者仅为0.6%。长期应用阿片类药物组患者似乎使用PCA的时间较长（分别为4 d和3 d），阿片类药物治疗相关的恶心和瘙痒发生率较低。与癌症患者相比，非恶性肿瘤性疼痛患者的阿片类药物消耗量较大，疼痛评分较高。焦虑和抑郁等较普遍地见于慢性疼痛人群，这些因素在这类患者术后疼痛较明显中也可能起到一定作用。当患者对手术产生消极情绪时，可能需要的镇痛药剂量较大[57]。除阿片类药物耐受和药效可能丧失外，采用阿片类药物治疗慢性疼痛的患者对手术可能持消极态度，这可加重焦虑和恐惧，并导致阿片类药物的消耗量增大。

长期使用阿片类药物的患者术后镇痛不足的一个原因是患者术前没有服用通常的基础剂量。某些患者在术后不能立刻口服用药，或者医护人员没有按常规方案执行这些医嘱。长期应用阿片类药物治疗的患者必须恢复其常规剂量的阿片类药物，因此患者住院期间宜继续服用基础水平量的药物。对于该原则例外的是通过手术可减轻其慢性疼痛的患者。大多数患者是阿片类药物依赖者，原先所用的透皮贴剂或者口服阿片类药物应在整个术后期间继续使用；如果患者不能口服用药，那么应将其口服阿片类药物的用药方案改为静脉阿片类药物的背景量，通常约为等效剂量的50%，必要时追加剂量。

阿片类药物依赖患者术后疼痛可能更加剧烈的另一个原因是其对阿片类药物耐受。耐受可能需要术中及术后给予较大剂量的阿片类药物，以预防疼痛。因此，对阿片类药物依赖患者可能需要应用基础剂量阿片类药物的同时间歇性给予较高剂量的阿片类药物，以达到镇痛。因为即使短期使用（数天或数周），阿片类药物也能发生耐受，所以即使术前短时间应用过阿片类药物的患者也应该监测其阿片类药物耐受的症状和体征。对阿片类药物耐受的患者术后更可能经历较剧烈的疼痛，更可能要求较高剂量阿片类药物来缓解疼痛[16]。某些患者可出现长期耐受，因此患者对阿片类药物的作用相对不敏感，即使患者已经停用该类药物数年。这种现象可能与神经元可塑性改变、NMDA受体和谷氨酸的激活作用以及一种内源性类阿片肽-脊髓强啡肽产生增多有关[16]。

如果患者在术后数小时内就能口服药物，那么应该恢复其长期口服阿片类药物治疗的基础剂量。此外，应该追加口服阿片类药物或静脉PCA系统。无论是经口服还是经静脉给药，因为阿片类药物耐受而可能需要间歇性给予较大剂量的阿片类药物，这能通过PCA装置来实施。为减轻耐受的影响，应用一种不同于患者既往使用的阿片类药物可能有益。由于个体之间对不同阿片类药物的反应存在差异，因此某些患者更换应用一种阿片类药物可能使镇痛效果更好，不良反应更轻[58]。

如果患者不能口服阿片类药物，那么应该将术前口服的阿片类药物剂量转换成等效静脉剂量，其中50%作为基础的持续静脉注射。如果必要，患者在术后可使用PCA系统来满足其对阿片类药物的额外需求量。这种技术可控制镇痛药作用的最佳使用速度，并减少与麻醉性镇痛药可能不足相关的用药延迟和焦虑。尽管有些担心使用PCA装置可能增强成瘾患者的奖赏行为[59]，但应用PCA能降低镇痛药用量不足的风险，而且这种方式引起成瘾的可能性低。一旦PCA中所用的预定剂量不足，就应该执行"补救"剂量程序。这种剂量能达到患者所需自控剂量的两倍。经护士评估后应该允许给患者反复调整该补救剂量。使用透皮贴剂镇痛的患者在术后应该继续使用该贴剂。由于高热能引起某些经皮用药物的吸收增加，因此证实术后发热的患者可能会意外地吸收较大剂量的阿片类药物，医护人员应该特别警觉这种可能性。

利用硬膜外或区域技术进行疼痛控制的患者对全身阿片类药物的需求量可能较少。应用低剂量局麻药持续滴注下，机体功能性活动可能得以改善。经蛛网膜下腔或硬膜外给予阿片类药物的作用效果也强于经口服或静脉内给药。因此，可能观察到其阿片类药物治疗的不良反应减少。但是，尚不明了围手术期应用区域阻滞技术或蛛网膜下腔阿片类药物是否可减少阿片类药物依赖患者对该药物的渴望感或药物成瘾的复发[10]。即使应用区域阻滞技术，这些患者可能仍需要继续使用术前的阿片类药物，至少应用其长期使用量的一部分，以防止戒断反应或可能存在于区域镇痛范围以外的慢性疼痛。如果允许长期应用阿片类药物的患者继续使用其通常剂量，那么可达到缓解疼痛的最佳效果。即使区域麻醉阻滞完善的情况下，完全停用阿片类药物可能引起患者主诉明显疼痛。若担心过度镇静，可给予约50%阿片类药物基础剂量，这种剂量下不可能发生戒断反应。任何情况下，可能都需要对这些患者进行经常性再次评估及调整药物剂量，以达到控制疼痛的最佳效果。

除区域麻醉技术外，术后应用辅助性药物能减少阿片类药物的需要量。非甾体类抗炎药能增强术后单独使用吗啡所获得的镇痛效果（尽管单独使用非甾体类抗炎药的镇痛效果通常不充分）。这类药物能有效地减少术后阿片类药物的使用量，因此阿片类药物相关不良反应的发生率较低。当然，这些药物对特殊类型的疼痛，如骨骼痛或肌肉骨骼痛患者，也具有镇痛作用。然而，非甾体类抗炎药的应用可能与胃肠道损伤、肾损害、出血性并发症、心血管并发症以及延迟骨愈合有关。氯胺酮已成功用于治疗某些对阿片类药物抵抗的顽固性疼痛患者[60]。一般认为NMDA拮抗剂氯胺酮能增强阿片类药物的镇痛作用，并能减轻患者对阿片类药物的耐受。术后谨慎使用苯二氮䓬类药物可能有利于对手术过度焦虑和恐惧的患者，但要注意避免过度镇静。

术后一旦患者胃肠功能恢复，就建议口服应用麻醉性镇痛药方案。而且，若患者既往一直服用阿片类药物缓释剂来治疗慢性疼痛，并且该慢性疼痛依然存在，则应该继续使用术前剂量。当患者需要额外用药来缓解疼痛时，可给予标准的短效阿片类药物如羟考酮、吗啡或氢吗啡酮。对阿片类药物耐受的患者在术后早期可能需要额外追加较高剂量的药物。对于这样的患者，应该根据疼痛水平和手术类型制定一项大致的渐进性疼痛治疗方案。

阿片类药物依赖患者术后疼痛治疗用药剂量应该与术前未使用过阿片类药物的患者术后一样。医护小组人员必须警惕异常觅药行为体征或者对合理使用镇痛药的失控行为。然而，阿片类药物耐受患者口服阿片类药物的剂量可能要高于以前未使用过阿片类药物的患者。可在门诊对出院后患者继续减少阿片类药物用量，直到该用量达到术前用于治疗慢性疼痛的基础剂量。该过程可能需要1～2个月。医护人员应避免增加治疗慢性疼痛的药物剂量作为术后阿片类药物的急需辅助剂量。应该执行一个限量处方，并制定合理的减药方案。应该给患者与疼痛管理中心约定出院后用药量减少过程的随访。较频繁的随访和监测可更好地评估恢复和药物使用情况，也可更好地评估是否发生更换或不当使用麻醉性镇痛药的情况。某些情况下，由一名家庭成员配发术后麻醉性镇痛药，可能降低药物滥用患者失控行为的发生几率。

药物成瘾患者的术后疼痛处理

成瘾药物的应用能导致大脑神经生物学永久性改变。这些改变能引起患者对成瘾药物的渴望，导致患者即使已经停止应用该药物数年后仍复发成瘾。这种病变可能使这些患者术后特别难以戒断阿片类药物。心理应激、与以前药物应用相关的环境刺激或者再次接触该药物本身就能引起成瘾行为的复发。不同患者之间以及不同药物之间，复发的可能性不同。随着阿片类药物的应用，发现脑内某些谷氨酸受体亚型水平的增高可能与成瘾复发有关[61]。长期使用吗啡治疗可能增加中脑结构内转录因子与基因的表达，从而导致对成瘾物质产生行为致敏作用[14,15]。总之，接触阿片类药物能引起脑内神经元的结构改变。阿片类药物产生的行为致敏作用以及神经生物学与结构的改变能够长期存在，并持续数月或数年。因此，有滥用药物史的患者在围手术期及手术后可能容易渴望这些药物，并且增加这些药物的使用。

择期手术前使一位对非法药物成瘾的患者处于稳定状态的一种方法是用长效剂型的药物替代短效药物，然后再长时间逐渐减少剂量。停用短效药物可能更常见不良反应症状，可能诱发对药物的渴望感，而停用长半衰期药物所产生的症状可能较少或较缓和。阿片类药物制剂的脱毒是一个长时间的过程；患者正在手术恢复期和存在术后疼痛时不可能成功地进行脱毒。然而，一旦患者术后疼痛已经缓解，机体正恢复良好时，可开始脱毒及停药。

对于使用阿片类药物拮抗剂如纳曲酮、混合激动-拮抗剂如纳布啡和布托啡诺（μ受体拮抗剂和κ受体激动剂）或部分激动剂-拮抗剂如丁丙诺啡（部分μ受体激动剂和κ受体拮抗剂）维持的患者来说，必须制定一项特殊方案。使用纯μ受体拮抗剂的患者，至少应在手术前24 h停止使用这类药物。否则，可能难以确定术后疼痛控制所需的阿片类药物用量；这类拮抗剂药物可能阻碍用于缓解疼痛所给μ激动剂的镇痛作用。对于应用混合激动剂-拮抗剂的患者，这类药物的镇痛作用有封顶效应。这类药物能竞争性结合μ受体（因为这类药物是μ受体拮抗剂），可阻滞术后所给予μ受体激动剂的μ受体兴奋作用。一些研究者报道，正在应用部分激动剂如丁丙诺啡（为部分μ受体激动剂，其对μ受体激动作用具有封顶效应）的患者，追加μ受体激动剂作为麻醉性镇痛药，结果对疼痛控制有一定的改善作用。尽管这种治疗方法对小手术后的患者可能有效，但是对于可能产生较严重疼痛的手术患者可能无效。一个更加谨慎可靠的方法是在术前约48～72 h内应用完全性μ受体激动剂来替代混合性激动-拮抗剂或部分μ受体激动剂，然后在度过手术恢复的急性期后，重新开始应用混合性药物。一般在重大手术后5～7 d内就能重新开始应用原先的药物。其目的应该是尽快使患者恢复到基础用药方案。

结论

所滥用药物对躯体与心理影响可能使围手术期处理药物依赖患者变得复杂化。遗憾的是，尚缺乏指导最佳临床实际的前瞻性研究。重要的是，避免对这些复杂患者治疗不足或治疗过度。

除了了解术后疼痛管理的基本概念外，人们还必须掌握成瘾的神经学与行为学基础知识。获取这些知识需要咨询成瘾医学和慢性疼痛方面的专家。还必须掌握药物的药理学知识，并反复评估患者。

（余喜亚译　杨　涛　邓小明校）

参考文献

1. Mao J: Opioid induced abnormal pain sensitivity: Implications in clinical opioid therapy. Pain 2002;100:213–217.
2. Compton P, Charavastra VC, Kintaudi K, et al: Pain responses in methadone-maintained opioid abusers. J Pain Symptom Manag 2000;20:237–245.
3. Laulin JP, Celerier E, Larcher A, et al: Opiate tolerance to daily heroin administration: An apparent phenomenon associated with enhanced pain sensitivity. Neuroscience 1999;89:631–636.
4. Collett B-J: Chronic opioid therapy for non-cancer pain. Br J Anaesth 2001;87:133–143.
5. Nissen LM, Tett SE, Cranoud T, et al: Opioid analgesic prescribing: Use of an audit of analgesic prescribing by general practitioners and the multidisciplinary pain center at Royal Brisbane Hospital. Br J Clin Pharmacol 2001;52:693–698.
6. Savage SR: Assessment for addiction in pain-treatment settings. Clin J Pain 2002;18(Suppl):S28–S38.
7. Volkow ND, Fowler JS, Wang GJ: Imaging studies on the role of dopamine in cocaine reinforcement and addiction in humans. J Psychopharmacol 1999;13:337–345.
8. Stoelting RK, Dierdorf SF: Anesthesia and Co-existing Disease, 2nd ed. New York, Churchill Livingstone, 1988, p 731.
9. McLellan AT, Lewis DC, O'Brien CP, Kleber HD: Drug dependence, a chronic medical illness: Implications for treatment, insurance, and outcomes evaluation. JAMA 2000;284:1689–1695.
10. May JA, White HC, Leonard-White A, et al: The patient recovering from alcohol or drug addiction: Special issues for the anesthesiologist. Anesth Analg 2001;92:160–161.
11. Nedeljkovic SS, Wasan A, Jamison RN: Assessment of efficacy of long-term opioid therapy in pain patients with substance abuse potential. Clin J Pain 2002;18:S39–S51.
12. McHugh P, Slavney P: Characteristics of motivated behaviors. In The Perspectives of Psychiatry. Baltimore, Johns Hopkins University Press, 1998, pp 165–177.
13. Koob GF, Le Moal M: Drug addiction, dysregulation of reward, and allostasis. Neuropsychopharmacology 2001;24:97–129.
14. Cami J, Farre M: Mechanisms of disease: Drug addiction. N Engl J Med 2003;329:975–986.
15. Nestler EJ: Molecular basis of long-term plasticity underlying addiction. Nat Rev Neurosci 2001;2:119–128.
16. Mitra S, Sinatra R: Perioperative management of acute pain in the opioid-dependent patient. Anesthesiology 2004;101:212–227.
17. Kieffer BL, Evans CJ: Opioid tolerance: In search of the Holy Grail. Cell 2002;108:587–590.
18. Jaffe JH, Martin WR: Opioid analgesics and antagonists. In Gilman AG, Nies AS, Rall TW, Taylor P (eds): Goodman and Gilman's The Pharmacological Basis of Therapeutics, 8th ed. New York, Pergamon, 1990, pp 485–521.
19. Sosnowski M, Yaksh TL: Differential cross-tolerance between intrathecal morphine and sufentanil in the rat. Anesthesiology 1990;73:1141–1147.
20. Kessler RC, McGonagle KA, Zhao S, et al: Lifetime and 12-month prevalence of DSM-III-R psychiatric disorders in the United States: Results from the National Comorbidity Survey. Arch Gen Psychiatry 1994;51:8–19.
21. O'Brien CP, McLellan AT: Myths about the treatment of addiction. Lancet 1996;347:237–240.
22. National Household Survey on Drug Abuse (NHSDA). Washington DC: Substance Abuse and Mental Health Services Administration (SAMHSA), 1999.
23. O'Connor PG, Schottenfeld RS: Patients with alcohol problems. N Engl J Med 1998;338:592–602.
24. Swift RML Drug therapy for alcohol dependence. N Engl J Med 1999;340:1482–1490.
25. Davis KM, Wu JY: Role of glutaminergic and GABAergic systems in alcoholism. J Biomed Sci 2000;8:7–19.
26. Lejoyeaux M, Solomon J, Ades J: Benzodiazepine treatment for alcohol-dependent patients. Alcohol Alcohol 1998;33:563–575.
27. Adinoff B: Double-blind study of alprazolam, diazepam, clonidine, and placebo in the alcohol withdrawal syndrome: preliminary findings. Alcohol Clin Exp Res 1994;18:873–878.

28. Weiss F, Porrino LJ: Behavioral neurobiology of alcohol addiction: Recent advances and challenges. J Neurosci 2002;22:3332–3337.
29. Kosten TR, O'Connor PG: Management of drug and alcohol withdrawal. N Engl J Med 2003;348:1786–1795.
30. Rickels K, DeMartinis N, Rynn M, et al: Pharmacologic strategies for discontinuing benzodiazepine treatment. J Clin Psychopharm 1999;19(Suppl 2):12S–16S.
31. Griffiths RR, Wolf B: Relative abuse liability of different benzodiazepines in drug abusers. J Clin Psychopharmacol 1990;10:237–243.
32. Janssen Pharmaceutical Company: Memo, received November 14, 2004.
33. Fishbain DA, Rosomoff HL, Rosomoff RS: Drug abuse, dependence, and addiction in chronic pain patients. Clin J Pain 1992;8:77–85.
34. Boot BP, McGregor IS, Hall W: MDMA (Ecstasy) neurotoxicity: Assessing and communicating the risks. Lancet 2000;355:1818–1821.
35. Lingford-Hughes A, Nutt D: Neurobiology of addiction and implications for treatment. Br J Psychiatry 2003;182:97–100.
36. Kampman KM, Volpicelli JR, Mulvaney R, et al: Effectiveness of propranolol for cocaine dependence treatment may depend on cocaine withdrawal symptom severity. Drug Alcohol Depend 2001;63:69–78.
37. Grabowski J, Roache JD, Schmitz JM, et al: Replacement medication for cocaine dependence: Methylphenidate. J Clin Psychopharmacol 1997;17:485–488.
38. Alterman AI, Droba M, Antelo RE, et al: Amantadine may facilitate detoxification for cocaine addicts. Drug Alcohol Depend 1992;31:19–29.
39. Solowij N, Stephens RS, Roffman RA, et al: Cognitive functioning of long-term heavy cannabis users seeking treatment. JAMA 2002;287:1123–1131.
40. Wesson DR, Ling W, Smith DE: Prescription of opioids for treatment of pain in patients with addictive disease. J Pain Symptom Manag 1993;8:289–296.
41. Daley DC, Marlatt GA: Relapse prevention. In Lowinson JH, Ruiz P, Millman RB (eds): Substance Abuse: A Comprehensive Textbook, 3rd ed. Baltimore, Lippincott Williams & Wilkins, 1997, pp 458–467.
42. Ascher JA, Cole JO, Colin JN, et al: Bupropion: A review of its mechanism of antidepressant activity. J Clin Psychiatry 1995;56:395–401.
43. Hobbs WR, Rall TW, Verdoorn TA: Hypnotics and sedatives, alcohol. In Hardman JG, Limbird LE (eds): Goodman and Gilman's The Pharmacologic Basis of Therapeutics, 9th ed. New York, McGraw-Hill, 1996, pp 361–398.
44. Gonzalez JP, Brogden RN: Naltrexone: A review of its pharmacodynamic and pharmacokinetic properties and therapeutic efficacy in the treatment of opioid dependence. Drugs 1988;35:192–213.
45. Mueller TI, Stout RL, Rudden S, et al: A double-blind, placebo-controlled pilot study of carbamazepine for the treatment of alcohol dependence. Alcohol Clin Exp Res 1997;21:86–92.
46. Donovan SJ, Nunes EV: Treatment of comorbid affective and substance use disorders: Therapeutic potential of anticonvulsants. Am J Addict 1998;7:210–220.
47. Chatterjee CR, Ringold AL: A case report of reduction in alcohol craving and protection against alcohol withdrawal by gabapentin. J Clin Psychiatry 1999;60:617.
48. Cornelius JR, Salloum IM, Ehler JG, et al: Fluoxetine in depressed alcoholics: A double-blind, placebo-controlled trial. Arch Gen Psychiatry 1997;54:700–705.
49. Kranzler HR, Burleson JA, Del Boca FK, et al: Buspirone treatment of anxious alcoholics: A placebo-controlled trial. Arch Gen Psychiatry 1994;51:720–731.
50. Kieffer BL: Opioids: First lessons from knockout mice. Trends Pharmacol Sci 1999;20:19–26.
51. Rasmussen K, Beitner-Johnson DB, Krystal JH, et al: Opiate withdrawal and the rat locus coeruleus: Behavioral, electrophysiological, and biochemical correlates. J Neurosci 1990;10:2308–2317.
52. Robbe D, Alonso G, Duchamp F, et al: Localization and mechanisms of action of cannabinoid receptors at the glutamatergic synapses of the mouse nucleus accumbens. J Neurosci 2001;21:109–116.
53. Helmus TC, Downey KK, Arfken CL, et al: Novelty seeking as a predictor of treatment retention for heroin dependent cocaine users. Drug Alcohol Depend 2001;61:287–295.
54. Kavanaugh DJ, McGrath J, Saunders JB, et al: Substance misuse in patients with schizophrenia: Epidemiology and management. Drugs 2002;62:743–755.
55. Rapp S, Ready B, Nessly M: Acute pain management in patients with prior opioid consumption: A case-controlled retrospective review. Pain 1995;61:195–201.
56. Hamilton J, Edgar L: A survey examining nurses' knowledge of pain control. J Pain Symptom Manag 1992;7:18–26.
57. Chapman CR, Cox GB: Anxiety, pain and depression surrounding elective surgery: A multivariate comparison of abdominal surgery patients with kidney donors and recipients. J Psychosom Res 21;1977:7–15.
58. Woodhouse A, Ward EM, Mather LE: Intra-subject variability in post-operative patient-controlled analgesia (PCA): Is the patient equally satisfied with morphine, pethidine and fentanyl? Pain 1999;80:545–553.
59. Beattie C, Umbricht-Schneiter A, Mark L: Anesthesia and analgesia. In Graham AW, Schultz TK (eds): Principles of Addiction Medicine, 2nd ed. Chevy Chase, Md: American Society of Addiction Medicine, 1998, pp 877–890.
60. Weinbroum AA: A single small dose of postoperative ketamine provides rapid and sustained improvement in morphine analgesia in the presence of morphine-resistant pain. Anesth Analg 2003;96:789–795.
61. Carlezon WA Jr, Nestler EJ: Elevated levels of GluR1 in the midbrain: A trigger for sensitization to drugs of abuse? Trends Neurosci 2002;25:610–615.

25 门诊手术的术后疼痛管理

NAVPARKASH SANDHU · SHYAMALA KARUVANNUR · DOMINIC HARMON

由于麻醉和外科技术的发展，以及降低医疗费用的需要，门诊手术量正逐渐增加[1]。2003年，北美70%的手术是在门诊完成的[2]。尽管门诊手术后大多数患者没达到中重度疼痛，但仍有大约5%~33%的患者有可能需要承受术后严重的疼痛[3,4]。疼痛是出院患者再次入院或进入急诊室最常见的原因[1,5]。

门诊外科正在日益扩大[6]。它不仅越来越复杂，而且患有慢性疾病如糖尿病、心绞痛的老年患者也逐渐增多。门诊外科术后的持续疼痛会导致很多不良反应。这对于长期患有慢性疾病的老年患者尤其有害[7]。本章基于循证医学，回顾了门诊患者的疼痛治疗，使医务人员能够对患者作出恰当的疼痛治疗选择。

门诊患者疼痛治疗的原则

患者教育

对患者的教育可以减轻焦虑和术后疼痛[8,9]。所有的知情同意书必须以口头形式说明并且要有书面记录。必须告知患者术后急性疼痛持续时间有限，使他们在心理上做好克服疼痛的准备。值得注意的是，文献报道门诊外科手术后的疼痛程度有差异[10]。因为各专科手术术后疼痛的评判标准还没有被系统地研究和报道过，所以文献报道结果不一致[10]。必须建立一个统一的门诊手术术后疼痛测量标准，从而可以告知患者术后有可能发生疼痛的程度。

患者必须熟悉疼痛管理概念，并懂得定期评价疼痛程度以修正疼痛治疗方案的必要性。必须告诉患者术后疼痛治疗所选择的方法，让他们与医师共同讨论治疗方案。必须向患者解释镇痛药选择的阶梯式方案（图25-1），告诉患者应该按时服药，而不是按需用药。患者应该知道如何发现家庭镇痛治疗时可能出现的问题[11]。例如，当发现药物不良反应或泵发生故障时，能够知道如何关闭家用输入装置。

医患双方均须掌握对方的联系信息，负责疼痛治疗的医师更必须获得一个详细的电脑文档，该文档包含接受家庭输注泵治疗的各种信息，如局麻药的输注速度及

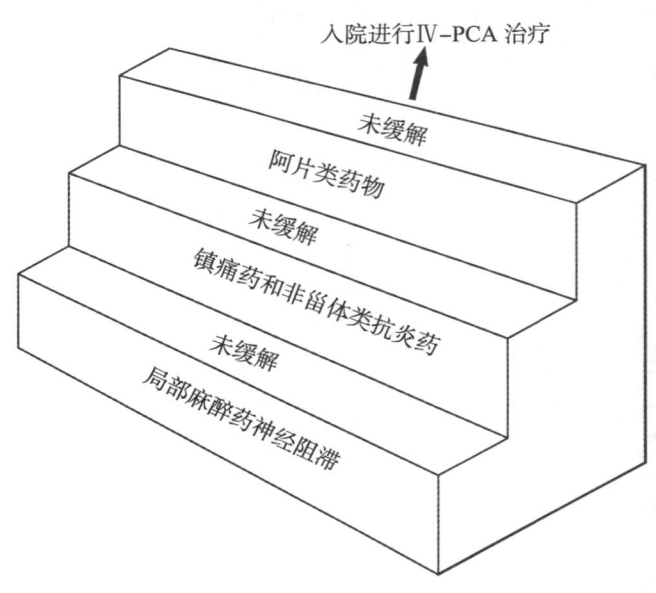

图25-1 非卧床患者的药物选择步骤。IV-PCA，静脉患者自控镇痛。

其他治疗处置、电话咨询后治疗所作的任何调整等。当患者遇到困难时，该文档能够保证患者在任何时候均可得到有效的指导。对接受持续神经阻滞的患者，应该每天通过电话了解输注情况，直至拔除导管后 1 天。

多模式镇痛

Kehlet 等[12]提出"通过单个药物或单一镇痛方法，如果不过分依靠仪器或监护系统，或不出现严重不良反应情况下，不能达到保证正常功能的完全或最佳镇痛"。多模式镇痛同样是"平衡止痛"，是联合使用对乙酰氨基酚、非甾体类抗炎药、阿片类药物和局部麻醉药。它通过药物的累积或协同效应达到最大止痛效果，而通过减小药物剂量和联合使用副作用不同的药物最大限度减少不良反应。多模式镇痛尤其适用于门诊手术。依据手术的类型、患者生理和心理特征、家庭的支持来选择特异性联合治疗方法。使用多模式镇痛的一个目的是减少阿片类药物在门诊手术时以及之后的使用量，从而防止镇静、烦躁、恶心、呕吐等不良反应的发生。

超前镇痛

超前镇痛是一种抗伤害性疼痛的治疗方法，它能预防神经中枢对疼痛传入信号的相应的处理整合，这种整合能够放大术后疼痛的程度[13]。实验研究有力地证实了超前镇痛的益处[14]。然而，临床研究却存在争议[15]。临床研究的困难在于所使用的超前镇痛概念不同[13]。超前镇痛能预防手术切割和围手术期炎症损伤所导致的中枢敏化。局部麻醉药阻断了疼痛刺激向中枢神经系统的传导，可减少术后镇痛药的需要量[16,17]。在手术前服用或经直肠使用非甾体类抗炎药对术后早期恢复有益。

程序化镇痛管理

程序化镇痛管理可以成为疼痛治疗标准化方案的有用工具（图 25-2）。程序化管理能改善术后疼痛治疗[18]。

全身和局部麻醉技术

依据患者和手术，选择不同的麻醉方法。门诊麻醉技术的进展包括短效麻醉剂的使用和区域麻醉比例的增加。全身麻醉的主要缺点是术后恶心、呕吐的发生率高以及中重度疼痛，这有可能导致患者延迟出院[19]。新药及药物的联合应用、新型设计的穿刺针和导管以及影像技术的介入提高了区域麻醉的质量和安全性。在初期研究中，志愿者皮内注射布比卡因脂质体可以延长麻醉时间长达 48 h[20,21]。广泛运用此类药物能够在单次注射后延长镇痛时间，将是对门诊患者疼痛治疗的重大改革。

在门诊手术中，一个有争论性的问题就是区域麻醉是否明显优于全身麻醉。一些公开发表的资料结果也不一致[22]。所有的全身及区域麻醉都各有优点与缺点（旁注 25-1 和 25-2）。这主要取决于外科医师、患者情况以及麻醉医师的专业知识。每个医疗单位根据其并发症的发生率、恢复室所需时间以及患者意见来选择方案至关重要。

局部麻醉技术包括皮下浸润、腔内和关节内滴注、区域阻滞、单个周围神经阻滞、神经丛或轴索的阻滞。区域麻醉可单用，也可以复合全身麻醉，为术中和术后提供镇痛治疗。周围神经阻滞能提供极好的麻醉效果，且副作用最小。手术前周围神经置管能延长术后的止痛治疗。神经轴索麻醉也是全麻之外的一个选择。缺点包括麻醉操作时间、等待阻滞起效时间长，还有少见的神经并发症。其他一些用于门诊手术的局部麻醉技术有静脉局部麻醉以及眼科手术的眼球周围、眼球后神经阻滞和表面麻醉。

持续外周输注麻醉技术允许调整给药速度，也便于调节药物的浓度和组成。家用的患者自控式局部麻醉是这个领域的重大进步。

有几个装置用于门诊患者的持续神经阻滞。一次性压力控制型装置能够按预先设定的速度释放局麻药。它比程序控制的泵更昂贵，但却不需要患者在家中进行程序设置。Accufuser（McKinley Medical，Wheat Ridge，Colo）可以 0.5、1、2、4、5、8 和 10 ml/h 的固定速度泵出液体，以锁定 15、30 和 60 min 的时间间隔给予 0.5、1 和 2 ml 的药物剂量。这是一个大容量的简单机械装置，能够持续 2~3 天（图 25-3）。

程序控制的泵，例如 Gemstar yellow（Hospira Inc.，Lake Forrest，Ill）（图 25-4）和 PainPump 2（Stryker，Kalamazoo，Mich），把 2~3 天用量的局麻药装在容器或者大袋中，这样可以为患者自控式给药提供更多给药速度的选择。

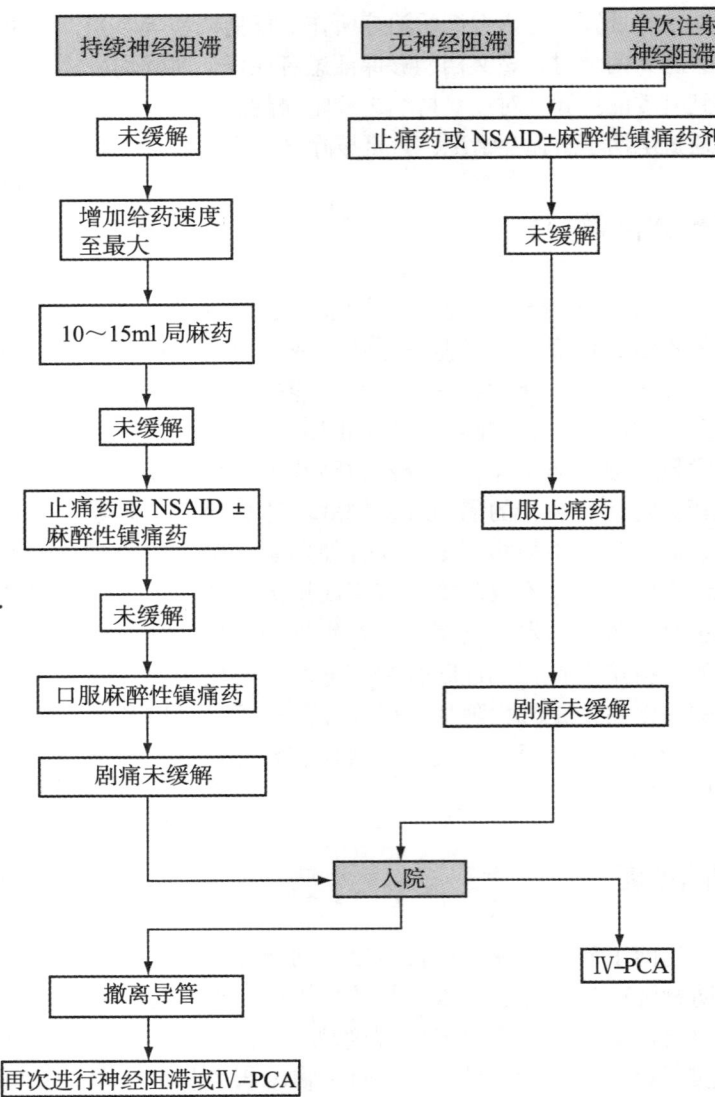

图 25-2 非卧床患者的疼痛治疗流程图。IV-PCA，患者自控静脉镇痛；NSAID，非甾体类抗炎药。

旁注 25-1	区域麻醉的优点

对患者的益处
- 避免全身麻醉
- 减轻疼痛
- 缩短痊愈时间
- 减少恶心和呕吐的发生

对外科医师的益处
- 使快速的术后评估成为可能

对医院的益处
- 快速恢复和早期出院
- 减少术后护理的工作量
- 减少意外入院

旁注 25-2	区域麻醉的缺点

- 起效时间较长
- 特殊的不良反应
- 延长阻滞可能会导致出院延迟
- 需要外科医师的合作
- 依赖专业知识
- 避免用于骨折合并巨大软组织肿胀患者，因为骨折后软组织肿胀会导致筋膜间隔综合征的发生。而疼痛是筋膜间隔综合征发生的早期警报，局麻药有可能会掩盖疼痛症状

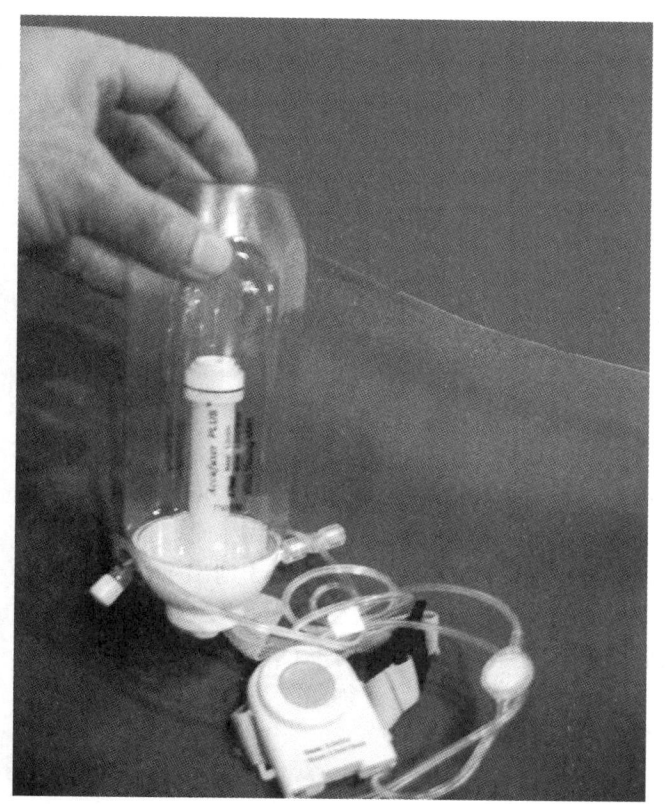

图25-3 Accufuser（人造橡胶泵）不需要电池，因有不同直径的导管可选，故背景和推注剂量有几种不同的选择。

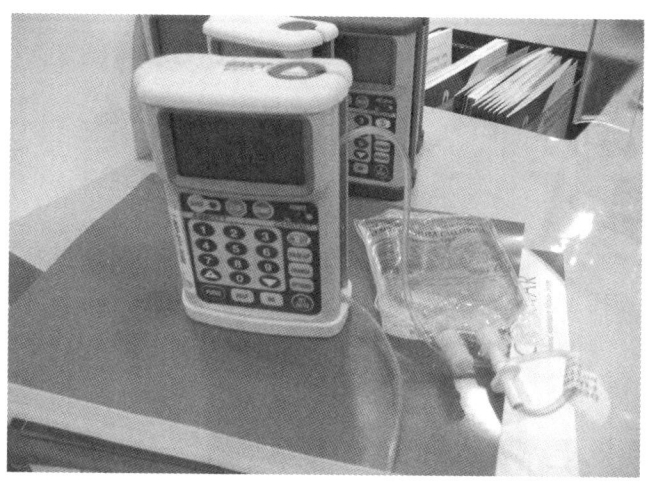

图25-4 Gemstar Yellow 是一种可重复利用、简洁、多用途的装置，它可以按程序泵出镇痛药。

对乙酰氨基酚

对乙酰氨基酚治疗轻度疼痛既价廉，又有效。它通过多重作用机制发挥镇痛作用[23]，与非甾体类抗炎药不同，它不刺激胃黏膜、影响血小板功能或导致肾功能不全。对乙酰氨基酚能显著减少阿片类药物的用量[24]。推荐的直肠使用剂量（高达 45 mg/kg）比口服剂量（15 mg/kg）大，主要是因为直肠吸收不完全。24 h 内儿童的最高用量是 90 mg/kg，成人 4g。对乙酰氨基酚也可与阿片类药物合用，治疗术后镇痛。非阿片类药物推荐剂量上限限制了复方药物用来治疗短期的轻中度疼痛（表 25-1）。

非甾体类抗炎药

除非有禁忌证，所有术后疼痛患者都可以使用 NSAID[25]。传统的 NSAID，被称为非选择性 NSAID，具有明显的胃肠道、血液系统和肾的不良反应，这些不良反应的发生是因为抑制了环氧合酶 I（Cox-I）。该类药物可减少阿片类药物的用量。例如阿司匹林、

表 25-1	镇痛药和 NSAID		
药物	成人的剂量和给药途径	儿童的剂量和给药途径	注意事项
乙酰胺基	500～1000mg/3～4h，PO 最大剂量 4000 mg/d	30～40mg/kg 负荷剂量； 10～15mg/kg/4～6h PO/PR 最大剂量是 90mg/(kg·d)	中毒剂量可导致肝毒性
阿司匹林	325～650 mg/4～6h，PO	12～20mg/kg/4～6h，PO	儿童总量 75mg/（kg·d） 可能引起 Reye 综合征、胃刺激
布洛芬	200～800 mg/6～8h，PO	4～10 mg/kg/6-8h，PO	胃刺激、血小板减少症（罕见）、皮疹、头痛、头晕、视物模糊和中毒性弱视
痛力克	负荷量 30 mg IM/IV 10mg/4～6h PO	0.5mg/kg/6～8h，PO 或 IM	使用不要超过 5 天，嗜睡、头晕、头痛、胃肠道的疼痛和消化不良

IM，肌内注射；IV，静脉注射；PO，口服；PR，经直肠给药。

表 25-2 Cox-2 抑制剂的推荐剂量及作用持续时间

药物	成人的剂量和给药途径	持续时间（hr）	Cox-2/Cox-1 的效能比
塞来昔布	100~400mg/12h，PO	4~8	8
艾托考布	60~240mg，PO	>24	106
帕瑞考昔	20mg，IM/IV	6~12	—
罗非昔布	25~50mg，PO	12~24	35
伐地考昔	20mg，PO	6~12	30

IM：肌内注射 IV：静脉注射 PO：口服

布洛芬、萘普生和双氯芬酸（见表 25-1）。对于有消化性溃疡病史的患者和有 Reye 综合征危险的儿童，必须避免使用阿司匹林。这些药物可以单独使用，也可以与阿片类药物或神经阻滞镇痛合用。依据患者的医疗条件来选择 NSAID 药物。

在抗炎和门诊手术镇痛方面，选择性 Cox-2 NSAID 与非选择性 NSAID 同样有效[26]，但胃肠道毒性作用却较少。选择性 Cox-2 NSAID 另外一个明显优点是在手术期间不会损害血小板功能[27]。帕瑞考昔是一种可注射使用的长效 Cox-2 选择性 NSAID，对门诊手术镇痛有效（表 25-2）[28]。罗非昔布已经停止生产，塞来昔布和伐地考昔也已被警告长期使用可能增加心肌梗死的发生率。

阿片类药物

通常，短效阿片类药物（例如芬太尼）术中即开始使用，以辅助全身麻醉。在麻醉恢复室，静脉用芬太尼或吗啡可缓解中到重度疼痛。门诊手术患者出院后，应用吗啡镇痛的不良反应比芬太尼大[29]。考虑到患者出院后有可能发生中重度术后疼痛，长效阿片类口服药可用作术后镇痛[30]。表 25-3 列出了用于术后镇痛的常见阿片类口服药。控释型羟考酮较控释型吗啡副作用小[31]。阿片类药物的不良反应有便秘、恶心呕吐、镇静和呼吸抑制。必须给予患者一些如何治疗这些副作用的合理建议。

非药理学技术

非药理学技术可用于门诊手术的疼痛治疗。因为电针镇痛技术可能发生电信号来源的偏移，以及很难定量是否为疗法本身的安慰作用，故其临床效能仍有争议[32]。其他用于手术期间辅助镇痛的非药理学技术有冷镇痛法、超声和催眠法。需要随机临床研究来证实门诊手术后这些方法的镇痛效应[33,34]。

表 25-3 术后口服阿片类药物

药物	成人的剂量和给药方式	儿童的剂量和给药方式	注意事项
吗啡	10~20mg/2~3h	每 3~4h 0.3mg/kg	哮喘患者慎用 可导致婴儿呼吸抑制
可待因	15~60mg/4~6h	每 3~4h 1mg/kg	用于中重度疼痛 可与对乙酰氨基酚合用
吗啡缓释片	15~30mg/6~8h	—	
哌替啶	50~150mg/3~4h	—	禁与单胺氧化酶抑制剂合用
氢吗啡酮	2~4mg/4~6h	每 3~4h 0.06mg/kg	
羟考酮	5~10mg/3~4h	每 3~4h 0.2mg/kg	
羟考酮缓释片	10~20mg/12h	—	

某些特定手术的镇痛处理

腹部外科

腹股沟疝

髂腹股沟神经可以通过两点式技术进行阻滞。在髂前上棘距离表面 2.5 cm 处注入 10ml 局麻药。即使在轴索麻醉或全身麻醉中，也可以沿着外科切口注射局部麻醉药。另一种方法是外科医师在切皮后或手术结束后沿切口注入 5～10 ml 0.25%的布比卡因。非甾体类抗炎药和（或）阿片类药物应该在麻醉结束前常规使用。患者在咳嗽或活动时可通过用手掌按压伤口来减少疼痛。脊髓周围神经阻断的镇痛效应与髂腹股沟神经阻滞以及手术切口的浸润麻醉相似[35]。

阑尾切除术

简单的阑尾切除术患者可以在手术当天回家。可以在手术伤口注入 5～10 ml 0.25%的布比卡因。术后早期使用非甾体类抗炎药及阿片类药物。

腹腔镜胆囊切除术

所有腹腔镜胆囊切除术的切口均可在手术切开前注射 0.5%利多卡因，在手术关闭切口后注入 2～3 ml 0.25%布比卡因。出院前还应给予非甾体类抗炎药。在患者能够服用口服药后就应立即给予对乙酰氨基酚/可待因复合物。口服羟考酮可以用于疼痛控制效果不佳的患者。

泌尿外科手术

成人行包皮环切术可以单独依靠阴茎神经阻滞完成。对于儿童和婴儿，可以选择全身麻醉，也可在背侧阴茎注射 0.1～0.2 ml/kg 的 0.25%布比卡因进行麻醉；它能持续 24 h 缓解疼痛。因为血管痉挛有引起坏疽的危险，故禁用肾上腺素。尽管局部使用 EMLA 乳膏（2.5%利多卡因+2.5%丙胺卡因）持续时间较阴茎背神经阻滞短，但疼痛缓解效果相当，易于在家中反复使用[36]。非甾体类抗炎药应该常规处方，同时加上阿片类药物。

在睾丸切除术、睾丸固定术或睾丸鞘膜积液修复术之前，可以捏住阴囊皮肤，用示指和拇指抓住精索，用 23 号针刺入精索。当排除穿刺针在血管内以后，注入 0.25%的布比卡因或 0.2%罗哌卡因（3～4 ml）。同时，也可以给予非甾体类抗炎药和阿片类药物。在切开阴囊皮肤前必须注射利多卡因。另一种方法是，外科医师可以在暴露完精索后注入 4～5 ml 0.25%的布比卡因。把睾丸用绷带或阴囊托保护好可以减轻术后疼痛。还有一种方法是靠近髂前上棘行髂腹股沟神经阻滞。

整形外科手术

乳房和腹部的整形外科手术可引起严重术后疼痛，这些手术患者的心理影响会加重疼痛。他们应该接受非甾体类抗炎药、阿片类药物和抗焦虑药治疗。0.5%布比卡因（0.3 ml/kg）或罗哌卡因进行周围神经阻滞，可以较长时间缓解术后乳房疼痛[37]。

耳鼻喉科手术

接受鼓室乳突手术的儿童，在手术当天进行颈浅丛的一个分支即耳大神经阻滞可以减轻手术疼痛。在胸锁乳突肌中点后缘皮下注射 2 ml 0.25%的布比卡因+肾上腺素 1∶2 000 000[38]。非甾体类抗炎药和阿片类药物可同时应用。

妇产科手术

可在手术结束时于手术切口用 0.25%的布比卡因（最大量 2 mg/kg）进行浸润麻醉，也可使用 NSAID 和阿片类药物。NSAID 对子宫痉挛特别有效[39]。

上肢手术

肩部手术

肩部及肘部手术重度疼痛的发生率为 25%[4]。

肌间沟阻滞 肌间沟阻滞适用于肩部周围的手术，可作为基本麻醉技术或全麻的辅助技术。肌间沟单次注射阻滞为手术期间提供了极好的麻醉效果，但是不利于出院后疼痛治疗[40]。通过神经刺激、找异感或超声引导技术进行中斜角肌阻滞，完成肩关节镜检查或肩袖修复术。通过肌间沟[41]、脊柱旁或后方[42]于颈神经根部或干部放置导管，利于术后疼痛治疗。

患者出院回家可携带一次性注射装置（例如 Accufuser 或镇痛泵）或可回收程序控制泵，如 Gemstar Yellow。必须有家庭护士的随访协作才能使用这些装置。然而，这些装置并不是能完全控制疼痛的[43]。患者可能不得不另外给予局麻药来控制疼痛。并发症包括少见的神经阻滞如膈神经阻滞、喉返神经阻滞和星状神经节阻滞，这些必须给患者解释清楚[43]。

肩胛上神经阻滞 可以注射 10 ml 长效局麻药，例如 0.25% 布比卡因或左布比卡因或 0.2% 罗哌卡因进行肩胛上神经阻滞，其优于肩胛中点平面的脊柱麻醉。尽管没有肌间沟阻滞有效，但肩胛上神经阻滞能够为患有严重肺部疾病的患者提供更佳选择，因为膈神经阻滞有可能影响呼吸。锁骨上神经阻滞能够很好地缓解术后疼痛[44]。

远端手臂的手术

锁骨下导管 锁骨下臂丛神经导管置入技术可以避免膈神经、喉返神经或星状神经节的阻滞。在这里放置导管更安全，导管渗漏罕见，也很少发生气胸。利用神经刺激器技术，通常采用垂直入路的神经阻滞。18 号绝缘 Touhy 针 (Contiplex, B. Braun Medical, Bethlehem, Pa) 插入肩胛骨喙突下。当通过 0.3～0.4 mA 的电流有手或前臂肌颤时，将 20 号导管穿过穿刺针。一种刺激导管 (Arrow International, Reading, Pa) 可以用来刺激神经丛，注药前应确定导管顶端的位置。如果没有反应，应调节导管，直至达到最佳肌颤。刺激导管对门诊患者作用有限。

在超声引导下，腋窝血管和臂神经丛显示在肩胛骨喙突区域锁骨的下方[45]。当神经束被很好地显示时，在皮肤上标记好传感器位置。进行局部消毒并铺无菌单。将涂有传导胶的无菌盖子装在超声探头上，将一 17 号 Touhy 穿刺针头向头侧进针 1～2cm。穿刺针方向朝着腋静脉和腋动脉之间，局麻药注入臂丛神经束中部，把针退入胸小肌，调节位置到腋动脉和外侧索。当确认穿刺针的位置后，注入局麻药。然后，穿刺针再进深一点，当没有压力时，将穿刺针的方向变得水平些，朝着后索和腋动脉之间的方向第三次注药，同时放入 20 号硬膜外导管[Flextip (Arrow International)]。

现在，确定导管的位置，然在超声引导下退回导管，使其顶端留在腋动脉后方（图 25-5 和 25-6）。导管在臂丛神经后束及中束之间弯曲，其位置在退回时容易鉴别。因为很难判断导管顶端的位置，可以通过导管注入 1～2 ml 的空气，当空气从顶端排出时，超声显示为高回声或是白色而容易被看到。假如空气向动脉的两个方向扩散，则导管的位置是令人满意的。当它向静脉扩散时，就需要退回导管继续空气试验。

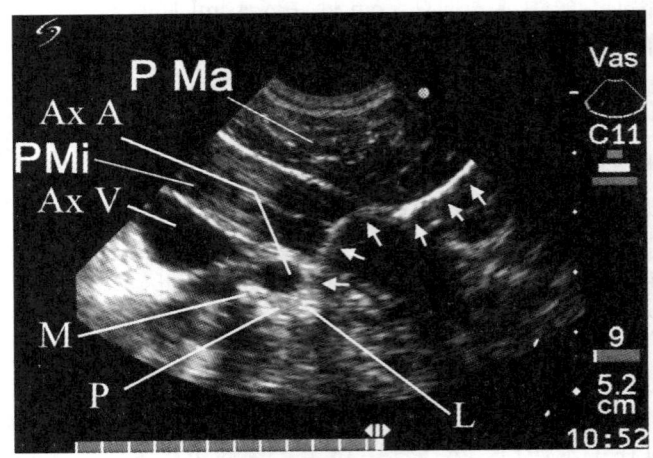

图 25-5 超声影像图所示的臂丛神经束和导管。L、M 和 P 分别标出了侧索、中索和后索。导管用白色箭头标出。AxA，腋动脉；AxV，腋静脉；PMa，胸大肌；PMi，胸小肌。

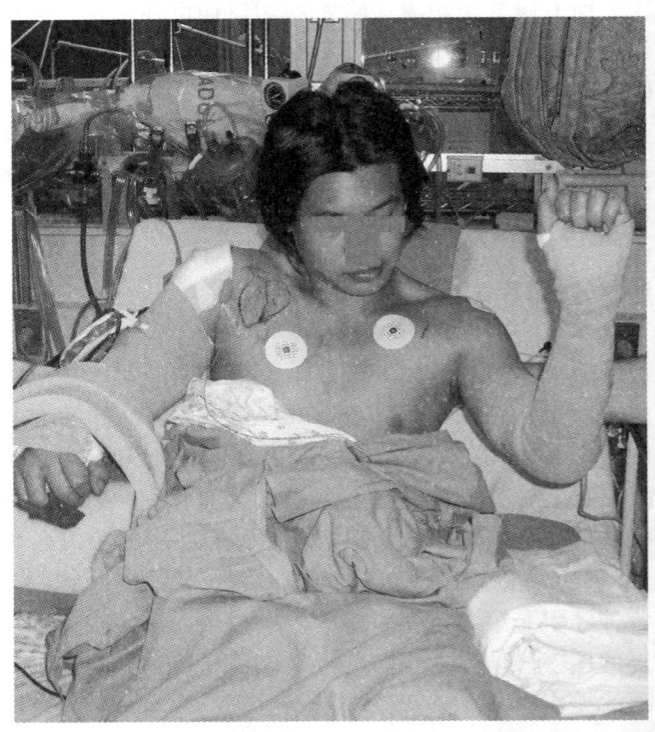

图 25-6 患者为 14 岁男性，右侧桡骨骨折切开复位内固定并修复左臂复杂撕裂伤手术，可以通过超声引导下同时双侧锁骨下神经阻滞完成。右侧导管用于术后镇痛。

当导管位置适合时，用透明贴固定导管。因为导管在行进中已弯曲数次，故不可能移位或渗漏。

腋窝导管 腋窝导管可以用于手、腕或肘部的手术后镇痛。因导管经潮湿部位（腋窝）进入，故易于感染。可以通过寻找压力落空感或电刺激技术来确认穿刺针位置。其导管的渗漏或移位比锁骨下导管更容易发生。以 4～6 ml/h 的速度注射 0.25% 布比卡因或 0.2% 罗哌卡因；辅加患者自控给药，可提高疼痛控制满意度[46]。

下肢手术

膝关节镜检查

膝关节镜是最普通的门诊下肢畸形矫正术，可以通过股神经和坐骨神经阻滞来完成。当使用中枢轴索阻滞或全身麻醉时，持续股神经阻滞适用于术后疼痛治疗。还有其他一些技术用于术后镇痛。股神经阻滞（图 25-7 和 25-8）或类似技术如髂筋膜阻滞，比关节内浸润麻醉更能缓解疼痛[47]。可以通过神经刺激器或超声引导技术放置一个 Cotiplex 或刺激导管。假如局麻药不能充分镇痛，可以加用 NSAID 和一种口服阿片类药物。必须告知患者有可能发生股四头肌无力，行走时要小心。进行腰肌间隔阻滞和导管置入技术（图 25-9），与腹股沟韧带下股动脉导管插管镇痛效果相同[48]。布比卡因可以单次注入关节腔内，也可以通过导管持续给予，但镇痛作用不如股神经阻滞[21]。

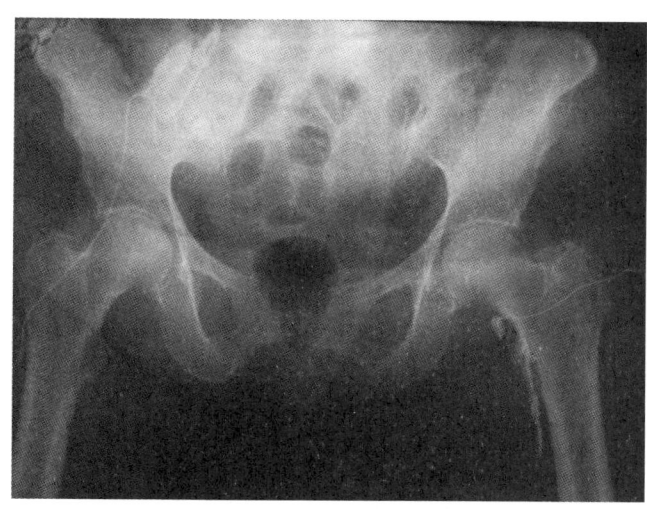

图 25-8　为图 25-7 患者 X 线片。右侧导管直接位于腰肌间隔，和造影剂混合的局麻药扩散在腰肌周围。左侧导管放在股神经后方，位于腹股沟韧带下方，见混有造影剂的局麻药向下扩散到未预期的位置。持续输注，两侧能达到同样满意的镇痛效果。

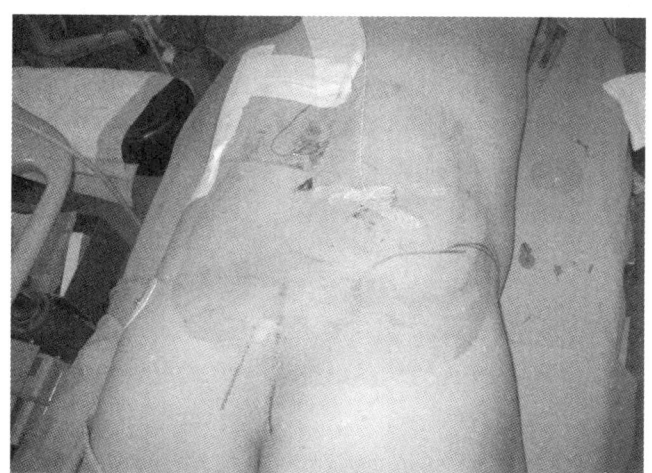

图 25-9　髋部手术患者，一个硬膜外导管放在 L2-3 水平，一个腰肌间隔的导管通过神经刺激器技术放在 L4 水平。

脚和踝部的手术

坐骨神经或其终末分支既可以通过单次注射，也可以通过导管持续注射来阻滞。使用这种阻滞方法可以减少术后 NSAID 和阿片类药物的用药量[49]。为了安全，固定导管必须穿过腘绳肌腱的侧面（图 25-10 和 25-11）。

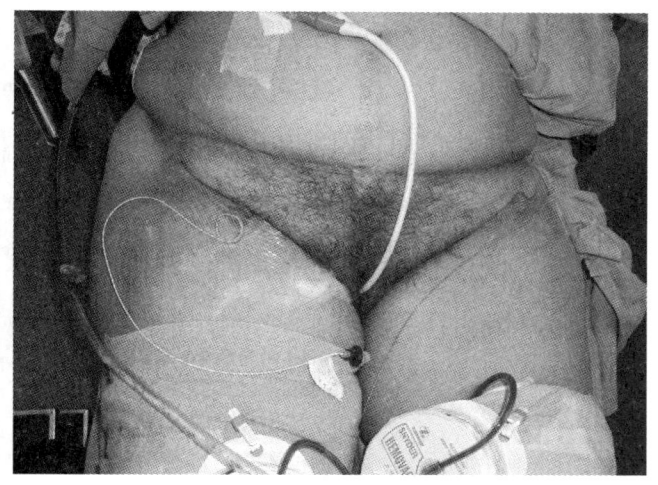

图 25-7　两侧股动脉导管麻醉为双侧膝关节手术提供了术后镇痛。

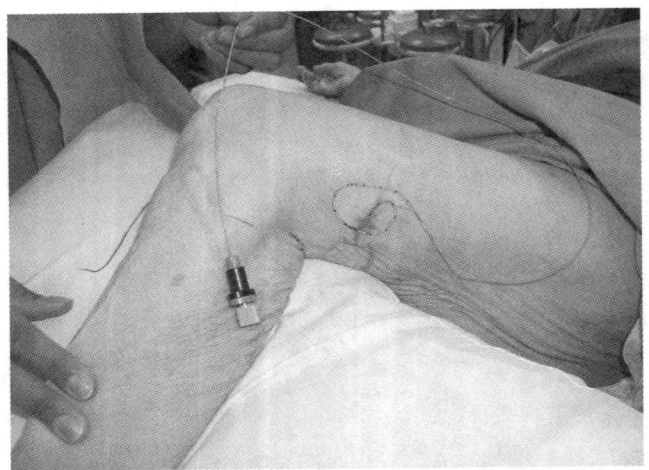

图 25-10　腘窝内放置导管用于手术麻醉和术后镇痛治疗。

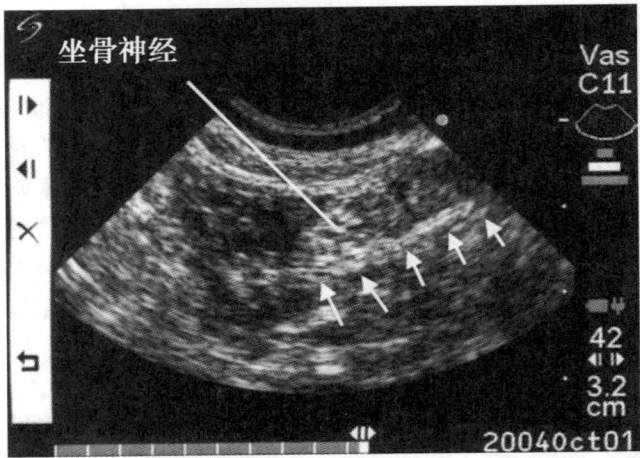

图 25-11　图 25-10 所示患者的腘窝导管以及坐骨神经的超声图像，利用超声引导，白色箭头指示放置在坐骨神经前面的导管。

小结

成功的门诊外科手术取决于有效镇痛、不良反应较小，并且出院回家后能够安全处理疼痛问题。大量研究表明：有相当比例的患者并未得到有效的术后镇痛治疗。除非有特殊禁忌证，超前镇痛应用于所有患者。根据每一患者期待的术后疼痛水平制定一个标准化、多模式的术后镇痛方案。通过电话随访患者，了解患者的手术是否导致轻度、中度甚至重度的术后疼痛，并确定疼痛治疗的效果。

（周英杰　毛燕飞译　熊源长校）

参考文献

1. Davies HTO, Crombie IK, Macrae WA, Rogers KM: Pain clinic patients in northern Britain. Pain Clinic 1992;5:129–135.
2. Crombie IK, Davies HTO, Macrae WA: Cut and thrust: Antecedent surgery and trauma among patients attending a chronic pain clinic. Pain 1998;76:167–171.
3. Macrae WA, Davies HTO: Chronic postsurgical pain. In Crombie IK, Linton S, Croft P, et al (eds): Epidemiology of Pain. Seattle, International Association for the Study of Pain 1999, pp 125–142.
4. Perkins FM, Kehlet H: Chronic pain as an outcome of surgery. Anesthesiology 2000;93:1123–1133.
5. Macrae WA: Chronic pain after surgery. Br J Anaesth 2001;87:88–98.
6. Richardson J, Sabanathan S, Mearns AJ, et al: Post-thoracotomy neuralgia. Pain Clinic 1994;7:87–97.
7. Polinsky ML: Functional status of long-term breast cancer survivors. Health Social Work 1994;19:165–173.
8. Tasmuth T, Blomqvist C, Kalso E: Chronic post-treatment symptoms in patients with breast cancer operated in different surgical units. Eur J Surg Oncol 1999;25:38–43.
9. Kroner K, Knudsen UB, Lundby L, Hvid H: Long term phantom breast syndrome after mastectomy. Clin J Pain 1992;8:346–350.
10. Vecht CJ, Van der Brand HJ, Wajer OJM: Post-axillary dissection pain in breast cancer due to a lesion of the intercostobrachial nerve. Pain 1989;38:171–176.
11. Jung BF, Ahrendt GM, Oaklander AL, Dworkin RH: Neuropathic pain following breast cancer surgery: Proposed classification and research update. Pain 2003;104:1–13.
12. Sindrup SH, Jensen TS: Efficacy of pharmacological treatments of neuropathic pain: An update and effect related to mechanism of drug action. Pain 1999;83:389–400.
13. Main CJ, Williams AC: Musculoskeletal pain. Br Med J 2002;325:534–537.
14. Woolf CJ, Mannion RJ: Neuropathic pain: Aetiology, symptoms, mechanisms, and management. Lancet 1999;353:1959–1964.
15. Villanueva L, Dickenson AH, Ollat H: The Pain System in Normal and Pathological States. Seattle, IASP Press, 2004.
16. Pons TP, Preston E, Garraghty AK: Massive cortical reorganisation after sensory deafferentation in adult macaques. Science 1991;252:1857–1860.
17. Ramachandran VS, Hirstein W: The perception of phantom limbs. Brain 1998;121:1603–1630.
18. Borsook D, Becerra L, Fishman S, et al: Acute plasticity in the human somatosensory cortex following amputation. NeuroReport 1998;9:1013–1017.
19. Knecht S, Henningsen H, Hohling C, et al: Plasticity of plasticity? Changes in the pattern of perceptual correlates of reorganisation after amputation. Brain 1998;121:717–724.
20. Dostrovsky JO: Immediate and long-term plasticity in human somatosensory thalamus and its involvement in phantom limbs. Pain Suppl 1999;6:S37–S43.
21. Halligan PW, Marshall JC, Wade DT: Three arms: A case study of supernumerary phantom limb after right hemisphere stroke. J Neurol Neurosurg Psychiatry 1993;56:159–166.
22. Devor M, Raber P: Heritability of symptoms in an experimental model of neuropathic pain, Pain 1990;42:51–67.
23. Seltzer Z, Wu T, Max MB, Diehl SR: Mapping a gene for neuropathic pain-related behaviour following peripheral neurectomy in the mouse. Pain 2001;93:101–106.
24. Turner JA, Ersek M, Herron L, et al: Patient outcomes after lumbar spinal fusions. JAMA 1992;268:907–911.
25. Chaturvedi N, Abbott CA, Whalley A, et al: Risk of diabetes related amputation in South Asians vs Europeans in the UK. Diabet Med 2002;19:99–104.
26. American Cancer Society: What are the risk factors for breast cancer? Available at www.cancer.org/docroot/CRI/content/CRI_2_4_2X_What_are_the_risk_factors_for_breast_cancer_5.asp?sitearea=/
27. Tasmuth T, von Smitten K, Hietanen P, et al: Pain and other symptoms after different treatment modalities of breast cancer. Ann Oncol 1995;6:453–459.

28. Smith WCS, Bourne D, Squair J, et al: A retrospective cohort study of post mastectomy pain syndrome. Pain 1999;83:91–95.
29. Kooijman CM, Dijkstra PU, Geertzen JH, et al: Phantom pain and phantom sensations in upper limb amputees: An epidemiological study. Pain 2000;87:33–41.
30. Wartan SW, Hamann W, Wedley JR, McColl I: Phantom pain and sensation among British veteran amputees. Br J Anaesth 1997;78: 652–659.
31. Jensen TS, Krebs B, Nielsen J, Rasmussen P: Immediate and long-term phantom limb pain in amputees: Incidence, clinical characteristics and relationship to pre-amputation limb pain. Pain 1985;21:267–278.
32. Kalso E, Perttunen K, Kaasinen S: Pain after thoracic surgery. Acta Anaesthesiol Scand 1992;36:96–100.
33. Larsson TJ, Bjornstig U: Persistent medical problems and permanent impairment five years after occupational injury. Scand J Soc Med 1995; 23:121–128.
34. Turk DC, Okifuji A: Perception of traumatic onset, compensation status, and physical findings: Impact on pain severity, emotional distress, and disability in chronic pain patients. J Behav Med 1996; 19:435–453.
35. Johnston M, Vogele C: Benefits of psychological preparation for surgery: A meta-analysis. Ann Behav Med 1993;15:245–256.
36. Nikolajsen L, Ilkjaer S, Kroner K, et al: The influence of preamputation pain on postamputation stump and phantom pain. Pain 1997;72: 393–405.
37. Keller SM, Carp NZ, Levy MN, Rosen SM: Chronic post thoracotomy pain. J Cardiovasc Surg 1994;35:161–164.
38. Wallace MS, Wallace AM, Lee J, Dobke MK: Pain after breast surgery: A survey of 282 women. Pain 1996;66:195–205.
39. Landreneau RJ, Mack MJ, Hazelrigg SR, et al: Prevalence of chronic pain after pulmonary resection by thoracotomy or video-assisted thoracic surgery. J Thorac Cardiovasc Surg 1994;107:1079–1086.
40. Callesen T, Kehlet H: Postherniorrhaphy pain. Anesthesiology 1997;87:1219–1230.
41. Stiff G, Rhodes M, Kelly A, et al: Long-term pain: Less common after laparoscopic than open cholecystectomy. Br J Surg 1994;81:1368–1370.
42. Perttunen K, Tasmuth T, Kalso E: Chronic pain after thoracic surgery: A follow-up study. Acta Anaesthesiol Scand 1999;43:563–567.
43. Houghton AD, Saadah E, Nicholls G, et al: Phantom pain: Natural history and association with rehabilitation. Ann Roy Coll Surg Engl 1994;76: 22–25.
44. Sherman RA, Sherman CJ: A comparison of phantom sensations among amputees whose amputations were of civilian or military origins. Pain 1985;21:91–97.
45. Smith J, Thompson JM: Phantom limb pain and chemotherapy in pediatric amputees. Mayo Clin Proc 1995;70:357–364.
46. Diatchenko L, Slade GD, Nackley AG, et al: Genetic basis for individual variations in pain perception and the development of a chronic pain condition. Hum Mol Genet 2005;14:135–143.
47. Katz J, Jackson M, Kavanagh BP, Sandler AN: Acute pain after thoracic surgery predicts long-term post-thoracotomy pain. Clin J Pain 1996; 12:50–55.
48. Tverskoy M, Cozacov C, Ayache M, et al: Postoperative pain after inguinal herniorrhaphy with different types of anaesthesia. Anesth Analg 1990;70:29–35.
44. Singlyn FJ, Lhotel L, Fabre B: Pain relief after arthroscopic shoulder surgery, a comparison of intraarticular analgesia, suprascapular nerve block and interscalene block. Anesth Analg 2004;99:589–592.
45. Sandhu NS, Capan LM: Ultrasound guided infraclavicular brachial plexus block. Br J Anaesth 2002;89:254–259.
46. Iskander H, Rakotondriamihary S, Dixmerias F, et al: Analgesia with continuous axillary block after severe hand trauma: Self-administration vs continuous infusion. Annales Francaises d'Anesthésie et de Réanimation. 1998;17:1099–1103.
47. Iskander H, Benard A, Ruel-raymond J, et al: Femoral blocks provide superior analgesia compared with intra-articular ropivacaine after anterior cruciate ligament repair. Reg Anesth Pain Med 2003;28:29–32.
48. Kaloul I, Guay J, Cote C, Fallaha M: The posterior lumbar plexus (psoas compartment) block provides similar postoperative analgesia after total knee replacement Can J Anaesth 2004;51:45–51.
49. Mendicino RW, Statler TK, Catanzariti AR: Popliteal sciatic nerve blocks after foot and ankle surgery: An adjunct to postoperative analgesia. J Foot Ankle Surg 2002;41:38–41.

26 术后慢性疼痛的预防

WILLIAM A. MACRAE

20世纪90年代，对疼痛门诊患者进行的流行病学研究显示，手术和创伤是慢性疼痛的主要病因[1,2]。从而引发了许多关于术后慢性疼痛文章的发表[3-5]。在此之前，术后慢性疼痛是一个被忽视的话题，即使有个别手术后疼痛的报道，但文献零散，不可能描述全面。本章不再赘述这一背景，而是探讨其机制，研究已知的危险因素，提出可能的预防措施。如欲阅读相关论文，可见所引述的参考文献。

术后慢性疼痛有多种形式和表现。同一种手术后可以发生几种不同类型的疼痛，而且有多种机制。例如，在开胸手术中，为了进入胸腔，术者必须切除一段肋骨或撑开肋骨。无论哪个操作都不可避免会造成肋骨或前后连接处关节的骨骼创伤。肋间神经紧位于肋骨下缘内侧，易被损伤，发生神经性疼痛。手术也影响肺或其他脏器，结果参与该神经性疼痛。胸腔引流常是疼痛的原因之一[6]。乳腺手术后，患者自述许多不适症状如麻木、刺痛、肿胀和敏感，可能导致疼痛样严重不适[7,8]。这种疼痛可能是幻痛[9]，肋间神经损伤引起的神经性疼痛[10]或者瘢痕性疼痛[11]。显然，即使某个手术并不存在任何一种术后疼痛综合征，也会有许多不同问题。

还要明确的是这些疼痛综合征并非是术后状态所独有，其他病因也可导致这些类似问题。因此，治疗措施也没有独特性。术后神经性疼痛综合征的治疗方法同其他任何神经性疼痛一样，如糖尿病性神经病变、创伤性或疱疹后神经痛[12]。术后机械性骨骼肌疼痛的治疗方法与其他骨骼肌疼痛一样[13]。

术后慢性疼痛的机制

任何手术都可能导致慢性疼痛。有许多不同的机制，但神经系统的变化是最重要的因素。

神经性疼痛复杂，有许多病因和机制[14]。显然，神经损伤如横断、牵张或压迫等均可导致神经性疼痛。但是重要的是要知道疼痛系统对其他组织的损伤也有反应[15]。一个例子就是广泛研究的皮肤热损伤，如日晒伤。过去认为日晒伤是由"皮肤损伤"所致。这种解释并不恰当，因为损伤不会增强感觉系统的敏感性；如眼损伤不会改善视觉敏感性。皮肤的热损伤可导致一系列级联性改变，如炎症介质从受损细胞中释放，将C与Aδ纤维的神经末梢包绕。这可通过降低伤害性感受器的阈值，增加其兴奋性而改变伤害性感受器。这种兴奋过度可发生在外周神经和脊髓中。结果以往无伤害性刺激成为疼痛性刺激（异常性疼痛），疼痛性刺激产生比平常更剧烈的疼痛（痛觉过敏）。正是对皮肤感觉神经的致敏化（由损害引起）而导致了疼痛。同样热损伤也引起致敏化，手术中不可避免的损伤也会引起这些变化，导致致敏化和痛觉过敏。

损伤对神经系统的改变不仅在外周与脊髓，而且也在大脑。1991年，有学者首次描述了去传入后感觉皮层的重新定位[16]。这种现象广泛发生于人类截肢手术后[17]。它在损伤后不久就可出现[18]，可随时间而变化[19]。适应性也发生在丘脑[20]。反常的是，大脑的损伤能造成周围神经的知觉错误，例如Halligan等报道一例患者脑卒中后感觉到有第三只手[21]。

许多不同的损伤都可造成包括周围与中枢神经系统的致敏化。这种超敏反应可能是进化而来的一种有益反应，它可防止受伤动物受到进一步损伤，鼓励休息，进而促进痊愈。这种敏感性在损伤愈合后应该恢复至正常水平，但并不总是如此。不能从这种损伤诱导的痛觉过敏状态恢复至正常水平可能是手术后慢性疼痛的主要原因之一。目前尚不明了为什么神经系统不能如此调整的原因。动物研究提示遗传因素与神经性疼痛的发生有关[22,23]。

了解手术后神经系统变化的程度和易发生慢性疼痛的机制对诸多方面都很重要。这种知识了解能改变人们对患者术后出现疼痛时的责难。手术不可能不对组织造成一定的损伤；不管手术怎样做，术后均可诱发痛觉过敏。正常情况下，随着伤口愈合，这种状态将恢复至正常，但并不总是如此。因此，一例患者是否发生术后慢性疼痛可能更多地取决于患者神经系统的"设置"，而不是手术者精细地做什么。当患者术后发生慢性疼痛时，推断外科医师一定做错什么或者加以责难都是不合适的。还应该明确的是过分简单化的治疗方案如简单的神经阻断或进一步手术，则不可能有利，并且可能引起进一步损伤，对患者不利。这种对神经系统变化程度的研究提示，药理学、心理学和行为学治疗可能比有创治疗对患者更加有益。

危险因素

大部分手术是因为患者疾病或损伤必须通过手术治疗才能得以改善。其他一些病例是患者进行美容整形手术以及社会因素的手术，如女性绝育术和输精管切除术。一些患者也接受了不适当的手术。不断有许多患者因背痛而手术，尽管证据表明手术对许多患者无助，实际上可能加重病情[24]。许多腹痛患者患有内脏痛觉过敏综合征，手术可能加重这些问题。这类患者可能因为幻想希望治愈或者因为前次手术的并发症而进入反复手术的恶性循环中。

因此，术后慢性疼痛的危险因素一定是起源于所导致手术的疾病的危险因素。为了预防截肢术后的幻肢痛和残肢痛，唯一最重要的方法就是戒烟和减肥，因为外周血管疾病和糖尿病是截肢的两大最常见原因[25]。乳腺癌等疾病的危险因素复杂，包括遗传学、人口统计学及生活方式因素[26]。筛查和早期检测将影响这些疾病的结局。如果我们要现实而全面地考虑术后慢性疼痛的各种危险因素，就不能忽视这些因素。

人口统计学及社会心理学因素

两项乳房手术后疼痛的研究报道了年龄的影响。Tasmuth 等[27]报道年龄越小，肿瘤越大，术后疼痛越强，疼痛时间越长。Smith 等[28]发现乳房切除术后慢性疼痛发生率在 70 岁以上者为 26%，在 50～69 岁者为 40%，在 30～49 岁者为 65%。该项研究还显示与年龄有关的其他人口统计学因素，如婚姻状态、居住条件及就业情况，均可能影响疼痛的发生。

在上肢或下肢截肢术后，年龄似乎不是幻肢痛的危险因素[29-31]。人口统计学因素对开胸手术后的疼痛似乎并不重要[6,32]。

许多研究显示疼痛是引起劳动能力丧失的重要原因[33]。无论客观体征如何，那些将疼痛归因于特殊创伤（如一次手术）的患者在情感痛苦、生活干扰以及疼痛程度方面明显重于那些疼痛隐匿性或自发性发作的患者[34]。这一发现使我们了解了如何对患者做一些术前准备工作，例如在手术知情同意前告知患者有关慢性疼痛的信息，以改变患者的感受，从而获得更好的结局[35]。

术前疼痛

Nikolajsen 等对截肢术前疼痛对截肢术后残肢痛和幻肢痛影响进行了一项详细的研究，结果截肢术前疼痛显著增高术后残肢痛和幻肢痛以及术后 3 个月时幻肢痛的发病率[36]。然而，患者在截肢术后 6 个月时过高评估了其截肢术前的疼痛程度（与其截肢术前评分相比较）；尽管患者陈述其幻肢痛的程度与其截肢前疼痛相近，但患者在截肢术前后的实际描述并不支持这些陈述。

在一项因乳腺癌行乳房切除术的女性研究中，Kroner 等[9]发现在乳房切除术前乳房痛与乳房幻觉痛以及无痛性乳房幻知之间有相关性[9]。

在因癌症进行开胸手术的患者中，开胸手术前用过麻醉性镇痛药的患者中有 48% 会出现开胸手术后慢性疼痛，而术前没用过麻醉性镇痛药的患者中只有 5% 会出现[37]。目前尚不能明确术后疼痛是术前疼痛的延续或是真正的术后疼痛综合征。

手术类型

术后慢性疼痛的发病率因手术类型和方式不同而异。例如，表26-1列举各种乳房手术后慢性疼痛的发病率。

一项来自芬兰的研究显示，在大手术量医疗单位行乳癌手术的女性患者慢性疼痛发生率低于在乳房手术经验较少的医院行手术的女性患者[8]。

很难确定乳房手术的原因是否影响慢性疼痛的发病率，因为恶性与良性病变所行的手术方式不同，而手术类型也确实影响疼痛的发病率[38]。

有关手术技术对开胸手术后疼痛影响的证据相互矛盾，有些文献表明有差异[6]，有些则显示无远期差别[39]。截肢的水平与类型对幻肢痛的发病率似乎没有影响[31]。

在关于疝修复术后疼痛的一篇综述中，Callesen和Kehlet[40]报道各种开放手术技术之间没有任何差异，但是腹腔镜疝修复术比开放手术疼痛轻、恢复期更短。对胆囊切除术患者，长期右上腹痛发生率在腹腔镜手术后为3.4%，而开腹手术是9.7%[41]。

芬兰的两项研究显示恶性与良性疾病开胸手术后慢性疼痛同样常见[32,42]。然而另一项研究表明，良性食管病变术后慢性疼痛比肺癌手术后更常见[6]。

截肢术的原因并不影响幻肢痛的发病率[31]。Houghton等[43]发现，创伤性与血管性截肢患者之间幻肢痛的发病率无任何差异。民间或军事原因而截肢的截肢者之间也无任何差异，这也证实了上述结果[44]。

表26-1　乳房手术后慢性疼痛的发生率

手术方式	发生率（%）
乳房缩小整形术	22
乳房切除术	31
乳房增大术	
硅胶	22
盐水	33
位于肌肉下	50
位于乳腺下	21
乳房切除及重建术	
无假体植入	30
有假体植入	53

Modified from Wallace MS, Wallace AM, Lee J, Dobke MK: Pain after breast surgery: A survey of 282 women. Pain 1996;66:195-205.

并行治疗

其他治疗的影响结果相互矛盾。一些研究显示放疗和化疗对慢性疼痛的发生率并无影响[9]。然而，其他研究则显示接受化疗和（或）放疗的患者慢性疼痛发病率较高[8,27]。Smith等认为难以解释不同治疗与疼痛之间的关系，因为存在许多复杂因素，如年龄[28]。

Smith和Thompson对Mayo诊所儿童因创伤或癌症行截肢术的研究显示，化疗可显著增加幻肢痛的危险（表26-2）[45]。

遗传因素

引人注意的问题是为何只是某些人发生术后慢性疼痛。显然，有许多因素决定个体易感性，遗传因素可能是部分原因。小鼠研究表明，遗传因素影响神经损伤后是否患慢性疼痛[22,23]。Diatchenko等发表了第一篇论文证实人类在基因多态性、疼痛敏感性与慢性疼痛发生危险性之间存在相关性[46]。研究显示一些人类疼痛综合征有遗传因素，该领域的研究者临床考虑的是这些条件中的部分能否成为损伤后更易发生慢性疼痛的标志物。这些条件包括偏头痛、纤维肌痛综合征、肠易激综合征、膀胱性尿频尿急以及雷诺现象[特别对称性，包括寒冷季节肢体末梢极度冰冷和红斑性肢痛病（"灼痛"足），通常在夜间]。

必须说明与这种遗传可能性不符的是，许多患者接受多次手术而只在某种特殊手术后发生慢性疼痛。某些患者接受双侧手术，但是只有一侧发生术后慢性疼痛综合征，而另一侧却没有。显然这是一个复杂而诱人的领域，有许多有趣的问题有待今后数年去解决。

表26-2　小儿截肢的幻觉痛

患者及处理	发生率（%）
创伤相关性截肢	12
肿瘤患者	48
截肢前或同时化疗	74
截肢后化疗	44
不化疗	12

Modified from Smith J, Thompson JM: Phantom limb pain and chemotherapy in pediatric amputees. Mayo Clin Proc 1995;70:357-364.

围手术期疼痛

围手术期疼痛是否为慢性疼痛的一项危险因素一直是许多研究的课题。这具有重大意义，因为围手术期疼痛是一项我们对其有一定控制的因素。早期研究结果混乱，受到患者对过去疼痛记忆的影响（一个众所周知、颇为微妙的话题）。研究表明，患者并不能对过去的疼痛进行准确分级。对过去疼痛的描述受到许多因素的影响，包括随后所患疼痛的强度，特别是在回忆当时。一些研究比较了围手术期记录的疼痛描述与术后数月患者对疼痛回忆的描述，结果发现两者相关性差。因此，进行前瞻性研究对围手术期疼痛的有效评估很重要。遗憾的是，几乎没有研究能满足这些标准；但是如果满足了这些条件，手术后慢性疼痛的发生率确实与手术后疼痛的强度相关[47]。

围手术期疼痛的正确治疗与术后慢性疼痛发生率低相关。两者是否存在因果相关性尚不清楚。然而，就目前所知，我们应该采取所有可能措施来尽可能减轻围手术期疼痛，以尽量避免长期问题。

减少慢性疼痛的麻醉与镇痛选择

很多研究探讨了麻醉技术对短期术后疼痛的影响。两项研究对随机接受局麻或全麻的患者术后10天内的疼痛进行了评估。Tverskoy等研究发现，疝修补术后2天内接受局麻＋全麻或椎管内麻醉的患者疼痛明显轻于单纯全麻者[48]。术后第10天，局麻＋全麻组的疼痛仍显著轻于单纯全麻组。

Jebeles等对儿童的扁桃体及增殖体切除术后疼痛进行的一项细致研究结果显示，术前接受局部浸润麻醉的儿童，到术后10天内不仅疼痛评分降低，而且吞咽功能也改善[49]。因此推测，在手术时给予局部麻醉药可避免术中及术后早期伤害性刺激大量集中传入神经系统。这种保护作用可避免引起慢性疼痛的致敏化。然而，不是所有比较区域麻醉与全身麻醉的研究都显示有这种有益作用[50]。

在一项剖宫产术后慢性疼痛的研究中，有慢性疼痛的患者更可能是接受全麻，而不是硬膜外麻醉，且术后剧烈疼痛的回忆率更高[51]。

输精管切除术后常见慢性疼痛，但局麻与全麻的结果却相反[52,53]。

术前预防

术前镇痛

术前及围手术期疼痛与手术后慢性疼痛的发病率较高有关，该发现使研究者试图在手术前给患者进行镇痛。动物研究提示，预先给予镇痛药可减少神经系统的变化，这形成了该方法的理论基础[54]。Bach等的一项研究被多次引用[55]，该研究对拟行下肢截肢术的患者在手术前72 h给予硬膜外局麻药及阿片类药物持续镇痛。该研究报道该方法可降低术后1年时幻觉痛的发生率，但存在方法学上的问题。随后，Nikolajsen等进一步对该问题进行了一项随机、双盲、对照研究，结果显示该方法并不能降低幻觉痛，也不能改变痛觉过敏、异常疼痛或抽紧样（wind-up-like）疼痛[57]。随后研究也不能确定截肢术或者其他手术形式之前治疗疼痛可防止远期疼痛。

许多研究显示，截肢术前的疼痛是慢性幻觉痛的一项危险因素。我们不能放弃这个重要的研究线索，因为幻觉痛一般是难以治疗的，因此预防是关键。然而，尽管已证实超前镇痛没有临床效果，我们应该看到围手术期合理治疗疼痛可能减少慢性疼痛的可能性。以前研究中所用的方法可能不合适，不足以减少伤害性刺激的传入。也许联合用药可能减少术后慢性疼痛。

一些研究已经探讨了术前给药来降低术后疼痛，这些药物包括加巴喷丁[58-61]、NSAID[62]、芬太尼和氯胺酮[63]、局麻药阻滞[64-66]、局麻药阻滞联合NSAID[67]以及可乐定和氯胺酮[68]。结果相矛盾，虽然不能低估方法学问题，但仍需进行大规模随机对照试验。

损伤后疼痛主要是一种痛觉过敏现象。有证据表明，利多卡因滴注可降低热损伤引起的继发性痛觉过敏，而不降低原发性痛觉过敏，推测可能通过脊髓而发挥作用[69]。也有证据表明，围手术期给予氯胺酮可降低术后痛觉过敏[68]。这都是值得进一步研究的方向。

高危患者的术前筛选

遗传危险因素的存在使筛选成为可能。被认为具有特别危险的患者可以优先接受最可能降低其危险的治疗。可能存在相关的遗传因素，许多在该领域工作的学者认为，患有其他疾病的患者更易发生术后慢性疼痛。Kalkman等研究了易发生术后严重疼痛的因素，结果显示,年龄较小、女性、术前疼痛较明显、切口较大以及手术类型(如开腹手术、矫形手术)都是独立预测因素[70]。另一项术前筛选方法是评估对热刺激的反应[71]。

如前所述,患者认为他们的疼痛原因与发作能影响疼痛的严重程度,并影响其生活。因此,术前宣教对于最大限度地减轻术后疼痛具有重要作用,尤其越来越明显的是,这种疼痛通常并不是外科医师的失误。

矫形手术后复杂性区域疼痛综合征发生率非常高。这是一个非常难以解决的问题,因此预防具有十分重要的意义。建议读者阅读 Reuben 关于该问题的综述[72]。

结论

因为术后慢性疼痛的治疗常常无效,因此预防第一。考虑到大多数发达国家用在手术治疗方面的资源总量,令人惊讶的是,更多资源并不是用于改善远期结局。迫切需要精心设计、合理组织的研究来为如何减轻术后慢性疼痛提供有效的数据。减少术后慢性疼痛数量的最简单方法或许是减少不必要手术的数量。

(王玮玮译　侯　炯　邓小明校)

参考文献

1. Davies HTO, Crombie IK, Macrae WA, Rogers KM: Pain clinic patients in northern Britain. Pain Clinic 1992;5:129–135.
2. Crombie IK, Davies HTO, Macrae WA: Cut and thrust: Antecedent surgery and trauma among patients attending a chronic pain clinic. Pain 1998;76:167–171.
3. Macrae WA, Davies HTO: Chronic postsurgical pain. In Crombie IK, Linton S, Croft P, et al (eds): Epidemiology of Pain. Seattle, International Association for the Study of Pain 1999, pp 125–142.
4. Perkins FM, Kehlet H: Chronic pain as an outcome of surgery. Anesthesiology 2000;93:1123–1133.
5. Macrae WA: Chronic pain after surgery. Br J Anaesth 2001;87:88–98.
6. Richardson J, Sabanathan S, Mearns AJ, et al: Post-thoracotomy neuralgia. Pain Clinic 1994;7:87–97.
7. Polinsky ML: Functional status of long-term breast cancer survivors. Health Social Work 1994;19:165–173.
8. Tasmuth T, Blomqvist C, Kalso E: Chronic post-treatment symptoms in patients with breast cancer operated in different surgical units. Eur J Surg Oncol 1999;25:38–43.
9. Kroner K, Knudsen UB, Lundby L, Hvid H: Long term phantom breast syndrome after mastectomy. Clin J Pain 1992;8:346–350.
10. Vecht CJ, Van der Brand HJ, Wajer OJM: Post-axillary dissection pain in breast cancer due to a lesion of the intercostobrachial nerve. Pain 1989;38:171–176.
11. Jung BF, Ahrendt GM, Oaklander AL, Dworkin RH: Neuropathic pain following breast cancer surgery: Proposed classification and research update. Pain 2003;104:1–13.
12. Sindrup SH, Jensen TS: Efficacy of pharmacological treatments of neuropathic pain: An update and effect related to mechanism of drug action. Pain 1999;83:389–400.
13. Main CJ, Williams AC: Musculoskeletal pain. Br Med J 2002;325:534–537.
14. Woolf CJ, Mannion RJ: Neuropathic pain: Aetiology, symptoms, mechanisms, and management. Lancet 1999;353:1959–1964.
15. Villanueva L, Dickenson AH, Ollat H: The Pain System in Normal and Pathological States. Seattle, IASP Press, 2004.
16. Pons TP, Preston E, Garraghty AK: Massive cortical reorganisation after sensory deafferentation in adult macaques. Science 1991;252:1857–1860.
17. Ramachandran VS, Hirstein W: The perception of phantom limbs. Brain 1998;121:1603–1630.
18. Borsook D, Becerra L, Fishman S, et al: Acute plasticity in the human somatosensory cortex following amputation. NeuroReport 1998;9:1013–1017.
19. Knecht S, Henningsen H, Hohling C, et al: Plasticity of plasticity? Changes in the pattern of perceptual correlates of reorganisation after amputation. Brain 1998;121:717–724.
20. Dostrovsky JO: Immediate and long-term plasticity in human somatosensory thalamus and its involvement in phantom limbs. Pain Suppl 1999;6:S37–S43.
21. Halligan PW, Marshall JC, Wade DT: Three arms: A case study of supernumerary phantom limb after right hemisphere stroke. J Neurol Neurosurg Psychiatry 1993;56:159–166.
22. Devor M, Raber P: Heritability of symptoms in an experimental model of neuropathic pain, Pain 1990;42:51–67.
23. Seltzer Z, Wu T, Max MB, Diehl SR: Mapping a gene for neuropathic pain-related behaviour following peripheral neurectomy in the mouse. Pain 2001;93:101–106.
24. Turner JA, Ersek M, Herron L, et al: Patient outcomes after lumbar spinal fusions. JAMA 1992;268:907–911.
25. Chaturvedi N, Abbott CA, Whalley A, et al: Risk of diabetes related amputation in South Asians vs Europeans in the UK. Diabet Med 2002;19:99–104.
26. American Cancer Society: What are the risk factors for breast cancer? Available at www.cancer.org/docroot/CRI/content/CRI_2_4_2X_What_are_the_risk_factors_for_breast_cancer_5.asp?sitearea=/
27. Tasmuth T, von Smitten K, Hietanen P, et al: Pain and other symptoms after different treatment modalities of breast cancer. Ann Oncol 1995;6:453–459.
28. Smith WCS, Bourne D, Squair J, et al: A retrospective cohort study of post mastectomy pain syndrome. Pain 1999;83:91–95.
29. Kooijman CM, Dijkstra PU, Geertzen JH, et al: Phantom pain and phantom sensations in upper limb amputees: An epidemiological study. Pain 2000;87:33–41.
30. Wartan SW, Hamann W, Wedley JR, McColl I: Phantom pain and sensation among British veteran amputees. Br J Anaesth 1997;78:652–659.
31. Jensen TS, Krebs B, Nielsen J, Rasmussen P: Immediate and long-term phantom limb pain in amputees: Incidence, clinical characteristics and relationship to pre-amputation limb pain. Pain 1985;21:267–278.
32. Kalso E, Perttunen K, Kaasinen S: Pain after thoracic surgery. Acta Anaesthesiol Scand 1992;36:96–100.
33. Larsson TJ, Bjornstig U: Persistent medical problems and permanent impairment five years after occupational injury. Scand J Soc Med 1995;23:121–128.
34. Turk DC, Okifuji A: Perception of traumatic onset, compensation status, and physical findings: Impact on pain severity, emotional distress, and disability in chronic pain patients. J Behav Med 1996;19:435–453.
35. Johnston M, Vogele C: Benefits of psychological preparation for surgery: A meta-analysis. Ann Behav Med 1993;15:245–256.
36. Nikolajsen L, Ilkjaer S, Kroner K, et al: The influence of preamputation pain on postamputation stump and phantom pain. Pain 1997;72:393–405.
37. Keller SM, Carp NZ, Levy MN, Rosen SM: Chronic post thoracotomy pain. J Cardiovasc Surg 1994;35:161–164.
38. Wallace MS, Wallace AM, Lee J, Dobke MK: Pain after breast surgery: A survey of 282 women. Pain 1996;66:195–205.
39. Landreneau RJ, Mack MJ, Hazelrigg SR, et al: Prevalence of chronic pain after pulmonary resection by thoracotomy or video-assisted thoracic surgery. J Thorac Cardiovasc Surg 1994;107:1079–1086.
40. Callesen T, Kehlet H: Postherniorrhaphy pain. Anesthesiology 1997;87:1219–1230.

41. Stiff G, Rhodes M, Kelly A, et al: Long-term pain: Less common after laparoscopic than open cholecystectomy. Br J Surg 1994;81:1368–1370.
42. Perttunen K, Tasmuth T, Kalso E: Chronic pain after thoracic surgery: A follow-up study. Acta Anaesthesiol Scand 1999;43:563–567.
43. Houghton AD, Saadah E, Nicholls G, et al: Phantom pain: Natural history and association with rehabilitation. Ann Roy Coll Surg Engl 1994;76: 22–25.
44. Sherman RA, Sherman CJ: A comparison of phantom sensations among amputees whose amputations were of civilian or military origins. Pain 1985;21:91–97.
45. Smith J, Thompson JM: Phantom limb pain and chemotherapy in pediatric amputees. Mayo Clin Proc 1995;70:357–364.
46. Diatchenko L, Slade GD, Nackley AG, et al: Genetic basis for individual variations in pain perception and the development of a chronic pain condition. Hum Mol Genet 2005;14:135–143.
47. Katz J, Jackson M, Kavanagh BP, Sandler AN: Acute pain after thoracic surgery predicts long-term post-thoracotomy pain. Clin J Pain 1996; 12:50–55.
48. Tverskoy M, Cozacov C, Ayache M, et al: Postoperative pain after inguinal herniorrhaphy with different types of anaesthesia. Anesth Analg 1990;70:29–35.
49. Jebeles JA, Reilly JS, Gutierrez JF, et al: Tonsillectomy and adenoidectomy pain reduction by local bupivacaine infiltration in children. Int J Pediatr Otorhinolaryngol 1993;25:149–154.
50. McCartney CJL, Brull R, Chan VWS, et al: Early but not long-term benefit of regional compared with general anesthesia for ambulatory hand surgery. Anesthesiology 2004;101:461–467.
51. Nikolajsen L, Sorensen HC, Jensen TS, Kehlet H: Chronic pain after Caesarean section. Acta Anaesthesiol Scand 2004;48:111–116.
52. McMahon AJ, Buckley J, Taylor A, et al: Chronic testicular pain following vasectomy. Brit J Urol 1992;69:188–191.
53. Paxton LD, Huss BK, Loughlin V, Mirakhur RK: Intra-vas deferens bupivacaine for prevention of acute pain and chronic discomfort after vasectomy. Brit J Anaesth 1995;74:612–613.
54. Woolf CJ, Chong M: Preemptive analgesia—treating postoperative pain by preventing the establishment of central sensitisation. Anesth Analg 1993;77:362–379.
55. Bach S, Noreng MF, Tjellden NU: Phantom limb pain in amputees during the first 12 months following limb amputation, after preoperative lumbar epidural blockade. Pain 1988;33:297–301.
59. Dirks J, Fredensborg BB, Christensen D, et al: A randomised study of the effects of single-dose gabapentin versus placebo on postoperative pain and morphine consumption after mastectomy. Anesthesiology 2002;97:560–564.
60. Rorarius MGF, Mennander S, Suominen P, et al: Gabapentin for the prevention of postoperative pain after vaginal hysterectomy. Pain 2004; 110:175–181.
56. Nikolajsen L, Ilkjaer S, Christensen JH, et al: Randomised trial of epidural bupivacaine and morphine in prevention of stump and phantom pain in lower limb amputation. Lancet 1997;350:1353–1357.
57. Nikolajsen L, Ilkjaer S, Jensen TS: Effect of preoperative extradural bupivacaine and morphine on stump sensation in lower limb amputees. Brit J Anaesth 1998;81:348–354.
58. Fassoulaki A, Patris K, Sarantopoulos C, Hogan Q: The analgesic effect of gabapentin and mexiletine after breast surgery for cancer. Anesth Analg 2002;95:985–991.
61. Dierking G, Duedahl TH, Rasmussen ML, et al: Effects of gabapentin on postoperative morphine consumption and pain after abdominal hysterectomy: A randomised, double blind study. Acta Anaesthesiol Scand 2004;48:322–327.
62. Priya V, Divatia JV, Sareen R, Upadhye S: Efficacy of intravenous ketoprofen for pre-emptive analgesia. J Postgrad Med 2002;48:109–112.
63. Katz J, Scmid R, Snijdelaar DG, Coderre TJ, et al: Pre-emptive analgesia using intravenous fentanyl plus low-dose ketamine for radical prostatectomy under general anesthesia does not produce short-term or long-term reductions in pain or analgesic use. Pain 2004;110:707–718.
64. Katz J, Clairoux M, Kavanagh BP, et al: Pre-emptive lumbar epidural anaesthesia reduces postoperative pain and patient-controlled morphine consumption after lower abdominal surgery. Pain 1994;59:395–403.
65. Aguilar JL, Rincon R, Domingo V, et al: Absence of an early pre-emptive effect after thoracic extradural bupivacaine in thoracic surgery. Br J Anaesth 1996;76:72–76.
66. Gill P, Kiani S, Victoria BA, Atcheson R: Pre-emptive analgesia with local anaesthetic for herniorrhaphy. Anaesthesia 2001;56:414–417.
67. Espinet A, Henderson DJ, Faccenda KA, Morrison LMM: Does pre-incisional thoracic extradural block combined with diclofenac reduce postoperative pain after abdominal hysterectomy? Br J Anaesth 1996;76:209–213.
68. De Kock M, Lavand'homme P, Waterloos H: Balanced analgesia in the perioperative period: Is there a place for ketamine? Pain 2001;92: 373–380.
69. Holthusen H, Irsfeld S, Lipfert P: Effect of pre- or post-traumatically applied lidocaine on primary and secondary hyperalgesia after experimental heat trauma in humans. Pain 2000;88:295–302.
70. Kalkman CJ, Visser K, Moen J, et al: Preoperative prediction of severe postoperative pain. Pain 2003;105:415–423.
71. Werner MU, Duun P, Kehlet H: Prediction of postoperative pain by preoperative nociceptive responses to heat stimulation. Anesthesiology 2004;100:115–119.
72. Reuben S: Preventing the development of complex regional pain syndrome after surgery. Anesthesiology 2004;101:1215–1224.